HANDBOOK OF PRESCRIPTIVE TREATMENTS FOR CHILDREN AND ADOLESCENTS

Related Titles of Interest

Ammerman and Hersen, *Handbook of Behavior Therapy with Children and Adults: A Developmental and Longitudinal Perspective*

Bellak, *The T.A.T., C.A.T., and S.A.T. in Clinical Use, Fifth Edition*

Finch, Nelson, and Ott, *Cognitive-Behavioral Procedures with Children and Adolescents*

Hersen and Last, *Handbook of Child & Adult Psychopathology: A Longitudinal Perspective*

Kratochwill and Morris, *The Practice of Child Therapy, Second Edition*

Meyer, *The Clinician's Handbook, Third Edition*

Teglasi, *Clinical Use of Story Telling: Emphasizing the T.A.T. with Children and Adolescents*

Van Hasselt and Hersen, *Handbook of Behavior Therapy and Pharmacotherapy for Children: A Comparative Analysis*

HANDBOOK OF PRESCRIPTIVE TREATMENTS FOR CHILDREN AND ADOLESCENTS

Robert T. Ammerman

Western Pennsylvania School for Blind Children

Cynthia G. Last

Nova University Center for Psychological Studies

Michel Hersen

Nova University Center for Psychological Studies

Editors

Allyn and Bacon

Boston London Toronto Sydney Tokyo Singapore

Copyright © 1993 by Allyn and Bacon
A Division of Simon & Schuster, Inc.
160 Gould Street
Needham Heights, Massachusetts 02194

Library of Congress Cataloging-in-Publication Data

Handbook of prescriptive treatments for children and adolescents /
    Robert T. Ammerman, Cynthia G. Last, Michel Hersen, editors.
        p.   cm.
        Includes bibliographical references and indexes.
        ISBN 0-205-14825-5
        1. Child psychiatry—Handbooks, manuals, etc. 2. Adolescent
    psychiatry—Handbooks, manuals, etc. 3. Behavior therapy for
    children—Handbooks, manuals, etc. 4. Behavior therapy for
    teenagers—Handbooks, manuals, etc.   I. Ammerman, Robert T.
    II. Last, Cynthia G.   III. Hersen, Michel.
        [DNLM: 1. Behavior Therapy—in adolescence—handbooks.
    2. Behavior Therapy—in infancy & childhood—handbooks. 3. Drug
    Therapy—in adolescence—handbooks. 4. Drug Therapy—in infancy &
    childhood—handbooks. 5. Mental Disorders—in adolescence—
    handbooks. 6. Mental Disorders—in infancy & childhood—handbooks.
    WS 39 H2368]
    RJ499.3.H366   1993
    618.92'689—dc20
    DNLM/DLC
    for Library of Congress   92-49080
                                                                  CIP

ISBN 0-205-14825-5
              H48259

Printed in the United States of America

10 9 8 7 6 5 4 3 2 1   97 96 95 94 93

To Patrick, Jonathan, and Nathaniel

CONTENTS

PREFACE

Until recently, treatment of children and adolescent psychopathology received scant empirical attention. Absence of a strong research literature necessitated implementation of interventions based solely on theoretical speculation and untested clinical practices. Happily, the past 20 years has seen a dramatic growth in both the quantity and quality of research on child and adolescent treatment. As reviewed in Chapter 1, recent meta-analyses confirm the effectiveness of psychotherapy for children and adolescents in general, and behavior therapy in particular. Clinicians who wish to adopt a prescriptive approach to treatment (that is, one that is guided by the extant empirical literature) now have a sizable body of research on which to base their interventions.

The primary objective of this book is to provide guidelines for treatment of children and adolescents that are derived from the empirical literature. An additional goal is to go beyond much of the available research and examine such issues as (1) potential impediments to treatment, (2) use of secondary interventions if the "treatment of choice" is unsuccessful, and (3) prevention of relapse.

The *Handbook of Prescriptive Treatments for Children and Adolescents* is divided into three parts. Part One consists of an introductory chapter examining the bases of a prescriptive approach to the treatment of children and adolescents. Part Two, which comprises the bulk of the book, is composed of chapters examining specific child and adolescent disorders. The format used within each chapter is highly specific and parallel across disorders.

Headings consist of Description of Disorder, Differential Diagnosis and Assessment, Treatment, Case Illustration, and Summary. The various case illustrations presented are actual treatment cases, hypothetical in some instances and a combination of the actual and hypothetical in yet other instances, in order to reflect the many complexities and issues so often faced in day-to-day clinical practice. The remaining chapters in Part Three are concerned with special issues in the treatment of children and adolescents: fire setting, sexual abuse, physical abuse and neglect, children of divorce, and chronic medical illness.

We acknowledge the support and assistance provided to us at each stage of bringing this book to fruition. We are especially grateful to the late Jerome Frank, our editor at Pergamon Press, who first accepted our proposal. We also extend our appreciation to his successor, Mary Grace Luke. In addition, we thank our editor at Allyn and Bacon, Mylan Jaixen, for his help and support. We also acknowledge the contributors to this volume for sharing their expertise with us. A number of others provided considerable assistance to us. Special consideration is due to Mary Jo Horgan and Ann Huber for their clerical support. Also, we thank Gretchen Boehm, Mary Anne Frederick, Jenifer McKelvey, Mary Newell, Kim Sterner, Melodi Parker, and Mary Trefelner.

R. T. A.
C. G. L.
M. H.

ABOUT THE EDITORS

Robert T. Ammerman (Ph.D., University of Pittsburgh, 1986) is Supervisor of Research and Clinical Psychology, Western Pennsylvania School for Blind Children, and Adjunct Assistant Professor of Psychiatry, Western Psychiatric Institute and Clinic, University of Pittsburgh School of Medicine. He is the recipient of grants from the National Institute on Disabilities and Rehabilitation Research (U.S. Department of Education) and the Vira I. Heinz Endowment to examine behavioral interventions for children and their families. Dr. Ammerman is the editor of seven books, including *Treatment of Family Violence* (with Michel Hersen) and *Children at Risk* (with Michel Hersen).

Cynthia G. Last (Ph.D., State University of New York at Albany, 1982) is Professor of Psychology and Director of the Child and Adolescent Anxiety Disorder Clinic in the Department of Psychology at Nova University. She is editor and founder of the *Journal of Anxiety Disorders*. She has coauthored and coedited eight books, including *Child Behavior Therapy Casebook, Handbook of Anxiety Disorders, Handbook of Child Psychiatric Diagnosis,* and *Anxiety Disorders in Children*. Dr. Last is the recipient of several research grants from the National Institute of Mental Health to study anxiety disorders in children and adolescents. She has published numerous journal articles and book chapters on the assessment, diagnosis, and treatment of anxiety disorders in both children and adults.

Michel Hersen (Ph.D., State University of New York at Buffalo, 1966) is Professor of Psychology at the Center for Psychological Studies, Nova University. He is Past President of the Association for Advancement of Behavior Therapy. He has coauthored and coedited 79 books, including *The Clinical Psychology Handbook* (second edition) and *Single Case Experimental Designs*. He has also published more than 180 scientific journal articles and is coeditor of several psychological journals, including *Behavior Modification, Clinical Psychology Review, Journal of Anxiety Disorders, Journal of Family Violence,* and *Journal of Developmental and Physical Disabilities*. He is coeditor of *Progress in Behavior Modification* and Associate Editor of *Addictive Behaviors*. Dr. Hersen is the recipient of several research grants from the National Institute of Mental Health, the Department of Education, the National Institute of Disabilities and Rehabilitation Research, and the March of Dimes Birth Defects Foundation.

ABOUT THE CONTRIBUTING AUTHORS

Sandra T. Azar (Ph.D., University of Rochester, 1984) is Associate Professor of Psychology in the Frances L. Hiatt School of Psychology at Clark University. She has published extensively in the area of child abuse and neglect and is currently conducting research in this area supported by the National Institute of Mental Health.

Lee Baer (Ph.D., Nova University, 1980) is Associate Professor of Psychology in the Department of Psychiatry, Harvard Medical School, Director of Research in the OCD Clinic, and Director of the Biostatistics Unit in the Department of Psychiatry at Massachusetts General Hospital. He is the author of more than 70 articles, books, and chapters, primarily in the area of behavioral and pharmacologic treatments for OCD and related disorders, and is coeditor of the textbook entitled *Obsessive Compulsive Disorders: Theory and Management* (second edition).

M. Susan Burns (Ph.D., George Peabody College of Vanderbilt University, 1983) is Assistant Professor of Psychiatry at the University of Pittsburgh School of Medicine and Applied Researcher at Theiss Health and Child Development Center. Her research and publication interests include dynamic assessment of children's "zones of proximal development"; the social roots of cognitive competence, including how parents, teachers, therapists, and more competent peers enhance development; and early intervention for young children at risk for academic failure, including children with psychiatric problems, those affected by substance abuse, and those in multiple foster placements.

John Christopher (Ph.D., University of Texas at Austin, 1992) is an Assistant Professor of Counseling Psychology at the University of Guam. Dr. Christopher has been working to develop models of the influence of early experiences on personality development and has published in this area. He has also pursued interests in cross-cultural psychology, philosophical psychology, theories of the self, psychological well-being, moral development, and psychopathology.

Edward R. Christophersen (Ph.D., University of Kansas, 1970) is Chief of the Behavioral Pediatrics Section at the Children's Mercy Hospital and Professor of Pediatrics at the University of Missouri at Kansas City School of Medicine. He has published seven books and over 130 articles and chapters. Dr. Christophersen is on the editorial board of the *Journal of Applied Behavior Analysis* and serves as Review and Special Article Editor for the *Journal of Developmental and Behavioral Pediatrics*. His current research and clinical interests are in behavioral pediatrics.

Paul M. Cinciripini (Ph.D., Auburn University, 1978) is Associate Professor in the Departments of Psychiatry and Medicine at the University of Texas Medical Branch, Galveston, Texas. He has published in the areas of smoking cessation, nicotine psychopharmacology, and cardiovascular reactivity. Dr. Cinciripini is currently doing work supported by the National Institute of Health and Ciba-Geigy Corporation on the efficacy of the transdermal nicotine patch and the effects of various precessation smoking schedules on smoking cessation outcome.

Judith A. Cohen (M.D., University of Pittsburgh, 1978) is a Board Certified Child Psychiatrist and Assistant Professor of Child Psychiatry at the University of Pittsburgh School of Medicine. She is Medical Director of the Child and Adolescent Sexual Abuse Clinic at the University of Pittsburgh. Dr. Cohen's research and clinical interests focus on the impact and treatment of child sexual abuse. She has many publications in this area, as well as a currently funded grant through the National Center on Child Abuse and Neglect.

Robert Cole (Ph.D., Cornell University, 1976) is Associate Professor of Psychiatry (Psychology) at the University of Rochester Medical Center and a Vice President of National Fire Service Support Systems, Inc. He has published extensively in the area of children at risk for major psychopathology. His interests include the development of prevention programs for children at risk for social and behavioral problems. Dr. Cole is a coauthor of the *Fireproof Children Handbook* and the *Fireproof Children Education Kit,* program guides for community agencies addressing the problem of juvenile fire play and fire setting.

Ronald Dahl (M.D., University of Pittsburgh, 1984) is Assistant Professor of Psychiatry and Pediatrics and Director of the Child and Adolescent Sleep Laboratory at the University of Pittsburgh School of Medicine. Dr. Dahl runs a large program (including both research and clinical work) covering a wide array of sleep problems in children and adolescents.

Margaret Dempsey (M.A., University of Texas at Austin, 1992) is a doctoral student in school psychology. Her primary areas of interest are in childhood depression, particularly from a developmental perspective, as well as its link to the family system.

Andrew R. Eisen (Ph.D., State University of New York at Albany, 1992) is Assistant Professor of Clinical Psychology at Fairleigh Dickinson University. He completed his clinical child psychology internship at the University of Mississippi Medical Center. Dr. Eisen's clinical and research interests are in the areas of assessment and treatment of anxiety and affective disorders in children and adolescents. His current research involves the prescriptive treatment of overanxious disorder.

Jack W. Finney (Ph.D., University of Kansas, 1983) is Associate Professor of Psychology and Director of the Child Study Center at Virginia Polytechnic Institute and State University. He is a clinical child psychologist whose research focuses on individual and family issues associated with children's health and use of primary and specialty health care services. Dr. Finney also studies behavioral processes associated with children's unintentional injuries, and is Chairperson of the Society of Pediatric Psychology's Task Force on Injury Control.

Daniel J. Fischer (M.S.W., University of Michigan, 1984) is a clinical social worker at the University of Michigan Medical Center Department of Child/Adolescent Psychiatry. He has published in the area regarding classification of anxiety disorders. His principal areas of interest have been diagnosis and behavioral treatment of children with disruptive behavior disorders and childhood anxiety disorders.

Greta Francis (Ph.D., Virginia Polytechnic Institute and State University, 1986) completed her predoctoral internship and a National Research Service Award postdoctoral research fellowship at Western Psychiatric Institute and Clinic at the University of Pittsburgh. She currently is Assistant Professor in the Department of Psychiatry and Human Behavior at Brown University. Dr. Francis is also a staff clinical psychologist in the Charles Badley Day Treatment Program and is the Director of the Anxiety Disorders Clinic at the Emma Pendleton Bradley Hospital. Her clinical and research interests include anxiety and affective disorders in children and adolescents.

Brian A. Glaser (Ph.D., Indiana State University, 1989) is Assistant Professor of Counseling Psychology at the University of Georgia. He is also on the faculty of the Marriage and Family

Certificate Program and is an Adjunct Fellow of the Center for Family Research, Institute for Behavioral Research, at the University of Georgia. Dr. Glaser serves on the editorial board of the *Journal of Addictions and Offender Counseling.* His principal area of interest is family interventions for disorders of conduct.

Wendy Grolnick (Ph.D., University of Rochester, 1987) is Assistant Professor of Psychology in the doctoral program in clinical psychology at Clark University. Dr. Grolnick's research focuses on children's motivation and adjustment with an emphasis on contextual factors that influence children's behavior. She has worked with the Rochester, New York, Fire Department's Fire Related Youth program and the New York City Fire Department's Juvenile Firesetters Intervention Program in her work on juvenile fire setting.

Lori A. Head (Pharm.D., Purdue University, 1989) is Clinical Assistant Professor in the College of Pharmacy at the Medical University of South Carolina, and Clinical Instructor in Psychopharmacology at the Institute of Psychiatry. Dr. Head is currently working in the area of child and adolescent psychopharmacology and is doing research on metabolism and pharmacokinetics of neuroleptics in children.

Joseph Himle (M.S.W., University of Michigan, 1984) is Lecturer in Psychiatry and Senior Social Worker at the University of Michigan Department of Psychiatry. He has published several articles regarding diagnosis, Axis-I comorbidity, and the cognitive-behavioral treatment of anxiety disorders. Mr. Himle is also a doctoral pre-candidate at the University of Michigan Schools of Social Work and Psychology.

Katherine Dowdell Hommerding (B.A., University of Pennsylvania, 1986) is an advanced graduate student in the doctoral program in clinical psychology at the University of Pittsburgh. Her research interests include parental conflict, infant attachment, and socioemotional development in children at risk.

John J. Horan (Ph.D., Michigan State University, 1970) is Professor of Counseling Psychology at Arizona State University. Most of his writing has focused on the experimental evaluation of cognitive-behavioral counseling strategies. Dr. Horan is a former faculty member of Pennsylvania State University.

Arthur M. Horne (Ph.D., Southern Illinois University, 1971) is Professor, Director of Training in Counseling Psychology, and Head of the Department of Counseling and Human Development Services at the University of Georgia. He is also an Associate of the Institute for Behavioral Research at the University of Georgia. Dr. Horne has published five books, including *Treating Conduct and Oppositional Defiant Disorders in Children* and *Troubled Families: A Treatment Manual,* as well as more than 50 articles and chapters. He has conducted a decade-long research project examining family interaction patterns in functional and aggressive families and his current interests include examining models of intervention with dysfunctional families.

Betsy Hoza (Ph.D., University of Maine, 1989) is Assistant Professor of Psychiatry at Western Psychiatric Institute and Clinic (WPIC). She completed postdoctoral training in clinical research at WPIC in the Attention Deficit Disorder Program in 1990. Her current research interests are peer relationships and cognitive-motivational factors in ADHD and nonproblem children.

Walter H. Kaye (M.D., Ohio State University, 1970) is Director of Western Psychiatric Institute and Clinic's Center for Overcoming Problem Eating (COPE) treatment program, an Associate Professor of Psychiatry at the University of Pittsburgh School of Medicine, and is trained in both psychiatry and neurology. Dr. Kaye was recruited to WPIC from the National Institute of Mental Health where, for seven years, he conducted research on appetite regulation, the effects of food on mood in humans, and improved treatment techniques for eating disorders. He is a nationally recognized expert in the field of eating disorders, a member of the editorial board of the

International Journal of Eating Disorders, and the author of numerous articles and publications.

Philip C. Kendall (Ph.D., Virginia Commonwealth University, 1977) is Professor of Psychology and head of the Division of Clinical Psychology at Temple University. He is editor of *Cognitive Therapy and Research* and associate editor of *Journal of Consulting and Clinical Psychology.* The author of numerous research papers and monographs, Dr. Kendall authored *Child and Adolescent Therapy: Cognitive-Behavioral Procedures* and *Coping Cat Workbook,* and has also coauthored *Clinical Psychology: Scientific and Professional Dimensions* (with Ford), *Cognitive Behavioral Therapy for Impulsive Children* (with Braswell), and *Anxiety Disorders in Youth: Cognitive-Behavioral Intervention* (with several coauthors). He was president of the Association for Advancement of Behavior Therapy. His interests lie in cognitive-behavioral assessment and treatment, especially with children and adolescents.

Gregory K. Lehne (Ph.D., Cornell University, 1978) is Assistant Professor of Medical Psychology in the Department of Psychiatry and Behavioral Sciences, Johns Hopkins University School of Medicine. He is on the faculties of the Psychohormonal Research Unit and the Sexual Disorders Clinic, and also in private practice specializing in evaluation and treatment of sexual and gender disorders. Dr. Lehne has published in the areas of homosexuality, as well as childhood, adolescent, and adult sexual disorders.

Lauren M. Loos (M.A., University of California, San Diego, 1991) is a doctoral student at the University of California, San Diego, teaching parents to implement behavior therapy with their children who have autism. Her research interests include assessing and teaching perspective-taking skills with individuals with autism.

Martin J. Lubetsky (M.D., Wayne State University School of Medicine, 1981) is an Assistant Professor of Child and Adolescent Psychiatry at Western Psychiatric Institute and Clinic,

University of Pittsburgh School of Medicine, and Director of the John Merck Multiple Disabilities Program. He has worked with children and adolescents who have developmental disabilities and psychiatric/behavioral problems. Dr. Lubetsky has authored and coauthored several articles and book chapters in the areas of mental retardation, abuse and neglect in the multihandicapped, medication trials, and other areas in developmental disabilities and child psychiatry.

Anthony P. Mannarino (Ph.D., Ohio State University, 1976) is Associate Professor of Child Psychiatry and Psychology at the Department of Psychiatry, University of Pittsburgh School of Medicine. His current research and clinical interests are the evaluation and treatment of sexually abused children and the short- and long-term impact of abuse. Dr. Mannarino currently has a research grant from the National Center on Child Abuse and Neglect to study the psychological impact of child sexual abuse.

Daniel S. Marullo (M.A., University of Houston, Clear Lake, 1987) is a doctoral candidate in the Medical Psychology program at the University of Alabama at Birmingham. His research has focused on parent and adolescent characteristics as they relate to adherence to chronic illness.

William E. Minichiello (Ed.D., University of Massachusetts at Amherst, 1971) is Assistant Professor of Psychology in the Department of Psychiatry, Harvard Medical School, Director of Psychological Clinical Services in the OCD Clinic, and Chief Psychologist of the Behavior Therapy Unit at Massachusetts General Hospital. He serves on the Scientific Advisory Board of the Obsessive Compulsive Foundation, and his primary area of interest is in behavioral treatments for OCD and related disorders. Dr. Minichiello is also coeditor of the textbook entitled *Obsessive Compulsive Disorders: Theory and Management* (second edition).

John Money (Ph.D., Harvard University, 1952) is Professor of Medical Psychology and Professor of Pediatrics, Emeritus, in the Department of

Psychiatry and Behavioral Sciences and the Department of Pediatrics, Johns Hopkins University School of Medicine. He has authored numerous books, including *Man and Woman, Boy and Girl, Lovemaps, Vandalized Lovemaps, Gay, Straight and In-Between,* and *The Kaspar Hauser Syndrome.* Dr. Money is the senior editor, with Dr. Herman Musaph, of the *Handbook of Sexology.* His research continues to be in psychoendocrinology and medical sexology.

Deborah Osgood-Hynes (Psy.D. candidate, Denver University) is a Clinical Fellow in Psychology in the Department of Psychiatry, Harvard Medical School and Massachusetts General Hospital. She recently completed a predoctoral internship in psychology in the Behavior Therapy Unit of the Massachusetts General Hospital, and, pursuing completion of her Psy.D. requirements, is currently in a fellowship specializing in behavioral treatment of OCD and related anxiety disorders, in addition to trichotillomania and tic disorders.

Renée Pearlmutter (M.S.W., University of Pennsylvania, 1990) is the research coordinator for the Family Interaction Study being conducted in the Frances L. Hiatt School of Psychology at Clark University. Her work involves coordinating research efforts on a study of child abuse.

William E. Pelham, Jr. (Ph.D., State University of New York at Stony Brook, 1976) is Associate Professor of Psychiatry and Psychology, University of Pittsburgh. He is author of more than 80 publications dealing with Attention-Deficit Hyperactivity Disorder (ADHD). His areas of ADHD study include peer relationships, pharmacological and behavioral treatment, and family distress. Dr. Pelham is a fellow of the American Psychological Association.

Aureen Pinto (Ph.D., University of Iowa, 1989) is Assistant Professor of Psychiatry (Psychology) in the Department of Psychiatry of the University of Rochester. She received internship and postdoctoral training at Yale and Brown Universities. Dr. Pinto's primary interests are in the diagnosis and phenomenology of affective and anxiety disorders in seriously disturbed children and adolescents.

Stephanie S. Rude (Ph.D., Stanford University, 1983) is Assistant Professor in the Department of Educational Psychology at the University of Texas at Austin. Dr. Rude is active in both clinical and research training and directs internship placement for the Counseling Psychology program at the University of Texas. Her primary research interests are cognitive aspects of depression and the role of client variables such as learned resourcefulness in psychotherapeutic outcome.

Floyd R. Sallee (M.D., Southern Illinois University, 1978; Ph.D., University of Pittsburgh, 1988) is Associate Professor of Child Psychiatry at the Medical University of South Carolina. He is the Director of the Tic and Tourette Disorder Program as well as the Molecular Neuropharmacology Laboratory. Dr. Sallee has published in the area of pediatric psychopharmacology with an emphasis on stimulant and neuroleptic treatments and their effect on the dopaminergic system. His current research focuses on the relative efficacy of haloperidol and pimozide in children suffering from Tourette disorder.

Regina Santelli (Ph.D., Duquesne University, 1988) is Assistant Director of Clinical Services at St. Francis Medical Center, Community Mental Health/Mental Retardation. Dr. Santelli has had extensive clinical experience, with particular emphasis in corrections, addictions, eating disorders, and the dually diagnosed. Her doctoral research was on compulsive overeating, and she was previously the Senior Psychiatric Clinician for the Inpatient Eating Disorders Unit at the University of Pittsburgh, Western Psychiatric Institute and Clinic.

Laura Schreibman (Ph.D., University of California, Los Angeles, 1972) is Professor and Chair of the Department of Psychology at the University of California, San Diego. She directs a federally funded research proposal focusing on the experimental analysis and treatment of autism. Her current research interests include experimental analysis of attention and language in autism, family intervention, family assessment, and generalization of behavior change. She has published over 85 articles, book chapters, and books in the areas related to the behavior analysis and treatment of autism.

Paul Schwartzman (M.S.–Counseling, University of Rochester, 1980) is President of National Fire Service Support Systems, Inc., an organization specializing in research, training, and program development addressing children and fire. Mr. Schwartzman is a coauthor of the *Fireproof Children Handbook* and the *Fireproof Children Education Kit,* program guides for community agencies addressing the problem of juvenile fire play and fire setting. He has published articles about his research regarding children and fire and other high-risk behaviors. Mr. Schwartzman maintains a private practice in Rochester, New York.

Mitsuko P. Shannon (Pharm.D., University of Kentucky, 1982; M.D., Marshall University, 1988) is a Fellow in Child and Adolescent Psychiatry at the Medical University of South Carolina, Charleston, South Carolina. Dr. Shannon's areas of interest include pediatric psychopharmacology, childhood post-traumatic stress disorder, and organic psychopathology.

Daniel S. Shaw (Ph.D., University of Virginia, 1988) is Assistant Professor of Psychology and Psychiatry at the University of Pittsburgh. He has published extensively on the effects of parental conflict on child outcome in married and divorced populations. Dr. Shaw also has been concerned with the adverse effects of other chronic family stressors on child outcome, including parental psychopathology, overcrowding, and low income. This focus on chronic family adversity has recently been directed to studying the precursors of antisocial behavior in high-risk populations, beginning when children are 1 to 2 years old.

Wendy K. Silverman (Ph.D., Case Western Reserve University, 1981) is Professor of Psychology at Florida International University. Dr. Silverman has published widely in the area of childhood anxiety. She has research grants from National Institute of Mental Health to evaluate the efficacy of various treatment interventions for childhood phobic and anxiety disorders.

Vaughan Stagg (Ph.D., George Peabody College of Vanderbilt University, 1983) is Assistant Professor of Psychiatry at the University of Pittsburgh School of Medicine and Clinical Administrator of the Theiss Health and Child Development Center. His research and publication interests include the role of social support networks of parents, assessment of low-incidence handicapping conditions, and psychopathology of child witnesses of violence. Currently Dr. Stagg is involved in the creation of clinical services for young children with psychiatric problems.

Aubyn C. Stahmer (M.A., University of California, San Diego) is a doctoral student at the University of California, San Diego, specializing in the study of children with autism. Her current research involves examining symbolic play in children with autism as it relates to social and language development.

Kevin D. Stark (Ph.D., University of Wisconsin, 1985) is Associate Professor of Educational Psychology at the University of Texas and Acting Director of the School Psychology Program. He serves on the editorial board of *School Psychology Review, School Psychology Quarterly, Behavior Modification,* and *Journal of Emotional and Behavioral Disorders.* Dr. Stark's principal areas of research and writing have been in cognitive-behavior therapy, depressive disorders among youth, and the delivery of mental health services in schools.

Jeannie Starzynski (M.S.W., University of Pittsburgh, 1982) is currently Coordinator of Staff Development at Western Psychiatric Institute and Clinic, University of Pittsburgh Medical Center. She has specialized in child development and mental health and has had extensive experience as a family therapist on adolescent and young adult inpatient psychiatric units, working for the past five years on the Eating Disorders Unit at WPIC. Ms. Starzynski has also participated in a longitudinal study of depression in children. She has published in the areas of affective disorders, delinquency, and eating disorders.

Bruce A. Thyer (Ph.D., University of Michigan, 1982) is Professor of Social Work and Adjunct Professor of Clinical Psychology at the University of Georgia, and Associate Clinical Professor of Psychiatry and Health Behavior at the Medical College of Georgia. Dr. Thyer is the founding editor of *Research on Social Work Practice* and serves on the editorial boards of the *Journal of Anxiety Disorders, Journal of Applied Behavior Analysis, The Behavior Analyst, Journal of Behavioral Education,* and *Journal of Behavior Therapy and Experimental Psychiatry.* Dr. Thyer has written over 120 journal articles and authored or edited six books. His major professional interest is in promoting behavior analysis with social work and the other human service professions.

Kimberli R. H. Treadwell (B.A., Miami University, 1989) is a doctoral candidate of clinical psychology at Temple University. Her dissertation examines cognitive distortions in anxious children. Ms. Treadwell is currently a diagnostician and therapist at the Child and Adolescent Anxiety Disorders Clinic at Temple University, a federally funded cognitive-behavioral treatment outcome study. Her interests include childhood internalizing disorders and their treatment.

Jan L. Wallander (Ph.D., Purdue University, 1981) is Associate Professor of Psychology at the Civitan International Research Center at the University of Alabama at Birmingham. He has published extensively in the area of pediatric psychology, especially on adjustment to chronic illness in children. Dr. Wallander is President of the Society of Pediatric Psychology (Section V, Division 12, American Psychological Association), Associate Editor of the *Journal of Pediatric Psychology,* and holds a Research Career Development Award from NIH/NICHD. He currently directs a NIH/NICHD-funded longitudinal study of stress, coping, and adjustment in adolescents with mild mental retardation.

Theodore E. Weltzin (M.D., University of Minnesota, 1984), is Assistant Professor of Psychiatry at the University of Pittsburgh. He is currently the Director of the Inpatient Eating Disorder Program, Center for Overcoming Problem Eating. His research, conducted jointly with Dr. Walter Kaye, focuses on the psychobiology of anorexia and bulimia nervosa. He has published several articles in the field of abnormal eating behavior and the effects of pharmacologic probes on eating behavior in anorexia and bulimia nervosa. Dr. Weltzin currently is involved in research grants examining the effects of reproductive function in women with bulimia nervosa and also the association between bulimia nervosa and alcohol abuse.

Cindy L. Wigg (M.D., St. Louis University, 1980) is Assistant Professor of Psychiatry and Behavioral Sciences at University of Texas Medical Branch. She is the Medical Director of the Adolescent Psychiatry Inpatient Unit and Associate Training Director for the General Residency Program. Dr. Wigg's interests include the presentation of affective disorders in children and adolescents, adolescent development, and medical student and resident education.

CHAPTER 1

A PRESCRIPTIVE APPROACH TO TREATMENT OF CHILDREN AND ADOLESCENTS

Robert T. Ammerman   Western Pennsylvania School for Blind Children
Cynthia G. Last   Nova University
Michel Hersen   Nova University

INTRODUCTION

After decades of relative neglect when contrasted with adults, child and adolescent psychopathology and treatment have become the focus of increased interest and research. This is evidenced in part by a dramatic rise in publications on the assessment and treatment of child and adolescent disorders. For example, two recent special issues of the *Journal of Consulting and Clinical Psychology* have been devoted to treatment of children and adolescents (Kazdin, 1990a; Morris & Kendall, 1991). Similarly, in 1989, the *American Psychologist* dedicated an entire issue to problems faced by children and youth (Horowitz, 1989). Also, a number of journals have been established in the last 20 years that are specifically devoted to children (e.g., *Journal of Abnormal Child Psychology* and *Journal of Child and Family Studies*), and several established journals have grown in prominence as they increasingly demonstrate high standards of methodological rigor (e.g., *Journal of the American Academy of Child and Adolescent Psychiatry*).

Growth in the quantity of research on children and adolescents and improvements in design and methodology have greatly expanded our knowledge base. Illustrative is our increased understanding of such areas as adolescent suicide, which has been elucidated by several large-scale research efforts (e.g., see Pfeffer, 1989). Similar advances have taken place in behavioral categorization and psychiatric diagnosis (see Last & Hersen, 1989). For example, significant strides have been made in differentiating the disruptive behavior disorders (attention deficit-hyperactivity disorder, conduct disorder, oppositional defiant disorder) (see Baum, 1989) and in delineating school phobia versus separation anxiety disorder (see Burke & Silverman, 1987). Theoretical advances have also occurred. It is now generally accepted that child and adolescent psychopathology must be considered in the context of normal cognitive, social, and emotional development. Also, physiological concomitants of a number of disorders such as obsessive-compulsive disorder (see Rapoport, 1986) have been identified.

Taken together, it is evident that the field has expanded both quantatively and in increased sophistication in experimental design. It is against this backdrop that an empirically driven, prescriptive approach to treatment is imperative. That is, now it is possible for clinicians to conduct assessments and select treatments while being guided by the extant scientific literature.

EFFECTIVENESS OF PSYCHOTHERAPY WITH CHILDREN AND ADOLESCENTS

What is child psychotherapy? How effective is it? What factors and characteristics are associated with positive outcome? All of these questions have generated considerable debate over the past half century and have been the subject of several reviews in the last decade (Kazdin, 1991). There is a general consensus that, relative to adult psychotherapy, research on child and adolescent psychotherapy is nascent. However, there has been an equally strong drive in recent years to take stock of the child and adolescent psychotherapy literature, and examine the overall effectiveness of psychotherapeutic interventions as well as identify parameters of positive outcome. Indeed, an empirically focused and prescriptive approach to treatment demands such information.

The first question (What is psychotherapy?) defies a simple resolution. Kazdin (1991) has estimated that there are over 230 approaches to *child psychotherapy,* which he broadly defines as

> an intervention designed to decrease distress, psychological symptoms, maladaptive behavior or to improve adaptive and psychosocial functioning. These ends are sought primarily through interpersonal sources of influence such as learning, persuasion, counseling, and discussion integrated into a specific treatment plan. The focus is on some facet regarding how clients feel (affect), think (cognition), and act (behavior). (p. 785)

Early reviews (e.g., Levitt, 1957) argued against the effectiveness of child psychotherapy relative to no treatment, although the literature on which these conclusions were based was scant and characterized by serious methodological limitations. Research conducted since these reviews appeared, although methodologically stronger, still suffers from shortcomings in design. Most prominent among these are failure to use control groups, unclear or poorly delineated subject populations, vague treatment protocols, failure to monitor treatment integrity, and use of inappropriate assessment strategies. An additional area of concern in many investigations to date has been the lack of statistical power to detect significant differences between treatments (rather than between treatment and no-treatment controls) (Kazdin & Bass, 1989).

The advent of meta-analysis (Glass, McGrow, & Smith, 1981) has permitted a quantitative examination of treatment outcome research. In meta-analysis, studies meeting previously determined criteria are aggregated and rated according to predetermined criteria, and main effects across studies are derived. Specifically, each study is quantified in such a way as to generate an *effect size,* which is defined as the difference between means of treatment and control conditions divided by the standard deviation of the control group. The effect size reflects overall treatment effectiveness and is further used to delineate factors associated with treatment outcome (e.g., type of treatment, subject characteristics implicated in positive outcome). The advantage of meta-analysis is that it is an objective approach to examining multiple studies rather than relying solely on the subjective judgment inherent in so-called traditional reviews.

However, meta-analysis is a correlational procedure, and within-study methodological limitations are not obviated through this statistical approach. That is, all studies have equal weight in a meta-analysis, regardless of design limitations. (It should be noted that the degree to which methodologically weak studies influence a meta-analysis is a matter of contention. Weiss and Weisz [1990] examined the influence of threats to internal and external validity on a meta-analysis of child psychotherapy. Results indicated that such factors accounted for only 7 percent of the outcome variance, compared with 11 percent for "substantive" variables [e.g., type of treatment, age]. Validity factors did not affect the pattern of findings in the meta-analysis, but rather they *reduced* overall effect size. This finding belies the concerns of several authors [e.g., Wilson & Rachman, 1983] that validity problems may contribute to an overestimation of effect size.)

Two recent meta-analyses (Casey & Berman, 1985; Weisz, Weiss, Alicke, & Klotz, 1987) have sought to determine the overall effectiveness of child and adolescent psychotherapy, and identify factors associated with positive outcome. Casey and Berman examined 75 studies (published between 1952 and 1983) of psychotherapy outcome in children and adolescents aged 3 to 15 years. Specific goals of the meta-analysis were to determine (1) whether or not some forms of psychotherapy were superior to others, (2) if the efficacy of psychotherapy varied as a function of outcome measures used, and (3) those child characteristics that mediate outcome. Studies reviewed had an average $N = 42$ at posttreatment, looked at children who were primarily male (60 percent) and had a mean age of 8.9 years, and included treatments that were carried out for an average of 9.5 weeks (range = 1 to 37 weeks). Behavior therapy was the most common form of treatment represented (56 percent); 21 percent of studies examined cognitive-behavior therapy. Client-centered therapy was evaluated in 28 percent of studies, and dynamic therapy was represented in 9 percent.

Results indicated an overall effect size of .71. In other words, children receiving psychotherapy had an outcome more than two-thirds of a standard deviation better than controls. This finding is consistent with meta-analyses of adult psychotherapy (e.g., Shapiro & Shapiro, 1982). Behavioral interventions were more effective than their nonbehavioral counterparts, with effect sizes of .91 and .40, respectively. No differences were found between play versus nonplay therapies, individual versus group approaches, parent-involved versus child-only interventions, or as a function of age. Treatment effectiveness was greater in children displaying impulsivity, phobia, and somatic problems (these were also most likely to

be targeted in those studies evaluating behavior therapy). Problems of social adjustment were less responsive to treatment.

Shapiro and Shapiro (1982) argued that the reltive superiority of behavior therapy was tempered by the fact that behavioral and nonbehavioral treatment outcome studies tended to target different problems. Moreover, they contended that assessment measures used in behavioral studies were often directly linked to treatment targets, as opposed to more global indices of functioning utilized in nonbehavioral studies. When these therapy-specific measures (which the authors believed led to an artificially inflated effect size for behavior therapy) were excluded from the analysis, behavior therapy was no longer superior to nonbehavioral interventions.

In a second meta-analysis, Weisz and colleagues (1987) examined 105 outcome studies (see Weiss & Weisz, 1990) of behavioral and nonbehavioral interventions with children and adolescents aged 4 to 18 years. Studies were selected only if they contrasted a treatment condition with a nontreatment or minimally treated (i.e., attention) control group. As in Casey and Berman (1985), the authors sought to identify overall treatment effectiveness as well as correlates of positive treatment outcome. However, Weisz and associates (1987) cogently argued that the close link between assessment to the treatment target in many behavioral evaluations is not necessarily a confound in determining effect size of behavior therapy versus nonbehavioral interventions. They pointed out that, for example, in the case of phobia, the most clinically meaningful indication of fear and its reduction is degree of approach to the feared stimulus (typically used to assess behavioral interventions for phobia). In this case, global measures of child adjustment are tangentially, not primarily, relevant. In their meta-analysis, Weisz and associates distinguished between outcome "measures similar to the training procedures [that] are appropriate and necessary for a fair test of treatment success" (1987, p. 546) and those assessments intricately linked to treatment that were deemed "unnecessary."

Findings revealed a mean effect size of .79 for treatment versus control comparisons. Once again, behavior therapy was found to be more effective than nonbehavioral interventions (.88 versus .44). This superiority remained when "appropriate and necessary" assessments were retained (.93 versus .45), but it disappeared when *all* therapy-like measures were eliminated. Overall effect size did not significantly change as a function of problem type (i.e., overcontrolled versus undercontrolled behavioral disorders). Children (ages 4 to 12) were more likely to improve when contrasted with adolescents (ages 13 to 18). Also, investigations using analogue samples obtained equivalent findings to those recruiting subjects from clinics. Finally, treatment gains were likely to be maintained at 6-month followup.

A third meta-analysis (Durlak, Fuhrman, & Lampman, 1991), albeit more circumscribed in scope, examined the effectiveness of and mediating factors in cognitive-behavior therapy for children. Specifically, 64 studies published between 1970 and 1987 were selected for analysis. Criteria for inclusion consisted of the use of a control group, treatment of behaviorally disordered children, and implementation of cognitive-behavioral treatment *without* concurrent family therapy or other form of treatment. Results indicated that treatment effectiveness was mediated by age and, presumably, level of cognitive development. The effect size was greater for children aged 11 to 13 years (.92) relative to children aged 5 to 10 years (.57 and .55). The authors concluded that cognitive-behavior therapy is more effective for children in the formal operations stage of cognitive development rather than in the preoperational and concrete operations stages. Other factors (e.g., type of problem, methodological features) did not emerge as significant influences on effect size.

The above meta-analyses yield several important conclusions. First, psychotherapy is an effective intervention for a variety of social, emotional, and behavioral problems in children and adolescents. Moreover, treatment effects are durable at short-term followup. Second, behavior therapy in particular is an especially effective type of intervention. And third, effect sizes are similar in meta-analyses of both the child and adult treatment literatures.

However, meta-analyses are constrained by the limitations of the studies subjected to evaluation. Indeed, there are a variety of critical issues in the treatment outcome literature for children and adolescents that require attention in future research (see Kazdin, 1990b, 1991). As the empirical literature evolves and expands, we will more closely approximate Paul's oft-quoted query: "*What* treatment, by *whom,* is the most effective for *this* individual with *that* specific problem, under *which* set of circumstances?" (1967, p. 111). Some of the needs that must be addressed (Kazdin, 1990b) in future research are:

- Increased evaluation of clinical samples
- Consideration of diagnostic comorbidity
- Evaluation of underresearched treatment modalities
- Evaluation of combined interventions
- Outcome measurement of both symptom reduction and increased prosocial functioning
- Determination of clinical versus statistical significance
- use of psychometrically strong and appropriate assessment instruments
- Monitoring of treatment integrity
- longer and more frequent posttreatment followup assessments
- Consideration of statistical power to detect differences between two or more treatments

FROM RESEARCH TO CLINICAL PRACTICE

The clinician searching for an empirically focused, prescriptive approach to treatment faces several impediments upon examining the literature. Aside from methodological problems that limit conclusions drawn from existing studies, there is a discrepancy between the focus of much of the research on treatment of children and adolescence and actual clinical practice. Kazdin, Bass, Ayers, and Rodgers examined the characteristics of 223 studies published between 1970 and 1985. They found that the bulk of these studies represented a restricted focus in terms of client, treatment, and outcome factors. For example, the majority of research emphasized treatment come independent of mediating influences, thus failing "to avoid the implicit view that a given treatment is likely to operate in a uniform fashion across all conditions" (1990, p. 737). Other tendencies in the literature were a disproportionate evaluation of behavioral versus other types of interventions, a preponderance of subject samples recruited from schools rather than clinics, treatment delivery in group rather than individual formats, almost exclusive use of brief treatments, and implementation of child treatment without participation of parents and/or teachers.

Paradoxically, a significant number of clinicians practice with a blatant disregard of the empirical literature (as evidenced by the popularity of psychodynamic and play therapies despite the demonstrated effectiveness of behavioral interventions). Conversely, there is an equal disregard in much of treatment outcome research for salient issues faced in clinical practice. In clinical settings, clients typically present with multiple problems and comorbid diagnoses, additional factors impinge on child and family functioning (e.g., family and neighborhood violence, poverty), treatment is individually or family based with concurrent involvement of other adult caretakers, and treatment is lengthy. Other issues clinicians face and that potentially interfere with treatment are client noncompliance, logistical difficulties (e.g., client transportation problems), multiple treatments and involvement of several clinicians, intermittent rather than regular contact, and relapse. Rarely are these issues addressed formally in treatment outcome research.

This is not to say that the more circumscribed focus of much treatment outcome research precludes generalization of findings to clinical settings. In fact, there is evidence to indicate that current clinical practice is largely ineffective. Weisz and Weiss (1989) used the Child Behavior Checklist to contrast children and adolescents treated at an outpatient clinic with dropouts from the same setting. No therapy effect was found at posttreatment or at 1-year followup. While at first glance, these results might appear to mitigate the more sanguine conclusions derived from the meta-analyses, it is also possible to interpret these findings as an endorsement for a prescriptive approach to treatment. Indeed, Weisz and Weiss pointed out that "child and adolescent psychotherapy can be effective when conditions of therapy are carefully arranged, as when specific targets of treatment are clearly delineated, when these are well matched to the type of therapy provided and when the therapists involved are well trained in the approach they use" (1989, p. 746).

THE EMERGENCE OF CHILD AND ADOLESCENT PSYCHOPHARMACOLOGY

Pharmacology treatment of psychiatric problems in children and adolescents is a recent development. Not surprisingly, therefore, controlled research in this area is sparse. However, as etiological models of child and adolescent psychopathology have increasingly emphasized the combined influences of social, psychological, and biological factors, pharmacological approaches have emerged as an important intervention. Indeed, although child and adolescent psychopharmacology as a whole suffers from a lack of empirical research, several drugs have been the focus of careful experimental evaluation. Recent examples include methylphenidate (Ritalin) for attention deficit-hyperactivity disorder (see Dulcan, 1985b) and clorimipramine (Anafranil) for obsessive-compulsive disorder. Table 1–1 presents a list of psychotropic medications and their established and possible indications for children based on a recent comprehensive review by Bukstein (in press).

Despite the increased use of pharmacological agents with children and adolescents, it must be emphasized that such interventions are always administered in conjunction with psychosocial treatment. As Dulcan pointed out, "Medication is almost never appropriate as the sole intervention for the entire therapeutic 'career' of a child or adolescent." She also warns against "piecemeal care, with medication over or under used and poorly integrated with psychosocial or educational interventions" (1985a, p. 64).

Table 1–1. Psychotropic Agents Used with Children

AGENT	ESTABLISHED INDICATION(S)	POSSIBLE INDICATION(S)
Antidepressants		
Imipramine	Enuresis	Major depression School refusal or phobia Panic disorder Obsessive-compulsive disorder Phobic disorders Dysthymic disorder
Amitriptyline		
Desipramine	Attention-deficit hyperactivity disorder	(as above) Conduct disorder Sleep terror disorder Sleep walk terror
Nortriptyline		Major depression
Fluoxetine		Major depression Obsessive-compulsive disorder
Neuroleptics		
Chlorpromazine	Acute Psychotic states Bipolar disorder Manic phase Schizophreniform disorder Drug-induced psychosis schizrenia	Dyscontrol Severe aggressive or agitated behavior
Thioridazine	Autistic disorder and Pervasive developmental disorder	(as above)
Trifluoperazine	Dyskinetic movement disorders Tourette's disorder	(as above)
Haloperidol	(as above) Chronic motor or vocalic disorder	
Thiothixene		
Pimozide		
Stimulants		
Dextroamphetamine	Attention-deficit hyperactivity disorder	ADHD in (a) Tourette's/Other tic disorders (b) Autistic disorder or pervasive developmental disorders (c) Head trauma
Methylphenidate	Attention-deficit hyperactivity disorder	(same as above)
Pemoline	Attention-deficit hyperactivity disorder	(same as above)
Propranolol		Hypertension Tachyarrhythmias Aggression Dyscontrol states Migraine headaches
Benzodiazepines		
Diazepam	Seizures Sleep walking Night terrors	Anxiety disorders Behavior disorders
Other Drugs		
Lithium carbonate	Bipolar disorder	Bipolar II Rapid cycling Aggressive behavior

Table 1–1. *(Continued)*

AGENT	ESTABLISHED INDICATION(S)	POSSIBLE INDICATION(S)
Clonidine	Hypertension	Tourette's disorder Attention-deficit hyperactivity disorder Manic episodes Aggressive behavior
Antihistamines		Anxiety Insomnia
Hydroxyzine		Drug-induced extrapyramidal reactions Agitation

Source: Adapted from Bukstein, O. G. (1993). Overview of pharmacological treatment. In V. B. Van Hasselt & M. Hersen (Eds.), *Handbook of behavior therapy and pharmacotherapy for children.* Boston: Allyn and Bacon.

SUMMARY

A prescriptive approach to the treatment of child and adolescent psychopathology necessitates clinical practice dictated by the empirical literature. Until recently, this literature has been sparse and methodologically weak. At this point, however, it is clear that psychotherapy for children and adolescents is effective. Behavior therapy stands out as especially efficacious for a variety of internalizing and externalizing disorders. In addition, psychopharmacological interventions have become increasingly important adjuncts to psychosocial treatment. Much research remains to be conducted, particularly taking into account several issues salient to practices that have not yet been addressed in the empirical literature.

REFERENCES

Baum, C. G. (1989). Conduct disorders. In T. H. Ollendick & M. Hersen (Eds.), *Handbook of child psychopathology* (2nd ed., pp. 171–196). New York: Plenum.

Bukstein, O. G. (in press). Overview of pharmacological treatment. In V. B. Van Hasselt & M. Hersen (Eds.), *Handbook of behavior therapy and pharmacotherapy for children.* Boston: Allyn and Bacon.

Burke, A. E., & Silverman, W. K. (1987). The prescriptive treatment of school refusal. *Clinical Psychology Review, 7,* 353–362.

Casey, R. J., & Berman, J. S. (1985). The outcome of psychotherapy with children. *Psychological Bulletin, 98,* 388–400.

Dulcan, M. K. (1985a). Psychopharmacology in childhood and adolescence. *Psychiatric Annals, 15,* 64.

Dulcan, M. K. (1985b). The psychopharmacologic treatment of children and adolescents with attention deficit disorder. *Psychiatric Annals, 15,* 69–86.

Durlak, J. A., Fuhrman, P., & Lampman, C. (1991). Effectiveness of cognitive-behavior therapy for maladapting children: A meta-analysis. *Psychological Bulletin, 110,* 204–214.

Glass, G. V., McGraw, B., & Smith, M. L. (1981). *Meta-analysis in social research.* Beverly Hills, CA: Sage.

Horowitz, F. D. (1989). Editor, Special Issue: Children and their development: Knowledge base, research agenda and social policy application. *American Psychologist, 44,* 95–445.

Kazdin, A. E. (1990a). Editor, Special Series: Research on therapies for children and adolescents. *Journal of Consulting Psychology, 58,* 681–740.

Kazdin, A. E. (1990b). Psychotherapy for children and adolescents. *Annual Review of Psychology, 41,* 21–54.

Kazdin, A. E. (1991). Effectiveness of psychotherapy with children and adolescents. *Journal of Consulting and Clinical Psychology, 59,* 785–798.

Kazdin, A. E., & Bass, D. (1989). Power to detect differences between alternative treatments in comparative psychotherapy outcome research. *Journal of Consulting and Clinical Psychology, 57,* 138–147.

Kazdin, A. E., Bass, D., Ayers, W. A., & Rodgers, A. (1990). Empirical and clinical focus of child and adolescent psychotherapy research. *Journal of Consulting and Clinical Psychology, 58,* 729–740.

Last, C. G., & Hersen, M. (Eds.). *Handbook of child psychiatric diagnosis.* New York: Wiley & Sons.

Levitt, E. E. (1957). The results of psychotherapy with children: An evaluation. *Journal of Consulting Psychology, 21,* 189–196.

Morris, R. J., & Kendall, P. C. (1991). Editors, Special Section: Clinical child psychology: Perspectives on child and adolescent therapy. *Journal of Consulting and Clinical Psychology, 59,* 763–860.

Paul, G. L. (1967). Outcome research in psychotherapy. *Journal of Consulting Psychology, 31,* 109–118.

Pfeffer, C. R. (1989). Suicide. In L. K. G. Hsu & M. Hersen (Eds.), *Recent developments in adolescent psychiatry.* New York: Wiley & Sons.

Rapoport, J. L. (1986). Childhood obsessive compulsive disorder. *Journal of Psychology and Psychiatry, 27,* 289–295.

Shapiro, D. A., & Shapiro, D. (1982). Meta-analysis of comparative therapy outcome studies: A replication and refinement. *Psychological Bulletin, 92,* 581–604.

Weiss, B., & Weisz, J. R. (1990). The impact of methodological factors on child psychotherapy outcome research: A meta-analysis for researchers. *Journal of Abnormal Child Psychology,* 639–670.

Weisz, J. R., & Weiss, B. (1989). Assessing the effects of clinic-based psychotherapy with children and adolescents. *Journal of Consulting and Clinical Psychology, 57,* 741–746.

Weisz, J. R., Weiss, B., Alicke, M. D., & Klotz, M. L. (1987). Effectiveness of psychotherapy with children and adolescents: A meta-analysis for clinicians. *Journal of Consulting and Clinical Psychology, 55,* 542–549.

Wilson, G. T., & Rachman, S. J. (1983). Meta-analysis and the evaluation of psychotherapy outcome: Limitations and liabilities. *Journal of Consulting and Clinical Psychology, 51,* 54–64.

CHAPTER 2

AUTISTIC DISORDER

Laura Schreibman   University of California, San Diego

Lauren M. Loos   University of California, San Diego

Aubyn C. Stahmer   University of California, San Diego

DESCRIPTION OF DISORDER

Autistic disorder, first described as early infantile autism in 1943 by Leo Kanner, has proven to be one of the most fascinating forms of childhood psychopathology challenging the talents of clinicians, teachers, and families. Over the past 30 years, behavioral researchers and clinicians have spent a tremendous amount of time and effort understanding the nature of the psychopathology and developing effective treatments.

It is quite likely that one of the reasons for the fascination with autism is the specific behavioral features that comprise the syndrome. Below is a brief description of the main behaviors associated with autistic disorder (for a more comprehensive description, see Schreibman, 1988).

Clinical Features

1. *Deficits in social behavior.* Perhaps the hallmark feature of children with autism is their profound and pervasive deficits in social attachment and behavior. There is a distinct failure to bond with parents or to attach emotionally with others. This is evident in failure to establish eye contact, resistance to being held, indifference to (or active avoidance of) the affectionate overtures of others, and otherwise general social unresponsiveness. Infants with autism typically do not cry for attention, do not like being held, and prefer to be alone. This preference for being alone typically persists as the child grows older. Such children are described as being "loners." They do not seek out or play interactively with peers. They do not come to their parents when hurt or frightened nor do they use their parents as a secure base in novel situations. Many parents report that they feel their child is not emotionally attached to them. Even a very high functioning, older individual with autism may exhibit social deficits such as not being responsive to the more subtle social cues of others.

2. *Deficits in speech and language.* Approximately 50 percent of children with autism do

The preparation of this chapter, and some of the research reported herein, was facilitated and supported by U.S.P.H.S. Research Grants MH 39434 and MH 28210 from the National Institute of Mental Health.

not develop functional language. Those who do speak typically exhibit speech that is qualitatively different from the speech of normal children and children with other language disorders. Speaking children with autism often exhibit a specific speech anomaly called *echolalia:* the repetition of words or phrases spoken by others. In *immediate echolalia,* the children repeat what they have just heard. For example, the child is asked "What is this?" to which she replies "What is this?" In *delayed echolalia,* the child repeats something heard in the past. For example, the child may be sitting at the dinner table and begin to repeat instructions from the teacher given earlier in the day or perhaps a television commercial heard several weeks earlier. Another distinctive speech anomaly is *pronominal reversal* wherein personal pronouns are reversed. The child may say "You want to go outside" or "Johnny go outside" instead of "I want to go outside." In addition, the speech of individuals with autism is often characterized by *dysprosody.* Thus the speech is inaccurate in pitch, rhythm, inflection, intonation, pace, and/or articulation such that even individuals with relatively sophisticated language skills often sound abnormal when they speak.

3. *Demand for sameness in the environment.* Kanner (1943) described children with autism as having a compulsive desire for the "preservation of sameness." Typically this behavior is evident when the child becomes distressed by changes in the environment (such as furniture arrangements), routes of travel, or daily routine. He or she may have very rigid play patterns, ritualistic preoccupations (e.g., memorizing bus schedules), or rituals such as insistence on eating particular foods, wearing only certain clothing, touching particular objects, or repeatedly asking the same question.

4. *Abnormalities in response to the sensory environment.* Many children with autism have histories of suspected, but unconfirmed, deafness or blindness. They may fail to respond to their name or to a loud sound. Similarly, they may not notice someone entering a room. However, such lack of responsivity is highly variable in nature. The child who does not respond to his name or a noise might cover his ears at the sound of a fire engine or repeat a television commercial. A child who fails to notice the presence of others may be able to spot a piece of candy several feet away or be fascinated by pieces of lint falling through a beam of light. Unusual responsivity is noted in other modalities as well. Children with autism might be over- or underresponsive to touch, pain, or temperature. They may lick, smell, or mouth objects or be fascinated by spinning objects such as fans.

5. *Self-stimulatory behavior.* Many children with autism engage in self-stimulatory behavior (also called stereotypy), which involves stereotyped, typically repetitive, nonfunctional behavior whose purpose seems to be primarily to provide sensory feedback. Common forms of self-stimulation include gross motor behaviors, such as body rocking, arm and/or hand flapping, head rolling, jumping, spinning, or clapping. Other behaviors include waving fingers in front of eyes, gazing from the side of the eye, repetitive vocalizations, gazing intently at spinning objects, or gazing into space.

6. *Self-injurious behavior (SIB).* SIB involves any behavior in which the individual inflicts damage to his or her own body. In individuals with autism the most common forms of SIB include head banging and self-biting of hands or wrists. Other behaviors are elbow or leg banging, hair pulling, face scratching, or self-slapping of sides of face. Such individuals may tear out their fingernails with their teeth, gouge their eyes, and bite off pieces of flesh. Self-injury may vary in intensity and therefore the amount of damage incurred can range from slight to life threatening.

7. *Unusual affect.* Individuals with autism may exhibit flattened, excessive, or otherwise inappropriate affect. Some seem totally placid, others may throw raging tantrums with the slightest of provocations, laugh hysterically or cry inconsolably for no apparent reason. Many of the children exhibit irrational fears (e.g., a certain picture, a certain television theme song, a specific food).

Associated Features

1. *Intellectual functioning.* Kanner (1943) originally believed children with autism to be intelligent; we now know, however, that the majority are in fact retarded. Current research estimates that approximately 60 percent of children with autism have measured IQs below 50, 20 percent between 50 and 70, while 20 percent measure 70 or above. Typically there is a discrepancy between scores on verbal and performance tasks. These children do better on performance tests and more poorly on verbal tests. As with other children, IQ in children with autism tends to remain stable throughout childhood and adolescence and tends to be predictive of future educational accomplishments. Thus, while autism and retardation are separate events, they often coexist in the same individual.

2. *Special skills.* Many children with autism exhibit isolated areas of normal or exceptional performance that are incongruous with their otherwise diminished functioning level. These abilities most commonly fall into the areas of memorization, mechanical abilities, or musical skills. An extremely small minority of these individuals are true "savants" (as in the movie *Rainman*), but many display exceptional skills of some kind.

Epidemiology

Existing studies show the prevalence of true autism to be between 3.1 and 5 per 10,000 live births. Most commonly the statistic is reported as 1 per 2,500 births. The disorder is heavily weighted toward the male such that for every 1 girl there are 4 boys with the disorder. The disorder is not differentially associated with any particular race, geographical location, or socioeconomic level.

Etiology

The etiology of autistic disorder is unknown. Earlier theories suggested that the disorder was psychogenic in origin and the parents, especially the mother, were implicated as causative agents (e.g., Bettelheim, 1967). However, the parent-causation hypothesis is no longer considered valid, and currently most believe that the disorder is organic in nature although the specific nature of the organic problem is unknown. It is quite possible that autism is a syndrome comprised of a set of behaviors differentially exhibited by subgroups of individuals whose disorder can be attributed to different etiologies. Thus some have hypothesized subgroups of autistic disorder with correlated genetic factors (e.g., August & Lockhart, 1984; Ritvo et al., 1985), neurochemical factors (e.g., Mesibov & Dawson, 1986; Sahley & Panksepp, 1987), and neuroanatomical factors (e.g., Bauman & Kemper, 1985; Murikami, Courchesne, Press, Yeung-Courchesne, & Hesselink, 1989).

DIFFERENTIAL DIAGNOSIS AND ASSESSMENT

DSM-III-R Categorization

The set of diagnostic criteria set forth in the DSM-III-R (American Psychiatric Association, 1987), based on consensus of clinical impressions, is the most widely used and accepted of the many available criteria. Autistic Disorder is a subcategory of Pervasive Developmental Disorder (the other is Pervasive Developmental Disorder, Not Otherwise Specified [PDD NOS]). The criteria for Autistic Disorder include:

1. Qualitative impairment in reciprocal social interaction as manifested by at least two of the following characteristics: (a) marked lack of awareness of the existence or feelings of others, (b) no or abnormal seeking of comfort at times of distress, (c) no or impaired imitation, (d) no or abnormal social play, and (e) gross impairment in the ability to make peer friendships.

2. Qualitative impairment in verbal and nonverbal communication, and in imaginative activity, as manifested by at least one of the following: (a) no mode of communication, such as communicative babbling, facial expression, gesture, mime, or spoken language; (b) markedly abnormal nonverbal communication, as in the use of

eye-to-eye contact, facial expression, body posture, or gestures to initiate or modulate social interaction; (c) absence of imaginative activity, such as play-acting of adult roles, fantasy characters, or animals, and lack of interest in stories about imaginary events; (d) marked abnormalities in the production of speech, including volume, pitch, stress, rate, rhythm, and intonation; (e) marked abnormalities in the form or content of speech, including stereotyped repetitive use of speech (e.g., echolalia), reversal of pronouns, idiosyncratic use of words or phrases, or frequent irrelevant remarks; and (f) marked impairment in the ability to initiate or sustain a conversation with others, despite adequate speech.

3. Markedly restricted repertoire of activities and interests, as manifested by at least one of the following: (a) stereotyped body movements, (b) persistent preoccupation with parts of objects or attachment to unusual objects, (c) marked distress over changes in trivial aspects of environment, (d) unreasonable insistence on following routines in precise detail, and (e) markedly restricted range of interests and a preoccupation with one narrow interest.

4. Onset during infancy or childhood (although the diagnosis of Autistic Disorder is usually reserved for those exhibiting features of the syndrome by the age of 36 months).

Differential Diagnosis

1. *Schizophrenia, childhood type.* Children who might fall into this category (formerly called childhood schizophrenia) share several features with children diagnosed with autistic disorder. These include sustained impairment in social relations, resistance to change, speech abnormalities, and constricted or inappropriate affect (e.g., Schreibman, 1988). However, there are important distinctions between the two populations. One distinction is age of onset. For a diagnosis of autistic disorder, the child must exhibit the main clinical features of the syndrome prior to the age of 3 years with no history of normal development. Schizophrenic children, on the other hand, typ-

ically have some period of normal development before onset of symptoms between the ages of 3 and 12 years. In addition, these children with later onset are more likely to exhibit the features of adult schizophrenia. In general, autistic disorder is differentiated by early onset, less common family history of mental disorder, normal or above-average motor development, more severe cognitive impairment, no period of normal development preceding the appearance of symptoms, good physical health, and failure to develop complex language and social skills. In contrast, children likely to be diagnosed as schizophrenic, childhood type, have a later onset of symptoms, family history of mental disorder, poor physical health, poor motor development, less cognitive impairment, periods of remissions and relapses (with a period of normal development prior to symptom onset), better language skills, and the presence of delusions and/or hallucinations (Schreibman, 1988). In addition, schizophrenic children may indulge in the creation of a fantasy life or inner world, whereas such behavior is not associated with autistic disorder (Clarizio & McCoy, 1983).

2. *Pervasive developmental disorder.* This diagnostic category is reserved for those children who neither manifest the behaviors of schizophrenia nor the specific features of autism. However, there are other differences between children with pervasive developmental disorder (PDD) and children with autistic disorder (e.g., American Psychiatric Association, 1987; Mesibov & Dawson, 1986). PDD children exhibit impairment in social relationships, however, the impairment may not take the form of unresponsiveness. The language impairments may be of different form and/or less severe than in autism. In addition, motor abnormalities and other behavioral oddities are more likely to be present in PDD children.

3. *Developmental aphasia.* Children with developmental aphasia fail to develop, or are delayed in the development of, comprehension and vocal expression of language. These children share some features with children with autism,

including echolalia, pronominal reversal, sequencing problems, and comprehension difficulty, however the language deficits in autism are more severe than in aphasia (e.g., Churchill, 1972; Rutter, Bartak, & Newman, 1971). As a consequence of language difficulties, many aphasic children acquire secondary problems in social relationships (Ornitz & Ritvo, 1976), although the social difficulties of aphasic children are not as pervasive or severe as those seen in autism. In contrast to children with autistic disorder, aphasic children generally make eye contact, achieve meaningful communication via gestures, exhibit emotional intent, engage in imaginative play, and are more likely to be of normal intelligence (e.g., American Psychiatric Association, 1987; Shea & Mesibov, 1985; Wing, 1976).

4. *Mental retardation.* Most children with autism are like children with mental retardation in that they display poor intellectual ability that persists throughout their lives. In addition, many children with retardation exhibit behaviors seen in autism, including echolalia, self-stimulation, SIB, and difficulties in attention. There are, however, several distinctions between the two disorders (Schreibman, 1988). First, most children with retardation exhibit appropriate social behavior. Second, children with retardation are more likely to be communicative even though their communicative abilities may be limited. Third, normal physical development is associated more with autism than with retardation. Fourth, while it is common for children with retardation to show impairments across a wide range of functioning, children with autism usually display a more variable pattern of deficits. Children with autism tend to perform better on tests measuring visuo-spatial abilities than on those assessing verbal skills. Additionally, they are more likely to display exceptional abilities in limited areas. In general, as discussed earlier, most children with autism also are retarded, in which case the child would receive a secondary diagnosis of retardation.

Assessment Strategies

Assessment procedures applied to children with autistic disorder can be divided into two categories that are not mutually exclusive: One type of assessment is used for diagnostic purposes in that it measures the presence or absence (or degree) of behaviors associated with the disorder. The other type of assessment seeks to provide information specifically related to the design and implementation of an appropriate treatment plan.

Diagnostic Assessments

These assessments are used primarily for diagnostic evaluations although they also may provide detail that will be useful in developing a treatment plan. Typically the diagnostic process begins with an initial screening, wherein the child is observed and parents and/or caregivers (or the child, if appropriate) are interviewed to gather information and to make a diagnostic evaluation (e.g., Schreibman & Charlop, 1987). Following such initial screening, the clinician has an array of behavior checklists and ratings scales from which to choose to help determine diagnosis. These ratings and checklists are designed to obtain measures of the child's birth and behavioral history, symptoms, speech, current behavioral characteristics, and other features diagnostic of autistic disorder (e.g., Schreibman & Charlop, 1987). The most frequently used of these assessments are Rimland's Diagnostic Checklist for Behavior Disturbed Children, Form E-2 (Rimland, 1971), the Childhood Autism Rating Scale or CARS (Schopler, Reichler, DeVellis, & Daly, 1980), the Behavior Observation Scale for Autism or BOS (Freeman, Ritvo, Guthrie, Schroth, & Ball, 1978), the Behavior Rating Instrument for Autistic and Atypical Children or BRIAAC (Ruttenberg, Dratman, Fraknoi, & Wenar, 1966), and the Autism Behavior Checklist (Krug, Arick, & Almond, 1979). Each of these instruments has its strengths and weaknesses and may be more applicable in particular situations and for particular needs. In a review of the psychometric properties of these assessments, Parks (1983) concluded that, with the exception of Rimland's Diagnostic Behavior Checklist, each has acceptable reliability and validity.

These rating scales and checklists are typically supplemented by assessments of the child's intellectual abilities, language abilities, and social and adaptive functioning. The instruments used for these assessments are typically the standardized measures used with other developmentally disabled or with nonhandicapped children. For more comprehensive discussions of these assessments as applied to the child with autism, see Schreibman and Charlop (1987).

Behavioral Assessment

Although diagnostic assessments are important, they are often of limited utility for the design of treatments. Because the diagnosis of autistic disorder is applied to a heterogeneous group of children, the identification of an individualized treatment plan is not usually facilitated by the diagnosis alone. Rather, assessment of the specific behavioral characteristics of a given child and an analysis of the environmental determinants of these behaviors are essential if an appropriate treatment plan is to be developed. Schreibman and Koegel (1981) suggested three steps in the behavioral assessment of autism. First, the specific behaviors of an individual child are operationally defined so they can be reliably measured. For example, a particular child's SIB might involve head banging on specific surfaces, self-biting of wrists, and hair pulling.

Second, environmental variables controlling these specific behaviors are identified. This is commonly referred to as a *functional analysis,* in that it seeks to demonstrate the function the behavior serves in terms of environmental changes. For example, a clinician would be interested in determining under what conditions the child engages in SIB and also under what conditions the child refrains from SIB (e.g., Touchette, MacDonald, & Langer, 1985; Iwata, Dorsey, Slifer, Bauman, & Richman, 1982). To illustrate, results of this analysis for our particular child might indicate that the child is more likely to engage in SIB when demands are placed upon him and less likely to engage in SIB when left alone. We might also discover that head banging is more frequent in one setting whereas self-biting is more frequent in another environment. In other words, once this information is acquired, it becomes possible to make more informed choices regarding treatment. Thus, for our child who engages in SIB, it appears that the behavior may serve as an avoidance/escape be-

havior to terminate demands. That is, the behavior is maintained by negative reinforcement. Given our understanding of learning principles, we are well equipped to determine how to reduce behaviors maintained by such contingencies. Thus we might choose to be certain the demands are not terminated when SIB occurs. Or, more likely, we may remove the demands in those situations where the SIB is more likely to occur and gradually introduce the demands, along with training the child more appropriate ways to communicate his desire to escape the situation (e.g., requesting help).

The third step in designing a treatment is to group specific behaviors in terms of common controlling variables. Thus we may determine that various SIB or self-stimulatory behaviors are controlled by the same variables. Economy of effort and effect may be achieved by manipulating those variables.

One uniquely behavioral assessment that assists the clinician in determining the specifics of the target behavior(s) and functional analysis is the behavioral observation (cf. Schreibman & Charlop, 1987). This is usually structured or semistructured wherein the child's behavior is observed under a variety of conditions in order to assess what the child does in what circumstances. Typically, these observations are scored (in vivo or on tape) according to predetermined, operationally defined behaviors that allow for objective quantification of behavior (see Lovaas, Koegel, Simmons, & Long, 1973, for an excellent example of this type of assessment).

Therefore, behavioral assessment is particularly appropriate for the behavioral treatment of autism in that it tells us, in precise terms, exactly what the child does and does not do, specifies the variables controlling these behaviors, and suggests what alterations in the environment might be most appropriate for treatment.

TREATMENT

Evidence for Prescriptive Treatment

Behavioral Therapy

Due to the heterogeneity of characteristics in people with autism, treatment must be flexible in its ability to deal with differences among individuals as well as differences in intensity of various behaviors. Because of its emphasis on the analysis of individual behaviors (or groups of behaviors) and their controlling environmental determinants, the behavioral approach to treatment is uniquely suited to address individual needs in diverse populations.

As suggested earlier, autism can be characterized by a set of behavioral excesses and deficits. However, the pattern of these behaviors may vary substantially across individual children. Within the behavioral treatment approach, it has been useful to categorize an individual's behavioral repertoire in this way. As a result, interventions addressing specific excesses and deficits have been developed on an individual basis.

Behavioral deficits in children with autism often include language and social skills, play behaviors, and self-help skills. Low or zero baseline rates of these behaviors have successfully been increased by using behavioral principles developed to strengthen behaviors or to create new behavioral repertoires. Thus, application of such procedures as positive reinforcement, negative reinforcement, prompting, shaping, and chaining have been used in various forms, and often in combination, to specifically target deficient behavioral repertoires in children with autism.

Behavioral excesses associated with autism include self-injurious behavior, self-stimulatory behavior, compulsive behavior, and noncompliance. In general, these behaviors can be decreased by using extinction (failure to present maintaining reinforcement), differential reinforcement of other behaviors (DRO), or time out. Time out and extinction are especially effective for decreasing behaviors inappropriately used to elicit attention and for noncompliance. Behaviors may also be decreased by reinforcing alternative behaviors or by punishing inappropriate responses. All of these techniques can be, and often are, combined in an effective intervention. Importantly, techniques based on positive programming procedures are being developed and refined to accentuate positive, rather than negative, aspects treatment for individuals with autism.

Early work in the behavioral treatment of autism typically focused on breaking down complex behaviors and teaching them individually. For example, Lovaas, Berberich, Perloff, and Schaeffer (1966) established imitation of simple vocal sounds (positively reinforced by bites of food) and gradually shaped those sounds into words, word combinations, and so on. Using similar applications of discrimination learning, other specific behaviors were established, including appropriate use of pronouns, prepositions, and other language concepts (Lovaas, 1966).

More recently, however, behavioral clinicians have attempted to treat behavioral deficits by addressing more complex and comprehensive behavioral repertoires. Such an emphasis holds promise for affecting behavioral change in a more economical manner. In this case, analysis of response classes in terms of environmental controlling variables is essential. For example, Carr (1977) isolated three basic motivational factors that seem to account for most cases of SIB. These include contingent positive reinforcement (e.g., attention, acquiescence to child's demands), negative reinforcement (e.g., escape from, or avoidance of, aversive situations such as difficult demands), and self-stimulation (i.e., the SIB is intrinsically enjoyable, presumably because of the sensory input it provides). Thus, SIB for an individual child might involve one or more of these motivating factors. Understanding of the complexities of environmental determinants allows for the design of more efficient and effective treatments.

Recent research has addressed two deficits affecting wide ranges of behavior in individuals with autism. These are deficits in *motivation* and *lack of responsivity to multiple cues* in the environment. Lack of motivation is indicated by temper tantrums, crying, noncompliance, inattention, or attempting to leave the situation (Koegel & Egel, 1979). Lack of responsivity to multiple cues has been called "stimulus overselectivity" and involves the failure to utilize all of the important cues in an educational setting (cf. Lovaas, Koegel, & Schreibman, 1979; Schreibman, 1988, for reviews). For example, an individual with autism may use only irrelevant cues, such as a piece of clothing or hairstyle, to identify a person.

Increasing motivation and reducing deficits in responsivity to multiple cues have far-reaching effects on the autistic individual's ability to learn (Koegel, O'Dell, & Koegel, 1987). A motivated person is more likely to attend to the learning situation, to generalize these newly acquired responses to new environments, and to maintain the behaviors over time. Although the individual must be motivated to attend to the learning situation, attention to relevant cues is required in order to ensure that appropriate learning occurs and that newly acquired knowledge will generalize. Targeting these two pivotal factors can be seen as a way of "normalizing" the individual's interaction with the environment and thus may be instrumental in ensuring global improvements. These issues are addressed in a treatment package developed by Koegel and colleagues.

This program, referred to as Pivotal Response Training, focuses on increasing language in children with autism. It includes components that increase motivation and specific procedures to increase responsivity to multiple cues. Motivation can be enhanced by (1) allowing the child to participate in choosing the activities in a teaching situation, (2) using direct response-reinforcer relationships, (3) interspersing maintenance tasks among acquisition tasks, (4) providing rewards immediately and contingently, and (5) reinforcing the individual's attempts to make the desired response. To reduce stimulus overselectivity, situations are created that require the child to use multiple cues (i.e., conditioned discriminations). For example, if the child chooses to work with a red crayon, the treatment provider presents several colors of crayons along with corresponding colored pencils. This forces the child to discriminate color and type of object, resulting in attention to two cues. Pivotal Response Training is currently being used for language training and in parent training programs, and preliminary data are very encouraging (Schreibman, Stahmer, & Loos, 1991).

Although previously discussed treatment strategies have been very successful in increasing appropriate behaviors in individuals with autism, all require the continued presence of the treatment provider. This dependence remains a limitation to the generalization of treatment effects. Optimally, the individual would generalize acquired behavioral repertoires across settings without the presence of supervision or continued instruction. Research with normally functioning as well as some physically and mentally handicapped individuals indicates that reliance on a therapist can be successfully decreased through the use of *self-management* programs (see Kopp, 1988; Browder & Shapiro, 1985, for reviews). Self-management typically involves the following components: self-evaluation of performance, self-monitoring, and self-delivery of reinforcement. Ideally, individuals learn to monitor and to maintain appropriate behavior in the absence of supervision.

Recently, children and adolescents with autism have been taught to use self-management to produce and maintain changes in their own behavior. Behaviors can be increased in using self-management by reinforcing periods of time in which the child behaves appropriately. Examples of behaviors that have been increased are independent work skills (Sainato, Strain, Lefebvre, & Rapp, 1990) and independent play behaviors in children and adolescents with autism (Stahmer & Schreibman, in press). Self-management can be used to decrease behavioral excesses as well. It is similar to DRO, as the client receives reinforcement for periods of time when the target behavior is *not* exhibited. For example, Koegel and Koegel (1990) taught adolescents with autism to reduce their own self-stimulation for extended periods of time by using a self-management treatment package.

The advantages of self-management programs for working with individuals with autism include the following: (1) minimizing dependence on the presence of the treatment provider (Sainato et al., 1990), (2) improved generalization and maintenance of behavior change, and (3) increasing independence for the individual which may lead to more positive interactions in the community. Self-management techniques are effective with high-functioning and relatively low-functioning children with autism (Koegel & Koegel, 1990). Initially, training an individual to use self-management may be time consuming. However, studies suggest that once the individual has learned the technique, it can be used across settings and across behaviors with relatively little additional intervention (Stahmer & Schreibman, in press; Koegel & Koegel, 1990).

Another recent trend in the field of behavioral treatment is the use of nonaversive techniques to solve behavior problems (e.g., Cohen, Donnellan, & Paul, 1987; Horner et al., 1990). Such change in emphasis in the field has come about due to ethical, legal, and social considerations. In the past, punishment was thought to be the easiest, most effective way to decrease behavioral excesses. Punishment, defined behaviorally, is the contingent administration of a consequence that results in a decrease in the target behavior. Unlike the colloquial use of the word *punishment,* in behavioral terms the consequence does not necessarily have to be generally painful or aversive. For example, if a child does not like candy, candy can serve as a punisher for that child. Punishment was one of the first techniques successfully used to decrease many of the dangerous self-injurious behaviors seen in individuals with autism (Lovaas & Simmons, 1969). However, continued research has led to the development of an increasing number of nonaversive treatment alternatives. Two examples of nonaversive interventions include differential reinforcement of other or alternative behaviors and functional equivalence training.

The differential reinforcement of other behaviors is the delivery of reinforcement after a specified interval in which the inappropriate target behavior is not exhibited. DRO has advantages over punishment. It does not require the delivery of a stimulus that is aversive to the individual and it is resistant to recovery after the termination of the intervention. A variation of DRO is teaching an alternative behavior. For example, instead of using extinction for nail biting, the child learns to use his or her hands to engage in drawing or appropriate toy play.

A particularly creative method of nonaversive behavior therapy is functional equivalence training (e.g., Carr & Durand, 1985). As mentioned earlier, SIB may frequently function as an escape behavior that allows the child to avoid demanding tasks. These researchers identified the specific social function maintaining the SIB (in this case, communication) and replaced the inappropriate behavior with a socially appropriate alternative. For example, the child was taught to elicit help from a teacher during a difficult task instead of engaging in inappropriate behavior. In this way, behavior problems can be reduced by teaching children alternative ways to communicate rather than by punishing the behavior.

The use of nonaversive techniques for decreasing behavioral excesses is relatively new and developing rapidly. The careful planning of school programs using these positive methods has contributed substantially to the move away from institutions and into community-based settings for individuals with autism (e.g., Cohen et al., 1987). These techniques can be helpful in reducing the high cost of institutions by helping handicapped people within the community setting.

Pharmacotherapy

Traditionally, the role of psychoactive agents in the treatment of autism has been to decrease the behavioral symptoms associated with the disorder and to promote more functional behavior. Pharmacotherapy is most often used in conjunction with other forms of treatment, such as behavior modification and school-based programs. Currently, no psychoactive drug has been shown to eliminate the behavioral symptoms or the intellectual deficits associated with autism. However, some psychoactive drugs have been shown to facilitate learning when used in conjunction with special education and behavior modification. Recent research in the area has focused on fenfluramine, antipsychotics such as haloperidol, opiate antagonists such as naltrexone, and vitamin B6.

Ritvo, Freeman, Geller, and Yuwiler (1983) issued a report on the use of fenfluramine in a sample of 14 children with autism, in which half of the children had hyperserotonemia. Fenfluramine is an anorexongenic agent that markedly decreases brain serotonin in animals. Blood serotonin levels fell an average of 51 percent in both normal and hyperserotonemic patients after one month of fenfluramine treatment and returned to baseline when the drug was discontinued. Behavioral improvements seen in these children included decreased motility disturbances, improved sleep patterns, increased eye contact, increased spontaneous use of language, and increased social awareness across subjects with and without hyperserotonemia. Adverse effects of the drug on behavior included weight loss, diminished appetite, and lethargy. However, more recent research indicates that the drug has minimal effects on cognitive performance and behavior, and these effects tend to be neutral or negative rather than positive. In a study of 15 children with autism by Sherman, Factor, Swinson, and Darjes (1989), no significant improvement was found on any measure for the fenfluramine group. In fact, marked differences in free play between the experimental and control groups were noted, but these differences favored the placebo condition. Unfortunately, after its initial success, fenfluramine has not proved to be a very effective drug for use in children with autism.

Antipsychotic drugs also have been used to improve behavior in children with autism. Haloperidol, a low-dose, high-potency neuroleptic, decreases the neurotransmitter dopamine and also has antiserotonergic effects. In a carefully designed study by Anderson and colleagues (1989), haloperidol had several beneficial effects for children with autism, including decreasing maladaptive behaviors (e.g., hyperactivity, temper tantrums, withdrawal, and stereotypies), increasing social relatedness, and possibly improving attentional mechanisms. Halperidol combined with language training was superior to haloperidol or language training alone. Untoward effects of the drug, depending on the dosage, included sedation, decreased attention span, and some withdrawal diskinesia.

Recent evidence indicating abnormalities in levels of endogenous opioids in subgroups of people with autism has sparked investigation of the use of opiate antagonists in the treatment of this disorder. In preliminary studies, naltrexone, an opiate antagonist, has reduced stereotypies, withdrawal, and hyperactivity, and increased verbal production in some individuals with autism (e.g., Campbell, Perry, Small, & Green, 1987). The only side effect appears to be slight sedation. However, further investigation of this drug is warranted.

Research using vitamin B6 and magnesium to treat autism began when Rimland, Callaway, and Dreyfus (1978) reported that 30 to 40 percent of the children with autism who were taking vitamin B6 showed significant behavioral improvement. Positive effects of the vitamin B6 and magnesium combination included increases in interaction with family members, increased awareness, increased speech production, and decreases in temper tantrums and disruptive behaviors. In a similar study, 14 percent of 91 subjects with autism improved markedly, 33 percent improved somewhat, 42 percent showed no improvement, and 11 percent worsened (Lelord et al., 1988). There is little information on the specific characteristics of the individuals for which treatment was most effective.

Unfortunately, no drug has been found that will "cure" autism. Given the heterogeneity in this population, it is unlikely that one drug will be effective for all individuals with autism. Currently, there are no conclusive diagnostic criteria to determine appropriate psychopharmacological treatment for particular individuals with autism. Unfortunately, the mechanism of action for many of the aforementioned drugs is unclear, and further research is needed to determine indications and contraindications of specific drugs used to treat individuals with autism.

Alternative Treatments

There are few alternative treatments available for autistic disorder. This is not to say that alternative therapies may not be effective, just that empirical evidence is lacking and thus it is difficult to draw conclusions regarding their efficacy.

The first treatment approach used with children with autism was based on a psychodynamic model. This model posited that autism resulted when the child withdrew from what he or she perceived as a hostile and threatening world. This dangerous environment was somehow communicated to the child via pathological parental responses to the child's growing autonomy. The resulting arrest in ego development was due to the child's need to expend energy to defend against the environment (Bettelheim, 1967).

Treatment based on this model typically involves separating the child from the parents and placing him or her in a substitute environment with a surrogate parent. This surrogate parent presumably provides the child with the warm, permissive, and nurturing environment in contrast to that provided by the real parents. In this environment the child is encouraged to explore the world and the self, and all attempts to do so are met with love, acceptance, and encouragement. In such an environment the child's sense of power over the world and autonomy are thought to be restored so the child can function in the world (Bettelheim, 1967). Other types of psychodynamic therapy emphasize sensory stimulation and play as a means to reach out to children with autism. These types of therapy, such as holding therapy, sensory integration therapy, and play therapy all claim to help the child overcome sensory deficits (Nelson, 1984). The goal of these therapies is to help the child learn to experience the world and respond to it a more normal manner.

Again, there is little or no empirical evidence to support any of these types of treatments with individuals with autism. Further, the etiological conceptions upon which many are based are erroneous. Research indicates, for example, that there is no validated support that parents of children with autism have greater pathology than parents of other handicapped children (e.g., Schreibman, 1988). The development of treatments, such as behavior therapy and psychopharmacological interventions, has opened new avenues for parents and other treatment providers.

Selecting Optimal Treatment Strategies

There are several variables treatment providers should consider when choosing optimal treatment strategies for individuals with autism. Some of these elements include the child's functioning level, age, and environment. All aspects of the child's ability and history should be taken into account, along with particular problem behaviors.

First, the treatment provider should assess the functioning level of the child. Language assessments for expressive and receptive language are an important first step in deciding what type of instruction may be most appropriate for a par-

ticular child. Also, nonverbal IQ must be taken into account. Some children, especially in the case of autism, have discrepant verbal and nonverbal skill levels. Motor skills are often assessed to determine whether or not some tasks are deficient due to motor difficulty. All of these areas can be measured by using standardized tests and clinical interviews and by observing the child's behavior in several environments. The individual's age must also be taken into account to ensure that the tasks are age appropriate.

Another important factor in choosing a treatment strategy is the feasibility of implementing treatment in the child's specific environment. For example, it is important to know if the parents are willing and/or able to participate in a parent training program. Often, schools have limitations on the types of interventions they can implement, thus making treatment consistency difficult. Various environments may also elicit different behaviors. A child may demonstrate noncompliance with a parent yet obey at school. This is why it is beneficial to look at the antecedents and consequences of behavior in different environmental circumstances.

All of these factors must be taken into account when choosing treatment options for any particular individual with autism. Also, the specific behaviors exhibited by an individual child will help determine treatment strategy. Obviously, SIB, aggression, or other severely disruptive behaviors require immediate attention and may take temporary precedence over other aspects of treatment. Because of the heterogeneity in the disorder and the great differences in environment for each child, treatments must be designed individually.

Problems in Carrying Out Interventions

Different variables can lead to the failure of a behavioral intervention. One common problem is inconsistent implementation of the treatment. Gaining compliance from treatment providers may be difficult. Because group homes and school environments are often understaffed, it is difficult for treatment providers to devote necessary attention to individual students. Parents, who often work very well as therapists, have other responsibilities and often cannot attend to their handicapped child consistently.

Many institutions, public schools in particular, are limited in the type of intervention they can use. For some schools even extinction is seen as too aversive. In some environments even the delivery of positive reinforcers is impractical or considered inappropriate (i.e., "bribery"). These schools must work even harder at being consistent and designing creative interventions.

A typical problem exhibited by children with autism is failure to generalize what they have learned to new settings and people, other than those associated with the training. Also, the responses these children learn are often rote responses that have minimal variability and involve little collateral change in behavior. In addition, once training is terminated, responses generally extinguish rather rapidly. These problems, if not adequately addressed in treatment, may lead to great difficulty and frustration to treatment providers and parents, and often limit the degree to which a person with autism can function in the community.

Relapse Prevention

All of the preceding problems are inherent in most treatment strategies utilized with individuals with autism. In the following section we will discuss particular strategies that can be incorporated into treatment to help minimize some of these problems. One very successful way to increase generalization and maintenance of treatment gains is by extending the treatment environments through parent training.

Teaching parents to provide treatment for their children with autism at home began in the late 1960s and early 1970s. As mentioned by Schreibman, Koegel, Mills, and Burke (1984), there are several advantages to parent training, including (1) parents are around the child more often than any teacher or clinician and can provide round-the-clock treatment, (2) having parents work with teachers and therapists to ensure continuity of treatment across environments, (3) enabling the

parents to become involved in their child's development, and (4) ensuring maintenance of skills learned long after therapy has been discontinued. Parent training also makes treatment more available, as it can be learned and implemented anywhere the family resides. Most parent training programs involve teaching the parents basic behavior modification techniques such as those described earlier. The training is usually accomplished through a combination of modeling, lectures, and behavioral rehearsal with feedback. The most important aspect of parent training programs is that they have been found to be necessary for the generalization and maintenance of treatment gains (Lovaas et al., 1973).

By training parents and, if possible, teachers to administer treatment programs, the child with autism can consistently receive treatment in many environments throughout every day. This comprehensive approach can increase generalization and ensure that treatment gains will maintain over time. Also, new treatment strategies, such as self-management and Pivotal Response Training, incorporate techniques designed to enhance generalization and maintenance. Thus, combination of extended treatment environments (i.e., teacher and parent training) and incorporation of interventions aimed at achieving more global change (i.e., Pivotal Response Training and self-management) hold great potential for achieving substantial and generalized improvement in functioning for individuals with autism.

CASE ILLUSTRATION

Case Description

Clark was an attractive 6-year-old boy referred to our behavioral treatment program. He was of average build with wavy brown hair and green eyes. He was the first of two children born to a middle-class family. He was the product of a full-term normal pregnancy with an uneventful labor and delivery. As an infant, Clark's mother described him as quiet and not demanding much attention. His physical and motor development appeared to be normal. The family's other child, a 2-year-old girl, appeared to be functioning normally in both verbal and social skills. Both parents had some college education and were currently employed. The father worked in sales and the mother was an officer in the local police department. Both parents were in good health, and there was no history of mental disorder on either side of the family. The family appeared to be open and friendly. Upon beginning participation in our program. Clark had received two independent diagnoses of autism, and the parents had accepted Clark's disorder and were anxious to learn new methods for controlling his behavior and increasing his learning.

On his first day of treatment, Clark walked in holding his mother's hand paying little attention to the new faces he had encountered. Upon entering the clinic, he ran for some crayons and immediately began drawing letters on a piece of paper, spelling out names of various automobile companies. Upon completion of each word, Clark immediately began to flap his hands rapidly for several seconds. During the initial interview for our program, Clark's parents discussed several of his behavioral problems. His preoccupation with automobile companies was exemplified by the crayon episode. Of greater concern to his parents was Clark's tendency to run away frequently. Besides these and various other behavioral problems, Clark's language was severely deficient. He rarely used any language spontaneously, yet he readily repeated immediately all or part of whatever was said to him. Clark's parents noted that it was nearly impossible to establish eye contact for any length of time and they additionally reported that he often exhibited inappropriate or very labile emotional behavior. For example, seemingly frustrating situations induced uncontrollable laughter and silliness.

Differential Diagnosis and Assessment

A third diagnosis of autism was made at our clinic based on behavioral observations and information provided by the parents. Clark was then admitted to our program. After acceptance, we completed a battery of behavioral, intellectual, and language assessments in order to determine Clark's behavioral excesses and deficits and to design an effective intervention based on this information.

First, behavioral observations were conducted in a setting unfamiliar to Clark. A room was set up not unlike a family room, with a sofa, coffee table, chairs, and various toys and books. Clark's behavior with each parent and then with a stranger (a person unknown to Clark) was videotaped through one-way mirrors in three separate sessions. These videotapes were then scored for appropriate (e.g., functional speech, social behavior such as affection, and appropriate use of toys) and inappropriate (self-stimulation, tantrums, inappropriate speech, and noncompliance) behaviors. As expected, appropriate behaviors were deficient and inappropriate behaviors were excessive.

Clark's use of speech was primarily limited to echolalia, although he exhibited some understanding of language by following simple directions (i.e., "Touch your nose" and "Bring me the green ball"). Clark showed little affection or appropriate social behavior and his play skills were limited. In the observational session with his mother, Clark attended to her only when she reached into her purse for a piece of gum. It was only at this point that he used spontaneous speech, saying "Gum." After his mother said "No," Clark proceeded to scream until she rather hurriedly got another piece out of her purse and gave it to him. Clark's use of toys was deviant as well. Rather than using the toys for their intended function, Clark lined objects into rows and/or repeatedly waved them in front of his eyes. Clark's initial reaction to being in a room with an unknown person was to attempt to leave. When he did not succeed in opening the door, he began to giggle while staring at his reflection in the one-way mirror.

Following these behavioral observations, we conducted standardized intellectual, social, and language assessments. Two measures of intellectual ability, the Leiter International Performance Scales and the Stanford-Binet, were used. Clark's performance on the Leiter, a nonverbal measure, yielded a standard score of 67. The Stanford-Binet includes both verbal and nonverbal assessments of intellectual ability. Clark's score on the quantitative or nonverbal portion of the Stanford-Binet was 63 and was 39 on the verbal section of the assessment. His composite score was 49, indicating moderate retardation with severe language deficits.

Scores on the Vineland Adaptive Behavior Scales, a standardized instrument used to evaluate proficiency in communication, self-help or daily living skills, and socialization, was administered via interview to Clark's mother. Clark received a composite score of 70, with most notable deficits occurring in the expressive communication and socialization domains.

In order to further assess Clark's understanding of language, the Peabody Picture Vocabulary Test (PPVT) and Assessment of Child Language Comprehension (ACLC) were given. These assessments are standardized with respect to population norms. Results showed some impairment in both understanding of language on the PPVT and in Clark's ability to attend to multiple relevant informational cues necessary to obtain correct answers on the ACLC.

Treatment Selection

Thus far, assessments and observations suggested a moderately functioning child with behaviors typical of autism. Based on these indications, we suggested a multifaceted program including behavioral management and language training. Because of Clark's language deficits, his difficulty in attending to multiple informational cues, and his characteristic lack of motivation, we emphasized Pivotal Response Training. In order to enhance generalization and maintenance of treatment gains, we implemented our program within a parent training paradigm.

Treatment Course and Problems in Carrying Out Intervention

During the course of our behavioral program, Clark and his mother maintained weekly clinic appointments of one and a half hours each. Clark participated in language training the entire time

either with a clinic therapist or with his mother. Clark's mother participated in one hour of parent training during each appointment. Half of the time was spent observing and practicing language training with Clark and half was spent one-on-one with a clinic therapist discussing and planning behavioral interventions to conduct at home.

Language Training

As mentioned before, Pivotal Response training was used to enhance Clark's language skills by increasing his motivation and his ability to respond to multiple environmental cues. Pivotal Response Training took place in either one of two therapy rooms. Each small room was equipped with a table and two chairs, various toys, and a tray of food and/or beverage reinforcers.

The Pivotal Response Training procedure was followed as described in the preceding section on behavior therapy. Clark sat across from the therapist beside a table. The table was previously set up with favored toys and food items. Clark preferred books, crayons and paper, and puzzles to other toys, and usually chose to eat bits of potato chips or peanuts. Clark was given his choice of activities unless he compulsively requested an item or used it inappropriately, in which case the object was removed from the room until the next session. For example, Clark had a favorite page in a particular book. Occasionally he refused to change pages and began laughing inappropriately when viewing the page. Whenever it became clear to the therapist that this was occurring, the book was removed from the room until a later session.

Although initially Clark disliked sitting in the chair and attempted to leave at the slightest opportunity, he soon appeared to be excited to begin sessions. When we began treatment, we often rewarded Clark for sitting appropriately in his chair with his hands on his lap. In order to improve his attention to the therapist, he was also rewarded for good eye contact independent of his use of language. Soon, Clark learned that it was worth his while to participate and attend to therapy, and after breaks he would lead the therapist by the hand back to the therapy room.

At the beginning of Pivotal Response Training,

Clark had very little expressive language. Initial responses included primarily one-word expressions such as "chip," "nut," "draw," and "book." Typical sessions consisted of the following: The therapist began by presenting a few different toys and food items on a lapboard in front of Clark and saying "Show me what you want." Clark usually responded by pointing to one of the items, which the therapist would pick up. The other items were then put aside. While holding the chosen object in Clark's view, the therapist waited for a few moments for an appropriate spontaneous response. When Clark emitted an appropriate word or a reasonable attempt, the therapist gave him access to the chosen object along with verbal praise as reinforcement. When Clark did not utter any words or appropriate attempts, the therapist used a prompt in order to elicit a response. For example, if the chosen reinforcer was a book and a short time had elapsed with no spontaneous use of language, the therapist, making sure Clark was attending, said "read," "book," or "look." Clark usually responded by repeating whatever the therapist said and was then immediately given access to the object. Occasionally, Clark did not respond to the prompt. This usually occurred if the prompt was for a difficult response or if Clark was not attending to the therapist. If this was the case, the problem was remediated by the therapist changing the prompt and/or further engaging Clark's attention. In order to model appropriate language and associated use of toys, the therapist took turns participating in activities with Clark. Whenever the therapist took a turn, he or she narrated the chosen activity and participated appropriately.

As language training proceeded, Clark's spontaneous use of words increased as did the number of different words he said. Along with this, he began to combine words such as "I want," and "chip please." Clark's interest in different toys also expanded to include a baby doll and bottle and a cooking set. Through therapist modeling, he learned more appropriate play skills.

Parent Training

Clark's mother learned to use Pivotal Response Training and behavioral management as we trained Clark. First, she was given two manuals—one for general behavior modification techniques and the other specific to Pivotal Response Training. After she read both manuals and exhibited understanding by correctly completing related written exercises, she participated in parent training. During language training, Clark's mother initially observed a therapist working with him from the observation room through a one-way mirror. Later, she joined the therapist to observe training in the therapy room. After one or two sessions of observation, Clark's mother was encouraged to work with him with the therapist still in the room providing feedback. As she became more proficient in implementing language training procedures, the therapist was gradually faded from the room.

The speed of parental acquisition of language training skills was moderate. Typical errors in carrying out Pivotal Response Training included use of noncontingent reinforcement and excessive parental control over activities. Although Clark's mother often reinforced appropriate use of language promptly and correctly, she occasionally offered rewards either too late after occurrence of the behavior or for an inappropriate response. Rather than allowing Clark to choose what to work with, his mother often directed his attention to an activity of her choice. As a result of these initial deviations in correct implementation of Pivotal Response Training, Clark frequently exhibited frustration and subsequent disruptive behavior. After approximately three months of training, Clark's mother became more consistent in her correct use of reinforcement and often remembered to allow Clark to choose most activities. She also began using our language training techniques virtually any time she was with Clark, including in the home and on outings. This resulted in Clark's increased communication ability, decreased disruptive and self-stimulatory behaviors, and decreased maternal stress. Clark's mother remarked how much easier her life had become and how her free time had increased because of the positive changes in Clark's behavior.

As another component of our parent training program, Clark's mother was given instruction in home management of her son's behavioral problems. For 30 minutes during each weekly session, she met with a therapist to discuss at-home interventions and progress. During the first training session, Clark's mother was asked to list behaviors that were problematic. These consisted of running away, laughing uncontrollably, not sitting at the dinner table, and having tantrums. Of these four behaviors, running away was initially targeted because it was potentially dangerous and thus required immediate intervention.

Once we identified the first target behavior, Clark's mother was instructed to keep data on frequency, time, and situation of occurrence of her son's running away. Results after the first week indicated that Clark ran away an average of three times per day. Occurrences usually took place either in a shopping area or at home. Even though his mother called him when he ran, he ignored her. We decided to teach him to come to his mother when she called him. The program that Clark's mother decided to implement with the consultation of the therapist consisted of the following: (1) Mother continued to record the frequency of the target behavior. (2) Mother attempted to motivate Clark to come when called by frequently giving him the opportunity to come when called followed by a positive reinforcer for approach behavior. During this intervention, Clark's mother planned to always carry a favored treat and intermittently say "Come here, Clark." She was to do this in various situations. To ensure Clark's success, she was instructed to make it easy for Clark to earn a treat by asking him to "come here" in low-risk situations then to gradually introduce the request in higher risk areas such as the shopping center and in their unfenced front yard. (3) Time out was used for noncompliance. After the first two weeks, Clark's behavior improved. Although he still attempted to run away, he usually promptly returned when his mother called him.

Interventions for the other three behaviors and for those that developed during the course of treatment were carried out in a similar fashion. First, Clark's mother kept a baseline record of the target behavior and then developed an appropriate intervention. Interventions were geared toward rewarding appropriate behaviors rather than punishment whenever possible. Clark's mother gradually became more independent of the therapists. In fact, she became highly proficient in developing and implementing behavioral programs completely by herself.

Outcome and Termination

After approximately five months, Clark's mother met our criteria for graduation from the parent training program. She had learned to correctly implement Pivotal Response Training and to effectively develop and carry out behavioral programs.

We measured Clark's progress using those assessments that had been used at pretreatment. We found improvements in his use of appropriate language and social skills. Additionally, his disruptive and inappropriate behaviors occurred less frequently and in some cases were replaced by those that were functional.

Followup and Maintenance

Following graduation, clinic visits were discontinued; however, Clark's mother was contacted by a therapist once a week to assess progress and to assist in dealing with any problematic behaviors. Problems that arose were not unlike those encountered in parent training. Occasionally, previously treated behaviors recurred. In most of these cases, it was effective for Clark's mother to simply reinstate the behavioral intervention she had used for the problem before.

After a three-month followup period. Clark's behaviors were again assessed. We found increases in his self-help skills and his understanding of language. The greatest gains in receptive language were found in the ACLC, where Clark made significant improvement in his understanding of items that required attention to more than one component. Our observations of Clark at this followup were positive. He appeared more social and more affectionate, especially with his mother, and his use of functional language had increased dramatically. Clark's family was pleased by his progress and they were able to enjoy more activities together because of the knowledge and skills they now had to deal with their son's behavior.

SUMMARY

Autistic disorder is a severe form of psychopathology characterized by deficits in social behavior, deficits in speech and language, excessive demands for consistency in the environment, abnormalities in sensory responsiveness, self-stimulatory behavior, self-injury, and unusual affect. The disorder is rather rare, occurring in approximately 1 per 2,500 births, yet it shares some features with other types of childhood psychopathology such as mental retardation, schizophrenia in childhood, and developmental aphasia. The etiology of autism is unknown, but prior conceptualizations of the etiology in terms of psychogenic origins have been largely abandoned in favor of the current view of autism as an organically based disorder of unknown cause.

Assessment strategies employed by researchers and clinicians fall into two general categories: those designed to determine diagnoses and those designed to provide information relevant for treatment. Behavioral assessment involves using a variety of strategies that allow for determining specific behaviors (excesses and deficits) exhibited by individual children and for identifying environmental factors that may serve to evoke, shape, and maintain such behaviors. Such an approach is ideally suited for designing behavioral treatments on an individual basis for a heterogenous group such as autism.

The behavioral approach to treatment typically involves assessing the controlling factors for specific behaviors of an individual child and applying the principles of learning to alter those behaviors in the desired direction. Early work in the area focused on the analysis and control of individual behaviors. While this early work demonstrated the potency of behavioral intervention, limited generalization of behavior change remained a concern. More recent research has focused on providing extended treatment and addressing more complex behavioral repertoires in an effort to enhance generalization. These efforts include parent training, teacher training, and teaching programs, such as functional equivalence training, Pivotal Response Training, and self-management.

Although behavioral treatment is the most commonly used treatment for autistic disorder, some have found various pharmacological agents useful for assisting in the control of specific behaviors exhibited by these individuals. In addition, alternative treatments based on psychodynamic and sensory models have been applied but lack empirical support for their effectiveness.

When selecting optimal treatment strategies for individuals with autism, it is essential that characteristics of the child and of that child's environment be considered. It is also essential to anticipate potential problems in the implementation of these strategies and to include procedures to prevent relapse.

REFERENCES

American Psychiatric Association. (1987). *Diagnostic and statistical manual of mental disorders* (3rd ed., rev.). Washington, DC: Author.

Anderson, L. T., Campbell, M., Adams, P., Small, A. M., Perry, R., & Shell, J. (1989). The effects of haloperidol on discrimination learning and behavioral symptoms in autistic children. *Journal of Autism and Developmental Disorders, 19,* 227–239.

August, G. J., & Lockhart, L. H. (1984). Familial autism and the fragile-X chromosome. *Journal of Autism and Developmental Disorders, 14,* 197–204.

Bauman, M. L., & Kemper, T. L. (1985). Histoanatomic observations of the brain in early infantile autism. *Neurology, 35,* 866–874.

Bettelheim, B. (1967). *The empty fortress.* New York: Free Press.

Browder, D. M., & Shapiro, E. S. (1985). Applications of self-management to individuals with severe handicaps: A review. *Journal of the Association for Persons With Severe Handicaps, 4,* 200–208.

Campbell, M., Perry, R., Small, A. M., & Green, W. H. (1987). Overview of drug treatment in autism. In E. Schopler & G. B. Mesibov (Eds.), *Neurobiological issues in autism* (pp. 341–355). New York: Plenum.

Carr, E. G. (1977). The motivation of self-injurious behavior: A review of some hypotheses. *Psychological Bulletin, 84,* 800–816.

Carr, E. G., & Durand, V. M. (1985). Reducing behavior problems through functional communication training. *Journal of Applied Behavior Analysis, 18,* 111–126.

Churchill, D. W. (1972). The relation of infantile autism and early childhood schizophrenia to developmental language disorders of childhood. *Journal of Autism and Childhood Schizophrenia, 2,* 182–197.

Clarizio, H. F., & McCoy, G. F. (1983). *Behavior disorders in children* (3rd ed.). New York: Harper and Row.

Cohen, D. J., Donnellan, A. M., & Paul, R. (1987). *Handbook of autism and pervasive developmental disorders.* New York: Wiley & Sons.

Freeman, B. J., Ritvo, E. R., Guthrie, D., Schroth, P., & Ball, J. (1978). The Behavior Observation Scale for Autism: Initial methodology, data analysis, and preliminary findings on 89 children. *Journal of the American Academy of Child Psychiatry, 17,* 576–588.

Horner, R. H., Dunlap, G., Koegel, R. L., Carr, E. G., Sailor, W., Anderson, J., Albin, R. W., & O'Neill, R. E. (1990). Toward a technology of "non-aversive" behavioral support. *Journal of the Association for Persons with Severe Handicaps, 15,* 124–132.

Iwata, B. A., Dorsey, M. F., Slifer, K. J., Bauman, K. E., & Richman, G. S. (1982). Toward a functional analysis of self-injury. *Analysis and Intervention in Developmental Disabilities, 2,* 3–20.

Kanner, L. (1943). Autistic disturbances of affective contact. *The Nervous Child, 2,* 217–250.

Koegel, R. L., & Egel, A. L. (1979). Motivating autistic children. *Journal of Abnormal Psychology, 88,* 418–426.

Koegel, R. L., & Koegel, L. K. (1990). Extended reductions in stereotypic behavior through self-management in multiple community settings. *Journal of Applied Behavior Analysis, 23,* 119–128.

Koegel, R. L., O'Dell, M. C., & Koegel, L. K. (1987). A natural language teaching paradigm for nonverbal autistic children. *Journal of Autism and Developmental Disorders, 17,* 187–200.

Kopp, J. (1988). Self-monitoring: A literature review of research and practice. *Social Work Research and Abstracts, 24,* 8–20.

Krug, D. A., Arick, J. R., & Almond, P. J. (1979). Autism Screening Instrument for Educational Planning: Background and development. In J. Gilliam (Ed.), *Autism: Diagnosis, instruction, management, and research* (pp. 64–78). Austin: Austin Press.

Lelord, G., Barthelemy, C., Martineau, N., Bruneau, J. P., Muh, G., & Callaway, E. (1988). Clinical and biological effects of vitamin B6 + magnesium in autistic subjects. In J. Leklem & R. Reynolds (Eds.), *Vitamin B6 responsive disorders in humans.* New York: Alan R. Liss.

Lovaas, O. I. (1966). A program for the establishment of speech in psychotic children. In J. K. Wing (Ed.), *Early childhood autism* (pp. 115–144). London: Pergamon.

Lovaas, O. I., Berberich, J. P., Perloff, B. F., & Schaeffer, B. (1966). Acquisition of imitative speech in schizophrenic children. *Science, 151,* 705–707.

Lovaas, O. I., Koegel, R. L., & Schreibman, L. (1979). Stimulus overselectivity in autism: A review of research. *Psychological Bulletin, 86,* 1236–1254.

Lovaas, O. I., Koegel, R. L., Simmons, J. Q., & Long, J. S. (1973). Some generalization and follow-up measures on autistic children in behavior therapy. *Journal of Applied Behavior Analysis, 6,* 131–166.

Lovaas, O. I., & Simmons, J. Q. (1969). Manipulation of self-destruction in three retarded children. *Journal of Applied Behavior Analysis, 2,* 143–157.

Mesibov, G. B., & Dawson, G. (1986). Pervasive developmental disorders and schizophrenia. In J. M. Reisman (Ed.), *Behavior disorders in infants, children, and adolescents* (pp. 117–152). New York: Random House.

Murakami, J. W., Courchesne, E., Press, G. A., Yeung-Courchesne, R., & Hesselink, J. R. (1989). Reduced cerebellar hemisphere size and its relationship to vermal hypoplasia in autism. *Archives of Neurology, 46,* 689–694.

Nelson, D. L. (1984). *Children with autism an other pervasive disorders of development and behavior: Therapy through activities.* Thorofare, NJ: Slack.

Ornitz, E., & Ritvo, E. (1976). The syndrome of autism: A critical review. *The American Journal of Psychiatry, 133,* 609–621.

Parks, S. L. (1983). The assessment of autistic children: A selective review of available instruments. *Journal of Autism and Developmental Disorders, 3,* 255–267.

Rimland, B. (1971). The differentiation of childhood psychoses: An analysis of checklists for 2,218 psychotic children. *Journal of Autism and Childhood Schizophrenia, 1,* 161–174.

Rimland, B., Callaway, E., & Dreyfus, P. (1978). The effects of high doses of vitamin B6 on autistic children: A double-blind crossover study. *American Journal of Psychiatry, 135,* 472–475.

Ritvo, E. R., Freeman, B. J., Geller, E., & Yuwiler, A. (1983). Effects of fenfluramine on 14 outpatients with the syndrome of autism. *Journal of the American Academy of Child Psychiatry, 22,* 549–558.

Ritvo, E. R., Spence, M. A., Freeman, B. J., Mason-Brothers, A. M., Mo, M., & Marazita, M. L. (1985). Evidence for autosomal recessive inheritance in 46 families with multiple incidences of autism. *American *Journal of Psychiatry, 142,* 187–192.

Ruttenberg, B. A., Dratman, J. L., Fraknoi, J., & Wenar, C. (1966). An instrument for evaluating autistic children. *Journal of the American Academy of Child Psychiatry, 5,* 453–478.

Rutter, M., Bartak, L., & Newman, S. (1971). Autism—A central disorder of cognition or language? In M. Rutter (Ed.), *Infantile autism: Concepts, characteristics and treatment* (pp. 148–171). London: Churchill-Livingstone.

Sahley, T. L., & Panksepp, J. (1987). Brain opioids and autism: An updated analysis of possible linkages. *Journal of Autism and Developmental Disorders, 17,* 201–216.

Sainato, D. M., Strain, P. S., Lefebvre, D., & Rapp, N. (1990). Effects of self-evaluation on the independent work skills of preschool children with disabilities. *Exceptional Children, 56,* 540–549.

Schopler, E., Reichler, R. J., DeVellis, R. F., & Daly, K. (1980). Toward objective classification of childhood autism: Childhood Autism Rating Scale (CARS). *Journal of Autism and Developmental Disorders, 10,* 91–103.

Schreibman, L. (1988). *Autism.* Newbury Park, CA: Sage.

Schreibman, L., & Charlop, M. H. (1987). Autism. In V. B. Van Hasselt & M. Hersen (Eds.), *Psychological evaluation of the developmentally and physically disabled* (pp. 155–177). New York: Plenum.

Schreibman, L., & Koegel, R. L. (1981). A guideline for planning behavior modification programs for autistic children. In S. M. Turner, K. S. Calhoun, & H. E. Adams (Eds.), *Handbook of clinical behavior therapy* (pp. 500–526). New York: Wiley & Sons.

Schreibman, L., Koegel, R. L., Mills, D. L., & Burke, J. C. (1984). Training parent-child interactions. In E. Schopler & G. B. Mesibov (Eds.), *The effects of autism on the family* (pp. 187–205). New York: Plenum.

Schreibman, L., Stahmer, A. C., & Loos, L. M. (1991, November). Pivotal response training for use with children with autism. Poster presented at the 25th Annual Association for the Advancement of Behavior Therapy Convention. New York, NY.

Shea, V., & Mesibov, G. B. (1985). The relationship of learning disabilities and higher-level autism. *Journal of Autism and Developmental Disorders, 15,* 425–435.

Sherman, J., Factor, D. C., Swinson, R., & Darjes, R. W. (1989). *Journal of Autism and Developmental Disorders, 19,* 533–543.

Stahmer, A. C., & Schreibman, L. (in press). Teaching children with autism appropriate play in unsupervised environments using a self-management treatment package. *Journal of Applied Behavior Analysis.*

Touchette, P. E., MacDonald, R. F., & Langer, S. N. (1985). A scatter plot for identifying stimulus control of problem behavior. *Journal of Applied Behavior Analysis, 18,* 343–351.

Wing, L. (1976). Diagnosis, clinical description and prognosis. In L. Wing (Ed.), *Early childhood autism: Clinical, educational and social aspects* (2nd ed.). Oxford: Pergamon.

CHAPTER 3

MENTAL RETARDATION

Martin J. Lubetsky   University of Pittsburgh

DESCRIPTION OF DISORDER

Clinical Features

Mental retardation is defined by the American Association on Mental Retardation (AAMR) (Grossman, 1983) as "significantly subaverage general intellectual functioning existing concurrently with deficits in adaptive behavior and manifested during the developmental period." A person who is mentally retarded has difficulty in coping with many of life's tasks that require adaptation, flexibility, understanding, problem solving, and social skills. The extent of coping or adaptive "ability" is related to the degree of intellectual capability. In other words, the coping or adaptive difficulty is related to the degree of intellectual impairment. The ability to cope is partly dependent on society's attitudes toward people with mental retardation and the services and funding provided to them (Baroff, 1986, 1991).

Intelligence has been viewed in many ways. Sternberg (1982) described *intelligence* as the ability to learn and profit from experience and to acquire knowledge in so doing, the ability to reason, the ability to adapt to changing conditions, and possibly affected by the motivation to succeed. Baroff (1986) has questioned whether it is the basic

mental capacities or the processes used in problem solving that determine intelligence or subaverage intellectual functioning. Baroff (1986, 1991) prefers the process approach as a dynamic model such as that of Piaget. This process involves the integration of many factors. Sternberg (1982) has stated that "an intelligent person learns from his interactions with the environment and uses his experience to a greater advantage, can infer relations between events, apply these to new situations, integrate information, and apply problem solving in decision making and investigating alternatives."

In addition to subaverage intelligence, the problems in adaptation can be viewed as difficulties in accomplishing the developmental tasks expected for one's chronological age (Baroff, 1986, 1991). In the preschool years, a mentally retarded child displays delays in motor skills, language, cognitive skills, self-help, and socialization. The gross and fine motor skills may have a noticeable delay, as seen in a 30 to 40 percent delay in Down's syndrome infants relative to normal infants (Share, 1975). In a parent survey by Abramson, Gravink, Abramson, and Sommers (1977) delayed or abnormal motor development was the second most common cause of suspicion of retardation (32 percent), with obvious physical abnormalities being the first (58 percent). Also, basic self-care skills such as feeding, toileting, dressing, and grooming may be delayed. This subjects the mentally retarded child to an increased dependency on the caretaker, which interferes with the development of autonomy. The mentally retarded child may appear younger than his or her age, behave immaturely, and play with younger age peers. Social integration is difficult due to the immaturity, delayed speech, attitudes of others, and need for more supervision. Family acceptance, grief, and parental expectations make adjustment even more problematic for the family and the child.

By school age, the mentally retarded child shows problems with academic achievement, social skills, autonomy, self-confidence, and judgment. These developmental gains or delays certainly interrelate with expectations of the environment, culture, and family. The school-aged mentally retarded child encounters academic chalenges in very diverse educational settings dependent on population size, funding, expertise, and parental advocacy. The social development is significant in that this is a time when autonomy, peer relationships, self-confidence, expansion in interests, and motor skills develop. In the teenager, same-sex and opposite-sex interests develop, often with limited understanding or coping skills in the mentally retarded. This is also a time for vocational planning and skill development. Choices and successes depend on the mentally retarded adolescent's basic academic skills, social skills, work habits, and personality style, as well as good adult guidance in a qualified training site.

Another component of social skills deficits is difficulty with social awareness and interpreting affect. Learning to problem solve and how to react or respond depends on understanding that information is transmitted by others and oneself through the spoken word and nonverbal facial expressions, gestures, and voice modulation or prosody of speech (Tanguay & Russell, 1991). This social nonverbal communication was tested recently by Hobson, Ouston, and Lee (1989) by studying the ability of mildly retarded adolescents to match photographs of sad, angry, happy, surprised, and disgusted faces with vocal expressions of the same emotions. The retarded adolescents performed lower than nonretarded adolescents. The same retarded adolescents performed better on nonemotional stimuli than on the emotional recognition tasks. In addition, the social communication skills, specifically pragmatic and prosodic speech functioning, are disturbed in mentally retarded children and adolescents (Tanguay, 1990). The pragmatic skills comprise social rules that govern language and the prosodic skills involve the melody of speech (i.e., rate, rhythm, tone).

Associated Features

Mental retardation has a multitude of causes, many of which are unknown. The associated features may relate to the cause or suspected etiology or the possible coexistence of other medical/sensory/behavioral/emotional problems. For example, Down's syndrome is the most common noninherited genetic cause of mental retardation. Children with Down's syndrome will have a spectrum of physical features present. In general, the more severe the mental retardation, the more likely a cause may be found and associated abnormalities will exist. These abnormalities may include seizures, visual or hearing impairment, ambulating and motor difficulties, speech and swallowing problems, and other organ system involvement. These abnormalities may further impair the mentally retarded child's functioning (American Psychiatric Association, 1987).

Also, behavioral disturbance may be an associated feature that correlates with the intellectual, adaptive, and developmental problems, as well as resultant difficulties that adults may have in working with the mentally retarded child. These behavioral symptoms range from passivity, isolation, dependency, low self-esteem, to low frustration tolerance, aggressiveness, poor impulse control, and stereotyped self-stimulating and self-injurious behavior (American Psychiatric Association, 1987). The behavioral problems may be a direct result of the physical cause of the mental retardation, such as self-biting in Lesch-Nyhan syndrome. In some children, the behaviors may be learned based on adult or child role models. The behaviors may be conditioned by environmental factors, such as that seen in avoidance or escape mechanisms and attention-seeking or comfort-seeking methods.

In addition, other mental disorders or psychiatric illness is at least three or four times greater in the mentally retarded as compared to the general population (American Psychiatric Association, 1987). According to Rutter, Graham, and Yule (1970) in the Isle of Wight Study, in 9- to 11-year-old mentally retarded children, 30 percent had emotional disorders as rated by a teacher questionnaire, and 42 percent by a parent questionnaire. This is compared to 8 percent and 10 percent in nonretarded children. Corbett (1979) found 47 percent of mentally retarded children under 15 years of age showing a psychiatric disorder. Some reasons given for this increased incidence of psychiatric disturbance in the mentally retarded includes the negative attitudes conveyed by others, social rejection experienced, sense of isolation, low self-esteem, and feeling less capable or inadequate in school (Tanguay, 1990).

Epidemiology

The prevalence of mental retardation is determined by where the cut-off point is placed on the IQ distribution curve (Tanguay & Russell, 1991). The American Association on Mental Retardation (AAMR) decided that the cut-off point would be placed at 2 standard deviations from the mean, below which 2.28 percent of the population is found. This is the ideal, but in reality the estimate from epidemiologic studies using IQ measures has shown a prevalence rate of approximately 3 percent of the population (Zigler & Hodapp, 1986). Mercer (1973), in a community study using both IQ and adaptive behavior test scores, found a prevalence of approximately 1 percent. A number of studies suggest that the proportion of persons meeting both criteria would be closer to 1 percent than 3 percent (Birch, Richardson, Baird, Horobin, & Illsley, 1970; Mercer, 1973; American Psychiatric Association, 1987).

According to the President's Committee on Mental Retardation (1967, 1978), 89 percent of all retarded persons fall in the mild range (DSM-III-R reports 85 percent), 7 percent in the moderate range (DSM-III-R reports 10 percent), 3 percent in the severe range, and 1 percent in the profound range. Mental retardation is more common among males, with a male to female ratio of approximately 1.5 to 1.0 (American Psychiatric Association, 1987).

Etiology

Etiologic factors may be organic/biologic/physical or psychosocial/environmental, or both. In approximately 30 to 40 percent of the mentally retarded, no clear etiology can be found on evaluation (American Psychiatric Association, 1987). Major causes can be categorized as follows: Genetic factors can account for approximately 5 percent of mental retardation. Examples of genetic causes include inborn errors of metabolism (e.g., Tay-Sachs disease), other single-gene abnormalities (e.g., tuberous sclerosis), and chromosomal aberrations (e.g., translocation Down's syndrome and Fragile-X syndrome). Early alterations of embryonic development make up approximately 30 percent; a few examples are chromosomal changes (e.g., trisomy 21 Down's syndrome) and prenatal damage due to toxins (e.g., maternal alcohol consumption, infections). Pregnancy and perinatal problems occur in approximately 10 percent of mental retardation, such as fetal malnutrition, prematurity, hypoxia, trauma, and environmental toxins (e.g., lead). Environmental influences and mental disorders comprise approximately 15 to 20 percent, such as deprivation of nurturance and stimulation, and complications of severe psychiatric disorders (e.g., a drop in adaptive functioning in a person with borderline intellectual functioning following early-onset schizophrenia).

DIFFERENTIAL DIAGNOSIS AND ASSESSMENT

DSM-III-R Categorization

The essential features needed to diagnose mental retardation, as stated in the DSM-III-R (American Psychiatric Association, 1987) include: (1) significantly subaverage general intellectual functioning, (2) significant deficits or impairments in adaptive functioning, and (3) onset before the age of 18. In addition, this diagnosis is made whether or not there is a coexisting physical or psychiatric disorder. Since by definition the age of onset is before age 18, it is not diagnosed as retardation if a similar presentation occurs for the first time after age 18. If a child with mental retardation has deterioration in functioning (e.g., brain damage in an automobile accident), then a dementia can be superimposed on mental retardation (American Psychiatric Association, 1987).

Degrees of severity of mental retardation have varied by a few IQ points, depending on the source. DSM-III-R (American Psychiatric Association, 1987) categorizes levels of mental retardation as follows:

Degree of Severity	IQ
Mild	50–55 to approximately 70
Moderate	35–40 to 50–55
Severe	20–25 to 35–40
Profound	Below 20 or 25

The diagnosis of Mental Retardation is included in Axis II — Developmental Disorders in DSM-III-R, rather than Axis I — Clinical Syndromes as in DSM-III. The DSM-IV Committee is still debating this issue of which axis is the most appropriate (Shaffer et al., 1989).

Differential Diagnosis

In order to achieve the proper diagnosis and assess the differential of other diagnoses, a comprehensive evaluation from a multidisciplinary team is necessary. In a child with mental retardation, comprehensive assessment reveals that there are general delays in development in many areas. However, in a child with a specific developmental disorder, there is a delay or failure of development in a specific area, but normal development in other areas (American Psychiatric Association, 1987). Specific developmental disorders are characterized by inadequate development in arithmetic, expressive writing, reading, expressive and receptive language, articulation, or coordination. Pervasive developmental disorders are differ-

ential diagnoses in which there is a qualitative impairment in reciprocal social interaction, verbal and nonverbal communication, and imaginative play and interests. This is not merely a generalized *delay* in development, but an *abnormality* in the development of these areas that occur in pervasive developmental disorder (e.g., autistic disorder or pervasive developmental disorder, not otherwise specified). Pervasive developmental disorder and mental retardation may also coexist.

Borderline intellectual functioning is a V-code given when the IQ is between 71 and 84. This is not in the range of mental retardation and is differentiated based on psychoeducational testing and adaptive functioning scales.

Other sensory or motor problems in a child may simulate mental retardation (Baroff, 1986). These lags in development may be due to hearing impairments, visual impairments, or neuromuscular disorders such as hypotonia or cerebral palsy, without mental retardation present. Also, severe behavioral problems can interfere with a child's development or present as a developmental delay but not prove to be mental retardation.

Finally, sociocultural/environmental factors have been implicated in deprivation as a cause of mental retardation, especially in the mild range (Tanguay, 1990; Tanguay & Russell, 1991). It was postulated that the caregiver's lack of sufficient intellectual and verbal stimulation, as well as appropriate role modeling were causative. This has been shown to be largely incorrect, since the majority of children from these environments are not mentally retarded, unless there are other factors involved, including genetic.

Assessment Strategies

Wodrich and Joy (1986) stated that for multidisciplinary assessment of children with mental retardation to be effective, the evaluation must contain mutually understood language, propose a common purpose, and serve both a diagnostic purpose and a treatment planning role to facilitate intervention and remediation (Reschley, 1980). The assessment can then be used to inform others and provide needed information for future planning. Wodrich and Joy (1986) also summarized two approaches to assessment: behavior analysis approach and modality preference approach. The behavior analysis approach focuses on a detailed appraisal of the current academic and adaptive skills, so that a behavioral plan can concentrate on modifying behaviors. The goal is to train by shaping behavior and developing methods to teach the deficient skill and include reinforcement procedures to provide feedback and to promote motivation. In contrast, the modality preference approach is directed at a detailed analysis of the mental processing abilities that will provide a pattern of cognitive strengths and weaknesses. These modality preferences can guide the teacher to avoid the child's weaknesses and build on his or her strengths, or to strengthen the child's deficits in order to achieve progress. A prime source of this information is through the use of detailed psychometric instruments.

Comprehensive assessment is a part of a problem-solving process in which history, observations, interviews, and testing are completed in order to collect data. Then, this information is synthesized into a formulation, differential diagnosis, and treatment plan. Bergan (1977) developed a four-stage model of problem solving that includes problem identification, problem analysis, plan implementation, and problem evaluation after treatment. This links assessment to intervention.

Furthermore, assessment practices should be objective, reliable, and valid (Wodrich & Joy, 1986). To be objective, the data should be quantifiable, linked to norms or external criteria, and related to observable and verifiable events. Both the testing procedure and the process of testing should be reliable (i.e., consistent, accurate, and reproducible). Validity refers to the extent to which a test fulfills the function for which it is being used. Wodrich and Joy (1986) also noted that a fourth criterion for assessment practices is norm referencing. This involves comparing a score from an individual child with a representative sample of children.

Next, assessment strategies will be reviewed and categorized as assessment of intellectual capacity, adaptive skills, achievement, neuropsychologic

processes, and behaviors (see Neisworth & Bagnato, 1987). First, mentally retarded children can be evaluated for intellectual or skill deficits in which academic skills have not or cannot be acquired. This is different from performance deficits in which an already acquired skill is not displayed due to behavioral or emotional reasons (Wodrich & Joy, 1986).

Initial testing usually involves *intellectual ability measures* such as on a general scale like the Stanford-Binet Intelligence Scale: Fourth Edition (Thorndike, Hagen, & Sattler, 1986), which is used for children ages 2 years to adult. The Stanford-Binet: Fourth Edition is loaded with verbal items and yields five scores to appraise verbal reasoning, quantitative reasoning, abstract/visual reasoning, short-term memory, and a composite score. In contrast, the Wechsler Intelligence Scale for Children-Revised (WISC-R) (Wechsler, 1974) has 12 subtests and yields a Verbal score, Performance score, and Full Scale IQ score. The WISC-R is used for ages 6 to 16 years and assesses areas of vocabulary, reasoning, perceptual-motor skill, and memory.

Another model of intelligence testing utilizes theory-based measures such as the Kaufman Assessment Battery for Children (K-ABC) (Kaufman & Kaufman, 1983) for ages 2½ to 12½ years. The K-ABC consists of a Sequential Processing Scale that reflects a child's ability to problem solve in a serial order, a Simultaneous Processing Scale in which problem solving occurs with many stimuli integrated in a parallel order, and an Achievement Scale.

In addition to intelligence testing, *adaptive behavior measures* are a vital part of both diagnosis and treatment planning for a mentally retarded child. One example of such a measure is the AAMD Adaptive Behavior Scale (ABS) (Lambert & Windmiller, 1981). One part has nine domains that evaluate independence and daily living skills. The second part assesses inappropriate or unacceptable behaviors. It is completed by parents, caregivers, or teachers who know the child. Another assessment of adaptive skills is the Vineland Adaptive Behavior Scales (Vineland) (Sparrow, Balla, & Cicchetti, 1984). The Vineland has eight categories of behavior related to social competence and has several forms that cover birth to 18 years of age.

A third form of assessment is through *achievement tests,* which can be used for purposes of (1) screening to identify students potentially eligible for remedial programming, (2) classification/ placement to ascertain specific academic deficiencies, (3) prescriptive intervention to make curriculum adjustments based on specific deficits, and (4) program evaluation to evaluate benefits of special programming (Katz & Slomka, 1990). Examples of achievement tests are the Woodcock Reading Mastery Tests (Woodcock, 1973) for kindergarten through twelfth grade, and the Key Math Diagnostic Arithmetic Test (Connolly, Nachtman, & Pritchett, 1971) for kindergarten through eighth grade. Another more common skill-learning inventory used in developmentally delayed children is the Brigance Diagnostic Inventory of Basic Skills and Essential Skills (Brigance, 1977, 1980) for kindergarten through sixth grade and secondary schools.

A fourth assessment modality is through *neuropsychological testing* used to provide information to guide instructional planning, to rule out specific neurological problems, and to assess other areas such as sensory-motor, self-control, and personality characteristics that relate to specific cortical functions (Dean, 1982). Neuropsychological testing in children is appropriate if inherent cognitive problems contribute to a child's behavioral/ psychiatric disturbance (Taylor & Fletcher, 1990). Taylor and Fletcher (1990) have reviewed the "biobehavioral systems" approach to neuropsychological evaluation in which a multifactorial framework is used to consider environmental, psychosocial, and developmental influences. They have emphasized that rather than attempting differential diagnosis of emotional versus organic disorders, the biobehavioral systems approach focuses on the evaluation of developing cognitive and behavioral skills associated with the disability in question (see Lubetsky, 1991). One example is the Luria-Nebraska Neuropsychological Test Battery (Golden, Hammeke, & Purisch, 1978).

A fifth assessment strategy is to investigate *performance deficits* in which a child has certain skills but does not display them. In this situation, the assessment may begin with physical/medical evaluation but should then proceed to learning environment and learning attitude for causes. The school setting may contribute to a child's difficulty in learning. In addition, the child's motivation, mood, anxiety level, behavior, personality style, and attitude may directly affect performance. Evaluation and observation by a school psychologist or special education diagnostician would aid in determining what variables affect the child. Also, objective personality measures such as the Personality Inventory for Children (PIC) (Goldman, Stein, & Guerry, 1983) may aid in differentiating characteristics that are aberrant (compared to a group norm in the nonretarded population). Furthermore, behavioral assessment and psychiatric evaluation would aid in investigating performance deficits.

The next assessment strategy to be reviewed is *behavioral evaluation* in which an empirical approach "based on observations or experience" is conducted (Woolf, 1977). This empirically based behavioral assessment is not dependent on any specific theory of etiology for the behavior (Achenbach & Edelbrock, 1989). Ollendick and Hersen (1984) expanded on the definition of *child behavioral assessment* as "an exploratory, hypothesis-testing process in which a range of specific procedures is used in order to understand a given child, group, or social ecology, and to formulate and evaluate specific intervention strategies." Ollendick and Greene (1990) have supported that child behavioral assessment must have a developmental, age-appropriate context; normative comparisons to ensure that change in behavior is related to treatment, not to normal developmental change; a knowledge of the context in which the child's behavior occurs and the function that it serves; and a multimethod assessment approach. Hersen (1973) noted a behavioral assessment trial of motoric, physiological, and self-report systems as an alternative for indirect measurement (see Lubetsky, 1991; Shapiro & Browder, 1990; Iwata, Vollmer, & Zarcone, 1990).

Direct behavioral observation in the natural environment or in a controlled simulated setting provides an informative accounting of target behaviors. The primary goal is to identify the behavioral problems and the environmental factors contributing to the problem. The best known strategies for conducting direct observational assessment are event sampling and time sampling procedures (Barrett, Ackles, & Hersen, 1986). Behavioral assessment is individualized, integrated into the intervention, and ongoing, in order to reassess, monitor, and evaluate the intervention and outcome. A behavioral observation format designed to operationally define the *B*ehavior, the *A*ntecedent, and *C*onsequent conditions is the A-B-C format (Bijou, Peterson, & Ault, 1968). This format is an essential component in the functional analysis of a problem behavior. It provides a structured means of communication for the parent, teacher, or behavior therapist in order to assess the reasons for occurrence or responses that perpetuate a behavior.

In addition, behavioral rating scales completed by others can be helpful since direct observation by the clinician cannot be accomplished at all times. One sample of a behavioral rating scale developed for the mentally retarded population is the Aberrant Behavior Checklist (ABC) (Aman & Singh, 1983). This checklist has five subscales of Irritability, Lethargy, Stereotypy, Hyperactivity, and Excessive Speech. Another rating scale was designed to assess mood disorders in developmentally disabled children and adolescents. The Emotional Disorders Rating Scale for Developmental Disabilities (EDRS-DD) (Feinstein, Kaminer, Barrett, & Tylenda, 1988) behaviorally defines a broad range of affect and mood and is designed to be completed by direct caretakers on both frequency and severity measures.

The final assessment strategy used in differentiating causes of cognitive change or behavioral disturbance is the *psychiatric evaluation*. The role of the child and adolescent psychiatrist is to assess, diagnose, and treat psychiatric disturbances, and to participate in large multidisciplinary teams designed to treat the mentally retarded child and adolescent (Lubetsky, 1986; Joy, 1986; Russell, 1985). The psychiatric evaluation includes history, medical/neurologic/laboratory evaluation findings, psychoeducational/neuropsychological testing results, observational data, rating scale data, and interactional interview with the child and

parent and child, based on the child's developmental level. The assessment should be designed to determine the coexistence of a DSM-III-R defined mental disorder along with mental retardation.

TREATMENT

Evidence for Prescriptive Treatments

Behavior Therapy

Behavior modification or applied behavior analysis is based on methodological requirements that focus on the control and manipulation of environmental variables (Cipani, 1989, 1990). Cipani (1990) described these methodological requirements to include an empirical focus based on observable behavior, an analytical orientation assessing the functional relationship between variables, and effective therapies based on operant behavioral principles (Skinner, 1957). The operant model utilizes three temporally ordered events: *A*ntecedent stimulus, operant *B*ehavioral response, and environmental *C*onsequent stimulus. The appropriateness of behavior therapies in the mentally retarded population is related to the fact that the mentally retarded child's impaired communication, social interactions, and skill development restricts other forms of intervention. Treatment is based on the premise that mentally retarded children have a slow acquisition of new skills and propensity to learn aberrant behavior (Corbett, 1985). Thus, the functional analysis of these skills leads the therapist to increase or reinforce skills that promote learning and to decrease or withhold reinforcement for aberrant behaviors that obstruct learning. Behavior therapies have had proven successful for years in many populations, especially in the mentally retarded (Foxx, 1982; Kazdin, 1975; Meyer & Evans, 1989; Matson, 1990).

Good behavioral objectives lead to effective behavior therapy. A behavioral objective describes the desired behavior, the measurement of the behavior or criterion level of performance, and the circumstances in which the behavior will be performed (Foxx, 1982). The shaping of the behavior and thus the skill learning is based on the teacher's consequence to the child's response to the stimulus provided. The consequence that will increase the likelihood of a response is either a positive reinforcement (produce a desirable stimulus) or a negative reinforcement (remove a desirable stimulus). A punisher (withdrawal or presentation of an undesirable stimulus) will decrease the likelihood of a response.

Evans and Meyer (1985) proposed an educative approach to address excess behaviors in the mentally retarded. Children with mental retardation may exhibit some of the following behaviors: aggression, tantrums, throwing, property destruction, self-injury, stealing, swearing, stereotypic behaviors, rituals, wandering away, and noncompliance. An aberrant behavior often serves a purpose for the individual as an adaptive strategy that will need to be replaced by a more powerful strategy in order to reduce or eliminate the behavior that is a problem for others (Meyers & Evans, 1989). The more powerful strategy should be designed to improve skills or to teach new skills in order to achieve the intended purpose in a more prosocial manner than the problem behavior.

Models of behavioral prescriptive treatment can be categorized as behavior induction or reduction procedures (Whitman & Johnston, 1987). Behavior induction procedures are used to prompt or induce the desired behavior when it does not occur frequently. Examples include verbal instruction, modeling, physical guidance, and shaping. Behavior reduction procedures are used to reduce or eliminate the maladaptive or excess behaviors seen in many mentally retarded children. Examples include extinction (withholding reinforcement or ignoring), differential reinforcement, and punishment (e.g., time out from positive reinforcement, response cost, restitution/positive practice overcorrection, and aversive stimuli). In addition, cognitive-behavioral procedures are used to augment learning experiences through self-regulation, problem solving, cognitive strategy, correspondence, and self-instructional training (Whitman, 1987; Whitman, Burgio, & Johnston, 1984).

Behavioral treatments are often evaluated using single-case designs (Hersen & Barlow, 1976; Kazdin, 1977). For example, self-help skill programs that have been implemented successfully with the mentally retarded child include toilet training (Foxx & Azrin, 1973) and self-feeding (Matson, Ollendick, & Adkins, 1980). Successful social skills training programs include conversational skills (Matson, Kazdin, & Esveldt-Dawson, 1980) and preschool peer social interactions (Odom, Hoyson, Jamieson, & Strain, 1985). Differential reinforcement programs have been successful in stereotypy reduction (Repp, Dietz, & Dietz, 1976).

Pharmacotherapy

The use of medications in the mentally retarded has been a controversial topic. Controversies have centered around issues regarding advocacy for least restrictive/invasive treatment, overuse of drug treatment to control aberrant behaviors, lack of well-designed studies, and single-treatment approaches (see Hersen, 1979; Aman & Singh, 1988a; Aman, 1987). More recently, pharmacotherapy has been based on better psychiatric evaluation of the mentally retarded and improving diagnostic clarification of symptoms and behaviors (Sovner, 1987; Menolascino, Ruedrich, & Kang, 1991; Donaldson, 1984). With the awareness of dual diagnosis (i.e., mental retardation and psychiatric disorder), pharmacotherapy can be more appropriately used. Rivinus, Grofer, Feinstein, and Barrett (1989) have stated that although medications cannot "cure" mental retardation, they often can alleviate symptoms of psychiatric disorder coexisting with mental retardation.

Szymanski and Doherty (1989) and others have reported that the prevalence of mental disorder in the mentally retarded is several times higher than in nonretarded populations, approximately 30 to 60 percent (Szymanski, 1980; Eaton & Menolascino, 1982; Rutter, Tizard, Yule, Graham, & Whitmore, 1976; Matson & Barrett, 1982). Higher vulnerability of the mentally retarded to psychopathology may be due to several factors, including communication deficits, adaptive behavior deficits, sensory deficits, rejection, frustration, low self-esteem, and impaired coping responses (Szymanski & Doherty, 1989; Sovner & Hurley, 1983). Reiss, Levitan, and Szyszko (1982) referred to the failure to see emotional disturbances in the mentally retarded due to the presence of intellectual and adaptive deficits as "diagnostic overshadowing."

Pharmacotherapy in child psychiatry has progressed rapidly with the development of DSM-III, improved methodology, and development of rating scales (Campbell & Spencer, 1988). The application of psychopharmacology from adult studies has led to medication trials for similar disorders in mentally retarded children. A brief categorization of some of these disorders and medications include attention deficit hyperactivity disorder (with and without oppositional-defiant disorder)—methylphenidate, dextroamphetamine, pemoline, desipramine, clonidine; depression—tricyclic antidepressants; bipolar disorder (and some intermittent explosive/aggressive disorders)—lithium carbonate, carbamazepine, valproic acid; anxiety—buspirone; obsessive-compulsive disorder—fluoxetine, clomipramine; psychosis—antipsychotics; severe aggression—beta-blockers (e.g., propranolol); severe self-injurious behaviors—opiate antagonists (e.g., naltrexone). One caveat is that mentally retarded children taking medication should be monitored closely for a paradoxical response or side effects.

Medication effect can be assessed by monitoring target symptoms, through utilizing rating scales, direct observations, self-report, and parent report (Rogoff, 1989; Aman & Singh, 1988a). Medication trials can be evaluated more accurately through double-blind, placebo-controlled trials (Sprague & Werry, 1971; Hersen & Barlow, 1976). Side effects can be followed by utilizing checklists, direct observations, and physiologic parameters (Aman & Singh, 1988a; Gadow & Poling, 1988).

Alternative Treatments

Other treatment modalities for problems that arise in mentally retarded children and their families include parent and paraprofessional staff training, family therapies (e.g., psychoeducational), group therapies (e.g., social skills, activity, sexuality), individual therapies (e.g., play, creative and expressive arts, interpersonal), and support groups (e.g., parents, siblings, grandparents). Treatment approaches are designed to include parents, families, and agency staff since

they are the consistent caretakers who need to carry out treatment recommendations in the community. One example is behavior management training/parent training in which treatment programs are explained, taught, and practiced (see Baker, 1989). Another example is psychoeducational family therapy in which parents are taught principles about the child's illness, disorder, or problems; coping mechanisms; ways to seek help; understanding of the many therapeutic interventions; and awareness of the impact on the family system (see Goldenberg, 1985; Seligman & Darling, 1989).

Furthermore, various psychotherapies for the mentally retarded child have been utilized based on the developmental level, verbal skills, and social skills. Individual psychotherapy has focused on interpersonal relationships, expression of feelings in a safe environment, and development of self-esteem (see Sigman, 1985; Szymanski, 1980). Group therapies have focused on adolescent adjustment, sexuality, acceptance by normal peers, development of autonomy, and social skills (see Sigman, 1985; Welch & Sigman, 1980).

Finally, treatment of a child with mental retardation must begin with an assessment of needs with regard to basic deficits in adaptive skills. Areas of skill training include activities of daily living, self-help skills, social and conversational skills, classroom survival skills, and sexuality and personal space awareness. In addition, prevocational and vocational training constitute a major part of preparation for independent living.

Selecting Optimal Treatment Strategies

The treatment plan is based on competent assessment and diagnosis of the mentally retarded child. Treatment planning should involve a multidisciplinary team approach as well as the parents and teachers. Comprehensive history, observational data, rating scales, testing results, medical evaluation results, and diagnostic formulation should be reviewed in order to select optimal treatment methods. Meyer and Evans (1989) described four intervention components that must be considered in a comprehensive treatment plan for behavioral problems. Such a plan includes procedures for (1) short-term prevention, (2) immediate consequences (including crisis management), (3) establishing adaptive alternatives, and (4) long-term prevention. According to this model, the first step is to attempt to effect environment or ecological changes that will reduce the maladaptive behavior, or to increase supervision, or to anticipate the behavior and intervene.

In order to establish therapeutic change, the appropriate treatment modality must be based on the mentally retarded child's developmental and intellectual level, adaptive and social skills, environmental and family considerations, availability of therapeutic services, and diagnostic issues. The behavioral approach is usually chosen first due to the learning-based model of behavioral theory and learning needs of the mentally retarded child, frequency of behavior problems as the initial presentation, and history of empirically designed and tested treatment methods. Pharmacotherapy is chosen as a treatment option based on psychiatric diagnostic indications and usually severity of symptoms. Researchers have reported that behavior modification and pharmacotherapy in combination may be more effective than either treatment alone (Shalock, Foley, Toulouse, & Stark, 1985).

In addition, mentally retarded children who display adequate levels of verbal and social skills may benefit from various forms of group therapy or individual therapy, based on the emotional or social skills problems and the specific goals outlined. Family therapy may be appropriate depending on the family's grief issues, lack of understanding of the child's needs, or intrafamily conflicts. Certainly the selection for treatment options depends on the skills of the clinician involved, but should not outweigh the needs of the mentally retarded child and his or her family.

Problems in Carrying Out Interventions

Successful intervention depends on accurate assessment, diagnosis, and treatment planning. If any of these components are inaccurate, incomplete, or unable to be performed, then the outcome is likely to be unsuccessful. The treatment team needs to assess the skills of the clinician, the cooperation of the parents, and the probability of consistency in treatment follow-through in all of the child's environments. Treatment failure may not be the failure of the treatment methods but in the planning, training, and monitoring steps. Problems in successful intervention may be found at any of these steps (Meyer & Evans, 1989): (1) identify priority problems, (2) describe target behaviors in objective and measurable terms, (3) identify the conditions and circumstances that predict when the behavior will/will not occur, (4) list possible functions of these behaviors, (5) team planning with a Wish list and a Now list, (6) design an intervention plan, and (7) identify procedures to evaluate intervention outcomes.

The clinician may choose optimal treatment strategies, but if the child and family do not attend treatment sessions, do not comply with medication trials, or inconsistently carry out behavior management, then the outcome will not be successful. Engaging the child, family, school, and agencies in a cooperative therapeutic alliance is vital for achieving success in working with a lifelong disability. The clinician must present interventions in a manner that can be easily understood by the parents. The complexity of multistep data collection and behavioral intervention should be simplified in order to facilitate further treatment efforts with intellectually limited or emotionally stressed families. Training of physical management techniques should be individualized to help achieve success with families who have the potential to physically abuse or have admitted to losing control with their child. The instruction should include stress reduction and coping skills. Another problem in carrying out interventions exists when the controversy over treatment selection prevents the use of potentially successful behavioral methods or medications.

Relapse Prevention

In order to prevent relapse, the treatment team needs to consider the strengths and weaknesses of the child, family, and school personnel. The strengths can be promoted or reinforced to gain a more successful outcome. The weaknesses can be monitored in order to predict areas of potential failure and to develop a prevention plan. For example, if the child requires a certain degree of supervision without which he or she fails, then a plan of fading the amount of supervision can be designed and parents and teachers can be prepared for the frequency of supervision needed. Another example of relapse prevention occurs when the treatment team knows that transportation needs to be planned and/or funded for a family without access to a car or without funds for a long bus ride. Also, booster therapy sessions can be planned during times of crisis or expected stress. Telephone calls from the clinician to the family can be made between treatment sessions, prior to vacations, or after a course of treatment has terminated. Regular telephone contact between the teacher and clinician may allow problems to be identified before they develop or worsen.

In addition, relapse prevention can include expanding the reinforcement menu before satiation of a limited number of reinforcers occurs. Another example is ensuring that parents and school staff can physically carry out physical management techniques or are permitted to use time-out procedures if the child changes caretakers or schools. Also, an important aspect of medication compliance is education for the child, parents, and school staff about the medication effects and side effects. This includes an explanation of the consequences of discontinuing the medication without psychiatric monitoring.

CASE ILLUSTRATION

Case Description

Tommy is a 6½-year-old white boy who was referred to a multidisciplinary evaluation team in a child psychiatric developmental disabilities program by his kindergarten teacher. Tommy had been in a regular kindergarten with 28 children and one teacher for only two weeks when the teacher requested assistance from her principal. Tommy's teacher reported that he appeared one to two years behind in play skills, social skills, self-help skills, language use, and fine motor abilities. The teacher noted that Tommy wet himself at least two times in a 3½-hour day, scratched other children, threw toys indiscriminately, called out impulsively, ran around the room as he chose, laughed when redirected or reprimanded, and was irritable when demands were placed. Tommy had never been in a formal school setting prior to kindergarten and was at home with his mother or grandmother. Tommy had never been seen by a mental health professional or diagnostician and saw a variety of clinic pediatricians for immunizations.

Tommy is an only child living at home with his 26-year-old mother and 25-year-old father. His mother now works part time as a grocery store clerk since his father was laid off from an auto parts store six months ago. Tommy and his family moved several times due to his father's employment changes and they returned to his mother's hometown six months ago. It was at this time that his maternal grandmother became involved in part-time babysitting, and she recommended starting him in kindergarten. Tommy's mother graduated from high school; his father dropped out in tenth grade after failing twice. There is no significant medical or psychiatric family history except for a maternal aunt and paternal uncle who were reported to be slow and had learning problems.

Tommy was the only birth to a healthy mother and father, and he had no perinatal complications. He fed well and developed according to normal milestones by his mother's best memories. She was not aware of any developmental delays until age 4 when he spoke fewer words than she expected, age 5 when he still had wetting accidents, and age 5½ when he did not play well with peers or scratched them. She thought that these behaviors were due to the family's several moves or the parents' arguing over finances. Tommy's mother explained that discipline was erratic and that she and her husband yelled and spanked Tommy at times, but also gave in to his tantrums. In addition, she reported that Tommy occasionally stared off into space when demands were placed and she thought that it was oppositional or avoidant behavior.

Differential Diagnosis and Assessment

Tommy's mother, father, grandmother, teacher, principal, and pediatric clinic provided past and present behavioral, educational, social, family, and medical histories. There was a clear lack of appropriate developmental and child-rearing expectations on the part of Tommy's parents, who had no previous children and did not live near their own parents for advice. Tommy's pediatric care was inconsistent due to several family moves and changes in pediatricians. Pediatric records noted developmental concerns by age 3½ and recommendations for more frequent appointments and assessment, but the father insisted that his son was normal. From this assessment it was clear that the parents did not agree on many issues and the maternal grandmother's advice was limited.

Physical examination revealed a healthy, normal for age height and weight for a 6½-year-old boy, with impulsivity and oppositionality. He was somewhat uncoordinated, rapid in motor pace, and spoke in an immature manner with articulation errors. At one time in the examination, he stared off into space for less than 10 seconds and was not interruptible but then resumed playing. There was a question of brief eyelid fluttering. Further medical testing revealed the following results: Hearing tested within normal limits on audiometry and tympanometry. Ophthalmologic exam revealed a mild myopia with a recommendation for corrective lenses. Sleep-deprived EEG was not indicative of a seizure tendency but no clinical signs were seen during the test. A variety of organic, metabolic, hematologic laboratory studies were normal, including normal chromosome study with no Fragile-X found.

Psychoeducational assessment revealed an impulsive, hyperactive boy with a Stanford Binet: Fourth Edition (Thorndike et al., 1986) IQ of 59. The Vineland Adaptive Behavior Scales (Sparrow et al., 1984) revealed a composite score of 58. The Development Test of Visual Motor Integration (Beery & Buktenica, 1967) age equivalent was 4.8 years for a chronological age of 6.6 years. Speech and language evaluation revealed expressive language age of 4.0–4.8 years, receptive language age of 4.9–5.2 years, and many articulation errors. Thus, Tommy displayed deficiencies in intellectual functioning, visual-motor integration, fine motor skills, adaptive social and self-help skills, and speech and language skills.

Behavioral and psychiatric assessment showed an impulsive, overactive, inattentive, distractible, oppositional, defiant, noncompliant, occasionally aggressive, and disruptive boy. His affect ranged from silly and happy to irritable to angry at times of tantrum behavior. He did not appear sad, anxious, or psychotic. He reportedly wet himself two to three times a day and nightly, but was rarely encopretic. He had difficulty sharing and playing with peers. He frequently made eye contact with adults when displaying inappropriate behavior, and had tantrums when he did not get his own way. Aberrant Behavior Checklist scores, Connors/Iowa Teachers Rating Scores, and Antecedent-Behavior-Consequent data reflected the same behavioral problems at significant rates. These were completed in the office setting, in the classroom by the teacher and psychologist, and by the mother at home. In addition, Tommy was observed to display the same behaviors during interactions with his mother, father, and grandmother.

In summary, Tommy presents as a 6½-year-old boy with developmental delays, behavioral problems, vague family history of learning problems versus mental retardation, parental conflict, multiple family moves, and a question of a seizure disorder based on clinical observation. The impact of nature (i.e., genetic, inherited) versus nurture (i.e., learned, environmental) is not a clear one but is significant. No clear organic etiology for retardation was found. Diagnostically, provisional diagnosis from DSM-III-R included Axis I: (1) attention deficit hyperactivity disorder, (2) oppositional-defiant disorder, (3) functional enuresis; Axis II: (1) mental retardation, mild, (2) developmental language and articulation disorders; Axis III: (1) ruleout seizure disorder, (2) myopia. In addition, family issues have an impact on Tommy and so would the neurobehavioral effects of partial complex seizures if this interfered with development, academic functioning, memory, and behavior.

Treatment Selection

Treatment selection is based on the multidisciplinary team, psychiatric, behavioral, medical, and social assessments as described previously. Following the evaluation and differential diagnosis, a treatment plan begins with issues of dangerousness and whether there is a need for inpatient hospitalization or outpatient treatment. Then selection of professional discipline or skill level of the clinician depends on the treatment recommendations. It is important to begin with least restrictive treatment methods and then advance to more restrictive therapies or placements only as lesser restrictive measures fail. In addition, medical/organic workup proceeds until negative results are obtained or diagnostic conclusions are made.

In Tommy's situation the multidisciplinary team included a child psychiatrist, behavioral psychologist, psychiatric social worker, developmental specialist (special educator), psychoeducational evaluator (school psychologist), and child neurologist. The first team recommendation was placement in a smaller, learning support classroom with a special education teacher and classroom aide, in a public school setting. This would provide Tommy with more supervision in a classroom in which treatment recommendations would be successfully tried. If this is not possible or would take a school year to process, then another possibility is to request a classroom aide in the present setting and train both the teacher and aide through modeling and rehearsal.

The initial treatment selection was based on a behavioral functional analysis that showed attention seeking and avoidance/escape as determinants for his tantrums, yelling, noncompliance, and out-of-seat behavior. One of the initial behavior shaping techniques used was positive reinforcement for prosocial and "teacher-pleasing" behaviors. This included a star card with 4 blocks for desirable behaviors (e.g., "good listening," "good talking," "staying in seat," "keeping hands to self") and 2 blocks to fill with a star or "smiley face" in each category. Once his card is filled, he can earn one of four items pictured at the top of the card. The items are chosen from his reinforcement menu and he can select his choice at the start of each card. As he becomes more successful, the number of star blocks can increase from 8 to 12. In addition, positive verbal praise and touch can be used at high rates initially both in combination with the star card and separately. As he becomes more successful, the frequency of praise and touch can be gradually reduced.

Another behavior program chosen was compliance training to promote compliance. Tommy was given a directive in a few clear, simple words with both visual and auditory cues and modeled once. He was given a specified time to comply and then when he did not comply, the directive was repeated in a firm voice and a contingency warning was given. If he still did not comply, then the directive was repeated while manually guiding him in a hand-over-hand fashion in order to educate him on how it should be done. Initially, tantrums may occur in spite of the above approaches. This behavior can be treated with systematic attention and planned ignoring (extinction).

At the same time as behavioral treatment began at home and at school, the Connors/Iowa Teachers Rating Scales and the Aberrant Behavior Checklist were used in the classroom to provide information on inattention, hyperactivity, impulsivity, oppositionality, irritability, and speech production. Then, treatment methods used in the classroom consist of a structured classroom setting, task selection based on developmental readiness, initial high frequency of reinforcement, consistent clarity of requests with modeling and practice, and initial high rates of supervision. These were a few developmental/educational approaches used to promote attention, in-seat behavior, and task completion.

Social skills training was a focus in the school setting. Tommy had no interactions with peers at home or in his neighborhood. The adults were asked to model simple toy play, sharing, turn taking, asking questions, and verbalizing requests rather than acting out, and then Tommy practiced these tasks. Positive reinforcement was used and higher-functioning peers acted as role models. These methods were also utilized in parent management training sessions in the clinic setting.

Furthermore, enuresis was initially quantified

during a baseline period. The treatment plan was to utilize a bedtime star chart to encourage compliance with toileting before bed, reduction in fluids before bed, and being dry upon wake up. When wetting occurred, it was to be treated by Tommy, who was instructed to clean himself up, change his clothes, and put them in the washer. In addition, daytime reminders to toilet every two to three hours were used initially.

As mentioned earlier, outpatient appointments consisted of parent management training from developmental, behavioral, and psychoeducational perspectives. Modeling, roleplay, and practice sessions were utilized. Supportive therapy was given with a focus on grief issues, marital conflicts, and community and family supports. Consultation with the school was also ongoing.

Treatment Course and Problems in Carrying Out Interventions

Throughout the course of treatment, it was necessary to have ongoing monitoring and evaluation of treatment response. Tommy showed an increase in compliance, a decrease in tantrums (after an initial extinction burst), and an increase in social interactions with adults and peers. As reported, he persisted in overactivity, difficulty in staying in his seat, poor attention span, and easy distractibility with behavioral treatment. His scratching of others and throwing objects reduced during baseline and even more with the positive reinforcement program, social skills training activities, and decreased tantrums. Enuresis decreased during baseline, most likely due to staff inadvertently providing him cues to schedule his toileting and the parents withdrawal of fluids after dinner. The enuresis decreased more when tantrums decreased and compliance increased. However, the toileting star chart, restitution, and overcorrection finally reduced the enuresis to one day per two weeks and one night per month. Improved sleep patterns occurred through instituting an earlier bedtime, reading and reinforcement rituals prior to bed, avoidance of naps during the day, and reduction in junk food (caffeine products) prior to bed. These procedures reduced daytime

sleepiness and partly lessened daytime staring and daydreaming.

In spite of these treatment modalities, Tommy was overactive and displayed a short attention span, impulsivity, and distractibility. The Conners/Iowa Teachers Rating Scale and Aberrant Behavior Checklist Hyperactivity Subscale scores were consistently at high rates. Therefore, the child psychiatrist, in consultation with the therapist, teacher, and parents, decided to begin a methylphenidate trial (see Helsel, Hersen, & Lubetsky, 1988). Effects and side effects were explained, handouts on the medication and attention deficit-hyperactivity disorder were reviewed and Tommy's parents consented to a double-blind placebo controlled trial. The capsules were initially given at 8:00 A.M. and noon, Monday through Friday, with dosage determined by Tommy's weight for low, medium, and medium-high doses. Effects were monitored with Connors/Iowa Teachers Rating Scales, Aberrant Behavior Checklist, and direct observations. Side effects were monitored with a rating scale based on the *Physician's Desk Reference* (PDR, 1991). Once the optimal dose was determined, methylphenidate was also given at 4:00 P.M. and on weekends, since these same behaviors were a major problem at home. The addition of methylphenidate improved Tommy's attention span and ability to stay in seat, and decreased his impulsivity and daydreaming without medication side effects.

Problems in carrying out interventions were numerous. During the parents' involvement in evaluation, history taking was difficult. They could not agree on many of the issues and denied that their child could be mentally retarded or have behavioral/psychiatric problems. It took many sessions of education, support, grief work, and diffusing anger to build a cooperative, therapeutic relationship. Tommy's behaviors worsened during this assessment/pretreatment phase, almost necessitating hospitalization when school suspended Tommy. Tommy's father walked out on his wife temporarily, and Tommy's mother spanked Tommy and then took him to Children's Hospital emergency room when she feared she was losing control. However, the parents, maternal grandparents, and a neighbor all worked together to provide mutual emotional support, transportation to outpatient appointments, and participation in parent management training. The treatment team engaged the special education coordinator of the school district, the local Association for Retarded Citizens Advocate, and the local mental health/ mental retardation case manager to work with the clinicians and family.

Outcome and Termination

Tommy was placed in a transitional kindergarten in a public school. His classroom had 12 children with mild speech, cognitive or behavioral problems, and developmental delays. However, Tommy's aberrant behaviors were reduced but not eliminated at home and in his previous classroom, prior to this change in placement. Tommy showed increased compliance to 75 percent occurrence, staying in seat 70 percent of the time in the classroom, increased attention span and on-task behaviors at a rate of 80 percent, and accuracy of task 75 percent of the time. Tantrums decreased to less than one per day, scratching dropped to zero rates, and enuresis was at zero rates of occurrence for daytime and twice a month at nighttime. Treatment lasted for eight months with two booster sessions at one month and three months. Booster sessions consisted of behavioral management training. Both parents, grandmother, and a neighbor participated. Marital conflict lessened but did not resolve. Tommy's mother followed treatment recommendations more consistently than the father, but the father was home more due to being unemployed while the mother was working. In addition, methylphenidate was discontinued for one week at school with worsening symptoms, and was then resumed. Monthly medication appointments continued until parents chose to stop the methylphenidate before school ended.

Followup and Maintenance

The treatment terminated after the second booster session and Tommy changed school placement for the last four months of school. The family called back when Tommy's behaviors worsened at the beginning of summer vacation. They did not follow through with our recommendations for a summer camp program and Tommy had no structured programming. Also, Tommy was off of methylphenidate for six weeks. Two booster sessions were held with one followup session two weeks later, which showed partial reduction of aberrant behaviors. A part-time summer program was obtained and this helped reduce parental stress as well as further reduction of problem behavior. Methylphenidate was then reinstituted, which reduced impulsivity and inattention further. Due to this deterioration, followup phone calls were made every two weeks for another three months. Medication appointments were monthly. One more booster session was held two weeks after school started and a school consultation visit was made by the psychologist at the same time. The plan was for further problems to be raised in monthly medication appointments or by telephone calls from the parents or the special education teacher, in which case further sessions would be scheduled.

SUMMARY

Mental retardation has been defined as the combination of subaverage intellectual functioning and adaptive behavior problems. There is a wide range of etiologic factors but most of the time no clear cause is found. There is also a wide scope of behavioral and psychiatric symptoms that can develop in the mentally retarded and these symptoms can frequently be diagnosed as resulting from a treatable disorder. It is therefore the role of the clinician to perform a comprehensive, multidisciplinary team assessment in order to prescribe appropriate treatments. These treatments may include behavioral approaches, pharmacotherapy, psychotherapy, and developmental/ educational therapies in combination and in the childs' natural settings as well as in the clinic or hospital setting.

As reviewed in this chapter, treatment goals need to be set and frequently reevaluated in order to adjust treatment interventions to fit the needs of the mentally retarded child and his or her family. Empirically supported treatment was reviewed and a case example was described in order to illustrate the complexity of assessment and multiple interventions, as well as to reflect the need for followup and maintenance treatment. A cooperative working relationship between family, school, community agencies and clinicians is vital in order to ensure a successful outcome.

REFERENCES

Abramson, P. R., Gravink, M. J., Abramson, L. M., & Sommers, D. (1977). Early diagnosis and intervention of retardation: A survey of parental reactions concerning the quality of services rendered. *Mental Retardation, 15,* 28–31.

Achenbach, T. M., & Edelbrock, C. (1989). Diagnostic, taxonomic, and assessment issues. In T. H. Ollendick & M. Hersen (Eds.), *Handbook of child psychopathology* (2nd ed., pp. 53–69). New York: Plenum.

Aman, M. G. (1987). Overview of pharmacotherapy: Current status and future directions. *Journal of Mental Deficiency Research, 31,* 121–130.

Aman, M. G., & Singh, N. N. (1983). *Aberrant Behavior Checklist.* Canterbury, New Zealand: University of Canterbury.

Aman, M. G., & Singh, N. N. (1988a). Patterns of drug use, methodological considerations, measurement techniques, and future trends. In M. G. Aman & N. N. Singh (Eds.), *Psychopharmacology of the developmental disabilities* (pp. 1–28). New York: Springer-Verlag.

Aman, M. G., & Singh, N. N. (Eds.) (1988b). *Psychopharmacology of the developmental disabilities: Disorders of human learning, behavior, and communication.* New York: Springer-Verlag.

American Psychiatric Association. (1987). *Diagnostic and statistical manual of mental disorders* (3rd ed., rev.). Washington, DC: Author.

Baker, B. (1989). *Parent training and developmental disabilities.* New York: Guilford.

Baroff, G. S. (1986). Predicting the prevalence of mental retardation in individual catchment areas. *Mental Retardation, 20,* 133–135.

Baroff, G. S. (Ed.) (1986). *Mental retardation: Nature, cause, and management* (2nd ed.). Washington: Hemisphere Publishing.

Baroff, G. S. (1991). Mental retardation. *In Developmental disabilities: Psychosocial aspects* (pp. 53–109). Austin, TX: Pro-Ed.

Barrett, R. P., Ackles, P. K., & Hersen, M. (1986). Strategies for evaluating treatment effectiveness. In R. P. Barrett (Ed.), *Severe behavior disorders in the mentally retarded: Nondrug approaches to treatment* (pp. 323–357). New York: Plenum.

Beery, K. E., & Buktenica, N. A. (1967). *Developmental test of visual-motor integration.* Chicago: Follett.

Bergan, J. R. (1977). *Behavioral consultation.* Columbus, OH: Merrill.

Bijou, S. W., Peterson, R. F., & Ault, M. H. (1968). A method to integrate descriptive and experimental field studies at the level of data and empirical concepts. *Journal of Applied Behavior Analysis, 1,* 175–191.

Birch, H. G., Richardson, S. A., Baird, D., Horobin, G., & Illsley, R. (1970). *Mental subnormality in the community: A clinical and epidemiological study.* Baltimore: Williams and Wilkins.

Brigance, A. (1977). *Brigance Inventory of Basic Skills.* North Billerica, MA: Curriculum Associates.

Brigance, A. (1980). *Brigance Diagnostic Inventory of Essential Skills.* North Billerica, MA: Curriculum Associates.

Campbell, M., & Spencer, E. K. (1988). Psychopharmacology in child and adolescent psychiatry: A review of the past five years. *Journal of the American Academy of Child and Adolescenty Psychiatry, 27* (3), 269–279.

Cipani, E. (Ed.). (1989). *The treatment of severe behavior disorders.* (Monographs of the American Association on Mental Retardation No. 12). Washington, DC: American Association on Mental Retardation.

Cipani, E. (1990). Principles of behavior modification. In J. L. Matson (Ed.), *Handbook of behavior modification with the mentally retarded* (2nd ed., pp. 123–138). New York: Plenum Press.

Connolly, A., Nachtman, W., & Pritchett, E. (1971). *Manual for the Key Math Diagnostic Arithmetic Test.* Circle Pines, MN: American Guidance Service.

Corbett, J. A. (1979). Psychiatric morbidity and mental retardation. In F. E. James & R. P. Smith (Eds.), *Psychiatric illness and mental handicap* (pp. 28–45). London: Gaskell Press.

Corbett, J. A. (1985). Mental retardation: Psychiatric aspects. In M. Rutter & L. Hersov (Eds.), *Child and adolescent psychiatry: Modern approaches* (pp. 661–678). Boston: Blackwell Scientific Publications.

Dean, R. S. (1982). Neuropsychological assessment. In T. R. Kratochwill (Ed.), *Advances in school psychology* (Vol. 2, pp. 171–218). Hillsdale, NJ: Erlbaum.

Donaldson, J. W. (1984). Specific psychopharmacological approaches and rationale for mentally retarded: Problems and issues. In F. J. Menolascino (Ed.), *Specific psychopharmacological approaches and rationale for mentally retarded-mentally ill children* (pp. 171–188). New York: Plenum.

Eaton, L. F., & Menolascino, F. J. (1982). Psychiatric disorders in the mentally retarded: Types, problems, and challenges. *American Journal of Psychiatry, 139,* 1297–1303.

Evans, L. M., & Meyer, L. H. (1985). *An educative approach to behavior problems: A practical decision model for interventions with severely handicapped learners.* Baltimore: Paul H. Brookes.

Feinstein, C., Kaminer, Y., Barrett, R. P., & Tylenda, B. (1988). The assessment of mood and affect in developmentally disabled children and adolescents: The Emotional Disorders Rating Scale. *Research in Developmental Disabilities, 9,* 109–121.

Foxx, R. M. (1982). *Decreasing behaviors of severely retarded and autistic persons.* Champaign, IL: Research Press.

Foxx, R. M. (1982). *Increasing behaviors of severely retarded and autistic persons.* Champaign, IL: Research Press.

Foxx, R. M., & Azrin, H. H. (1973). *Toilet training the retarded.* Champaign, IL: Research Press.

Gadow, K. D., & Poling, A. G. (1988). *Pharmacotherapy and mental retardation.* Boston: Little, Brown.

Golden, C. J., Hammeke, T. A., & Purisch, A. D. (1978). Diagnostic validity of a neuropsychological battery derived from Luria's neuropsychological tests. *Journal of Consulting and Clinical Psychology, 46,* 1258–1265.

Goldenberg, I. (1985). Family therapy with the dual disability client. In M. Sigman (Ed.), *Children with emotional disorders and developmental disabilities: Assessment and treatment* (pp. 315–324). New York: Grune and Stratton.

Goldman, J., Stein, C. L. E., & Guerry, S. (1983). *Psychological methods of child assessment.* New York: Brunner/Mazel.

Grossman, H. J. (Ed.). (1983). *Classification in mental retardation.* Washington, DC: American Association of Mental Deficiency.

Helsel, W. J., Hersen, M., & Lubetsky, M. J. (1988). Stimulant drug use in children and adolescents with mental retardation: A review. *Journal of the Multihandicapped Person, 4,* 251–269.

Hersen, M. (1973). Self-assessment and fear. *Behavior Therapy, 4,* 241–257.

Hersen, M. (1979). Limitations and problems in the clinical application of behavioral techniques in psychiatric settings. *Behavior Therapy, 10,* 65–80.

Hersen, M., & Barlow, D. H. (1976). *Single case experimental designs: Strategies for studying behavior change.* New York: Pergamon.

Hobson, R. P., Ouston, J., & Lee, A. (1989). Recognition of emotion by mentally retarded adolescents and young adults. *American Journal of Mental Retardation, 93,* 434–443.

Iwata, B. A., Vollmer, T. R., & Zarcone, J. R. (1990). The experimental (functional) analysis of behavior disorders: Methodology, applications, and limitations. In A. C. Repp & N. N. Singh (Eds.), *Perspectives on the use of nonaversive and aversive interventions for persons with developmental disabilities* (pp. 301–330). Sycamore, IL: Sycamore Publishing.

Joy, J. E. (1986). Psychiatric assessment. In D. L. Wodrich & J. E. Joy (Eds.), *Multi-disciplinary assessment of children with learning disabilities and mental retardation* (pp. 227–246). Baltimore: Paul H. Brookes.

Katz, L. J., & Slomka, G. T. (1990). Achievement testing. In G. Goldstein & M. Hersen (Eds.), *Handbook of psychological assessment* (2nd ed., pp. 123–147). New York: Pergamon.

Kaufman, A. S., & Kaufman, N. L. (1983). *Interpretative manual for the Kaufman Assessment Battery for Children.* Circle Pines, MN: American Guidance Service.

Kazdin, A. E. (1975). *Behavior modification in applied settings.* Homewood, IL: Dorsey.

Kazdin, A. E. (1977). Assessing the clinical or applied significance of behavior change through social validation. *Behavior Modification, 1,* 427–452.

Lambert, N., & Windmiller, M. (1981). *AAMD Adaptive Behavior Scale, School Edition.* Monterey, CA: CTR/McGraw-Hill.

Lubetsky, M. J. (1986). The psychiatrist's role in the assessment and treatment of the mentally retarded child. *Child Psychiatry and Human Development, 16* (4), 261–273.

Lubetsky, M. J. (in press). Psychiatric assessment and diagnosis: Children. In A. S. Bellack & M. Hersen (Eds.), *Handbook of behavior therapy in the psychiatric setting.* New York: Plenum.

Matson, J. L. (1990). *Handbook of behavior modification with the mentally retarded* (2nd ed.). New York: Plenum.

Matson, J. L., & Barrett, R. P. (Eds.) (1982). *Psychopathology in the mentally retarded.* New York: Grune and Stratton.

Matson, J. L., Kazdin, A. E., & Esveldt-Dawson, K. (1980). Training interpersonal skills among mentally retarded and socially dysfunctional children. *Behavior Research and Therapy, 18,* 419–427.

Matson, J. L., Ollendick, T. A., & Adkin, J. (1980). A comprehensive dining program for mentally retarded adults. *Behaviour Research and Therapy, 18,* 107–112.

Menolascino, F. J., Ruedrich, S. L., & Kang, J. S. (1991). Mental illness in the mentally retarded: Diagnostic clarity as a prelude to psychopharmacological interventions. In J. J. Ratey (Ed.), *Mental retardation: Developing pharmacotherapies* (pp. 19–33). Washington, DC: American Psychiatric Press.

Mercer, J. R. (1973). The myth of 3 per cent prevalence. In G. Tarjan, R. K. Eyman, & C. E. Meyers (Eds.), *Sociobehavioral studies in mental retardation.* Washington, DC: Monographs of the American Association on Mental Deficiency.

Meyers, L. H., & Evans, I. M. (1989). *Nonaversive intervention for behavior problems: A manual for home and community.* Baltimore: Paul H. Brookes.

Neisworth, J. T., & Bagnato, S. J. (1987). Developmental retardation. In V. B. Van Hasselt & M. Hersen (Eds.), *Psychological evaluation of the developmental and physically disabled* (pp. 179–212). New York: Plenum.

Odom, S. L., Hoyson, M., Jamieson, B., & Strain, P. S. (1985). Increasing handicapped preschoolers' peer social interactions: Cross-setting and component analysis. *Journal of Applied Behavior Analysis, 18,* 3–16.

Ollendick, T. H., & Greene, R. (1990). *Behavioral assessment of children.* In G. Goldstein & M. Hersen (Eds.), *Handbook of psychological assessment* (2nd ed., pp. 403–422). New York: Pergamon.

Ollendick, T. H., & Hersen, M. (Eds.). (1984). *Child behavioral assessment: Principles and procedures.* New York: Pergamon.

Physician's Desk Reference. (1991). Oradell, NJ: Medical Economies Company.

President's Committee on Mental Retardation. (1967). *A first report on the nation's progress and remaining great needs in the campaign to combat mental retardation.* Washington, DC: U.S. Government Printing Office.

President's Committee on Mental Retardation. (1978). *Mental retardation: The leading edge.* Washington, DC: U.S. Government Printing Office, Publication Office (OHDS) 79-21018.

Reiss, S., Levitan, G. W., & Szyszko, J. (1982). Emotional disturbance and mental retardation: Diagnostic overshadowing. *American Journal of Mental Deficiency, 86* (6), 567–574.

Repp, A. C., Dietz, S. M., & Dietz, D. E. D. (1976). Reducing inappropriate behavior in classrooms and in individual sessions through DRO schedules of reinforcement. *Mental Retardation, 14,* 11–15.

Reschley, D. J. (1980). School psychologists and assessments in the future. *Professional Psychology, 11,* 841–848.

Rivinus, T. M., Grofer, L. M., Feinstein, C., & Barrett, R. P. (1989). Psychopharmacology in the mentally retarded individual: New approaches, new directions. *Journal of the Multihandicapped Person, 2* (1), 1–23.

Rofogg, M. L. (1989). Psychotropic medication. In I. L. Rubin & A. C. Croker (Eds.), *Developmental disabilities: Delivery of medical care for children and adults* (pp. 348–354). New York: Lea & Febriger.

Russell, A. T. (1985). The mentally retarded, emotionally disturbed child and adolescent. In M. Sigman (Ed.), *Children with emotional disorders and developmental disabilities: Assessment and treatment* (pp. 111–135). New York: Grune and Stratton.

Rutter, M., Graham, P., & Yule, W. (1970). *A neuropsychiatric study in childhood.* London: Spastics International Medical Publications and Heinemann.

Rutter, M., Tizard, J., Yule, W., Graham, P., & Whitmore, K. (1976). Research report: Isle of Wight Studies, 1964–1974. *Psychological Medicine, 6,* 313–332.

Schalock, R. L., Foley, J. W., Toulouse, A., & Stark, J. A. (1985). Medication and programming in controlling the behavior of mentally retarded individuals in community settings. *American Journal of Mental Deficiency, 89,* 503–509.

Seligman, M., & Darling, R. B. (1989). *Ordinary families special children.* New York: Guilford.

Shaffer, D., Campbell, M., Cantwell, D., Bradley, S., Carlson, G., Cohen, D., Denckla, M., Frances, A., Garfinkel, B., Klein, R., Pineus, H., Spitzer, R. I., Volkmar, F., & Widiger, T. (1989). Child and adolescent psychiatric disorders in *DSM-IV:* Issues facing the work group. *Brief Communication,* 830–835. American Psychiatric Association Task Force: American Academy of Child and Adolescent Psychiatry.

Shapiro, E. S., & Browder, D. M. (1990). Behavioral assessment. In J. L. Matson (Ed.), *Handbook of behavior modification with the mentally retarded* (2nd ed., pp. 93–122). New York: Plenum.

Share, J. B. (1975). Developmental progress in Down's syndrome. In R. Koch & F. de la Cruz (Eds.),

Down's syndrome (mongolism): Research prevention and management. New York: Brunner-Mazel.

Sigman, M. (1985). Individual and group psychotherapy with mentally retarded adolescents. In M. Sigman (Ed.), *Children with emotional disorders and developmental disabilities* (pp. 259–276). New York: Grune and Stratton.

Skinner, B. F. (1957). *Verbal behavior.* New York: Appleton-Century-Crofts.

Sovner, R. (1987). Behavioral psychopharmacology. In J. Stark, F. J. Menolascino, M. Albarielli, & V. Gray (Eds.), *Mental retardation and mental health: Classification, diagnosis, treatment, services.* New York: Springer-Verlag.

Sovner, R., & Hurley, A. D. (1983). Do the mentally retarded suffer from affective illness? *Archives of General Psychiatry, 40,* 61–67.

Sparrow, S. S., Balla, D. A., & Cicchetti, D. B. (1984). *The Vineland Adaptive Behavior Scales: A revision of the Vineland Social Maturity Scale by E. A. Doll.* Circle Pines, MN: American Guidance Services.

Sprague, R. L., & Werry, J. S. (1971). Methodology of psychopharmacological studies with the retarded. In N. R. Ellis (Ed.), *International review of research in mental retardation* (Vol. 5, pp. 147–210). New York: Academic Press.

Sternberg, R. J. (1982). The nature of intelligence. *New York University Education Quarterly, 12,* 10–17.

Szymanski, L. S. (1980). Individual psychotherapy with retarded persons. In L. S. Szymanski & P. E. Tanguay (Eds.), *Emotional disorders of mentally retarded persons* (pp. 131–149). Baltimore, MD: University Park Press.

Szymanski, L. S., & Doherty, M. B. (1989). Behavioral and psychiatric disorders. In I. L. Rubin & A. C. Croker (Eds.), *Developmental Disabilities: Delivery of medical care for children and adults* (pp. 334–366). Philadelphia: Lea & Febiger.

Tanguay, P. E. (1990). Mental retardation. In B. D. Garfinkel, G. A. Carlson, & E. B. Weller (Eds.), *Psychiatric disorders in children and adolescents* (pp. 291–305). Philadelphia: Saunders.

Tanguay, P. E., & Russell, A. T. (1991). Mental retardation. In M. Lewis (Ed.), *Child and adolescent psychiatry: A comprehensive textbook.* Baltimore: Williams & Wilkins.

Taylor, H. G., & Fletcher, J. M. (1990). Neuropsychological assessment of children. In G. Goldstein & M. Hersen (Eds.), *Handbook of psychological assessment* (2nd ed., pp. 228–255). New York: Pergamon.

Thorndike, R. L., Hagen, E. P., & Sattler, J. M. (1986). *Technical manual, Stanford-Binet Intelligence Scale: Fourth Edition.* Chicago: Riverside Publishing.

Wechsler, D. (1974). *Manual for the Wechsler Intelligence Scale for Children-Revised.* San Antonio: Psychological Corporation.

Welch, V. O., & Sigman, M. (1980). Group psychotherapy with mentally retarded, emotionally disturbed adolescents. *Journal of Clinical Child Psychology, 9,* 209–210.

Whitman, T., Burgio, L., & Johnston, M. B. (1984). Cognitive behavior therapy with the mentally retarded. In A. Myers & E. Craighead (Eds.), *Cognitive behavior therapy with children* (pp. 193–227). New York: Plenum.

Whitman, T. L. (1987). Self-instruction and mental retardation: Theoretical, research and educational perspectives. *American Journal of Mental Deficiency, 92,* 213–233.

Whitman, T. L., & Johnston, M. B. (1987). Mental retardation. In M. Hersen & V. B. Van Hasselt (Eds.), *Behavior therapy with children and adolescents: A clinical approach* (pp. 184–223). New York: Wiley & Sons.

Wodrich, D. L., & Joy, J. E. (1986). *Multi-disciplinary assessment of children with learning disabilities and mental retardation.* Baltimore: Paul H. Brookes.

Woodcock, R. W. (1973). *Woodcock Reading Mastery Tests.* Circle Pines, MN: American Guidance Service.

Woolf, H. B. (Ed.) (1977). *Webster's new collegiate dictionary.* Springfield, MA: Merriam.

Zigler, E., & Hodapp, R. M. (1986). *Understanding mental retardation.* New York: Cambridge University Press.

CHAPTER 4

SPECIFIC DEVELOPMENTAL DISORDERS

Vaughan Stagg   University of Pittsburgh
M. Susan Burns   University of Pittsburgh

DESCRIPTION OF DISORDER

In many ways, summarizing such a broad topic as specific developmental disorders is problematic. Although clinicians, researchers, and educators generally agree that such disorders exist, there is considerable disagreement concerning their definitions, diagnosis, and treatment regimens. Children and adolescents with specific developmental disabilities display inadequate development of particular language, academic learning, and/or motor skills. Children with such inadequate development do not have demonstrable physical or neurological disorders, global mental retardation, severe environmental deprivation, or deficient educational opportunities.

What DSM-III-R (American Psychiatric Association, 1987) delineates as specific developmental disorders are often considered in a more global definition by other professional and policy groups. One example is the definition of *specific learning disability* presented in U.S. Public Law 92-142, where specific learning disabilities are defined as a disorder in understanding or using language. The result of this language disorder may be impaired ability to listen, think, speak, read, write, spell, or do mathematical calculations. There is a close relationship between language and learning disorders. Children who have language disorders in the preschool often have subsequent learning problems in school years (Baker & Cantwell, 1989).

Clinical Features

A brief description of each of the specific developmental disorders is presented below. All of the disorders have their origin in childhood and each type varies widely in severity.

Developmental Coordination Disorder

This is the only motor skills disorder included in the specific developmental disorder section of DSM-III-R. This disorder is characterized by a marked impairment of gross (playing ball) or fine (zipping, handwriting) motor coordination not attributable to mental retardation or physical disorder. This impairment must interfere with academic achievement or daily living.

Language and Speech Disorders

Both receptive and expressive functioning tend to be affected in language-disordered children, but the disorder may be primarily one of reception or expression (Stark, 1987). Language-impaired children represent a heterogeneous population (Bliss, 1985).

Developmental Articulation Disorder

Developmental articulation disorder is defined as a consistent failure to make correct articulations of speech sounds. Children show misarticulations, substitutions, or omissions of speech sounds. This disorder is not attributable to pervasive developmental disorder, mental retardation, or physical or hearing impairment.

Developmental Expressive Language Disorder

Developmental expressive language disorder is defined by children having limitations in vocabulary size and word retrieval, word substitutions, functional descriptions, overgeneralizations, and overuse of jargon (Baker & Cantwell, 1989). There is controversy about the separation of expressive and receptive language disorders. However, clinical evidence leans toward a distinction between the two.

Developmental Receptive Language Disorder

Developmental receptive language disorder is defined as specific impairment of language comprehension skills. The areas of comprehension affected can include comprehension of vocabulary (word meaning), grammatical units, word ordering, discourse (recognizing multiple meanings that words have), and language usage (comprehending the subtle aspects of language) (Baker & Cantwell, 1989). More severe cases are recognizable by age 2. However, mild cases may not be identified until children are in elementary school.

Academic Skills Disorders

Academic skills disorders are not usually evident until children are in school. They vary in severity. Included are developmental arithmetic disorder, developmental expressive writing disorder, and developmental reading disorder.

Developmental Arithmetic Disorder

Developmental arithmetic disorder is defined in DSM-III-R as "marked impairment in the development of arithmetic skills that is not explainable by mental retardation, inadequate schooling, or hearing or visual defects." The diagnosis is made only if this impairment significantly interferes with academic achievement or with activities of daily living that requires arithmetic skills. The term *dyscalculia* is often used to represent mathematics disabilities.

Developmental Expressive Writing Disorder

Developmental expressive writing disorder is defined as impairment in the development of expressive writing skills that interferes with academic achievement or daily living. The impairment cannot be explained by mental retardation, poor schooling, visual or hearing defects, or a neurologic disorder (as per DSM-III-R). Impairment can include spelling errors, grammatical errors, punctuation errors within sentences, and poor paragraph organization. With mild cases of mental retardation, a child might exhibit a significant deviation in expressive writing that would indicate a concurrent diagnosis of this developmental disorder.

Developmental Reading Disorder

Developmental reading disorder is defined as impairment in the development of word recognition skills and reading comprehension that interferes with academic achievement or daily living. The impairment cannot be explained by mental retardation, poor schooling, visual or hearing defects, or a neurologic disorder. Oral reading is often slow and includes omissions, substitutions, and distortions of words. With mild cases of mental retardation, a child might exhibit a significant deviation in reading that would indicate the additional disorder.

Associated Features

Features associated with specific disabilities are presented in Table 4–1. Notice that many of the disorders are associated with each other as indicated in the overlap in the upper part of the table. The specific developmental disorders are also differentially associated with other difficulties such as behavior problems and delays in other developmental milestones.

Epidemiology

Obtaining sound epidemiological estimates for specific developmental disorders is a difficult task. Definitions (Hammill, 1990) generally focus on discrepancies between aptitude and achievement (as is true of DSM-III-R). However, how such discrepancies are operationalized governs the numbers of children classified (Keogh, 1990). In addition, measurement tools for determining discrepancies are often technically (Salvia & Ysseldyke, 1981) and clinically (Shepard, 1983) inadequate, and are sometimes weakened by institutional constraints (Christenson, Ysseldyke, & Algozzine, 1982). Sociocultural context is also associated with prevalence. For example, in countries where there is a low literacy rate, learning disabilities are not an educational problem (Schroeder et al., 1978). Specifically, because of lack of consensus in terms of definitions and diagnostic procedures, estimates differ widely. Thus, the following statistics should be viewed with caution.

Developmental Coordination Disorder

Estimates of this disorder occur infrequently in the literature. Approximately 5 percent of the elementary school-aged population can be characterized by the "clumsy child syndrome" (Gubbay, 1975; Gubbay, Ellis, Walton, & Court, 1965). Estimates generated in the 1960s of choreoform movement syndrome range from 2 to 20 percent of elementary children, with boys outnumbering girls by 3 to 1 (Silver & Hagin, 1990).

Language and Speech Disorders

Communication disorders represent the largest handicap found in the public schools of the United States. Over 1 million children with speech or language impairments were served in the schools according to a recent report to the Congress (U.S. Department of Education, 1987). This is considered to be an underestimate since this count was based on primary handicapping condition. Communication disorders are more frequently found in boys than girls.

In terms of language disorders, Wiig (1982) estimated that 3 million children between the ages of 3 and 17 years have a developmental language disorder. Baker (1990) reported that between 1 and 13 percent of children have some type of developmental language disorder.

Articulation disorders are more common than language disorders. Estimates range between 2 and 30 percent of children are affected. Extremely deviant phonological disorders are present in about 2 percent of children between the ages of 5 and 17 years (Hull, Mielke, Timmons, & Willeford, 1976).

Academic Skills Disorders

As Silver and Hagin (1990) have noted, it is surprising that realistic estimates of the prevalence of learning disorders have not appeared with any frequency. U.S. Department of Education's (1987) Office of Special Education figures indicate that 4.8 percent of all elementary-aged children received special services for learning disabilities. Hynd, Obrzut, Hayes, and Becker (1986) indicated that learning disabilities are prevalent in 2 to 3 percent of children. Overviews of prevalence data conclude that earlier held assumptions of lower prevalence of arithmetic and mathematics disabilities than reading or writing disabilities are false (Hallahan, Kauffman, & Lloyd, 1985).

Prevalence data for developmental reading disorder range from 2 to 8 percent (see DSM-III-R; American Psychiatric Association, 1987). Two-thirds of all learning disabilities' referrals are diagnosed as having developmental reading disorder (Schroeder et al., 1978). This disorder is more prevalent in boys than girls. Ratios of 2 or

Table 4–1. Associated Disorders (Common and Less Common)

	SPECIFIC DEVELOPMENTAL DISORDERS						
	Coordination	Articulation	Expressive Language	Receptive Language	Arithmetic	Expressive Writing	Reading
Coordination	—	1	1	1	1	1	
Articulation	1	—	1	1			
Expressive language	1	1	—	1	1	1	1
Receptive language	1	1		—	1	1	1
Arithmetic				1	—	1	
Expressive writing				1	—	—	1
Reading		1		1	1	1	—
Delays & other developmental milestones	1	1	1				
Functional enuresis		1	1				
Emotional problems			1, 2				
Social problems			1, 2	1			
Behavior problems			1, 2	1		1	1
Attention problems				1	1		3
Hyperactivity				1			3
EEG abnormalities				1			
Memory problems					1		

Sources:
[1] American Psychiatric Association. (1987) *Diagnostic and statistical manual of mental disorders* (3rd ed., rev.). Washington, DC: Author.
[2] Baker, L. (1990) Specific communication disorders. In B. D. Garfinkel, G. A. Carlson, & E. B. Weller (Eds.), *Psychiatric disorders in children and adolescents.* Philadelphia: Saunders.
[3] Schroeder, C. S., Schroeder, S. R., & Davine, M. A. (1978). Learning disabilities: Assessment and management of reading problems. In B. B. Wolman, J. Egan, & A. O. Ross (Eds.), *Treatment of mental disorders in childhood and adolescence.* Englewood Cliffs, NJ: Prentice Hall.

3 to 1 are found in the literature (Badian, 1983; Rutter & Yule, 1973).

Prevalence data for developmental expressive writing disorder are not available but are expected to be similar to incidence of developmental reading disorder. In terms of arithmetic, Fleischner and Garnett (1987) estimate that 6 percent of the school-aged population has serious difficulties in this area.

Etiology

Causes of specific developmental disorders can be categorized as intrinsic and extrinsic in nature. Intrinsic factors include neurobiological, biochemical, and genetic disturbances. Extrinsic factors are those imposed on the child by the environment, specifically the perinatal environment.

Neurological

Clinical evidence indicates a neurobiological process, though not necessarily a brain function, being responsible for learning disabilities (Tylenda, Hooper, & Barrett, 1989). This perspective originated from studies of brain-injured adults and the various learning/speech problems that they often exhibit.

Recent research has identified electrophysiological differences between dyslexics and normals. Hughes (1985) reviewed a number of studies and found an overall mean of 45 percent of abnormal electroencephalograms (EEGs) in dyslexics. The percentage of abnormal EEGs ranged from 7 to 29 percent in control groups.

Electrophysiologic studies have been criticized on a number of methodological grounds (Connors, 1987; Hughes, 1985; Taylor, 1987). Despite shortcomings, abnormal EEG findings do appear to be more frequent in reading-disabled individuals than in controls. What also is clear from the literature is that EEG patterns associated with reading disability are quite heterogenous. Studies employing event-related potentials have begun to probe differences between reading-disabled and normal children (Silver & Hagin, 1990). These hold promise for uncovering the relationship between central nervous system (CNS) activity and learning/language disorder.

A recent review of neuroimaging (computerized tomography and magnetic resonance imaging) studies by Hynd and Semund-Clikeman (1989) reached three conclusions. First, few abnormalities in gross morphology of brains in developmental dyslexics have been uncovered by computerized tomography or magnetic resonance imaging techniques. Second, significant deviations from normal in terms of brain symmetry and asymmetry have been found in dyslexics. Third, unusual patterns of brain asymmetry appear to be related to deficient expressive language functions.

Autopsy studies have been carried out on a limited number of developmental dyslexics (Drake, 1968; Galaburda & Kemper, 1979; Galaburda, 1989). Differences in symmetry were observed by Galaburda (1989). In addition, he observed unexpected ectopias (clusters of cortical cells where they should not be) and dysplasias. These unusual morphological features were located in the anterior language area.

Biochemical Disturbances

Biochemical disturbance have been put forth as causal mechanisms for specific disorders. Vitamin deficiencies and food allergies have been cited as the most common reasons for biochemical disturbances (Brenner, 1982; Mayron, 1979; Weiss, 1982). Raiten (1990) has cautioned that claims for effectiveness of megavitamin supplements have not been substantiated empirically. Furthermore, he noted that there have been reports of toxicity with large doses of vitamins.

The food allergy hypothesis has been controversial. As proposed by Feingold (1975), food additives, food colorings, preservatives, and salicylates were responsible for some cases of learning difficulty. The National Advisory Committee on Hyperkinesis and Food Additives of the Nutritional Foundation (1980) reviewed a select body of studies. This advisory committee concluded that further funding of the Feingold hypotheses was not warranted. Even though these and other studies (Weiss, 1986) are flawed, there appears to be a small percentage of children who may be affected by such additives.

Genetic Contributions

Heritability plays a role in specific developmental disorders. Evidence supporting a genetic component of learning disabilities has been supplied by family and twin studies (Smith & Pennington, 1987). The familial nature of reading disability has been demonstrated in one of the largest projects designed to study the genetics of reading disability—the Colorado Family Reading Study (Decker & Defries, 1981; Defries, 1985; Defries & Baker, 1983). Parental self-report of reading difficulty is a risk factor for the development of reading disability in their children. The risk of developing a reading disorder is increased by a factor of 4 to over 13 if either parent had difficulty in learning to read (Volger, Defries, & Decker, 1984).

More recently, data from four samples of families were combined (Pennington et al., 1991). Support was found for probable dominant transmission in one of the samples and semidominant or additive transmission in two of the remaining three samples.

Further evidence for a genetic component is provided by twin studies. Pennington and Smith's (1983) review found higher concordance rates for dyslexia in monozygotic twins than in dizygotic twins. The Colorado Family Reading Study (Decker & Vanderberg, 1985; Defries, Fulker, & La Buda, 1987) report significantly higher concordance rates for reading disorders in monozygotic than in dizygotic pairs.

Current findings are summarized by Silver and Hagin:

> While family and twin studies point to a familial prevalence for a specific reading disability, the genetic mode of transmission is still elusive. Overall findings point to a heterogeneous mode of transmission, with evidence for a polygenetic, multifactorial, autosomal-dominant mode and in female probands, a possible autosomal-recessive mode. (1990, p. 331).

Extrinsic Factors

A number of extrinsic factors have been associated with specific developmental disorders. They include perinatal exposure to infection or toxins (i.e., alcohol, cocaine, smoking), severe early deprivation, exposure to lead, perinatal brain injury or insult, and early nutritional deprivation. Environmental factors such as poverty, large family size, and recurrent otitis media underlie at least some cases of developmental language delay. Environmental factors are not the sole cause of language delay but if the child is already at risk, such factors are significant (Baker & Cantwell, 1989).

In many cases of specific developmental disorders, a number of the previously mentioned problems contribute to its cause. These are often established in an anecdotal fashion, not establishing a generalizable cause (Arnold, 1990). In a number of cases the etiology is unclear.

DIFFERENTIAL DIAGNOSIS AND ASSESSMENT

DSM-III-R Categorization and Differential Diagnosis

Assessment of all specific developmental disorders involves the use of formal standardized tests and informal clinical assessment. Differential diagnosis can be difficult in that diagnosis is to a large extent determined by exclusion. The current DSM-III-R definitions require that the child should be significantly below age expectancy in the particular area of disorder. Extensive assessment is needed to exclude or rule out other conditions such as mental retardation, pervasive developmental delay, and sensory or other physical impairment. There is also the need to assess associated conditions. For example, in a behaviorally disordered child with language difficulty, the clinician must determine the relative contribution of each condition to performance during the child's assessment. Table 4–2 summarizes criteria used to rule out specific diagnoses.

Assessment Strategies

Traditional static tests have been regularly used to diagnose children suspected of having specific developmental disorders. These tests are usually given in a single testing session in which instruction

Table 4–2. Differential Diagnosis of Specific Developmental Disorders

DIAGNOSIS TO BE RULED OUT	CRITERIA FOR RULING OUT DIAGNOSIS
Mental retardation	Normal results on standardized testing *and* normal adaptive behavior
Neurological disorder	Normal results on neurology exam
Visual impairment	Normal results on visual testing
Hearing impairment	Normal results on audiometric testing
Organically based communication disorders (i.e., cleft palate, apraxia, cerebral palsy)	Absence of facial deformities, neuromuscular or cerebral abnormalities
Elective mutism	Use of speech/language does not vary significantly depending on setting
Low achievement due to inadequate schooling	School history/records inadequate; indicate few absences, few changes in schools, or little disruption in schooling experience
Other health impairment (i.e., sickle cell anemia, arthritis, muscular dystrophy multiple sclerosis, or other chronic condition)	Health history indicates absence of conditions that affect strength, vitality, or alertness
Pervasive developmental disorder	Absence of gross abnormalities in nonlinguistic areas (play, object use, adaptive behavior)

Source: Adapted from Baker (1990).

is not provided. The tests can be domain general or domain specific. The tests are based on norms and the reference group is usually a national sample or some specialized group (i.e., deaf-blind). Test items are assigned an age ranking based empirically on what children usually achieve at that particular age.

To determine the specific disorder, a two-stage assessment process is undertaken. First, a child's general developmental skills (i.e., cognitive development) are assessed and compared to population or developmental norms. Next, the child is then assessed in the area of suspected developmental difficulty. Results of this phase of the assessment process are compared to the first to determine if specific aspects of the child's development differ significantly from the child's general development.

An alternative to using general domain tests such as an IQ test is using domain-specific tests. Children are given a standardized test within the specific domain of suspected impairment (e.g., Stanford Diagnostic Reading Tests) and the individual child's performance is compared with children of the same age to see if there is a signifi-

cant delay. Siegel (1989) and Ripens, Van Yperen, and Van Duijn (1991) argued that IQ is not needed for determination of expected performance level and proposed using the domain-specific expected performance level.

Traditional tests are often criticized because they give no specific suggestions for dealing with the student having trouble. Even though domain-specific tests give information about a student's performance within a specific content area, they do not indicate what is needed instructionally.

Dynamic assessment is suggested as an alternative to traditional assessment. In dynamic assessment, assistance designed to influence performance is given during the assessment as an indicator of receptivity/potential for change. Within the assessment, the examiner assesses children's thinking processes used while addressing the task and they specify types of instruction that work with the child (Campione, 1989). The contrast between traditional and dynamic assessment strategies are summarized in Table 4–3. This table was adapted from information by Campione and Brown (1987), Feuerstein (1980), Gamlin (1989), and Lidz (1991).

Table 4–3. Contrasts Between Dynamic Assessment and Static Assessment Strategies

STATIC STRATEGIES	DYNAMIC ASSESSMENT STRATEGIES
Norm referenced	Learner referenced
Focus is generally on diagnosis/identification	Prescriptive focus
Product based or assesses for past learning/achievement	Assess for ability to profit from instruction, responsiveness to new material, and ability to transfer or generalize from original learning situation to new problem types
Generally assumes that all children have generally comparable backgrounds and opportunity to acquire needed information	Posits that test performance is the result of prior environmental and educational experience
Assumes assessment results are valid over extended time periods; test results represent relatively permanent characteristics	Assumes that individual is modifiable and that assessment findings need to be updated

Source: Adapted from "Issues in Dynamic Assessment/Instruction" by P. Gamlin, 1989, *International Journal of Dynamic Assessment and Instruction, 1,* p. 16. Copyright 1989 by Captus Press. Used with permission.

TREATMENT

Evidence for Prescriptive Treatment

Treatment of specific developmental disorders generally takes place outside of a medical setting. Intervention agents have a number of options in remediating developmental and learning disorders. In the following section we will present both traditional and novel approaches to treatment.

Behavior Therapy

Correction of specific developmental disorders via applied behavior analysis and related approaches has been demonstrated empirically (Koorland, 1986). Approaches developed from this paradigm emphasize direct skill instruction. Such interventions are characterized by task analysis (breaking down complex tasks into component skills), frequent practice, use of corrective feedback and reinforcement, and regular measurement of how well the student is progressing. Precision teaching (Lindsley, 1964), and direct instruction (Stephens, 1977) are two examples.

However, there are problems with the behavioral approach to remediation of learning disabilities. One problem is that lower learning task skills are taught before higher skills, when these skills are not separable. Children often mis-

understand the global task being taught; for example, they think that reading is decoding. In addition, higher-level strategies are rarely taught (Campione, 1989).

Pharmacotherapy

Pharmacotherapy as a treatment modality for specific developmental disorders is an area of controversy. "At present there is no psychoactive drug that is specifically recognized by the Food and Drug Administration for the treatment of learning disabilities" (Gadow, 1991, p. 351).

Psychopharmacologic interventions with academic performance difficulties have been largely restricted to psychostimulant drugs. It should also be noted that few drug studies have addressed learning disabilities in the absence of hyperactivity. Pelham's (1986) review concluded that long-term outcome studies of the impact of psychopharmacologic treatment on academic achievement are flawed and no conclusions can be drawn. With short-term, well-designed studies, positive effects have been found. Psychostimulants appear to have positive effects on memory and attention. Several reviews have noted that academic productivity can be positively affected by medication. Effects, as measured by standardized achievement tests (Gadow & Swanson, 1986), have been noted with far less frequency.

A novel class of CNS agents has been labeled

as *nootropic* (from the Greek *noos* = mind, *tropein* = toward) by Giurgea (1978). This class of drugs is said to enhance CNS efficiency and facilitate learning and memory. In a series of investigations (DiLanni et al., 1985; Chase & Tallel, 1987; Helgott, Rudel, Koplewicz, & Krieger, 1987; Wilsher, 1987) one of the first drugs (piracetam) of this class was investigated. Reading-disabled children were the target population. As compared with controls, improvement in reading comprehension was found in piracetam-treated children. This conclusion is tempered by the fact that these studies provided little information about other concurrent reading interventions. Despite indications that this nootropic drug may have an effect on verbal processing, further research is warranted. As Silver and Hagin noted, "Piracetam is not ready for use as a therapeutic modality in the treatment of specific language disability. Educational intervention is still the way to go" (1990, p. 238).

Alternative Treatments

Dietary treatments. Dietary treatments and vitamin supplements have also been used to treat developmental disorders. Popular interventions have included regimens free of refined sugar and other food additives. Aman and Singh (1988) reviewed the impact of various vitamin and dietary treatments on the developmentally disabled. They concluded that well-designed studies essentially disproved claims of effectiveness on behavior or learning. Meta-analysis of some 23 diet modification studies (Kavale & Forness, 1985, 1987) support this conclusion.

Process training approaches. Process training approaches assume that learning-disabled children have deficits in basic psychological processes (i.e., visual perception, auditory perception, motor learning) that underlie academic achievement. Process training models were the first remedial techniques to be employed with the learning disabled. Programs such as the Frostig-Horne Visual Perception Training Program (Frostig & Horne, 1964), Kirk and Kirk's Visual Perceptual Training Approach (Kirk & Kirk, 1971), Newell Kephart's Approach (Kephart, 1960, 1971), and

Barsch's Movigenic Curriculum (Barsch, 1967) are examples of well-known process training approaches. As Hallahan and associates (1985) have noted, process remediation has been the most controversial area in the field of learning disabilities. Controversies have centered on (1) the reliable and valid measurement of perceptual and perceptual-motor abilities, (2) the causal relationship between process disabilities and academic difficulty, and (3) the role of other possible causes of learning disorders. Perhaps the most telling criticism is the general lack of effectiveness of process training approaches. Researchers (Hallahan & Cruickshank, 1973; Myers & Hammill, 1982; Lloyd, 1984; Kavale & Forness, 1985, 1987; Kavale, 1990) have not convincingly demonstrated that process training has an impact on academic functioning. Despite negative evidence, process training models undoubtedly will continue to be employed because of clinical tradition and their historical position in the field of learning disabilities (Kavale, 1990).

Cognitive training approaches. Cognitive training approaches assume that learning disabilities are the result of information processing or thinking disabilities. From this perspective, learning disorders are not the result of misperception, but rather they stem from inefficient use of learning strategies for selecting, remembering, and comparing information. Specific examples of curricula employing cognitive training include Instrumental Enrichment (Feuerstein, 1980) for older children and Cognitive Education (Haywood, Brooks, & Burns, 1991) for younger children. Both programs emphasize cognitive strategies that are applicable across academic or developmental domains. More recently, educators have employed this approach with language and emergent literacy development (Burns & Casbergue, 1991) and areas of reading and mathematics development (Brown & Campione, 1986).

Selecting Optimal Treatment Strategies

Our review suggests that both perceptual process approaches and dietary strategies have little value. A case for psychopharmacology has not yet been proven with academic skills. An approach specific to the academic skill to be remediated in combination with cognitive training or a generalizable form of behavior therapy appears best. One would select the appropriate treatment by assessing the resources in the child's ecology. This would include an assessment of family, classroom, school, and community resources. For example, some interventions would require transportation, parental literacy, school district or parental financial ability, or specialized teacher training. In evaluating resources, consideration must be given to these pragmatic concerns in addition to psychiatric issues. It is our experience that barriers other than the condition itself often interfere with the successful implementation of a treatment program.

Our experience also leads us to conclude that specific developmental disorders do not occur in isolation but are accompanied by a number of other psychosocial problems. In treating the child with multiple interventions, one has to be sure to maintain the integrity of each approach. This implies that solid communication must take place between the intervention agents. Concerns of the family system must also be addressed. Should optimal intervention approaches fail, several steps should be considered. Reassessment of the child and the child's ecology may need to occur. This may reveal that the initial treatment was not carried out due to barriers external to the child or that the initial treatment targets were in error.

Problems in Carrying Out Interventions

The differences between educational and medical/clinical definitions possibly create an initial misunderstanding between practitioners who address the needs of children with specific developmental disorders. Profound philosophical differences exist between researchers and intervention agents aligned with the various intervention technologies. These differences can have an impact on the translation of intervention strategies recommended by one setting to another. Other im-

pediments to treatment include lack of available resources (e.g., expensive materials, appropriately trained personnel, noncompliance on the part of parents or other agents, and the many associated features [see Table 4–1]).

Several factors should be examined if interventions fail. These include an examination of staff/child ratios. In some cases, a more individualized (1 to 1) approach may be necessary. One may need to reexamine the expectancies one has for child progress. One may also need to reexamine the procedures and the fidelity with which these procedures are applied. As mentioned earlier, external factors such as transportation, health, attendance, nutrition, and sleep habits should be examined to determine if they are contributing to failure.

Relapse Prevention

With specific developmental disorders, relapse is not the issue one faces with many Axis I conditions (i.e., the child does not "unlearn" reading). Rather, the issue is one of keeping the child from falling behind others as peer development proceeds normally. Frequent monitoring of the child's status is a must. Frequent monitoring appears to be a hallmark of all successful interventions. Coordination of services for children with specific developmental disorders is also essential. As Table 4–1 illustrates, these children can often have complex service needs.

CASE ILLUSTRATION

Case Description

Sally is a 3½-year-old female living in a neighborhood that consists of 1,700 units of government subsidized housing. Her parents are in their mid-thirties and both are living at home. Also living at home is a 7-year-old brother.

Presenting Problems

Sally's mother complains that Sally is "not talking," does not "socialize" with other children her age, and throws tantrums at home. The mother was first concerned when Sally was 18 months old and received intervention through general preschool programs. At this time, the mother continues to seek care because "she still slurs her speech and doesn't say enough words for her age." The mother denies that Sally has any sleep, appetite, or mood disturbances at home.

Developmental History

Sally was the 4-pound, 3-ounce product of a planned pregnancy. Her mother had wanted a girl after having a boy, so she was very pleased. The pregnancy was uneventful and the mother received regular prenatal care. Sally was born at 8 months' gestation by natural, vaginal childbirth. Labor was normal. Due to her low birth weight, Sally was in an incubator for 3 days and went home in 7 days. She was bottle fed without complications. She was an alert, cuddly baby. She sat at 6 months, crawled at 8 months, walked alone at 18 months, said her first word at 2 years, was toilet trained for day at 22 months, and was toilet trained for night at 6 months.

Medical History

Sally's immunizations are up to date; she sees a pediatrician regularly. There is no history of head trauma, ear infection, or other medical problems. Hearing is normal.

Family History

Sally's father stutters and her maternal uncle has mental retardation.

Differential Diagnosis and Assessment

Child Interview and Mental Status Exam

Sally is a well-kept, attractive, 3½-year-old girl who is tall for her age and has good eye contact. She was very cooperative throughout the interview and seemed to relate well to the examiner. She had poor articulation and only spoke single words ("Mommy," "Pop," and a few letters.) Otherwise she was very quiet. There were no stereotypies and no evidence of psychotic disorder. Her mood was slightly anxious. Her affect was appropriate and of normal range. She was oriented to person, place, and time, and memory seemed grossly intact. Cognition could not be adequately assessed due to her being so quiet.

When her mother left the room, Sally did not cry or try to go after her. Instead, she periodically called "Mommy" throughout the sessions. She smiled slightly at the interviewer most of the time. She spontaneously identified letters on blocks with which we were playing. She played quietly and could stack 10 blocks in a tower. However, anytime she was required to speak, she either would not or could not do so.

Developmental Testing

The Battelle Developmental Inventory (BDI) was administered to Sally at age 3 years, 11 months. The following is a summary of Sally's performance of the five domains of the BDI. In the *personal social domain,* she scored below the second percentile, indicating behavior below that of most children her age. In the *adaptive domain and motor domains,* she scored in the low average range. In the *receptive and expressive communication and cognitive domains,* she scored below the second percentile.

Impressions

Sally is a shy 3½-year-old who has had severe difficulty interacting with peers during the last year in preschool. She has continued to be extremely shy and even fearful of other children in the classroom setting. She also has significant speech delay. Her mother denies significant problems at home, but also admits knowing little about normal child development. There is no evidence of any trauma in her life that could play a role in her symptoms.

DSM-R Diagnosis

Axis I

1. Avoidant disorder of childhood
2. R/O Separation anxiety disorder

Axis II

1. Developmental expressive language disorder

2. R/O Developmental receptive language disorder
3. R/O Pervasive developmental disorder NOS
4. R/O Mild mental retardation

Axis III
None

Axis IV
Severity of Psychosocial Stressors — 2 — mild-mother unsure of her parenting skills

Axis V
Global Assessment of Functioning — current: 50 (Serious Symptoms); past: 50–60 (Serious to Moderate Symptoms)

Recommendations
1. Admit to therapeutic preschool
2. Developmental testing to rule out developmental disorder.
3. Is already in speech therapy through Public School Early Education.
4. Attend therapeutic preschool half time and Public School Early Education.

Treatment Selection

Treatment selection was carried out by Sally's treatment team. The team was headed by a child psychiatrist and consisted of representatives from psychology, education, social work, and the child's family. In addition, a representative from the local school system's special education programs actively participated. After examining developmental history, psychiatric and developmental evaluations, and recommendations, the team selected the following treatment: First, the child was admitted to the partial day hospital for half days and arrangements were made for a half-day language intervention program.

Sally participated in a morning program that emphasized a developmentally appropriate preschool program based on a cognitive training model. Within this model, Sally received problem-solving and thinking skills instruction that was applied to all areas of development, including

social/emotional and language development. Teachers encouraged Sally to use verbal expressive language to get her needs met and to interact successfully with her peers. The teacher to child ratio was 1 to 5. Sally was one of seven special needs children in a classroom with eight additional normally developing children. Another peer in the class was recruited and trained to engage Sally in social interaction during structured and free play. Health and nutrition needs were also met by the morning program. The second part of Sally's day was spent at a communication-based language enrichment program, which was consistent with her morning program and provided in-depth concentration on expressive language. Each program lasted approximately 3 hours and both were provided daily, five days a week.

Treatment Course and Problems in Carrying Out Interventions

Within the first week of entering the treatment program, Sally's eye contact with adults and peers improved. She did not interact with peers and did not verbalize with peers or adults. During the first month she had frequent absences. She began interacting nonverbally with peers toward the end of the first month of treatment. At this time she also began using words to request additional food from adults at lunch. Her receptive language was functional.

Around the beginning of her second month of treatment, Sally had poor hygiene and was absent frequently. After the parent was consulted on this matter, hygiene and attendance improved. For several weeks she was nonverbal, then again used words to ask for food. In addition, she began to verbalize to peers but the verbalizations were softly spoken and often unintelligible. She continued to play along side of peers. Toward the end of the second month, she made an intelligible initiation to a peer, saying "Mine" when a peer took a toy with which she was playing.

Toward the beginning of the third month of treatment, Sally started participating in structured group activities, answering in one-word answers those questions that were asked of her. She initiated a few interactions during peer play and said "Leave me alone" when she didn't want to interact. Her hygiene was improved.

In the fourth month of treatment, Sally had marked improvements in interaction and in expressive language. She played imaginative games with peers such as "going to McDonalds in a car" and was using three-word sentences when asking for food and toys and when interacting with peers.

In the fifth month of treatment, Sally began using more words, especially ones that more precisely conveyed a meaning. She used more and more labels, moving from identifying objects by function to identifying them by proper label. Her commands to others were expanded. She began to ask "WH" questions. She was interacting with peers in an age-appropriate manner. In the sixth month, Sally was discharged to a regular preschool program.

During the course of treatment several problems that impeded treatment appeared. Family discord arose during the course of treatment. This was reflected in Sally by a three-week return to a more withdrawn state in the second month of treatment.

Erratic transportation of the child between the two half-day programs occurred during the first month of treatment. This problem was solved with a meeting of both treatment programs in which the child's schedule was altered slightly.

The child's hygiene was also a problem. She frequently came to the partial program disheveled, unwashed, and, on occasion, smelly. This created social acceptance difficulties for Sally. The problem was addressed by meeting with the child's parents to reinforce the need for frequent baths and clean clothes.

The child was also subject to frequent illnesses, which meant that her attendance was inconsistent. Once the child was enrolled in the pediatric clinic and received regular visits, her health became better.

Hygiene, illness, and family discord issues were exacerbated by the income level of the family. With an income well below the poverty level, the family often had too few resources to meet the needs of the child and family.

Outcome and Termination

Marked improvement in language development was seen by the end of treatment in the partial program. More specifically, there was an increase in spontaneous use of communication of both social and preacademic contexts and an increase in mean length of utterance. Although significant improvement was noted, language development is not yet at age expectancy, particularly in the area of expressive vocabulary. Sally will need continued support if she is to continue the same rate of gains.

Marked improvement in social interaction with peers was also noted. By the end of treatment, she could participate in cooperative play activities and could engage in age-appropriate interpersonal problem solving. She readily made eye contact with peers and adults and showed appropriate affect during peer interactions. Because of her improvement in this domain, regular high-quality preschool was recommended with continued support in the language area. In planning for termination, the team felt it was important that her gains could best be sustained by continuity in her preschool programming. Therefore, the team recommended that she continue in her half-day language stimulation program and attend a regular preschool program for the remainder of the day.

In scheduling termination, a meeting of the treatment agents at the treatment program, the language stimulation program, and parents was held. Intervention techniques/methods were discussed and goals were set for the next phase. A step-by-step plan for transition from the partial to the preschool were laid out. They included short visits to the preschool, communication with the receiving teacher, and emotional support for Sally while she was meeting her new friends.

Followup and Maintenance

We feel that Sally's progress will be maintained and enhanced by her continued participation in preschool and in the language stimulation program. As the initial agency of treatment, we will follow up on the progress at 1-, 3-, and 6-month periods, communicating with parents and receiving agencies. We will assist with summer placement if necessary.

SUMMARY

In summary, a brief description of the specific developmental disorders delineated in DSM-III-R was presented. We have indicated that many of the disorders are associated with each other, as well as with various social/emotional and behavioral problems. Prevalence data indicate that approximately 5 percent of young children have specific developmental disorders, although estimates vary from a low of 1 percent to a high of 20 percent. Both intrinsic and extrinsic causes of specific developmental disorders were reviewed.

Diagnostic and treatment procedures were also covered. A case study was presented to illustrate specific developmental disorders with young children. This report was drawn from a psychiatric setting; case studies drawn from educational settings might look quite different.

This review is limited in scope for several reasons. This is an extraordinarily broad topic that is compounded by the fact that several different disciplines study, assess, and treat such disorders. The lack of operational definitions of these disorders makes comprehensive coverage difficult. Lack of agreement between disciplines affects reporting of prevalence data, etiology, and diagnosis. What is clear from this review is that these disorders affect large numbers of children. It is also evident that despite decades of intervention research with children and adolescents with these disorders, consensual agreement as to what works does not exist at this time.

REFERENCES

Aman, M. G., & Singh, N. N. (1988). Vitamin, mineral, and dietary treatments. In M. G. Aman & N. N. Singh (Eds.), *Psychopharmacology of the developmental disabilities* (pp. 168–196). New York: Springer-Verlag.

American Psychiatric Association. (1987). *Diagnostic and statistical manual of mental disorders* (3rd ed., rev.). Washington, DC: Author.

Arnold, L. E. (1990). Learning disorders. In B. D

Garfinkel, G. A. Carlson, & E. B. Weller (Eds.), *Psychiatric disorders in children and adolescents* (pp. 237–256). Philadelphia: Saunders.

Badian, N. A. (1983). Dyscalculia and nonverbal disorders of learning. In H. R. Myklebust (Ed.), *Progress in learning disabilities* (Vol. 5, pp. 235–264). New York: Grune & Stratton.

Baker, L. (1990). Specific communication disorders. In B. D. Garfinkel, G. A. Carlson, & E. B. Weller (Eds.), *Psychiatric disorders in children and adolescents* (pp. 257–270). Philadelphia: Saunders.

Baker, L., & Cantwell, D. P. (1989). Specific language and learning disorders. In T. H. Ollendick & M. Hersen (Eds.), *Handbook of child psychopathology* (2nd ed.). New York: Plenum.

Barsch, R. H. (1967). *Achieving perceptual-motor efficiency.* Seattle: Special Child Publications.

Bliss, L. S. (1985). A symptom approach to the intervention of childhood language disorders. *Journal of Communication Disorders, 18,* 91–108.

Brenner, A. (1982). The effects of megadoses of selected B complex vitamins on children with hyperkinesis: Controlled studies with long term follow-up. *Journal of Learning Disabilities, 15,* 258–264.

Brown, A. L., & Campione, J. C. (1986). Cognitive science and learning disabilities. *American Psychologist, 41,* 1059–1068.

Burns, M. S., & Casbergue, R. M. (1991). *Families and classrooms together: Early literacy collaboration.* New Orleans: Tulane University.

Campione, J. C. (1989). Assisted assessment: A taxonomy of approaches and an outline of strengths and weaknesses. *Journal of Learning Disabilities, 22,* 151–165.

Campione, J. C., & Brown, A. L. (1987). Linking dynamic assessment with school achievement. In C. S. Lidz (Ed.), *Dynamic assessment: An interactional approach to evaluating learning potential* (pp. 82–111). New York: Guilford.

Chase, C., & Tallal, P. (1987). Piracetam and dyslexia. In D. Bakker, C. Wilsher, H. Debruyne, & N. Bertin (Eds.), *Developmental dyslexia and learning disorders* (pp. 140–147). Basel: Karger.

Christenson, S., Ysseldyke, J., & Algozzine, B. (1982). Institutional constraints and external pressures influencing referral decisions. *Psychology in the Schools, 19,* 341–34.

Connors, C. K. (1987). Event related potentials and quantitative EEG brain-mapping in dyslexia. In D. Bakker, C. Wilsher, H. Debruyne, & N. Bertin (Eds.), *Developmental dyslexia and learning disorders* (pp. 9–21). Basel: Karger.

Decker, S. N., & Defries, J. C. (1981). Cognitive ability profiles in families of reading disabled children. *Developmental Medicine and Child Neurology, 23,* 217–227.

Decker, S. N., & Vanderberg, S. (1985). Colorado twin study of reading disability. In D. B. Gray & J. F. Kavanaugh (Eds.), *Behavioral measures of dyslexia* (pp. 123–136). Parton, MD: York Press.

Defries, J. C. (1985). Colorado reading project. In D. B. Gray & J. F. Kavanaugh (Eds.), *Behavioral measures of dyslexia* (pp. 107–122). Parton, MD: York Press.

Defries, J. C., & Baker, L. A. (1983). Colorado Family Reading Study: Longitudinal analysis. *Annals of Dyslexia, 33,* 153–162.

Defries, J. C., Fulker, D. W., & La Buda, M. C. (1987). Evidence for a genetic etiology in reading disability of twins. *Nature, 329,* 537–539.

DiLanni, M., Wilsher, C. R., Blank, M. S., Conners, C. K., Chase, C. H., Funkenstein, H. H. Helgott, E., Homes, J. M., Lougea, L., Maletta, G. J., Milewski, J., Pirozzolo, F. J., Rudel, H. G., & Tallal, P. (1985). Effects of piracetam in children with dyslexia. *Journal of Clinical Psychopharmacology, 49,* 307–309.

Drake, W. E. (1968). Clinical and pathological findings in a child with a developmental learning disability. *Journal of Learning Disabilities, 1,* 486–502.

Feingold, B. F. (1975). Hyperkinesis and learning disabilities linked to artificial food flavors and colors. *American Journal of Nursing, 75,* 797–803.

Feuerstein, RT. (1980). *Instrumental enrichment.* Baltimore: University Park Press.

Fleischner, J. E., & Garnett, K. (1987). Arithmetic difficulties. In K. A. Kavale, S. R. Forness, & M. Bender (Eds.), *Handbook of learning disabilities, Vol. 1: Dimensions and diagnosis* (pp. 189–209). Boston: Little, Brown.

Frostig, M., & Horne, D. (1964). *The Frostig program for the development of visual perception: Teacher's guide.* Chicago: Follett.

Gadow, K. D. (1991). Psychopharmacological assessment and intervention. In H. L. Swanson (Ed.), *Handbook on the assessment of learning disabilities: Theory, research, and practice* (pp. 351–372). Austin, TX: Pro-Ed.

Gadow, K. D., & Swanson, H. L. (1986). Assessing drug effects on academic performance. In K. D. Gadow & A. Poling (Eds.), *Advances in learning and behavioral disabilities, Supplement 1: Methodological issues in human psychopharmacology* (pp. 247–279). Greenwich, CT: JAI Press.

Galaburda, A. M. (1989). Ordinary and extraordinary brain development: Anatomical variation in developmental dyslexia. *Annals of Dyslexia, 39,* 67–80.

Galaburda, A. M., & Kemper, T. C. (1979). Cytoarchitectonic abnormalities in developmental dyslexia: A case study. *Annals of Neurology, 6,* 94–100.

Gamlin, P. J. (1989). Issues in dynamic assessment/instruction. *International Journal of Dynamic Assessment and Instruction, 1,* 13–25.

Giurgea, C. (1978). Pharmacology of nootropic drugs. In B. Deniker, C. Radouco-Thomas, A. Villaneuva, D. Baronet-LaCroix, & F. Gersin (Eds.), *Neuropsychopharmacology* (pp. 67–72). New York: Pergamon.

Gubbay, S. S. (1975). *The clumsy child: A study of developmental apraxia and agnostic ataxia.* Philadelphia: Saunders.

Gubbay, S. S., Ellis, E., Walton, J. N., & Court, S. D. (1965). Clumsy children: A study of apraxic and agnostic defects in 21 children. *Brain, 88,* 295–312.

Hallahan, D. P., & Cruickshank, W. W. (1973). *Psychoeducational foundations of learning disabilities.* Englewood Cliffs, NJ: Prentice Hall.

Hallahan, D. P., Kauffman, J. M., & Lloyd, J. W. (1985). *Introduction to learning disabilities* (2nd ed.). Englewood Cliffs, NJ: Prentice Hall.

Hammill, D. D. (1990). On defining learning disabilities: An emerging consensus. *Journal of Learning Disabilities, 23,* 74–84.

Haywood, H. C., Brooks, P. B., & Burns, M. S. (1991). *Cognitive curriculum for young children.* Watertown, MA: Charlesbridge Press.

Helgott, E., Rudel, R. G., Koplewicz, H., & Krieger, J. (1987). In D. Bakker, C. Wilsher, H. Debruyne, & N. Bertin (Eds.), *Developmental dyslexia and learning disorders* (pp. 110–122). Basel: Karger.

Hughes, J. R. (1985). Evaluation of electrophysiological studies on dyslexia. In D. B. Gray & J. Kavenaugh (Eds.), *Behavioral measures of dyslexia* (pp. 71–86). Parton, MD: York Press.

Hull, F., Mielke, P., Timmons, R., & Willeford, J. (1976). *National Speech and Hearing Survey* (OE Project 50978. Bureau of Education for the Handicapped, Office of Education, HEW). Fort Collins: Colorado State University.

Hynd, G. W., Obrzut, J. E., Hayes, F., & Becker, M. G. (1986). Neuropsychology of childhood learning disabilities. In D. Wedding, A. M. Horton, & J. Webster (Eds.), *The neuropsychology handbook: Behavioral and clinical perspectives* (pp. 456–485). New York: Springer-verlag.

Hynd, G. W., & Semrud-Clikeman, M. (1989). Dyslexia

and brain morphology. *Psychological Bulletin, 106,* 447–482.

Kavale, K. A. (1990). Variances and verities in learning disabilities interventions. In T. E. Scruggs & B. Y. L. Wong (Eds.), *Intervention research in learning disabilities* (pp. 3–33). New York: Springer-Verlag.

Kavale, K. A., & Forness, S. R. (1985). *The science of learning disabilities.* San Diego: College-Hill Press.

Kavale, K. A., & Forness, S. R. (1987). The far side of heterogeneity: Analysis of empirical subtyping in learning disabilities. *Journal of Learning Disabilities, 20,* 374–382.

Keogh, B. K. (1990). Learning disabilities. In M. C. Wang, M. C. Reynolds, & H. J. Walberg (Eds.), *Special education: Research and practice: Synthesis of findings* (pp. 119–142). Oxford: Pergamon.

Kephart, N. C. (1960). *The slow learner in the classroom.* Columbus, OH: Merrill.

Kephart, N. C. (1971). *The slow learner in the classroom* (2nd ed.). Columbus, OH: Merrill.

Kirk, S. A., & Kirk, W. (1971). *Psycholinguistic learning disabilities: Diagnosis and remediation.* Urbana: University of Illinois Press.

Koorland, M. A. (1986). Applied behavior analysis and the correction of learning disabilities. In J. K. Torgessen & B. Y. L. Wong (Eds.), *Psychological and educational perspectives on learning disabilities* (pp. 297–328). Orlando, FL: Academic Press.

Lidz, C. S. (1991). *Practitioner's guide to dynamic assessment.* New York: Guilford.

Lindsley, O. R. (1964). Direct measurement and prosthesis of retarded behavior. *Journal of Education, 147,* 62–81.

Lloyd, J. W. (1984). How should we individualize instruction – Or should we? *Remedial and Special Education, 5,* 7–16.

Mayron, L. W. (1979). Allergy, learning, and behavior problems. *Journal of Learning Disabilities, 12,* 41–49.

Myers, P., & Hammill, D. (1982). *Learning disabilities: Basic concepts, assessment practices, and instructional strategies.* Austin, TX: Pro-Ed.

National Advisory Committee on Hyperkineses and Food Additives. (1980). *Final report to the Nutrition Foundation.* New York: Nutrition Foundation.

Pelham, W. E. (1986). The effects of psychostimulant drugs on learning and academic achievement in children with attention-deficit disorders and learning disabilities. In J. K. Torgensen & B. Y. L. Wong (Eds.), *Psychological and educational perspectives on learning disabilities* (pp. 259–295). Orlando, FL: Academic Press.

Pennington, B. F., Gilger, J. W., Pauls, D., Smith, S. A., Smith, S. D., & Defries, J. C. (1991). Evidence for major gene transmission of developmental dyslexia. *Journal of the American Medical Association, 266,* 1527–1534.

Pennington, B. F., & Smith, S. D. (1983). Genetic influences on learning disabilities and speech and language disorders. *Child Development, 54,* 369–387.

Raiten, D. J. (1990). The medical basis for nutrition and behavior. In B. D. Garfinkel, G. A. Carlson, & E. B. Weller (Eds.), *Psychiatric disorders in children and adolescents* (pp. 410–427). Philadelphia: Saunders.

Ripens, J., Van Yperen, T. A., & Van Duijn, G. A. (1991). The irrelevance of IQ to the definition of learning disabilities: Some empirical evidence. *Journal of Learning Disabilities, 24,* 434–438.

Rutter, M., & Yule, W. (1973). Specific reading retardation. In L. Mann & D. Sabatino (Eds.), *The first review of special education.* Philadelphia: J. S. E. Press.

Salvia, J., & Ysseldyke, J. E. (1981). *Assessment in special and remedial education* (2nd ed.). Boston: Houghton Mifflin.

Schroeder, C. S., Schroeder, S. R., & Davine, M. A. (1978). Learning disabilities: Assessment and management of reading problems. In B. B. Wolman, J. Egan, & A. O. Ross (Eds.), *Treatment of mental disorders in childhood and adolescence.* Englewood Cliffs, NJ: Prentice Hall.

Shepard, L. A. (1983). The role of measurement in educational policy: Lessons from the identification of learning disabilities. *Educational Measurement: Issues and Practice, 2,* 4–8.

Siegel, L. S. (1989). IQ is irrelevant to the definition of learning disabilities. *Journal of Learning Disabilities, 22,* 469–478.

Silver, A. A., & Hagin, R. A. (1990). *Disorders of learning in childhood.* New York: Wiley & Sons.

Smith, S. D., & Pennington, B. F. (1987). Genetic influences. In K. A. Kavale, S. R. Forness, & M. Bender (Eds.), *Handbook of learning disabilities: Dimensions and diagnosis* (Vol. 1, pp. 49–76). College Hill Press.

Stark, R. E. (1987). Receptive and expressive language disorders. In M. I. Gottlieb & J. E. Williams (Eds.), *Textbook of developmental pediatrics.* New York: Plenum.

Stephens, T. M. (1977). *Teaching skills to children with learning and behavior disorders.* Columbus, OH: Merrill.

Taylor, H. G. (1987). The meaning and value of soft signs in the behavioral sciences. In D. E. Tupper (Ed.), *Soft neurological signs* (pp. 297–335). Orlando, FL: Grune & Stratton.

Tylenda, B., Hooper, S. R., & Barrett, R. P. (1989). Developmental learning disorders. In C. L. Frame & J. L. Matson (Eds.), *Handbook of assessment in childhood psychopathology: Applied issues in differential diagnosis and treatment evaluation.* New York: Plenum.

U.S. Department of Education. (1987). *Ninth Annual Report to Congress: 1987.* Washington, DC: U.S. Government Printing Office.

Volger, G., Defries, J. C., & Decker, N. (1984). Family history as an indicator of risk for reading disability. *Journal of Learning Disabilities, 17,* 616–619.

Weiss, B. (1982). Food additives and environmental chemicals as sources of childhood behavior disorders. *Journal of the American Academy of Child Psychiatry, 21,* 144–152.

Weiss, B. (1986). Food additives as a source of behavioral disturbances in children. *Neurotoxicology, 7,* 197–208.

Wilig, E. H. (1982). Communication disorders. In N. G. Haring (Ed.), *Exceptional children and youth* (pp. 81–108). Columbus, OH: Merrill.

Wilsher, C. R. (1987). Treatment of specific reading disabilities (dyslexia). In D. Bakker, C. Wilsher, H. Debruyne, & N. Bertin (Eds.), *Developmental dyslexia and learning disorders* (pp. 99–109). Basel: Karger.

CHAPTER 5

ATTENTION-DEFICIT HYPERACTIVITY DISORDER

Betsy Hoza   Western Psychiatric Institute and Clinic
William E. Pelham, Jr.   Western Psychiatric Institute and Clinic

DESCRIPTION OF DISORDER

Over the past several decades, a myriad of names have been assigned to the childhood syndrome that is currently labeled attention-deficit hyperactivity disorder (ADHD). These names have included minimal brain damage, minimal brain dysfunction, hyperkinetic reaction of childhood, hyperkinetic-impulse disorder, hyperactivity, and attention deficit disorder (with and without hyperactivity). The changes in terminology roughly parallel changes in beliefs regarding the core deficit of the disorder. An excellent historical review outlining the evolution of beliefs regarding the disorder may be found in Barkley (1990). The clinical features of the disorder have remained the same and are outlined below.

Clinical Features

The core symptoms of ADHD are inattention, impulsivity, and hyperactivity. Typical manifesta-tions of the inattention dimension of ADHD include problems with completing tasks or persisting at a play activity, difficulty concentrating on tasks requiring sustained attention (e.g., seatwork, homework), distractibility, and not attending to instructions. The impulsive features of ADHD include disruptive acts that represent acting without thinking, such as blurting out in class, barging into an ongoing game, problems with taking turns, and difficulty regulating behavior without external controls. Finally, the hyperactivity dimension involves excessive movement, including fidgeting, being out-of-seat at school, and excessive running and climbing (American Psychiatric Association, 1980, 1987).

Typically, the symptoms are evident by the time the child enters school, although a formal diagnosis may not be made until later in childhood. According to DSM-III-R (American Psychiatric Association, 1987), the symptoms must be present by age 7 and be of at least 6 months' duration. The degree of symptoms present must be excessive given the child's mental age, although considerable variability in symptomatology may be seen across settings, with complete absence of symptoms reported in some settings—most typically when the children are engaged in an activity in which they are very interested or when they are in a one-to-one setting. For this reason, "doctor's office diagnosis" is not possible. Instead, information regarding a child's behavior in the natural environment across multiple settings must be gathered from multiple informants (see Assessment below).

Associated Features

Whereas the clinical features of ADHD represent the defining features of the disorder, the associated features, to a large extent, represent the functional problems experienced by ADHD children. The most common associated features of ADHD are academic failure or underachievement, social maladaptation, and conduct problems.

Academic problems are common in ADHD children (Campbell & Werry, 1986; Lambert & Sandoval, 1980; Shaywitz & Shaywitz, 1988). About half of ADHD children may be considered underachievers, and over 40 percent have IQ/achievement discrepancies indicative of a possible learning disorder (Lambert & Sandoval, 1980). Further, recent studies (Mattison et al., 1986; Mattison, Humphrey, Kales, & Wallace, 1986) have shown that many children who are placed in classrooms for children with behavior disorders have ADHD. Finally, the academic problems of ADHD children are often not limited to the school setting. Clinicians who work with parents of ADHD children are often called on to help parents address problems related to homework completion and homework responsibility (i.e., keeping track of assignments, returning homework to school).

The social maladaptation problems of ADHD children are often pervasive, extending across settings (e.g., school versus home) and social groups (family, peers, school staff). With regard to peer relationships, peer informants report that ADHD children are socially rejected by peers, are aggressive toward peers, and engage in a high rate of annoying, disruptive behaviors (e.g., bother-ing others, bossing) (Carlson, Lahey, Frame, Walker, & Hynd, 1987; Pelham & Bender, 1982). In short, ADHD children exhibit a variety of disruptive behaviors in group or game settings that make them difficult playmates. In adult-child interactions, ADHD children show different, but equally serious, difficulties. These most often include defiant and noncompliant behaviors that create considerable family stress such as talking back, refusing to do what is asked, arguing, and temper outbursts. These oppositional behaviors often lead parents of ADHD children to implement negative and controlling parenting strategies (see Barkley, 1990; Campbell & Werry, 1986; and Mash & Johnston, 1990, for summaries of parent-child interactions associated with ADHD) and result in a very high comorbidity between ADHD and oppositional defiant disorder (Pelham, Gnagy, Greenslade, & Milich, 1992).

Conduct problems represent the more serious social transgressions associated with ADHD. Conduct problems, as defined in the DSM-III-R category of conduct disorder, include behaviors such as stealing, lying, physical fighting, fire setting, truancy, and destruction of property (American Psychiatric Association, 1987). These behaviors are observed at such a high rate in ADHD children that a number of recent papers have focused on the relationship between ADHD and the other disruptive behavior disorders (see review by Hinshaw, 1987).

Epidemiology

ADHD is the most commonly diagnosed childhood behavior disorder. Nonetheless, prevalence estimates vary widely, with most falling in the 3 to 5 percent range (see, e.g., Pelham et al., 1992). Shaywitz and Shaywitz (1988) recently argued, however, that this figure is a gross underestimate of the actual prevalence of ADHD in the general population, reflecting instead only children diagnosed by a professional. Boys are more commonly diagnosed than girls, with a mean ratio of 6 to 1 noted for clinic samples (Barkley, 1990). Recently, it has been argued that boys are more often referred than girls because ADHD boys exhibit more "noticeable" behaviors (e.g., aggression) as compared with girls (Barkley, 1990; Shaywitz & Shaywitz, 1988). While this may account for some of the difference in referral rates, it is unlikely to account entirely for the well-documented difference in prevalence rates for boys versus girls (see Barkley, 1990, for a discussion of this point).

Etiology

The cause of ADHD is not known, although the general consensus is that it is of biological origin. The current leading speculation is that ADHD is due to underfunctioning in parts of the brain controlling attention and impulsivity. No direct evidence for this viewpoint exists, largely due to the obvious difficulties in measuring directly brain function in children. A recent study by Zametkin and colleagues (1990), however, found reduced cerebral glucose metabolism, both globally and in specific areas of the brain involved in attention, in ADHD adults engaged in a task requiring attention.

The fact that ADHD tends to run in families suggests that there may be a genetic predisposition for ADHD (Biederman, Faraone, Keenan, Knee, & Tsuang, 1990). Indeed, there is a high occurrence of ADHD in offspring of parents with problems such as alcoholism (Pihl, Peterson, & Finn, 1990) that are thought to be, in part, biologically based. To date, however, adequate research (e.g., twin and adoption studies) to address directly possible genetic factors in ADHD has not been conducted. Nonetheless, a wide variety of biologic factors have been studied in the quest to better understand ADHD. These have included, for example, diet, neurochemical mechanisms, prenatal and perinatal events, and maternal alcohol consumption. An exhaustive review of these factors may be found in Shaywitz and Shaywitz (1988). Unfortunately, research has not identified a single etiologic factor implicated in the development of ADHD. They have, however, served to clarify what does *not* cause ADHD. As Barkley has recently noted, "Little if any evidence supports the notion that ADHD can arise purely out of social or environmental factors, such as poverty, family chaos, diet, or poor parent man-

agement of children" (1990, pp. 104–105). In summary, then, there is no single identifiable cause for ADHD at the present time.

DIFFERENTIAL DIAGNOSIS AND ASSESSMENT

DSM-III-R Categorization

DSM-III-R (American Psychiatric Association, 1987) diagnostic criteria differ from those of DSM-III (American Psychiatric Association, 1980) in that the presence of any 8 of 14 symptoms listed in the DSM-III-R are considered diagnostic of ADHD, regardless of the number of core symptom areas represented. In contrast, in the DSM-III, criteria had to be met in each of three core symptom areas (inattention, impulsivity, and hyperactivity) in order to receive a diagnosis of attention deficit disorder with hyperactivity. In addition, in the current DSM-III-R nomenclature, children who are primarily inattentive but show few symptoms of hyperactivity are classified as ADHD if at least 8 symptoms of ADHD are present. If fewer than 8 symptoms are present, they are classified as undifferentiated attention deficit disorder. In DSM-III such cases were placed in the category attention deficit disorder without hyperactivity if hyperactivity was never present, or attention deficit disorder, residual type, if hyperactivity was previously present.

As others have noted (e.g., Shaywitz & Shaywitz, 1988), the changes that occurred from DSM-III to DSM-III-R were decided primarily on the basis of agreement among experts, as opposed to being based on empirical studies. In the formulation of criteria for DSM-IV, there appears to be a thrust for changes to be based on empirical studies rather than consensus among experts (Shaffer et al., 1989). Given that recent factor-analytic studies (Lahey et al., 1988; Pelham et al., 1992) have demonstrated clearly that attention deficit symptoms are best described bidimensionally, with symptom clusters representing (1) inattention and (2) impulsivity/hyperactivity emerging, recently investigators have recommended that DSM-IV require symptoms in both of these areas for a diagnosis of ADHD (Pelham et al., 1992). In addition, attention deficits that are manifested primarily as inattention, without accompanying hyperactivity, may be diagnosed separately in DSM-IV as attention deficit disorder without hyperactivity (American Psychiatric Association, 1991; Shaffer et al., 1989).

Differential Diagnosis

There is a large degree of overlap between ADHD, oppositional defiant disorder (ODD), and conduct disorder (CD) (Hinshaw, 1987; Pelham et al., 1992). Indeed, in a normative sample of children recently studied by Pelham and associates (1992) using teacher rating scales, 85 percent of the children who met criteria for CD also met criteria for ADHD, and 53 percent of those who met criteria for ODD also met criteria for ADHD. The children who met criteria for a concurrent diagnosis of oppositional or conduct disorder constituted 46 percent of children who were identified as having ADHD. Further, in a study by Milich, Widiger, and Landau (1987), it was found that some of the classic symptoms of ADHD (e.g., "doesn't listen") operated better as exclusionary criteria for conduct disorder than as inclusionary criteria for ADHD, when positive and negative predictive power of individual symptoms were considered.

Guidelines in the DSM-III-R indicate that a CD diagnosis should be made when both ODD and CD criteria are met (American Psychiatric Association, 1987), but no such guidelines exist for overlap between ADHD and ODD or ADHD and CD. Thus, diagnoses of both ADHD and ODD *or* CD should be made when both apply. Although this lack of clarity over primary diagnosis may seem problematic from a diagnostic standpoint, it does not present difficulties from a treatment perspective. As noted below, it is the child's functional deficits that should be targeted in intervention, and these are not diagnosis specific. On the other hand, the nature and type of a child's concurrent problems may be prognostically important. Recent studies have indicated that children with concurrent conduct problems (e.g., aggression) appear to have worse outcomes (Hinshaw, 1987).

Assessment Strategies

Evaluation for ADHD should involve multiple informants from multiple settings, as ADHD symptomatology is not evident in all settings and situations, even for clinically diagnosed children. Symptoms are often absent in the doctor's office situation, rendering invalid the notion of doctor's office diagnosis. An excellent description of the situational variability of the disorder may be found in the DSM-III (American Psychiatric Association, 1980):

> Because the symptoms are typically variable, they may not be observed directly by the clinician. . . . Symptoms typically worsen in situations that require self-application, as in the classroom. Signs of the disorder may be absent when the child is in a new or a one-to-one situation. (p. 43)

Further, there is no single attention task that is diagnostic of ADHD, despite the marketing of technical devices for pediatricians and child psychiatrists to assess attention (Milich, Pelham, & Hinshaw, 1986; Pelham & Milich, 1991). In our own work, we have found useful an approach that utilizes standardized parent and teacher rating scales, in combination with a structured diagnostic clinical interview with the child's primary caretaker. Emphasis is placed on teacher ratings, given teachers' greater knowledge of age-appropriate behavior. Teacher ratings should never be the only criterion for diagnosis, however, given that they may be subject to negative halo effects (Abikoff, Courtney, Koplewicz, & Pelham, 1991).

The battery of rating scales that we currently employ includes the parent and teacher version of (1) the Disruptive Behavior Disorders Rating Scale (Pelham et al., 1992); (2) the SNAP Rating Scale (Atkins, Pelham, & Licht, 1985); (3) the Child Behavior Checklist (CBCL; Achenbach & Edelbrock, 1983, 1986); (4) the Conners Abbreviated Symptom Questionnaire (Goyette, Conners, & Ulrich, 1978); and (5) the Iowa Conners Teacher Rating Scale (Loney & Milich, 1982; Pelham, Milich, Murphy, & Murphy, 1989). Normative data are available for the teacher versions of all of these rating scales, and for the parent version of the CBCL and the Conners Abbreviated Symptom Questionnaire. Additional rating scales useful in the assessment of ADHD are available and are described in Atkins and Pelham (1991) and Barkley (1990).

It is important to bear in mind, however, that an assessment that includes the preceding procedures may be sufficient for the diagnosis of ADHD children but it is not sufficient for the identification of treatment targets. These traditional assessment tools provide information regarding the core symptoms of the disorder, but these core symptoms are not necessarily the focus of treatment. Instead, treatment focuses on identifying the problems in daily life functioning with which the child presents and then developing interventions to modify them (Atkins & Pelham, 1991; Pelham & Hinshaw, 1992). This can be accomplished by using a variety of techniques, including interviews and direct observations to define target behaviors, analyzing their antecedents and consequences, and obtaining baseline data. In addition, where social problems are a primary concern, peer measures such as positive and negative nomination procedures, peer rating scales, and/or peer reputation measures are useful in providing important information about the extent and types of peer problems (see Atkins & Pelham, 1991; Bukowski & Hoza, 1989; and Pelham & Bender, 1982; for discussions of peer measures).

TREATMENT

Given that the associated features of ADHD represent the problems of daily dysfunction that ADHD children experience, it is typically these associated features, rather than the core symptoms, that are targeted in treatment. As noted earlier, the areas of dysfunction most reported are social maladjustment, academic problems, and conduct problems. As there is tremendous variability from child to child in symptoms exhibited, it is important to take an individualized approach in determining treatment. One good rule of thumb is to make certain that the intervention brings about maximal improvement in the child's most

problematic areas of functioning. This point will be discussed in greater detail below.

Evidence for Prescriptive Treatment

The standard prescriptive treatments for ADHD are behavior modification, pharmacotherapy with stimulants such as methylphenidate (MPH), and the combination of behavior modification and stimulants. Alternative treatments such as cognitive therapy have also been employed, although with much less success. Each of these treatments will be discussed in greater detail here. Finally, it should be noted that more traditional forms of therapy, such as child-focused play therapy, are not effective in the treatment of ADHD and therefore will not be considered.

Behavior Therapy

Behavior management approaches to treating ADHD differ primarily in terms of who is outlining the contingencies and providing the consequences for the child. For a large number of ADHD children who attend regular schools with or without special services (e.g., "resource room" tutoring, learning disorder classroom), clinical behavior therapy is employed. This approach involves having the primary adults (parents, teachers) in the child's life implement an intervention with the assistance of a behavior therapist, who teaches the parents and teachers behavior management skills and thereby serves in a consultant role. For school problems (academic or social), it can be either the teacher or the child's parents who outline the contingencies and provide consequences for the child. In either case, however, the teacher's cooperation in monitoring the child's behavior is necessary. For home problems, it is typically the child's parents who implement the intervention.

In more restrictive settings, such as clinical treatment facilities and special education classrooms, direct contingency management is possible. This involves implementation of the behavioral procedures directly by a trained behavior therapist. Whereas the latter setup is advantageous in that closer monitoring by a trained behavior therapist occurs, often allowing for more intensive interventions, it is not always feasible or cost effective. In addition, training parents and teachers to serve as behavior change agents may increase the likelihood that cross-setting implementation of behavior management procedures will occur and that treatment effects will be maintained after termination. Regardless of who implements the intervention, however, the intervention strategies are essentially the same.

Manipulation of social consequences. With less severe problem behaviors, basic manipulation of positive and negative social consequences contingent on the child's behavior may be sufficient. This involves the adult giving praise for positive behaviors, ignoring minor inappropriate behaviors, and providing reprimands for negative behaviors. These basic behavior management techniques, and studies examining their effectiveness, are described elsewhere (Carlson & Lahey, 1988; Patterson, Reid, Jones, & Conger, 1975; Pfiffner & O'Leary, in press). However, administered alone, these procedures are rarely sufficient for ADHD children (Pelham & Murphy, 1986). Powerful back-up consequences in the form of tangible rewards and privileges that can be awarded or costed contingent on behavior and used in combination with other intensive procedures such as time out, are often necessary (Pelham, Carlson et al., in press; Hoza, Pelham, Sams, & Carlson, 1992). Thus, it is these more powerful interventions that we will describe below.

Manipulation of privileges and tangible consequences. Point or token systems are a common means of manipulating privileges and tangible consequences with ADHD children. Implementation of these systems involve identifying relevant positive and negative target behaviors and consequating these behaviors with the assignment or removal of points or tokens that can be traded later for privileges or tangible rewards. The privileges or rewards that the child will earn or lose must be powerful motivators in order for the intervention to be effective, and thus a "menu" approach for rewards is often desirable (Pfiffner &

Barkley, 1990). To date, a large number of studies have been conducted that document the effectiveness of point/token systems with ADHD children (see reviews by Carlson & Lahey, 1988; Pfiffner & O'Leary, in press). Both systems that reward good behavior with privileges and those that consequate poor behavior with loss of privileges have been shown to be effective. As Pfiffner and O'Leary (in press) have noted, recent empirical studies demonstrate that less deterioration of behavior occurs with the withdrawal of negative consequences (e.g., during fading of response cost procedures) than during withdrawal of rewards. Thus, response cost procedures may be considered an important component of treatment for ADHD children.

For school-based problem behaviors, a daily report card (O'Leary, Pelham, Rosenbaum, & Price, 1976) is a simple, easy-to-administer alternative to point or token systems. This approach involves having the child's teacher provide ratings or feedback to the child and his or her parents on a number of preestablished target behaviors. Parents then provide home-based rewards for school performance on the target behaviors. Rewards may be provided on a daily or a weekly basis, depending on the child's age and level of dysfunction.

Selection of target behaviors. As noted earlier, it is the child's problems in daily functioning, rather than the core symptoms of ADHD, that should be targeted in interventions for ADHD children. At the present time, however, there is disagreement in the literature as to whether problems in classroom behavior should be targeted directly in the form of consequences for inappropriate behavior or indirectly through consequences for poor academic performance. Whereas current literature documents that academic performance targets are sometimes accompanied by behavioral improvement in the classroom, the reverse may not be true (see Carlson & Lahey, 1988).

Thus, it appears that targeting academic performance directly is necessary to bring about notable change in academic targets. For ADHD children who also exhibit disruptive behavior, however, targeting academic performance will not be sufficient and classroom behavioral targets will need to be used as well (Hoza et al., 1992). Most studies of classroom behavioral interventions for ADHD employ concurrent consequences for both academic and behavioral targets. In two recent investigations, we employed the prototypic strategy of using rewards for academic targets (earning points for completing work accurately), and response-cost for behavioral targets (losing points for violations of classroom rules) (Carlson, Pelham, Milich, & Dixon, 1992; Pelham, Carlson et al., in press).

With regard to social behavior problems, behavioral targets should be set both to eliminate excessive or annoying behavior (e.g., teasing, interrupting) and to promote prosocial behavior (e.g., giving compliments, initiating a conversation). By balancing out negative with positive targets, the child is taught what to do, as well as what not to do (e.g., Fleischman, Horne, & Arthur, 1983). In addition, given recent empirical evidence that aggressive behavior is both stable over time and predictive of long-term negative outcomes (Huesmann, Eron, Lefkowitz, & Walder, 1984), aggression should always be targeted for intervention when it is present. In addressing ADHD children's peer problems, however, it is important to set reasonable goals. It is probably unrealistic to also try to make a severely rejected child actually *popular* with peers. A more reasonable goal might be to reduce aggression (e.g., through the use of time out) and to help the child learn to make one or two close friendships (see Furman & Robbins, 1985, and Hoza, 1989, for discussions of friendship).

In light of the negative peer reputation of many ADHD children (Pelham & Bender, 1982), and the fact that negative peer reputation tends to be stable over time (Coie & Dodge, 1983), benefit may be gained by involving the peer group in an intervention targeting peer problems. This may be done by targeting the behavior of the group in an attempt to treat an individual child. For example, in treating a socially withdrawn child who was ignored by peers, the first author recommended a group reward for the class each day that all children in the class were included in a game at recess.

Alternatively, group interventions may target the behavior of an individual child toward the group. A second child, who had a severe problem with teasing others, was treated by the first author in this manner in the context of a summer treatment program. Specifically, all children in a peer group were instructed to report instances of teasing from a particular child to adult counselors, who kept a tally. When the child successfully stayed within a predesignated number of teasings permitted for two consecutive days, the whole group was rewarded with ice cream. This intervention appeared to decrease dramatically the number of teasings performed by the target child while improving peer status. These successful applications of group contingencies to peer problems are consistent with results reported for group contingencies in the control of academic and disruptive classroom behaviors (see Hayes, 1976).

Determining the "dosage" of behavior therapy. One issue that is often neglected in the development of behavioral treatments for ADHD is that of determining the appropriate "dosage" of behavior therapy to employ. Some behavior modifiers recommend always starting with a minimal intervention and moving to more powerful ones only after the minimal one has proven insufficient. Recent work by O'Leary and colleagues (Futtersak, O'Leary, & Abramowitz, 1989, cited in Pfiffner & O'Leary, in press) addressing the effectiveness of differing intensity levels of reprimands with ADHD children indicates that use of immediate and continued strong reprimands is more effective than use of reprimands of increasing intensity. Unfortunately, however, in most studies of the effectiveness of behavior therapy, and typically in clinical practice, only one level of treatment is employed, with conclusions regarding the effectiveness of behavior therapy being based on that single trial.

As Hoza and associates (1992) have pointed out, however, there are problems with this approach. First, studies of the effectiveness of behavior therapy report vastly different results, depending on the potency of the intervention employed. For example, studies employing less potent procedures such as a daily report card

(O'Leary et al., 1976) lead to less promising outcomes than those using powerful response-cost procedures (Rapport, Murphy, & Bailey, 1982). When these two types of procedures are compared directly (Atkins, Pelham, & White, 1989), they differ vastly in their effectiveness. Indeed, one study employing a single-subject design (Hoza et al., 1992) compared multiple levels of behavior therapy and found a potent contingency involving loss of a highly desired activity to be much more effective than a standard response-cost procedure. Thus, level of potency of the behavioral intervention should be considered in developing a behavioral intervention.

For severely disturbed ADHD boys (e.g., those with concurrent ODD or CD), standard outpatient clinical behavior therapy may be insufficient, regardless of the potency of the consequences. In such cases direct contingency management may be necessary. For the past decade we have dealt with such children by enrolling them in an intensive treatment program that is conducted every summer. The program is described in some detail in the case study that follows. The program has proven to be a very effective short-term intervention for ADHD (Pelham, 1991).

Pharmacotherapy

CNS stimulants including methylphenidate (MPH, e.g., Ritalin), dextroamphetamine (e.g., Dexedrine), and pemoline (e.g., Cylert) are the most commonly prescribed medications for ADHD. MPH has been the most widely studied. MPH has been shown to improve classroom on-task behavior and academic performance, decrease classroom disruptive behavior, improve compliance with adult requests/commands, decrease the number of controlling commands adults direct to the child, and improve peer relationships (reviews by Gittelman & Kanner, 1986; Pelham, 1986; Whalen & Henker, 1991). The effects of dextroamphetamine and pemoline have been less widely studied, although studies that have directly compared these drugs to MPH have shown similar effects (e.g., Pelham et al., 1990). Although antidepressant medications have been used to treat hyperactivity, particularly for children who do not respond adequately to CNS stimulants (Bieder-

man, Baldessarini, Wright, Knee, & Harmatz, 1989), they are less effective than psychostimulants and have a higher side-effect profile (Rapoport, Quinn, Bradbard, Riddle, & Brooks, 1974). Given that antidepressant medications have been less widely used for ADHD, and are not well-studied in comparison with MPH, they are best tried after all three stimulants have failed to produce therapeutic effects. Thus, our discussion below will focus on the CNS stimulants.

Unlike behavior therapy, which only a minority of ADHD children receive, pharmacotherapy is administered to most ADHD children (80 to 90 percent) at some point in childhood (Bosco & Robin, 1980). Often it is administered as the sole treatment for ADHD, despite recommendations by both drug manufacturers (*Physician's Desk Reference,* 1991) and ADHD experts (DuPaul & Barkley, 1990; Pelham & Milich, 1991) that it be part of an integrated treatment package including psychosocial treatments. In addition, the decision to prescribe and/or maintain a child on CNS stimulants is often made in a subjective, unsystematic way (Copeland, Wolraich, Lindgren, Milich, & Woolson, 1987). Unfortunately, such unsystematic practices can result in erroneous decisions regarding whether or not to medicate a child. Our position is that a double-blind, placebo-controlled, clinical medication assessment should always be conducted before a decision is made to medicate a child with psychostimulants.

Furthermore, as Pelham and Milich (1991) have noted, a medication assessment should only be conducted if behavior therapy has been tried and has proven insufficient. When this occurs, the medication assessment should be conducted concurrently with an ongoing behavioral intervention. Such a medication assessment is essentially a single-subject study, whereby the effects of manipulating medication dosage is studied by using multiple dependent variable measures, including ratings by adults (e.g., teachers, parents, counselors) who are kept blind to the medication dosage information. When conducting such an assessment, it is important to evaluate whether improvement is seen in the child's *most problematic* behaviors (Pelham & Milich, 1991), since the best dose for one problem behavior may not be the best dose for another (Shaywitz & Shaywitz, 1988). Step-by-step descriptions of how to conduct such an assessment in a summer treatment program (Pelham & Hoza, 1987) and in a standard outpatient setting (Pelham & Milich, 1991), including recommendations regarding dosage and selection of target behaviors to be used in the assessment, are available elsewhere.

Concurrent behavior therapy and pharmacotherapy. In recent years, it has been argued that concurrent treatment with medication and behavior therapy is preferable to the singular use of either treatment (Pelham, 1989; Pelham & Murphy, 1986). This position has derived from empirical studies demonstrating that children treated with either intervention alone tend to continue to be more deviant than normal children, and show positive effects of treatment only during active treatment time (i.e., while medication is active, while the behavior program is being implemented). Furthermore, neither treatment is effective for all children (about one-third of treated children fail to respond to each type of treatment) and neither has been demonstrated to produce long-term effects. Thus, for cases for which behavior therapy proves insufficient, our recommendation is to take a "double-barrelled approach," since for many ADHD children concurrent behavior therapy and MPH produce maximal improvement (see Pelham & Murphy, 1986).

Alternative Treatments

A common alternative treatment for ADHD is cognitive training. As noted by Abikoff, "The central goal of [cognitive training] is the development of self-control skills and reflective problem-solving strategies, both of which are presumed to be deficient in children with ADHD" (1991, p. 205). Cognitive training for children includes methods such as those popularized by Meichenbaum (e.g., see Meichenbaum, 1977), which were thought to hold considerable promise as a treatment for ADHD. A review of studies conducted over the past 10 years, however, indicates that cognitive training treatments for ADHD, either alone or in combination with psychostimulant medication, have produced disappointing results (Abikoff,

1991). Although cognitive therapy procedures may deserve further investigation as a procedure to be employed *after* a lengthy, intensive, and successful *behavioral* intervention, they cannot be considered a leading intervention for ADHD at the present time.

Selecting Optimal Treatment Strategies

Given the heterogeneity among ADHD children, treatment planning must proceed on a case-by-case basis. However, we have found the following steps to be useful.

First, do a functional analysis of the child's problems by using multiple sources of information collected across multiple settings. Then prioritize the child's problem behaviors, selecting the two or three most debilitating functional problems for intervention. Take a baseline measure of the target behaviors, using measures appropriate to the behaviors selected (e.g., percentage of classroom assignments completed, frequency counts of aggression). Implement a standard behavioral program such as a daily report card or point system and monitor progress.

If sufficient progress is seen, continue the intervention and adjust as needed over time. If sufficient progress is not seen, consider a treatment change. If the child's parents and/or teachers are willing to participate in fairly complex behavioral programming, with assistance from a trained behavior therapist, this program change may reflect an increase in the potency of the behavioral intervention. If increased complexity is impractical or unfeasible, consider a double-blind, placebo-controlled medication assessment to evaluate combined effects of medication and standard behavior therapy. (See Pelham & Milich, 1991, for detailed instructions on how to conduct an outpatient medication assessment.) Only in rare circumstances do we recommend a medication trial in the absence of a behavioral intervention. Such a rare circumstance might be a situation in which a school is unwilling to participate in a behavioral intervention and parents are unable to successfully carry out a home-based intervention (e.g., due to severe maternal depression that must be addressed as a separate treatment issue).

Problems in Carrying Out Interventions

A number of problems can interfere with the effectiveness of the treatments described above. The primary problems to be discussed include noncompliance with treatment (or inconsistent implementation of treatment), parent or family pathology that limits treatment effectiveness, lack of cooperation from key persons (e.g., school personnel), child objections due to embarrassment regarding the intervention, problems of timing, and nonresponsiveness to treatment.

Noncompliance with Treatment (or Inconsistent Treatment Implementation)

Failure of adults (e.g., teachers, parents) to implement treatment for an ADHD child consistently, or in entirety, is a serious threat to the effectiveness of any intervention, and this problem has been noted repeatedly in the intervention literature (e.g., Atkins et al., 1989). Noncompliance with treatment can take the form of not administering medication as prescribed and/or failure to carry out behavioral programs and/or assignments. It has been our observation that optimal compliance is achieved when the persons implementing the program are provided with structure (e.g., written instructions) and ready-made materials (e.g., data sheets). Frequent contact with a trained therapist to troubleshoot is also helpful in increasing compliance, as noncompliance often occurs as a result of frustration or a belief that the treatment is not working. Booster sessions and followup phone calls for a period of time following initial treatment success and/or termination have also been employed (e.g., Fleischman et al., 1983).

Parent and/or Family Pathology

Sometimes parent and/or family pathology can interfere with treatment. For example, parental depression, substance abuse, and/or marital dif-

ficulties between the parents can influence family environment and affect implementation of treatment (Anastopoulos & Barkley, 1990; Mash & Johnston, 1990). If it is the clinician's judgment that these problems are sufficiently severe to prevent successful treatment of the child, the parents should be referred for appropriate treatment for themselves prior to (or concurrent with) treatment for their child.

One parent problem that we have only recently begun to study systematically is residual ADHD that interferes with the parents' ability to implement treatment for their child. In a recent case study (Evans, Vallano, & Pelham, in press), it was found that treating a mother's ADHD symptoms with pharmacotherapy significantly enhanced her ability to manage her son's behavior. The reader who is interested in learning more about treating ADHD in adults is referred to a recent chapter by Kane, Mikalac, Benjamin, and Barkley (1990).

Achieving Cooperation from School Personnel

Sometimes school personnel are reluctant to cooperate with outside consultants, or exert minimal or inconsistent effort such that treatment is eventually sabotaged. Although we have no absolute solution to these problems, we have found that maximal success is achieved when the behavior therapist's (consultant's) commitment to working with school personnel on an ongoing basis is evident through regular contacts. It is worth noting that all *studies* of behavior therapy efficacy in school settings involve multiple teacher-therapist contacts—at least weekly over an 8- to 16-week period (e.g., Gittelman et al., 1980; O'Leary & Pelham, 1978; Pelham et al., 1988; Pelham, Schnedler, Bologna, & Contreras, 1980). In *clinical practice,* therapists may try to get away with only a few visits. Lack of teacher follow-through may result from this approach, especially if teachers are left to resolve on their own treatment problems that arise—a task for which most teachers have little training. If frequent school visits are made, however, and teacher cooperation still is not obtained, parents may wish to have a meeting with the principal, with the therapist present, to request change.

In addition to regular school visits, it is important that behavior therapists use social reinforcement to reward teacher effort. This is especially important in the beginning stages in order to get the teacher to comply with treatment. As time goes on, improvement seen by the teacher in the target child should help to sustain teacher effort. Parents may wish also to provide material rewards (e.g., a dinner gift certificate for a cooperative teacher).

Often, however, difficulties associated with implementing an intervention in the school setting are compounded by the fact that a child has multiple teachers who may differ in their levels of interest in, or cooperation with, the intervention. Under these circumstances, we have found it helpful to have a meeting at the child's school of all the child's teachers prior to implementation of an intervention. This allows the teachers the opportunity to (1) meet the therapist, (2) hear a brief rationale for the procedures to be implemented, (3) ask questions, (4) give input for the establishment of target behaviors, (5) voice concerns about managing the program, and (6) decide not to participate. These goals can often be accomplished in a 30 to 45-minute session with up to 10 persons present. With regard to the final point pertaining to teacher participation, in a recent case treated by the first author, a small subset of the child's teachers elected not to participate in the daily report card program that was implemented for him. Because those teachers who did participate were enthusiastic about the intervention, the intervention was successful nonetheless. In cases such as this one, excluding teachers who prefer not to be involved can sometimes allow a program to run more smoothly.

Child Embarrassment Regarding the Intervention

With education of school personnel about the sensitivity of children to public knowledge about their intervention, and with careful planning that emphasizes confidentiality, situations that cause ADHD children to feel embarrassed about their treatment can often be avoided. In some instances, however, despite the best attempts, children will be made to feel uncomfortable (e.g., having an announcement made over the loudspeaker that it is time for the child to take her pill). In these situations, teaching the child some coping strategies and emphasizing that the treatment will be helpful can ease the child's discomfort. It would also be appropriate in such a situation for the behavior therapist to request a followup meeting with school personnel to discuss how the treatment is going and to address the problem at that time.

It is worth noting that elementary school classrooms are typically quite diverse in makeup, and many children will have special programs of some type. A skillful teacher can deal with individual differences in class discussions when necessitated by departures from standard classroom routines for the targeted ADHD child, or for any other child with special needs.

Problems of Timing

Before concluding that a treatment is not working for a given child, the clinician should consider problems related to timing. As Pelham and Milich (1991) have noted, in conducting an evaluation of medication effectiveness, it is important to make certain that the child's active medication time corresponds to those times of the day when the child has the most difficulty. For example, if a child from an LD placement is mainstreamed each day for social studies at 11:00 A.M., and experiences his or her most difficulty at this time, a standard breakfast dose of short-acting Ritalin at 7:00 A.M. is likely to have little impact, as the dose is largely worn off by this time. Similarly, there may be little likelihood that an overwhelmed, single mother with few resources will implement a complex behavioral program throughout the entire day (Wahler, 1980). Focusing the intervention at least initially on one specific problematic time of day (e.g., bedtime), rather than the entire day, may make the program manageable and effective.

Nonresponsiveness to Treatment

Nonresponsiveness to a well-implemented treatment is the most difficult challenge facing the clinician. When this occurs, a change in treatment type or potency is indicated. Often, following the steps listed earlier (see Selecting Optimal Treatment Strategies) can prevent problems with nonresponsiveness to treatment. In some instances, however, and despite the best planning, a child does not respond. At these times, a systematic approach of altering one component of treatment at a time is best. Sometimes, however, the severity of the situation requires drastic alterations in treatment. The case illustration in this chapter depicts how one might approach such a difficult case.

Relapse Prevention

Because ADHD is now widely conceptualized as a lifelong disorder, *relapse prevention* with regard to ADHD refers primarily to maintenance of treatment gains rather than relapse following cure. Rather than implementing short-term treatments, professionals working with ADHD children should begin to develop an approach to treatment not unlike that advocated for other chronic disorders, such as alcohol abuse (Marlatt & Gordon, 1985). That is, the focus needs to be not only on effective short-term interventions but also on how acute gains can be maintained over time. Unfortunately, there are no systematic, long-term followup studies comparing relapse in children treated with behavior therapy, medication, and concurrent behavior therapy and medication. Our recommendations pertaining to maintenance of short-term gains or prevention of relapse, therefore, must be considered speculative.

First, it is our best guess that treatment gains are best maintained when cross-setting consistency in treatment implementation is achieved (e.g., when behavioral programs are implemented both at home and at school). Further, consistent with popular parent training approaches (e.g., Fleischman et al., 1983; Patterson et al., 1975), it seems reasonable to assume that children treated with behavior therapy programs that teach appropriate behavioral responses, either alone or in combination with medication, will do better in the long run than those whose treatments suppress negative behaviors without teaching appropriate alternative behaviors.

Second, strategies that provide followup treatment and support beyond termination of initial therapy are likely to be more effective than those that do not. As noted earlier, these strategies may include followup parent training on an "as needed" basis, getting parents involved in parent-run support groups and equipping parents to monitor and modify school interventions (i.e., a daily report card) after termination of therapy by involving them in the therapist's meetings with the teacher. Further, it is likely that family variables such as presence versus absence of parental psychopathology, and parental compliance with treatment recommendations, will interact with child variables in determining child outcome.

Given the predictive value of peer relationships for later outcome (Cowen, Pederson, Babigian, Izzo, & Trost, 1973), it may be that peer relationships will prove to be a critical determinant, if not a mediator, of outcome for ADHD children. Thus, intervention followup for children with peer problems should always include recommendations that will continue to provide the child with opportunities for constructive interaction with peers. This may take the form of "booster" social skills training and/or structured community activities involving peers (e.g., Boy Scouts, sports teams). These recommendations should involve strategies for ensuring the child's success. These strategies might involve a behavior report system similar to the school daily report card that provides structure and home-based rewards for good behavior during these activities, and if necessary, a third dose of MPH to assist the child in behaving appropriately.

Finally, the behavior therapist and parents should always bear in mind the importance of having realistic goals for the ADHD child's peer relations and should bear these goals in mind in determining followup recommendations. For example, expecting peer group popularity is unrealistic for many ADHD children, and employing strategies to promote popularity (e.g., large birthday parties) may lead to failure. Instead, keeping goals realistic by focusing on promoting individual friendships with a few children (e.g., by trips to the movies, baseball game, etc.) are more likely to be successful and to promote self-esteem. These speculations await investigation.

We provide a case illustration of how to approach treating an ADHD child. This particular case was selected for presentation because of the many problems we encountered during the course of treatment. As such, it is not meant to be a textbook illustration of the "perfect approach" to treatment. On the contrary, it is meant to encourage clinicians who deal with extremely challenging children to continue to persist in modifying treatment until an effective approach is found.

CASE ILLUSTRATION

Case Description

Ted was a 10-year-old, white male with a history of continuing problems both at home and school. Ted's parents reported that these problems were evident by age 3 or 4, at which time Ted was expelled from daycare for being very destructive and for aggression toward other children. These problems escalated further when Ted entered kindergarten at age 5. In the first grade, Ted was formally diagnosed as having an attention deficit disorder, and Ritalin (5 mg, b.i.d.) was recommended. Ted's mother reported that, after 9 months on Ritalin, the effectiveness of the medication was unclear, due to problems with medication administration at school. At age 8, due to continuing and persistent problems, a trial of imipramine (20 mg/day) was implemented, which, according to Ted's mother, led to severe mood swings and increasingly destructive behavior. As a result of this deterioration in Ted's status, he was hospitalized for 32 days and later taken off imipramine. During this period, he was additionally diagnosed with conduct disorder. Approximately three weeks prior to our first contact with Ted at age 9, he had been put back on Ritalin at a dose of 15 mg b.i.d. Additional treatments that had been tried for Ted in the past included individual counseling, parent counseling, and behavioral parent management training.

At the time of Ted's initial contact with our program, Ted's mother reported problems with impulsivity, temper outbursts, swearing, aggression, defiance, difficulty completing assigned tasks, and inattention. Ted received treatment through our 1989 Children's Summer Day Treatment Program (STP) and our 1989–90 Saturday Treatment Program. Despite these interventions, severe difficulties remained. Therefore Ted was admitted to the 1990 STP for further intervention. At the time of the intake update for the 1990 STP, Ted's mother reported that he was currently "extremely hyperactive, argumentative, and noncompliant." She also reported that Ted's oppositional behavior was a severe problem, especially with regard to active defiance of adult commands. Ted's teacher reported that he exhibited extremely disruptive behavior in the classroom, was vindictive, and had used a weapon (a screwdriver) when fighting. Ted was suspended from school for a total of nine days during the previous school year for fighting.

During his first summer with the STP, Ted had received a clinical medication assessment and methylphenidate (MPH) was determined to be an essential component of treatment. Ted's teacher considered him to be completely unmanageable when off medication, as indicated in the following written description sent to our clinic:

> He was totally out of control. He didn't care what he said or did. He swore, put a plastic bag over his head, cut his jacket with scissors, ripped his behavior report, threw notebook and pencils in the hall, threatened to jump down a whole flight of steps, and refused to listen to the principal. After being put on his van [home], he wrote obscene words on the windows. . . . The day described . . . was half a day.

He was already in a full-time SED (socially and emotionally disturbed) placement and his school was recommending an even more restrictive placement for him.

Differential Diagnosis and Assessment

Ted met criteria for DSM-III-R diagnoses of attention deficit hyperactivity disorder, oppositional defiant disorder, and conduct disorder based on a structured parent interview, and parent and teacher rating scales. Since a diagnosis of conduct disorder supersedes a diagnosis of oppositional defiant disorder when criteria for both are met, Ted was assigned only ADHD and CD as diagnoses on Axis I. On Axis II, Ted was assigned diagnoses of developmental reading disorder and developmental expressive writing disorder, because of IQ/achievement discrepancies in excess of 15 standard score points in these areas. Rating scale scores and subject characteristics are summarized in Table 5–1.

Treatment Selection

The STP is an 8-week, intensive treatment program that resembles a summer camp to the treated child but is a licensed partial hospitalization program. The treatments implemented include a powerful token economy/point system, a time-out program, social skills and problem-solving training, and parent training.

A typical child's day in the STP lasts from 8:00 A.M. until 5:00 P.M. and is divided into the following activities: an academic classroom period and a computer-assisted classroom period, each staffed by a special education teacher and an aide; an art class; swimming; three outdoor recreational periods; and lunch. For most nonclassroom activities, one graduate student counselor and four undergraduate counselors supervised 12 children grouped by age. The point system, time out, and other behavioral treatments were implemented

throughout the day (see Pelham, 1990, for a comprehensive description of the program). The treatment thus focused on changing parenting skills, modifying children's behavior toward adults (e.g., reducing noncompliance), and developing appropriate socialization skills in a peer group setting. In addition, special behavioral programs were developed on an individual basis to meet the treatment needs of children who did not respond to the standard intervention of the point system and time out.

Medication

For the first two weeks of the program, children were not medicated so that observations of each child's response to behavior therapy in the absence of medication could be made. Medication assessments were conducted beginning in the third week for children whose behavior during the first two weeks of the program indicated the need for such an assessment, and for whom such an assessment was not medically contraindicated. Although Ted had a medication assessment in the previous STP and had been determined to be a responder to Ritalin, the severity of his behavior problems and his extreme oppositional behavior while on medication at school led to two primary concerns. The first had to do with whether another dosage or type of medication might be more appropriate for him (e.g., slow-release Ritalin). The second was a concern that he would eventually start refusing to take his medication, given his extreme oppositional behavior.

As such, it appeared critical to try to identify behavioral interventions that were effective for him in the absence of medication. Thus, a decision was made to repeat his placebo-controlled, double-blind, clinical medication assessment using slow-release Ritalin, and to include placebo days as well as a no-medication baseline of two weeks prior to the start of the medication assessment. During the no-medication and placebo days, the effectiveness of behavioral interventions could be tested. As noted below, however, Ted's medication assessment could not be completed and no data are thus reported due to extreme aggressive and self-destructive behavior when he was off medication, and due to the need to use an isolation

Table 5–1. Patient Characteristics

MEASURE	TED
Age in years	10.17
Abbreviated Conners Rating Scale	
Teacher	27
Parent	22
Iowa Conners Teacher Rating Scale	
Inattention/Overactivity	15
Aggression	11
DSM-III-R Structured Interview for Parents	
ADHD items endorsed	12
Oppositional Defiant items endorsed	9
Conduct items endorsed	3
Wechsler Intelligence Scale for Children-Revised—Full Scale IQ	113
Woodcock-Johnson Achievement Test	
Reading	89
Mathematics	111
Written language	92

Note: Rating scale scores reflect *un*medicated behavior.

room with him in which meaningful systematic data could not be collected. Thus, he was maintained on medication from the sixth week on.

Behavioral Interventions

We planned to begin treatment with the standard behavioral intervention package, including a point system, time out, a daily report card system, and parent management training, and to add additional individualized programs as needed (see below).

Treatment Course and Problems in Carrying Out Interventions

Weeks 1–2

During the first two weeks of the program, Ted was not medicated and standard behavior therapy including a point system, time out, and a daily report card (DRC) was applied (DRCs began in week 2). He spent almost the entire first day of the program in a single time out that was continuously escalated because he refused to serve it appropriately, and he was clearly "testing" the counselors. Subsequent to the first day, his compliance with the time-out procedure improved in that the daily average length of his time outs ranged from 10 to 45 minutes for the remainder of the two weeks. Despite his increased compliance with time out, however, Ted continued to exhibit high rates of negative behaviors such as verbal abuse to staff and interrupting.

Weeks 3–4

During week 3, with the beginning of medication administration, Ted's behavior improved. His behavior on his one placebo day during week 3, however, was consistent with his off-medication behavior during the two weeks prior to medication. During week 4, however, Ted's behavior began to deteriorate. On the first day of week 4, he served two time outs that were escalated to an average of 79 minutes in length. On his scheduled placebo day, he had to be medicated due to having assaulted three staff members and exhibiting self-destructive behavior. This included dragging

the classroom teacher out of the room by her hair while he was being removed from the classroom by another staff member to serve a time out. Ted's aggressive and self-destructive behavior appeared to be at least in part a response to the use of physical restraint by staff to enforce compliance with time out—a procedure that was necessary because of Ted's refusal to serve his time outs. Since time out with restraint was the most restrictive intervention typically used in our setting, and since it was clearly not working for Ted, a modification of his treatment was necessary before considering rehospitalization for him. Thus, with his parents' permission, a special program was designed for Ted to begin in week 5.

Week 5

On the second day of week 5, a level system was implemented for Ted that allotted different restrictions and/or privileges at each level. For example, at Level One, Ted was restricted to a single room for the entire day, except for one hour that was spent in the academic Learning Center classroom. At each successive level, additional privileges were earned. At the highest level, Level Four, Ted earned both special trips off-grounds and the right to select some of his daily activities. Ted's level placement was determined by the number and type of negative behaviors he exhibited the previous day (see Table 5–2). In order to move to the next level, Ted had to meet the criteria for the next level for an entire day (8:00 A.M. to 5:00 P.M.) before moving to that level. If Ted was at Level Two upon arrival, for example, he would have to meet the criteria for moving to Level Three for the entire day in order to move to Level Three the following day. If Ted violated the limits of his current level, however, he was immediately dropped to the level warranted by his behavior. Although Ted continued to be awarded points while on the level system, primarily so that it was not obvious to the other children that he was on a "special program," all of his privileges were determined by his level rather than his point total.

Ted was permitted to start at Level Three of the program on the first day that it was implemented, but a fully escalated time out (i.e., a time out he refused to serve appropriately) on the

Table 5–2. Ted's Special Program

LEVEL	RESULTS FROM	DAILY ROUTINE
1	Forty or more negative behaviors or a fully escalated time out that is not served appropriately (i.e., does not start immediately or has to be restarted)	No off-grounds privileges or field trips No recreational activities Academic classroom only Room restriction all day
2	Less than 40 negative behaviors and no time outs longer than 90 minutes	No off-grounds privileges or field trips On-site recreational activities only All classrooms Room restriction when group is off grounds
3	Less than 30 negative behaviors and no fully escalated time outs	Off-grounds privileges for recreation but no field trips All classrooms No room restriction
4	Less than 20 negative behaviors and no time outs longer than 10 minutes	Off-grounds privileges and field trips All classrooms No room restriction

Note: Criteria for the next level must be met for a full day before Ted can move to that level. Any time Ted violates limits of his current level, he drops immediately to the appropriate level and remains there until he meets criteria for movement to the next level (i.e., one full day of behavior that meets criteria for the next level).

first day resulted in his being dropped to Level One (room isolation) immediately. He worked his way up one level each day subsequent to that, so that by the end of week 5 he was at the highest level. It appeared initially, then, that the level system was working very well.

Week 6

Ted began week 6 at Level Four, the highest level, because he had earned Level Four privileges the previous week. Because the first day of week 6 was designated as a placebo day, the true effectiveness of the behavioral intervention could be tested. In the morning of the first day of week 6, however, Ted allegedly intentionally swallowed a pushpin from a bulletin board while being removed from the classroom for a time out. As a result, he was taken to the hospital for medical treatment. Once at the hospital, Ted told his father that he had not swallowed the pushpin but had only pretended that he had, and his parents elected to forego medical treatment. As a consequence for this behavior that had caused considerable distress to his parents and summer program staff, Ted was assigned to Level One privileges. Ted became extremely angry and verbally and physically abusive toward staff. He had to be restrained by a coun-

selor in the isolation room because he was damaging the walls and carpeting and physically assaulting the counselor who was assigned to sit with him in isolation. He refused to take any medication, even when it was determined necessary for him. His behavior was so extreme that it was decided to discontinue any further placebo days and a meeting was called with his parents to discuss possible expulsion from the program and the possible need for an inpatient hospitalization.

Because Ted's parents were extremely cooperative, however, and typically followed through on recommendations made by staff, it was decided to institute a home-level system that provided consequences at home for Ted's behavior at the program. This was possible due to the close relationship that Ted had with his mother. Indeed, his mother's attention was so reinforcing to him that it was an excellent motivator. She also reported fewer compliance problems with Ted than other adults. Thus, according to the home-level system, at Level One Ted was required to do "work chores" from the time that he arrived home after the summer program until bedtime, with no privileges of any kind. At the highest level, as a reward for a specified number of days at Level Four (the highest level) at the summer program, Ted could earn special weekend trips with his parents to his favorite places. Once this program was running concurrently with the STP level system, Ted's behavior began to improve dramatically. In fact, of the 13 remaining days of the summer program following implementation of the home-level system, Ted was at Level Four for all but 1 day. Thus, with concurrent home and STP-level systems in place, Ted's rate of prosocial behaviors increased, while his rate of negative behaviors and time outs decreased significantly. Finally, following implementation of both level systems and the elimination of nonmedication days from his medication schedule, the frequency and intensity of Ted's aggression decreased rather dramatically.

Outcome and Termination

Given the effectiveness of the level-system approach for Ted, a recommendation was made to Ted's parents upon termination of the summer program that he be placed in a partial hospitalization program that employs a level-system approach. They followed through with this recommendation and obtained such a placement for him for the following school year. He also continued to take Ritalin (20 mg slow-release Ritalin upon arrival at school combined with an early morning dose of 15 mg short-acting Ritalin prior to his bus ride to school).

Followup and Maintenance

Fourteen months after termination of the summer treatment program, Ted's mother reported that he continued to do well with the combination of a highly structured level system at school and psychostimulants. In fact, his early morning dose of Ritalin had been reduced from 15 mg to 10 mg. At home, she reported inconsistent use of a home back-up level system, depending on the degree of problems at home. She noted, however, that whenever the home-level system was in place, Ted did very well.

SUMMARY

ADHD is a common childhood behavior disorder characterized by inattention, impulsivity, and hyperactivity. These core symptoms, however, rarely occur alone. The most common associated features are peer problems, learning problems, and conduct problems. These associated features, or areas of dysfunction, are most typically what is targeted in intervention.

Both pharmacotherapy with a stimulant and behavior therapy are commonly employed treatments for ADHD. Behavior therapy should be tried first, with MPH added if behavior therapy proves insufficient. MPH should never be used alone in treating ADHD. Controlled double-blind, placebo-controlled medication assessments are recommended for determining appropriateness of a particular type and dosage of medication for ADHD. Similarly, multiple "doses" of behavior therapy should be tried in order to maximize treatment effects. In determining a final treatment regimen, practical considerations (e.g., ability of family or teacher to carry out the intervention) should always be taken into account. Finally, as the case study illustrates, despite the best planning and most controlled circumstances, treatment course does not always proceed as predicted. Thus, the challenge to the clinician is to respond flexibly to problems and alter treatment as needed.

REFERENCES

Abikoff, H. (1991). Cognitive training in ADHD children: Less to it than meets the eye. *Journal of Learning Disabilities, 24,* 205–209.

Abikoff, H., Courtney, M., Koplewicz, H. S., & Pelham, W. E. (1991, June). *The influence of halo effects on teachers' ratings of behavior problems.* Presented as a poster at the annual meeting of the Society for Research in Child and Adolescent Psychopathology, Zandvoort, Holland.

Achenbach, T. M., & Edelbrock, C. S. (1983). *Manual for the Child Behavior Checklist and Revised Child Behavior Profile.* Burlington: University of Vermont, Department of Psychiatry.

Achenbach, T. M., & Edelbrock, C. S. (1986). *Manual for the Teacher's Report Form and Teacher Version of the Child Behavior Profile.* Burlington: University of Vermont, Department of Psychiatry.

American Psychiatric Association. (1980). *Diagnostic and statistical manual of mental disorders* (3rd ed.). Washington, DC: Author.

American Psychiatric Association. (1987). *Diagnostic and statistical manual of mental disorders* (3rd ed., rev.). Washington, DC: Author.

American Psychiatric Association. (1991). *DSM-IV options book: Work in progress.* Washington, DC: Task force on DSM-IV.

Anastopoulos, A., & Barkley, R. A. (1990). Counseling and training parents. In R. A. Barkley (Ed.), *Attention deficit hyperactivity disorder: A handbook for diagnosis and treatment* (pp. 397–431). New York: Guilford.

Atkins, M. S., & Pelham, W. E. (1991). School-based assessment of attention deficit-hyperactivity disorder. *Journal of Learning Disabilities, 24,* 197–204.

Atkins, M. S., Pelham, W. E., & Licht, M. (1985). A comparison of objective classroom measures and teacher ratings of attention deficit disorder. *Journal of Abnormal Child Psychology, 13,* 155–167.

Atkins, M. S., Pelham, W. E., & White, K. J. (1989). Hyperactivity and attention deficit disorders. In M. Hersen (Ed.), *Psychological aspects of developmental and physical disabilities: A casebook* (pp. 137–156). Beverly Hills: Sage.

Barkley, R. A. (1990). *Attention deficit hyperactivity disorder: A handbook for diagnosis and treatment.* New York: Guilford.

Biederman, J., Baldessarini, R. J., Wright, V., Knee, D., & Harmatz, J. S. (1989). A double-blind placebo controlled study of desipramine in the treatment of ADD: I. Efficacy. *Journal of the American Academy of Child and Adolescent Psychiatry, 28,* 777–784.

Biederman, J., Faraone, S. V., Keenan, K., Knee, D., & Tsuang, M. T. (1990). Family-genetic and psychosocial risk factors in DSM-III attention deficit disorder. *Journal of the American Academy of Child and Adolescent Psychiatry, 29,* 526–533.

Bosco, J., & Robin, S. (1980). Hyperkinesis: Prevalence and treatment. In C. Whalen & B. Henker (Eds.), *Hyperactive children: The social ecology of identification and treatment.* New York: Academic Press.

Bukowski, W. M., & Hoza, B. (1989). Popularity and friendship: Issues in theory, measurement, and outcome. In T. J. Berndt & G. W. Ladd (Eds.), *Peer relationships in child development* (pp. 15–45). New York: Wiley.

Campbell, S. B., & Werry, J. S. (1986). Attention deficit disorder (hyperactivity). In H. Quay & J. Werry (Eds.), *Psychopathological disorders of childhood* (3rd ed., pp. 111–155). New York: Wiley.

Carlson, C. L., & Lahey, B. B. (1988). Conduct and attention deficit disorders. In J. C. Witt, S. M. Elliott, & F. M. Gresham (Eds.), *The handbook of behavior therapy in education* (pp. 653–677). New York: Plenum.

Carlson, C. L., Lahey, B. B., Frame, C. L., Walker, J., & Hynd, G. W. (1987). Sociometric status of clinic-referred children with attention deficit disorders with and without hyperactivity. *Journal of Abnormal Child Psychology, 15,* 537–547.

Carlson, C. L., Pelham, W. E., Milich, R., & Dixon, M. J. (1992). Single and combined effects of methylphenidate and behavior therapy on the classroom behavior, academic performance and self-evaluations of children with attention deficit-hyperactivity disorder. *Journal of Abnormal Child Psychology, 20,* 213–232.

Coie, J. D., & Dodge, K. A. (1983). Continuities and changes in children's social status: A five-year longitudinal study. *Merrill-Palmer Quarterly, 29,* 261–282.

Copeland, L., Wolraich, M., Lindgren, S., Milich, R., & Woolson, R. (1987). Pediatricians' reported practices in the assessment and treatment of attention deficit disorders. *Journal of Developmental and Behavioral Pediatrics, 8,* 191–197.

Cowen, E. L., Pederson, A., Babigian, H., Izzo, L. D., & Trost, M. A. (1973). Long-term follow-up of early detected vulnerable children. *Journal of Consulting and Clinical Psychology, 41,* 438–446.

DuPaul, G. J., & Barkley, R. A. (1990). Medication therapy. In R. A. Barkley (Ed.), *Attention deficit hyperactivity disorder: A handbook for diagnosis and treatment* (pp. 573–612). New York: Guilford.

Evans, S. W., Vallano, G., & Pelham, W. E. (in press). Attention deficit hyperactivity disorder. In V. B. Van Hasselt & M. Hersen (Eds.), *Handbook of adolescent psychopathology: A guide to diagnosis and treatment.*

Fleischman, M. J., Horne, A. M., & Arthur, J. L. (1983). *Troubled families: A treatment program.* Champaign, IL: Research Press.

Furman, W., & Robbins, P. (1985). What's the point? Issues in the selection of treatment objectives. In B. H. Schneider, K. H. Rubin, & J. E. Ledingham (Eds.), *Children's peer relations: Issues in assessment and intervention* (pp. 41–54). Springer-Verlag.

Gittelman, R., Abikoff, H., Pollack, E., Klein, D. F., Katz, S., & Mattes, J. (1980). A controlled trial of behavior modification and methylphenidate in hyperactive children. In C. K. Whalen & B. Henker (Eds.),

Hyperactive children: The social ecology of identification and treatment (pp. 221–243). New York: Academic Press.

Gittelman, R., & Kanner, A. (1986). Psychopharmacotherapy. In H. Quay & J. Werry (Eds.), *Psychopathological disorders of childhood* (3rd ed., pp. 455–495). New York: Wiley and Sons.

Goyette, C. H., Conners, C. K., & Ulrich, R. F. (1978). Normative data on revised Conners parent and teacher rating scales. *Journal of Abnormal Child Psychology, 6,* 221–236.

Hayes, L. A. (1976). The use of group contingencies for behavioral control: A review. *Psychological Bulletin, 83,* 628–648.

Hinshaw, S. P. (1987). On the distinction between attentional deficits/hyperactivity and conduct problems/aggression in child psychopathology. *Psychological Bulletin, 101,* 443–463.

Hoza, B. (1989). *Development and validation of a method for classifying children's social status based on two types of measures: Popularity and chumship.* Unpublished doctoral dissertation, University of Maine.

Hoza, B., Pelham, W. E., Sams, S. E., & Carlson, C. L. (1992). An examination of the "dosage" effects of both behavior therapy and methylphenidate on the classroom performance of two ADHD children. *Behavior Modification, 16,* 164–192.

Huesmann, L. R., Eron, L. D., Lefkowitz, M. M., & Walder, L. O. (1984). Stability of aggression over time and generations. *Developmental Psychology, 20,* 1120–1134.

Kane, R., Mikalac, C., Benjamin, S., & Barkley, R. A. (1990). Assessment and treatment of adults with ADHD. In R. A. Barkley (Ed.), *Attention deficit hyperactivity disorder: A handbook for diagnosis and treatment* (pp. 613–654). New York: Guilford.

Lahey, B. B., Pelham, W. E., Schaughency, E. A., Atkins, M. S., Murphy, H. A., Hynd, G., Russo, M., Hartdagen, S., & Lorys-Vernon, A. (1988). Dimensions and types of attention deficit disorder. *Journal of the American Academy of Child and Adolescent Psychiatry, 27,* 330–335.

Lambert, N. M., & Sandoval, J. (1980). The prevalence of learning disabilities in a sample of children considered hyperactive. *Journal of Abnormal Child Psychology, 8,* 33–50.

Loney, J., & Milich, R. (1982). Hyperactivity, inattention, and aggression in clinical practice. In M. Wolraich & D. K. Routh (Eds.), *Advances in developmental and behavioral pediatrics* (Vol. 3, pp. 113–147). Greenwich, CT: JAI Press.

Marlatt, G. A., & Gordon, J. R. (1985). *Relapse prevention: Maintenance strategies in the treatment of addictive behaviors.* New York: Guilford.

Mash, E. J., & Johnston, C. (1990). Determinants of parenting stress: Illustrations from families of hyperactive children and families of physically abused children. *Journal of Clinical Child Psychology, 19,* 313–328.

Mattison, R. E., Humphrey, F. J., Kales, S. N., Handford, H. A., Finkenbinder, R. L., & Hernit, R. C. (1986). Psychiatric background and diagnoses of children evaluated for special class placement. *Journal of the American Academy of Child Psychiatry, 25,* 514–520.

Mattison, R. E., Humphrey, F. J., Kales, S. N., & Wallace, D. J. (1986). An objective evaluation of special class placement of elementary schoolboys with behavior problems. *Journal of Abnormal Child Psychology, 14,* 251–262.

Meichenbaum, D. H. (1977). *Cognitive-behavior modification: An integrative approach.* New York: Plenum.

Milich, R., Pelham, W. E., & Hinshaw, S. P. (1986). Issues in the diagnosis of attention deficit disorder: A cautionary note on the Gordon Diagnostic System. *Psychopharmacology Bulletin, 22,* 1101–1104.

Milich, R., Widiger, T. A., & Landau, S. (1987). Differential diagnosis of attention deficit and conduct disorders using conditional probabilities. *Journal of Consulting and Clinical Psychology, 55,* 762–767.

O'Leary, K. D., Pelham, W. E., Rosenbaum, A., & Price, G. (1976). Behavioral treatment of hyperkinetic children: An experimental evaluation of its usefulness. *Clinical Pediatrics, 15,* 510–515.

O'Leary, S. G., & Pelham, W. E. (1978). Behavior therapy and withdrawal of stimulant medication with hyperactive children. *Pediatrics, 61,* 211–217.

Patterson, G. R., Reid, J. B., Jones, R. R., & Conger, R. E. (1975). *A social learning approach to family intervention: Vol. 1. Families with aggressive children.* Eugene, OR: Castalia.

Pelham, W. E. (1986). What we know about stimulant drug effects. *Journal of Children in Contemporary Society, 19,* 99–110.

Pelham, W. E. (1989). Behavior therapy, behavioral assessment, and psychostimulant medication in treatment of attention deficit disorders: An interactive approach. In J. Swanson & L. Bloomingdale (Eds.), *Attention deficit disorders IV: Current concepts and emerging trends in attentional and behavioral disorders of childhood* (pp. 169–195). London: Pergamon.

Pelham, W. E. (1990). *Children's summer day treatment program 1990 program manual.* Unpublished manuscript, University of Pittsburgh School of Medicine, Western Psychiatric Institute and Clinic, Pittsburgh.

Pelham, W. E. (1991, November). Intensive summer day treatment for ADHD: Behavioral and pharmacological treatments. Paper presented in W. E. Pelham (Chair), *Behavioral interventions for attention deficit hyperactivity disorder: New directions for a chronic disorder.* Symposium presented at the annual meeting of the Association for the Advancement of Behavior Therapy, New York.

Pelham, W. E., & Bender, M. E. (1982). Peer relationships in hyperactive children: Description and treatment. In K. Gadow & I. Bialer (Eds.), *Advances in learning and behavioral disabilities* (Vol. 1, pp. 365–436). Greenwich, CT: JAI Press.

Pelham, W. E., Carlson, C., Sams, S. E., Vallano, G., Dixon, M. J., & Hoza, B. (in press). Separate and combined effects of methylphenidate and behavior modification on the classroom behavior and academic performance of ADHD boys: Group effects and individual differences. *Journal of Consulting and Clinical Psychology.*

Pelham, W. E., Gnagy, E. M., Greenslade, K. E., & Milich, R. (1992). Teacher ratings of DSM-III-R symptoms for the disruptive behavior disorders. *Journal of the American Academy of Child and Adolescent Psychiatry, 31,* 210–218.

Pelham, W. E., Greenslade, K. E., Vodde-Hamilton, M. A., Murphy, D. A., Greenstein, J. J., Gnagy, E. M., Guthrie, K. J., Hoover, M. D., & Dahl, R. E. (1990). Relative efficacy of long-acting stimulants on children with attention deficit-hyperactivity disorder: A comparison of standard methylphenidate, sustained-release methylphenidate, sustained-release dextroamphetamine, and pemoline. *Pediatrics, 86,* 226–237.

Pelham, W. E., & Hinshaw, S. (1992). Behavioral intervention for attention deficit-hyperactivity disorder. In S. M. Turner, K. Calhoun, & H. E. Adams (Eds.), *Handbook of Clinical Behavior Therapy* (2nd ed., pp. 259–283). New York: Wiley & Sons.

Pelham, W. E., & Hoza, J. (1987). Behavioral assessment of psychostimulant effects on ADD children in a Summer Day Treatment Program. In R. Prinz (Ed.), *Advances in behavioral assessment of children and families* (Vol. 3, pp. 3–34). Greenwich, CT: JAI Press.

Pelham, W. E., & Milich, R. (1991). Individual differences in response to ritalin in classwork and social behavior. In L. Greenhill & B. P. Osman (Eds.), *Ritalin: Theory and patient management* (pp. 203–221). New York: MaryAnn Liebert, Inc.

Pelham, W. E., Milich, R., Murphy, D. A., & Murphy, H. A. (1989). Normative data on the IOWA Conners teacher rating scale. *Journal of Clinical Child Psychology, 18,* 259–262.

Pelham, W. E., & Murphy, H. A. (1986). Attention deficit and conduct disorders. In M. Hersen (Ed.), *Pharmacological and behavioral treatment: An integrative approach* (pp. 108–148). New York: Wiley and Sons.

Pelham, W. E., Schnedler, R. W., Bender, M. E., Miller, J., Nilsson, D., Budrow, M., Ronnei, M., Paluchowski, C., & Marks, D. (1988). The combination of behavior therapy and methylphenidate in the treatment of hyperactivity: A therapy outcome study. In L. Bloomingdale (Ed.), *Attention deficit disorders III: New research in attention, treatment and psychopharmacology* (pp. 29–48). London: Pergamon.

Pelham, W. E., Schnedler, R., Bologna, N., & Contreras, A. (1980). Behavioral and stimulant treatment of hyperactive children: A therapy study with methylphenidate probes in a within-subject design. *Journal of Applied Behavior Analysis, 13,* 221–236.

Pfiffner, L. J., & Barkley, R. A. (1990). Educational placement and classroom management. In R. A. Barkley (Ed.), *Attention deficit hyperactivity disorder: A handbook for diagnosis and treatment* (pp. 498–539). New York: Guilford.

Pfiffner, L. J., & O'Leary, S. G. (in press). Psychological treatments: School-based. In J. L. Matson (Ed.), *Hyperactivity in children: A handbook.* Des Moines, IA: Allyn and Bacon.

Physician's desk reference (45th edition). (1991). Oradell, NJ: Medical Economics.

Pihl, R. O., Peterson, J., & Finn, P. (1990). Inherited predisposition to alcoholism: Characteristics of sons of male alcoholics. *Journal of Abnormal Psychology, 99,* 291–301.

Rapoport, J. L., Quinn, P. O., Bradbard, G., Riddle, D., & Brooks, E. (1974). Imipramine and methylphenidate treatments of hyperactive boys. *Archives of General Psychiatry, 30,* 789–793.

Rapport, M. D., Murphy, H. A., & Bailey, J. S. (1982). Ritalin vs. response cost in the control of hyperactive children: A within-subject comparison. *Journal of Applied Behavior Analysis, 15,* 205–216.

Shaffer, D., Campbell, M., Cantwell, D., Bradley, S., Carlson, G., Cohen, D., Denckla, M., Frances, A., Garfinkel, B., Klein, R., Pincus, H., Spitzer, R. L., Volkmar, F., & Widiger, T. (1989). Child and adolescent psychiatric disorders in DSM-IV: Issues facing the work group. *Journal of the American Academy of Child and Adolescent Psychiatry, 28,* 830–835.

Shaywitz, S. E., & Shaywitz, B. A. (1988). Attention deficit disorder: Current perspectives. In J. F. Kavanagh & T. J. Truss (Eds.), *Learning disabilities: Proceedings of the national conference.* Parkson, MD: York Press.

Wahler, R. G. (1980). The insular mother: Her problems in parent-child treatment. *Journal of Applied Behavior Analysis, 13,* 207–219.

Whalen, C. K., & Henker, B. (1991). Social impact of stimulant treatment for hyperactive children. *Journal of Learning Disabilities, 24,* 231–241.

Zametkin, A. J., Nordahl, T. E., Gross, M., King, A. C., Semple, W. E., Rumsey, J., Hamburger, S., & Cohen, R. M. (1990). Cerebral glucose metabolism in adults with hyperactivity of childhood onset. *The New England Journal of Medicine, 323,* 1361–1366.

CHAPTER 6

CONDUCT DISORDERS

Arthur M. Horne   University of Georgia
Brian A. Glaser   University of Georgia

DESCRIPTION OF DISORDER

Clinical Features

Conduct disorders in children and adolescents represent a predominant childhood referral problem, accounting for the majority of presenting concerns to child and family agencies. Conduct disorders are among the more enduring dysfunctions of children and, if left untreated, frequently result in high personal and emotional — as well as financial — costs to the child, family, and society.

The term *antisocial behavior* has been used to describe children who commit aggressive acts, steal, lie, and engage in other activities that are major social rule violations and who make up the conduct disorder (Kazdin, Esveldt-Dawson, French, & Unis, 1987). Kazdin and associates reported that the clinical significance of antisocial behaviors is reflected in their relatively high prevalence and clinical referral rates, their stability and poor prognosis over the course of development, and their continuity within families and across multiple generations. Further, conduct-disordered children show serious dysfunction in their interactions in and out of the home. Most children demonstrate some of the characteristics of conduct-disordered children at some time in their development, but the high rate of aggressiveness and the violation of others' rights characterizes conduct-disordered children. Fighting, lying, school problems, physical aggression, and legal confrontations are typical of these children.

Associated Features

Conduct-disordered behavior involves a high rate of violation of family, school, and societal rules. Youths engaging in these behaviors also frequently exhibit concomitant problems, such as social incompetence, peer rejection, and other mental health disorders, including substance abuse, academic failure, suicidal behavior, and a higher probability of physical injury and premature death. Thus, the extent of the problems challenges personal, family, school, and community resources. Furthermore, once conduct-problem behaviors become chronic, they are quite refractory to intervention, as demonstrated by the high rates of recidivism of juvenile delinquents and the failure of treatment programs to maintain change in serious adolescent antisocial behavior (Henggeler, 1989; Kazdin, 1987).

Such behavior is also associated with a variety of maladaptive cognitive processes (e.g., deficits in problem-solving skills, attributing hostile intent to others). For example, Reeves, Werry, Elkind, and Zametkin (1987) found that deficits in cognitive skills may be expected when aggressive behavior in children is encountered.

Patterson, Reid, Jones, and Conger (1975) reported that aggressive 10- to 12-year-old children exhibited a behavior pattern more typical of normal 3-year-olds. Their conclusion was based on naturalistic observations conducted in the homes of aggressive and average children. They concluded that an aggressive child's process of socialization appeared to be severely inhibited, and that aggressive children did not learn the social skills necessary to function effectively in their family or in peer relationships. In fact, they found that conduct-disordered children were likely to receive three times as much punishment from their peers as nonaggressive children (Patterson et al., 1975). They reported that aggressive children tended to have greater difficulty mastering academic tasks, learned at a slower pace, did not spontaneously improve without a specific intervention, and experienced severe adjustment problems as adults.

Physical abuse has also been associated with conduct disorders in children. Lahey, Hartdagen, Frick, and McBurnett (1988) found that parental antisocial personality disorder is directly linked to both parental divorce and child-conduct disorder, but that divorce and conduct disorder are not directly related. That is, the often cited association between parental divorce and child conduct problems may be confounded because antisocial personality disorder is common among the parents of children with conduct disorder, and divorce is very frequent for adults with this disorder.

A longitudinal study of comorbidity of depressive disorders and conduct disorders suggested that children with depressive disorders had a 36 percent estimated risk of developing conduct disorder by age 19 (Kovacs, Paulauskas, Gatsonis, & Richards, 1988). Moreover, a relationship among depression, aggression, and suicidal behavior has been established (Apter, Bleich, Plutchik, & Mendelsohn, 1988; Cairns, Peterson, & Neckerman, 1988). The symptoms of impulsivity, depression, lack of fatigue, and suicidal ideation (when both affective disorder and conduct disorder are present) result in high risk for suicidal behavior (Marriago, Fine, Moretti, & Haley, 1986).

In summary, conduct-disordered children tend to exhibit high levels of aversive interactions with family members and peers, experience peer rejection, misattribute hostile intentions to others, and have early and chronic academic problems. Conduct disorder is also associated with attention-deficit hyperactivity disorder and with depression (McMahon & Forehand, 1988). Co-occurrence of conduct disorder and attention-deficit hyperactivity disorder is associated with a more serious form of conduct disorder (Walker, Lahey, Hynd, & Frame, 1987).

Epidemiology

Chronic and serious conduct problems during childhood and early adolescence present a major and costly problem for society. In 1989, for example, there were 2,611,664 juvenile arrests, 78,000 of which were for violent crimes, 515,000 for property crimes, 90,000 for vandalism, 190,000 for drug abuse and liquor law violations, and 180,000 for curfew and running away violations (Federal Bureau of Investigation, 1990, Table 2, p. 181). The cost to society includes not only the funds required for the repair and/or replacement of material goods and the health services necessary for victims but also the one billion dollars per year necessary to maintain the juvenile justice system (Feldman, Caplinger, & Wodarski, 1983). And, of course, the number of antisocial acts resulting in monetary loss and/or victim suffering committed by children and adolescents far exceeds the number of reported crimes. It is estimated that about 4 percent of boys under age 18 exhibit diagnosable disorders of conduct, and approximately two-thirds of those will continue to display antisocial behavior into adulthood (American Psychiatric Association [APA], 1987). The aggressive behavior of problem children is a prevalent and relatively stable childhood condition that frequently requires extended therapeutic attention.

Etiology

A conceptual framework developed by Horne, Norsworthy, Forehand, and Frame (1990), presented in Figure 6–1, addresses the development of conduct disorders and intervention points to help prevent antisocial behavior from developing.

The center line represents the developmental period from birth through adolescence. The model can be broken into two broad components. First, the child's developmental progression is presented. It depicts the child as having certain genetic predispositions, cognitive potential, and temperament, which may lead to initial conduct problems directly or indirectly through the development of coercive parent-child interactions. If a coercive interactional style is maintained, the child develops only weak bonding to conventional societal norms, increasing the probability of rejecting, and being rejected by, normal peers. At the same time, the child's conduct problems develop into displays of poor social competence (including attributional bias of hostility toward peers, lack of perspective taking, failure to consider alternative solutions to social problem situations, selection and enactment of inappropriate behaviors), which also result in the child being rejected by normal peers. When peer rejection is sustained over several years, the child will seek a commitment to a deviant peer group in early adolescence. If the child also has failed to develop appropriate academic skills over the grade-school years due to time spent off-task (and perhaps preceding cognitive deficits), by the time she or he reaches adolescence the student will not be invested in school nor will there be a success experience there. The combination of academic failure and association with a deviant peer group provides the final impetus for serious antisocial and illegal behavior.

The second component, represented in the bottom half of the figure, illustrates the environmental and systemic factors that influence families. Parental and family factors may further contribute to the development of chronic conduct disorder in youth, such as existing psychopathology, poor family management practices, economic stressors, and marital conflict.

The prevention model has been depicted in a linear fashion in order to illustrate the developmental nature of conduct problems. In actuality, the factors that contribute to the development of delinquency do not develop linearly. Rather, they are interactive in nature and acting at different levels of intensity at different times. These factors occur across time, conditions, and family characteristics and may differentially influence the child's development in various ways at different times.

DIFFERENTIAL DIAGNOSIS AND ASSESSMENT

DSM-III-R Categorization

Conduct disorders are divided into three types: group, solitary aggressive, and undifferentiated. As the names imply, group conduct disorders are most commonly evident when the person is with peers, whereas the solitary aggressive type usually manifests itself as aggressive physical behavior toward adults or peers but not as a function of group of gang activity. The undifferentiated type represents a mixture of clinical characteristics. The DSM-III-R defines conduct disorder as

> a persistent pattern of conduct in which the basic rights of others and major age-appropriate societal norms or rules are violated. The behavior pattern typically is present in the home, at school, with peers, and in the community. The conduct problems are more serious than those seen in Oppositional Defiant Disorder. . . . Physical aggression is common. Children or adolescents with this disorder usually initiate aggression, may be physically cruel to other people or to animals, and frequently deliberately destroy other people's property. . . . They may engage in stealing with confrontation of the victim, as in mugging, extortion, or armed robbery. At later ages, the physical violence may take the form of rape, assault, or, in rare cases, homicide. (APA, 1987, p. 53)

Often conduct-disorder problems are preceded by other problems, including oppositional defiant disorder, attention-deficit hyperactivity disorder,

Figure 6–1. Conceptual framework for development and prevention of serious conduct disorders in children

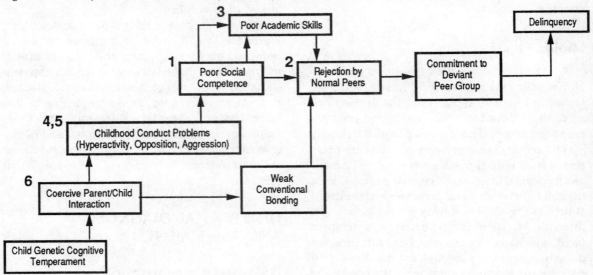

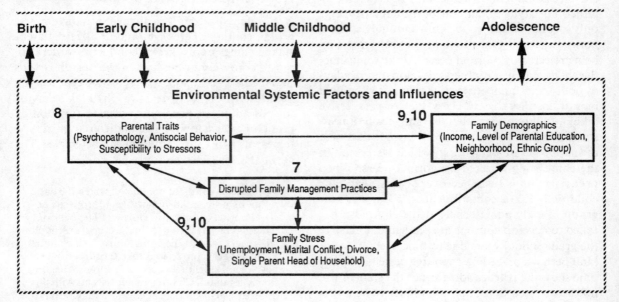

Potential Interventions:

1. Social Competence Enhancement (Four Levels)
2. Peer Counseling
3. Academic Remediation
4. Behavioral Self-control Strategies
5. Training Teachers/Educators in Behavior Management Strategies

6. Parent Training in Child Management Skills
7. Social Learning Family Therapy
8. Parent Individual Therapy
9. Couple/Single Parent Counseling
10. Parent Education / Career-vocational / Financial

Source: From *Family Counseling and Therapy* (2nd ed.) by A. Horne, K. Norsworthy, R. Forehand, & C. Frame (1990), Itasca, IL: Peacock Publishers. Reprinted by permission.

and family dysfunction. The diagnostic criteria for conduct disorder are:

A disturbance of conduct lasting at least six months in which at least three of the following have been present:

1. Has stolen without confrontation of a victim on more than one occasion
2. Has run away from home overnight at least twice while living in parental or surrogate home
3. Often lies
4. Has deliberately engaged in fire setting
5. Is often truant from school
6. Has broken into someone else's house, building, or car
7. Has deliberately destroyed others' property
8. Has been physically cruel to animals
9. Has forced someone to have sexual activity with him or her
10. Has used a weapon in more than one fight
11. Often initiates physical fights
12. Has stolen with confrontation of a victim
13. Has been physically cruel to people. (APA, 1987, p. 55)

Differential Diagnosis

Rather than attempt to separate children's behavior by diagnostic categories presented in the DSM-III-R, Patterson (1982) explained that children's antisocial behaviors are a heterogeneous set of symptoms. In his extensive review of the development of coercive behavior in children, he reported that there is considerable overlap among the various dysfunctional behavior patterns that children develop. Rather than attempt to narrowly define the behavior as attention deficit disorder, oppositional defiant disorder, or conduct disorder, Patterson stated that it would be better to examine the behavior in the context of the situation and learn what conditions permit or contribute to the clinical picture. There is good justification for using broader terms for behavioral problems of children, for whereas the DSM-III-R presents the categories distinctly, in practice there is considerable overlap. Werry, Reeves, and Elkind (1987), for example, have reported that the coexistence of attention deficit and conduct disorders is common. Coexistence of these disorders in-

creases the degree of disability, and it is these children who are more likely to be referred for treatment. Thus, Werry and colleagues argue that the dispute as to whether the child's diagnosis should be attention deficit or conduct disorder is not very important because most cases seen in clinics will have both disorders as defining characteristics.

Reeves and colleagues (1987) stated that conduct disorder seems to be a disorder with an early onset marked by egocentricity, aggressiveness, poor interpersonal relationships, and an adverse child-rearing environment. They suggested that oppositional defiant disorder and conduct disorder may well be the same condition, except that oppositional defiant disorder may be more common in girls, which suggests that it may be a less severe form of conduct disorder. In a study assessing the diagnoses of 108 children using DSM-III-R criteria, Reeves and associates (1987) found only 4 children with a conduct disorder diagnosis unaccompanied by any other diagnosis, and only 2 children had an oppositional defiant disorder diagnosis alone. Comparing clinically diagnosed children and a control group of normal children, Reeves and associates (1987) found that children with attention-deficit hyperactivity disorder and conduct disorder had a much higher frequency of adverse family backgrounds and were characterized by fathers with lower education levels, family alcoholism, and fathers with antisocial personalities. It may be that there is an interaction between the cognitive impairment condition of attention-deficit hyperactivity disorder and psychosocial environmental factors that contribute to conduct disorders. This interaction may result in clinical cases warranting attention because of the difficulties caused in classrooms, conflict in families, and the personal pain that children with this condition experience.

Assessment Strategies

There are many approaches to the assessment of conduct disorders in children and adolescents (Achenbach, 1985; Horne & Sayger, 1990; Kazdin, 1987; Martin, 1988; Ollendick & Hersen, 1984). Two common methods are the clinically derived and the multivariate approach. The clinical approach relies on observations in a clinical setting to develop an understanding of the syndrome being studied. Clinical diagnosis identifies which symptoms are present or absent from observed behaviors (the DSM-III-R [APA, 1987] is an example of such an assessment approach). Multivariate approaches, on the other hand, describe the degree to which a condition exists, and is determined by using factor-analytic studies of large groups. Assessments of children and adolescents have been variable and have not provided for careful delineation of disorders. The presence or absence of a disorder and the level or extent of the disorder is often difficult to determine. Further, there is often little convergence among diverse measures and there is often little agreement among persons providing the data (children and parents frequently have different perceptions of the child's behavior). Discrepancies in assessment methods for conduct disorders is common. As Kazdin stated, "There is at present no object measure of conduct disorder that is free of some source of bias, artifact, or judgment. The use of several different measures is essential to overcome the limitations of any single modality or scale" (1987, p. 51).

Four primary areas for assessment of conduct disorder include the (1) child, (2) family, (3) school, and (4) community. Cross-setting, multiple observer approaches are recommended and representative assessment procedures are presented in Table 6-1. Not all approaches should be utilized with each case.

Child Information

Child information may include a semistructured interview with the child, any of several inventories to obtain the child's perceptions of problems (Youth Self-Report Form, Children's Version of the Family Environment Scale, Children's Depression Inventory), and observations of the child as he or she interacts with other family members, the interviewer, or in other social contexts.

Family Information

Demographic data may be gathered in two ways. First, intake forms provide substantial information regarding family structure, and family genograms give a diagrammatic view of the family structure. Second, standardized instruments provide information about family dynamics (Family Environment Scale, Child Behavior Checklist, Parent Daily Report, Locke-Wallace Marital Adjustment Inventory) and provide data about the role of the child in the family.

School Information

School data include descriptive materials (school records, truancy information, teacher observations) as well as objective measures (Daily Behavior Checklist, Teacher Report Form). Ideally, observations of the child within the school environment are an integral part of data collection.

Community Information

Community information includes medical reports, court and police records, data from police or court documents, and child protective services or group home information.

TREATMENT

Treatment of conduct disorders may take a variety of forms, depending on the mission and setting of the service provider (private practice, school, court, community mental health center, child protective service). Common models of intervention include individual therapy, group therapy, behavior therapy, problem-solving skills training, pharmacotherapy, residential treatment, family therapy, parent training, or community-wide interventions (Kazdin, 1987). Conduct disorder is very stable and difficult to change, so a variety of interventions are called for. The existence of so many interventions reflects the experimentation and diversity of approaches to a most difficult problem, but is also indicative of the lack of a clearly defined intervention that has been demonstrated to be consistently effective with a high rate of success. For some treatment providers only one approach will be used, but in general there is considerable overlap among the interventions and in most situations a combination

Table 6–1. Summary of Assessment Approaches

AREA	INSTRUMENT/ PROCEDURE	SOURCE	PURPOSE	AUTHOR
Family Information	Family Intake Form	Family	Standard	Horne & Sayger, 1990
	Factors Contributing to Change Scale (FCCS)	Family	Standard	Horne & Sayger, 1990
	Therapist Termination Report	Family	Standard	Horne, 1989
	Genogram	Family	Clinical judgment	
	Parents Rating Form	Parent	Standard	Horne & Sayger, 1989b
	Family Environment Scale	Parent	Standard	Moos, 1974; Moos & Moos, 1984
	Family Problem-Solving Behavior Coding System	Video	Research	Nickerson, Light, Blechman, & Gandelman, 1976
	Beavers-Timberlawn Family Evaluation Scale	Video	Research	Lewis, Beavers, Gossett, & Phillips, 1976
	Child Behavior Checklist	Parent	Standard	Achenbach & Edelbrock, 1983
	Parent Daily Report	Parent	Standard	Patterson, Reid, Jones, & Conger, 1975
	Dyadic Adjustment Scale	Parent	Standard	Spanier, 1979; Spanier & Thompson, 1982
	Locke-Wallace Marital Adjustment Scale	Parent	Clinical judgment	Locke & Wallace, 1959
	Beck Depression Inventory	Parent/ child	Standard	Beck, 1967, 1972
	Symptom Checklist 90-R	Parent	Standard	Derogatis, 1983
Child Information	Youth Self-Report Form	Child	Standard	Achenbach & Edelbrock, 1987
	Semistructured Clinical Interview for Children	Child	Clinical judgment	Achenbach & McConaughy, 1989
	Children's Version of the Family Environment Scale	Child	Clinical judgment	Pino, Simons, & Slawinowski, 1984
	Children's Depression Inventory	Child	Standard	Kovacs, 1981
School Information	Teacher Interview	Teacher	Standard	
	Academic Performance	School	Standard	
	Daily Behavior Checklist	Teacher	Standard	Prinz, Conner, & Wilson, 1981
	Teacher Report Form	Teacher	Standard	Achenbach & Edelbrock, 1986
Community and Social Agencies Information	Medical Records	Agency	Standard	
	Court and Police Records	Agency	Standard	
	Child Protective Services Reports	Agency	Standard	

of approaches will be used. At the core of effective interventions is a behavioral focus.

Evidence for Prescriptive Treatment

Behavior Therapy

Behavior therapy has been the intervention of choice in the majority of empirically based evaluations of treatment programs focusing on conduct disorders. Behavior therapy emphasizes the learning of new behaviors and the reduction of maladaptive ones through reinforcement of successive approximations to the desired outcome, and other extinction or punishment for dysfunctional behaviors. Structure for the learning experience has ranged from maximum security in a tightly controlled correctional environment utilizing token economies and elaborate systems of punishment, to group and individual interviews in clinic or school settings utilizing social reinforcement and roleplaying.

Extensive reviews of the effectiveness of behavioral intervention programs have been written. Summaries of early work in a variety of settings have been provided by Costello (1972), Braukmann and Fixsen (1974), Burchard and Harig (1976), and Stumphauzer (1973). These reviews provided information about the effectiveness of behavior therapy, primarily in structured settings with close control over the delivery of services and the general environment. An example included Achievement Place in Lawrence, Kansas, a community setting program of group foster care for adjudicated juveniles. The system utilizes professionally trained teaching parents who attempt to correct behavioral deficits through modeling, practice, and instruction, using a token system. While these early systems of behavioral intervention demonstrated effectiveness of behavior change while clients were involved in the system, there were several drawbacks to the approach. First, the process was frequently quite expensive and required the development of a delivery service that provided for control and security. Second, the behavior changes that occurred frequently did not generalize beyond the treatment center.

In reviewing the treatment programs completed through 1975, Patterson and colleagues (1975) found behavioral/social learning family therapy approaches to be effective for reducing conduct-disorder behaviors of the child identified as the problem in the family, and treatment also had generalized to other family members, including siblings. Further, parents began to see their child's behavior as more positive, and parents became more effective at providing rewards for appropriate behavior and punishments for acting-out behavior. Overall, mothers seemed more satisfied with their children and rated the family as happier, and fathers developed a more influential role in the family by controlling coercive actions of the child.

In the years since, Patterson has continued to examine treating families with antisocial children, including examining specific treatment conditions. He has conducted carefully controlled studies to examine the effects of treatment versus control group outcome, and treatment versus placebo controls in working with families with stealers and other forms of deviant behavior (Patterson, 1982). In addition, other researchers have carried out programs to replicate his research with equally positive results (Fleischman & Horne, 1979; Sayger, Horne, Passmore, & Walker, 1988), and some have extended his work by addressing additional components of treatment and evaluation (Fleischman, Horne, & Arthur, 1983; Horne & Sayger, 1990; Kazdin, 1987). Other major contributors in the area of treating families in a social learning family therapy model have included Anthony Graziano, Rex Forehand, Daniel and Susan O'Leary, Robert Wahler, Elaine Blechman, and Ron Prinz.

Attempts to intervene during adolescence have resulted in minimal success. While some treatment programs targeting early to late adolescents have shown some initial success, followup results have been less encouraging (Kazdin, 1987; Patterson, 1986). Interventions that have demonstrated more effectiveness have been those that aim at influencing children at an earlier age and address others involved in the child's life: parents, teachers, and sometimes peers (Fleischman et al., 1983; Forehand, Wells, & Griest, 1980; Patterson et al., 1975).

Although the picture looks rather discouraging for changing well-established patterns of antisocial behavior in older adolescents, research in the last decade has provided some grounds for optimism about our ability to prevent the development of full-blown chronic conduct disorder in young children. First, well-designed empirical research studies have provided information about the developmental progressions likely to result in chronic conduct disorder, as well as correlates of the developing disorder. They have also identified clear markers of high-risk status in children. Second, a number of researchers have demonstrated the efficacy of several interventions in making at least short-term changes in specific types of conduct problems and antisocial behaviors.

Attempts to treat conduct problems in children and adolescents can be categorized into three major areas: individual child characteristics, behavior and learning problems of the child in the academic setting, and family management.

Individual child characteristics. In treating the individual child, the five areas of social competence outlined by Dodge, Pettit, McClaskey, and Brown (1986) (encoding of social problem, interpretation, response search, response decision, and behavioral enactment) have been primary targets of intervention. Chalmers and Townsend (1990) demonstrated that perspective-taking skills could be successfully taught to conduct-disordered girls. Attempts to teach social problem-solving strategies have been successful, with decreases in antisocial behavior maintained for up to one year (Guerra & Slaby, 1990; Kazdin, Bass, Siegel, & Thomas, 1989; Lochman, Burch, Curry, & Lampron, 1984). Guerra and Slaby's (1990) study also involved cognitive behavior modification of the youth's outcome expectancies for antisocial behavior and their value or importance to the youth. Lochman and Curry (1986) and Kazdin and associates (1989) showed that these children can benefit from learning strategies for controlling their anger. On the other side, increasing social

skills has not always been accompanied by reductions in antisocial behavior (Kazdin, 1987), and maintenance of learned prosocial behavior beyond a year has not been widely documented.

Focusing on a peer approach, Feldman and colleagues (1983) demonstrated that involving conduct-disordered youth with well-adjusted boys in social activities that stressed group participation resulted in decreased antisocial behavior. Bowman and Myrick (1987) also reported positive effects of a peer facilitation program in reducing behavior problems in middle childhood children.

Academic setting. Interventions in the academic setting have shown mixed results. Some evidence suggests that academic remediation is associated with decreased levels of conduct problem behavior (MacMillan & Kavale, 1986). Wilson and Herrnstein (1985) have noted that although academic skills may improve, antisocial behavior is not always reduced. However, instructing teachers in behavior management strategies has been effective both in reducing problem behaviors and improving academic performance (Kelley, 1989).

Family management. Treatments aimed at helping parents manage and discipline their problem children and at altering systemic functioning of the family have shown positive levels of success in decreasing oppositional and conduct-problem behaviors in preschool and elementary school-aged children (Kazdin, 1987; McMahon, Forehand, & Griest, 1981). In fact, Forehand and Long (1988) determined that their treated subjects were indistinguishable from normal controls at a seven and one-half year followup during adolescence. Sayger and colleagues (1988) demonstrated the effectiveness of a family intervention utilizing social learning family therapy, which resulted in positive behavioral changes in conduct-problem children and improvement in family relationships, family environment, problem solving, and other systemic factors.

Recent research has provided valuable information about specific causal, correlational, and risk factors for chronic antisocial outcome and has set the stage for an even more sophisticated approach to the problem. It is apparent that models of the development of chronic conduct disorder must consider not only the developmental trajectory of the child but the possible impact of various parental and family characteristics on each point in that trajectory. Figure 6–1 presented a schematic drawing of such a multidimensional model of conduct-problem development.

Each point in the model is proposed to be amenable to intervention, as indicated in Figure 6–1, resulting in many possible treatments. However, in contrast to previous research that has tended to concentrate on one specific problem area, it is proposed that every one of the areas in which a child and his or her family exhibit difficulties must be treated, in order to reduce the risk of chronic antisocial behavior beyond only temporary time periods. It must be noted, however, that to maximize the probability of detecting treatment efficacy, children and their families should receive treatment only for those areas in which they demonstrate deficits. In addition, the timing of the intervention must be such that the problem has been consistently present for some time, to minimize the probability of the false positive identification (a costly error in this type of intervention), but such that the problem has existed for a short enough time to keep the probability of effecting change high. In this model, it would appear imperative, then, to intervene with children who have repeatedly been identified as showing conduct problems in the home and school *before* they finish the fourth grade, when such behaviors appear to become firmly entrenched through association with deviant peers.

Previous research has further demonstrated two problems that must be addressed for an intervention to be successful: (1) generalization of treatment effects to the home and school environment and (2) long-term maintenance of treatment gains. One method for enhancing generalization of treatment effects is to train the desired behaviors in the natural setting. Thus, home-based and school-based interventions appear to be more useful than clinic-based programs. Second, given the resistance of conduct-problem behavior to change, it would appear to be necessary to adopt the chronic disease model of treatment suggested by Kazdin (1987). In this case, the child and his or her family are asumed to require "booster" intervention

treatment sessions on a regular basis to prevent recurrence of past problems and the development of new ones.

In summary, the existing research on the causes and correlates of, and interventions with conduct disorder in children and adolescents has been utilized to develop a multidimensional model of the development of chronic antisocial behavior. Based on this model, a multifaceted, flexible intervention program is recommended. The intervention utilizes treatment components previously demonstrated to be effective for each of the problems of academic characteristics, individual child characteristics, family factors, and social resources. The intervention components are empirically based, are carefully timed to occur after risk has been established but before antisocial behavior patterns have become entrenched, and are designed to enhance generalization across settings and time.

Pharmacotherapy

Psychopharmacology has also been used as an approach or an adjunct to treatment of conduct-disordered children, but results have not been promising. Lithium has been used with children who display sporadic unprovoked physical aggression and are refractory to usual treatment (Siassi, 1982). However, some research has suggested that certain children who have responded to lithium may have a variant form of bipolar disorder (DeLong & Aldershof, 1987). Gittelman and Kanner, in summarizing research on psychopharmacology with conduct-disordered children, reported:

> In summary, there is no well-established pharmacotherapy of conduct disorders except for the single satisfactory study of lithium. . . . Further research is required to provide clear estimates of drug efficacy in children with pure conduct disorders and in those who also suffer from ADDH [Attention Deficit Disorder with Hyperactivity] or from depression. (1986, p. 474)

Alternative Treatments

The behavioral characteristics of conduct disorder have been around much longer than have organized psychotherapy treatment models. Incarceration has long been the standard intervention for conduct-disordered youth, but the sole use of a deterrence/incarceration model has been judged to be a failure (e.g., see Goldstein, 1991). Consequently, a large number of explanations for the disorder have been developed, and from these theoretical models have come interventions designed to treat the problem.

The oldest model, and the one most prevalent into the 1960s, was the psychodynamic explanation and treatment for behavior disorders. Under this approach, the behavior observed was explained through inner life conflicts resulting in emotional disturbance, which was manifested in dysfunctional behavior. The primary mode of intervention was the analysis of unconscious conflict experienced by the child through interpretation by the therapist. This approach is very costly in terms of child and therapist time and, from an empirical stance, is an unproven methodology.

From the psychodynamic arena a number of other interventions have evolved. One that has been quite popular in correctional and school settings is *reality therapy,* an approach developed by William Glasser. Glasser developed reality therapy while working as a psychiatrist with the Ventura (California) Girl's School, and the intervention was designed to change irresponsible (acting-out) behavior on the part of the incarcerated girls. The approach emphasizes developing a trusting relationship with the client, and then engaging in a series of steps designed to help the client identify decision-making steps that will lead to positive behavior choices rather than delinquent behavior. Briefly, the steps involve the following:

- Establish a relationship.
- Examine the current activity ("What are you doing now?").
- Examine whether the current activity is working ("Is it working, is what you're doing helping you?").
- Help the client establish a plan.
- Use no punishment; let natural and logical consequences take their toll.
- Never give up.

The reality therapy approach has been found to be helpful in school settings where teachers and counselors have been able to develop an environment conducive to helping students take responsibility for their behavior and allowing considerable support and encouragement for their efforts. The approach has been more helpful than incarceration without the development of a therapeutic environment, but has not developed extensive empirical support. Just as much of the theoretical background of reality therapy developed from earlier models (primarily Adlerian or individual psychology approaches), so many of the steps of reality therapy have been incorporated into current social learning treatment programs. See, for example, in the model presented in this chapter, the section on helping children identify whether or not their current efforts are effective.

Selecting Optimal Treatment Strategies

Selection of the optimal treatment strategy will be based on completing a careful analysis of the behavior: What are the antecedents and consequences? What maintains the behavior? What function does the behavior serve in the family/classroom/group environment? What is the level of intervention necessary to impact the behavior of the conduct-disordered youth? What resources are available? The intervention should be based on the developmental level of the child, the stage of the problem, and the degree of cooperation that may be obtained from a variety of sources (parents, siblings, teachers, peers).

Problems in Carrying Out Interventions

The greatest difficulty in implementing effective treatment procedures includes having access to and cooperation from the parties involved. Early research that demonstrated effectiveness of behavioral interventions in restricted environments had control over environmental factors so that change was within the control of the therapist. In the natural environment, on the other hand, cooperation from other parties is frequently not available: (1) parents may attribute the problem to the child and refuse to cooperate, (2) parents may be so severely debilitated that they are unable to cooperate with therapeutic interventions, (3) teachers are overextended and may not be invested in assisting in change programs, (4) courts or juvenile centers may see their role as punitive rather than therapeutic and refuse to cooperate with treatment plans, and (5) treatment programs may be so limited in time that effective change is not viable.

On the other hand, one of the weaknesses of early studies where control was possible was lack of generalization to the natural environment once the student was released back into the community. If therapists are able to work with the child in the natural environment and effect change, it is more likely to be maintained.

Relapse Prevention

Relapse prevention occurs best when the natural environment supports the prosocial behaviors developed, which is why systemic, environmental change is important. "Nastiness begets nastiness," and so families that engage in coercive, painful interactions will not support positive changes made by the identified patient independent of the family. Rather, the coercive interchange must change in the social structure, usually the home. Similarly, when children experience failure in school, they will not adhere to positive social conduct; the school must be a place to find support and success.

Once change has been effected, followup is crucial. "Booster sessions" with telephone calls or personal visits to the home, school, or community agency are important. Improvements seem to begin to erode after about three months and a visit or "booster session" at this point is effective for helping people maintain their positive change.

CASE ILLUSTRATION

Case Description

Bobby was referred to the university clinic by the Child Protective Services (CPS) office of the local welfare department. He had been placed in a foster home under the supervision of CPS by the juvenile court system.

Bobby

Bobby was 13 years old. He was in the sixth grade but was functioning at a very low level academically and had been placed in a class for the severely emotionally disturbed. At school he would fight, argue, talk back, and refuse to do his school work. Temper outbursts were common. He was in frequent altercations on the playground and in the cafeteria, and in recent months he had been molesting girls by grabbing them and on two occasions he had forced a girl to the ground and attempted to remove her underclothes. Bobby had been picked up by the police for committing vandalism to the school (shooting windows with a BB gun), for being out late at night walking the streets, and for suspicion of slashing car tires. On each occasion he was remanded to the custody of his mother.

Kelly (Mother)

Kelly had been married twice but was divorced. She currently lived with Jake, who was unemployed. She had three other children (Dusty, Nick, Terri). Kelly was overweight, intellectually slow, and received aid for dependent children (ADC) to provide for the children and herself. She had been arrested for prostitution on several occasions. Kelly indicated that she drank alcohol quite heavily but did not use illegal drugs.

Jake

Jake lived with Kelly but was out of the home when Bobby was referred for treatment; he had been arrested for house burglary. While in jail awaiting trial, Jake attempted suicide and was removed to the state hospital for observation and treatment.

Other Family Members

Bobby had two brothers (Dusty, Nick) and a sister (Terri) who lived in the home. Dusty and Nick were in school and both were similar to Bobby—they experienced academic difficulties, were not working at grade level, and were in frequent fights and other conflicts with other students. The grandmother, Jean, was a widow who lived two blocks away. She had little contact with the family and she and Kelly argued a lot;

Kelly had even physically struck Jean a number of times when they argued. Jean would provide the family with money to cover expenses when necessary, but she lived on widow's benefits and had little extra money.

Differential Diagnosis and Assessment

Bobby met the DSM-III-R criteria for conduct disorder: He stole, ran away from home, lied, was truant from school, had broken into a neighbor's house, destroyed others' property, had been cruel to animals, attempted forced sexual activity, and initiated fights.

Child Information

Bobby completed a clinical interview, the Youth Self-Report Form, the Children's Depression Inventory, and a self-concept inventory. These measures indicated he had low self-esteem, poor self-concept, experienced depression, and saw himself as a violent, angry person who deserved to have revenge against those whom he perceived had "wronged" him.

Family Information

Kelly completed a family intake form, the Child Behavior Checklist, the Family Environment Scale, and the Beck Depression Inventory. The Child Behavior Checklist scores clearly placed Bobby in the clinical area for delinquency, aggression, hyperactivity, and depression. The Family Environment Scale reflected a family low in cohesion and high in conflict. Kelly's score on the Beck Depression Inventory was in the clinically depressed range.

School Information

Bobby had been assessed using the WISC-R and the Peabody Individual Achievement Test (PIAT) and his scores on those measures indicated he had limited intellectual abilities (full-scale IQ = 72), though the psychologist reported that he had been very uncooperative and likely was much brighter than the scores would indicate. The Teacher Report Form of the Child Behavior

Checklist was consistent with the parent's report. The teacher provided information on the Daily Behavior Checklist over several weeks and Bobby clearly engaged in a high rate of aggressive acts within the classroom setting.

Treatment Selection

Bobby

Individual sessions were scheduled with Bobby to provide several specific interventions:

1. *Anger control.* Feindler and Ecton (1986) have described a detailed program for teaching adolescents effective anger control, both in groups and individually. It was decided to use that model during individual twice-weekly sessions. Included in the treatment program was stress management (relaxation training), cognitive challenges to irrational thinking, and assertiveness.
2. *Social skills training.* Matson and Ollendick (1988) have provided detailed instructions for teaching social skills to children, and Goldstein, Sprafkin, Gershaw, and Klein (1980) have developed a structured learning program of social skills development for adolescents. An intervention combining qualities of both programs was developed.
3. *Career and vocational training.* Steps were taken to assist Bobby in considering vocational plans and begin developing career goals.

Family

Family intervention included the following:

1. *Parent training.* Usiang the Fleishman, Horne, and Arthur model presented in *Troubled Families* (1983), a parent training intervention was planned. This model includes teaching parental self-control skills, setting up for success, and communication patterns for effective parent-child interactions.
2. *Family therapy.* Once-a-week family sessions were developed to provide all members of the family with the opportunity to share, examine

family issues and dynamics, and develop more effective family communications skills.

3. *Family support.* Steps were taken to assist Kelly to develop more structure in her lifestyle, to work with home visitors from the welfare department who came weekly to teach home-making skills, and to become involved in a local private industry council employment program.

School

In the school setting the following steps were taken:

1. *Teacher training.* The teacher met weekly with the therapist to review classroom management procedures, monitor Bobby's behavior, and discuss ways of structuring the learning activities in smaller steps so that Bobby could experience success.
2. *Peer program.* Bobby was placed in a counseling group at his school. In the group, students were assigned counseling peers — fellow students who had received training in peer counseling and had volunteered to provide support and encouragement to fellow students.

Treatment Course and Problems in Carrying Out Interventions

Bobby

The weekly sessions teaching Bobby anger control and social skills went well. He was picked up immediately after school twice a week by a caseworker from CPS and delivered to the university clinic office. Refreshments were always available and he seemed to enjoy the attention and the snacks. Bobby argued that he knew all we were covering, but he was not able to demonstrate the skills when we would ask him to show us on videotape. When confronted, he would report he hated to see us, but then would immediately break out laughing and say, "I got you, didn't I? You thought I really hated you." The biggest difficulty was in presenting the rationale for disputing irrational thoughts and for developing assertive rather

than aggressive behavior. To cope with that problem, we used models who were of the same socioeconomic background and used the same language as Bobby to do some of our roleplays.

Family

The parent training program and family therapy intervention did not go well at first. Kelly would fail to show for sessions or would come inebriated. Approximately two weeks into treatment, the children who were still in the home (Bobby was in a foster home) were removed from the home and placed in foster care after Kelly was arrested for prostitution and disorderly conduct. The foster parents (two sets — one had the three boys, one had the girl) agreed to participate in parent training and to use the parenting skills with the children at home. As part of each week's session, the children were seen as a group for dealing with family issues.

When Kelly returned home, she was court ordered to attend an alcohol treatment program and to attend parenting classes with the children and the foster parents. After two months, the children were returned to their home and Kelly and the children continued to attend parenting classes.

School

The special education teacher stayed quite involved in the therapy intervention and was an excellent support person. She was able to provide a high level of classroom structure and developed a token program for all students involved. The peer counselor did not work well because of social class distinctions and the school was unable to provide a peer counselor with a social background similar to Bobby's. Instead, arrangements were made for him to go several times each week to the local Boys Club where he received intensive athletic training in basketball and other sports.

Outcome and Termination

Treatment lasted nine months. At the end of treatment, Bobby was moved from the special education class to a mainstream academic program. He continued to have arguments with other students but had ceased fighting and other acts of violent behavior.

Followup and Maintenance

Bobby and his family were seen once a month at the university clinic for six months after termination. A caseworker from CPS provided transportation and assured that they would arrive. Kelly continued to receive financial support to attend the private industry council job-training program and she was escorted to AA meetings weekly. Jake never returned to the home. Bobby was seen weekly at his school by the school counselor who provided encouragement and support for problems he experienced. Bobby also continued at the Boys Club. He was not a good enough athlete for school teams. At the end of one year of followup posttreatment, Bobby remained out of legal trouble, though he and Kelly argued at least weekly.

SUMMARY

Children and adolescents who engage in a variety of acts such as vandalism, running away, fire setting, truancy, fighting, and other acts that violate the rights of others are referred to as conduct disordered. While all children engage in some of these behaviors some of the time, the high rate of engagement of conduct-disordered adolescents cause them to result in high personal and emotional—as well as financial—costs to the child, the family, and to society in general. The dysfunction is one of the more enduring problems children may have and accounts for a major portion of referrals for mental health and correctional services.

A number of approaches have been developed for treating childhood aggression, and of those, behavioral interventions have demonstrated the greatest efficacy and utility. Interventions need to be designed to impact conduct-disordered children based on developmental stage and level of dysfunction. A broad intervention program that addresses problems across settings and circumstances is recommended. Individual, family, and school involvement is essential.

REFERENCES

Achenbach, T. (1985). *Assessment and taxonomy of child and adolescent psychopathology.* Newbury Park, CA: Sage.

Achenbach, T., & Edelbrock, C. (1983). *Manual for the Child Behavior Checklist and Revised Child Behavior Profile.* Burlington: University of Vermont, Department of Psychiatry.

Achenbach, T., & Edelbrock, C. (1986). *Manual for the Teacher's Report Form and Teacher Version of the Child Behavior Profile.* Burlington: University of Vermont, Department of Psychiatry.

Achenbach, T., & Edelbrock, C. (1987). *Manual for the Youth Self-Report and Profile.* Burlington: University of Vermont, Department of Psychiatry.

Achenbach, T., & McConaughy, S. (1989). *Semistructured clinical interview for children aged 6–11.* Burington, VT: University of Vermont Department of Psychiatry.

American Psychological Association. (1987). *The diagostic and statistical manual of psychiatric diagnoses* (3rd ed., rev.). Washington, DC: Author.

Apter, A., Bleich, A., Plutchik, R., & Mendelsohn, S. (1988). Suicidal behavior, depression, and conduct disorder in hospitalized adolescents. *Journal of the American Academy of Child and Adolescent Psychiatry, 27,* 696–699.

Beck, A. (1967). *Depression: Clinical, experimental, and theoretical aspects.* New York: Harper & Row.

Beck, A. (1972). *Depression: Causes and treatment.* Philadelphia: University of Pennsylvania.

Bowman, R. P., & Myrick, R. D. (1987). Effects of an elementary school peer facilitator program on children with behavior problems. *The School Counselor, 34,* 369–378.

Braukman, C. J., & Fixsen, D. L. (1974). Behavior modification with delinquents. In M. Hersen, R. M. Fisher, & P. M. Miller (Eds.), *Progress in behavior modification.* New York: Academic Press.

Burchard, J. D., & Harig, P. T. (1976). Behavior modification and juvenile delinquency. In H. Leitenberg (Ed.), *Handbook of behavior modification and behavior therapy* (pp. 405–452). Englewood Cliffs, NJ: Prentice Hall.

Cairns, R. B., Peterson, G., & Neckerman, H. (1988). Suicidal behavior in aggressive adolescents. *Journal of Clinical Child Psychology, 17,* 298–309.

Chalmers, J., & Townsend, M. (1990). The effects of training in social perspective taking on socially maldjusted girls. *Child Development, 61,* 178–190.

Costello, J. (1972). *Behavior modification and corrections.* The Law Enforcement Assistance Administration. National Technical Information Service, #PB 223-629/A5.

DeLong, R. G., & Aldershof, A. L. (1987). Long-term experience with lithium treatment in childhood: Correlation with clinical diagnosis. *Journal of the American Academy of Child and Adolescent Psychiatry, 26,* 389-394.

Derogatix, L. R. (1983). *SCL-90-R administration, scoring, and procedures manual—II.* Towson, MD: Clinical Psychometric Research.

Dodge, K. A., Pettit, G. S., McClaskey, C. L., & Brown, M. (1986). Social competence in children. *Monographs of the Society for Research in Child Development, 51,* (Serial No. 213).

Federal Bureau of Investigation. (1990). *Uniform crime reports: Crime in the United States, 1989.* Washington, DC: Author.

Feindler, E. L., & Ecton, R. B. (1986). *Adolescent anger control: Cognitive-behavioral techniques.* Elmsford, NY: Pergamon.

Feldman, R. A., Caplinger, T. E., & Wodarski, J. S. (1983). *The St. Louis conundrum: The effective treatment of antisocial youths.* Englewood Cliff, NJ: Prentice Hall.

Fleischman, M., & Horne, A. (1979). Working with families: A social learning approach. *Contemporary Education, 50,* 66-71.

Fleischman, M., Horne, A., & Arthur, J. (1983). *Troubled families: A treatment program.* Champaign, IL: Research Press.

Forehand, R., & Long, N. (1988). Outpatient treatment of the acting out child: Procedures, long term follow-up data, and clinical problems. *Advances in Behavior and Research Therapy, 10,* 129-177.

Forehand, R., Wells, K., & Griest, D. (1980). An examination of the social validity of a parent training program. *Behavior Therapy, 11,* 488-502.

Gittelman, R., & Kanner, A. (1986). Psycho-pharmacotherapy. In H. Quay & J. Werry (Eds.), *Psychopathological disorders of childhood* (3rd ed., pp. 455-494). New York: Wiley & Sons.

Goldstein, A. P. (1991). *Delinquent gangs.* Champaign, IL: Research Press.

Goldstein, A. P., Sprafkin, R. P., Gershaw, N. J., & Klein, P. (1980). *Skillstreaming the adolescent: A structured learning approach to teaching prosocial skills.* Champaign, IL: Research Press.

Guerra, N. G., & Slaby, R. G. (1990). Cognitive mediators of aggression in adolescent offenders: 2. Intervention. *Developmental Psychology, 26,* 269-277.

Henggeler, S. (1988). *Delinquency in adolescence.* Newark Park, CA: Sage.

Horne, A. M. (1989). *Therapist termination report.* Unpublished document. Athens, University of Georgia.

Horne, A. M., & Sayger, T. V. (1989b). *Parent rating form.* Unpublished document. Athens: University of Georgia.

Horne, A. M., & Sayger, T. V. (1990). *Treating conduct and oppositional defiant disorders in children.* New York: Pergamon.

Horne, A., Norsworthy, K., Forehand, R., & Frame, C. (1990). *A delinquency prevention program.* Unpublished manuscript. Athens: University of Georgia.

Kazdin, A. (1987). *Conduct disorders in childhood and adolescence.* Newbury Park, CA: Sage.

Kazdin, A. E., Bass, D., Siegel, T., & Thomas, C. (1989). Cognitive-behavioral therapy and relationship therapy in the treatment of children referred for antisocial behavior. *Journal of Consulting and Clinical Psychology, 57,* 522-535.

Kazdin, A. E., Esveldt-Dawson, K., French, N. H., & Unis, A. S. (1987). Problem-solving skills training and relationship therapy in the treatment of antisocial child behavior. *Journal of Consulting and Clinical Psychology, 55,* 76-85.

Kelley, M. L. (1989). *School-home notes: A behavioral intervention for parents and teachers.* New York: Guilford.

Kovacs, M. (1981). Rating scales to assess depression in school-aged children. *Acta Paedopsychiatrica, 46,* 305-315.

Kovacs, M., Paulauskas, S., Gatsonis, C., & Richards, C. (1988). A longitudinal study of comorbidity with and risk for conduct disorders. *Journal of Affective Disorders, 15,* 205-217.

Lahey, B. B., Hartdagen, S. E., Frick, P. J., & McBurnett, K. (1988). Parsing the confounded relation to parental divorce and antisocial personality. *Journal of Abnormal Psychology, 97,* 334-337.

Lewis, J., Beavers, W., Gossett, J., & Phillips, V. (1976). *No single thread: Psychological health in family systems.* New York: Brunner/Mazel.

Lochman, J. E., Burch, P. R., Curry, J. F., & Lampron, L. B. (1984). Treatment and generalization effects of cognitive-behavioral and goal-setting interventions with aggressive boys. *Journal of Consulting and Clinical Psychology, 52,* 915-916.

Lochman, J. E., & Curry, J. F. (1986). Effects of social problem-solving training and self-instruction training with aggressive boys. *Journal of Clinical Child Psychology, 15,* 159-164.

Locke, H., & Wallace, K. (1959). Short marital-adjustment and prediction tests: Their reliability and validity. *Marriage and Family Living, 21,* 251–255.

MacMillan, D. L., & Kavale, K. A. (1986). Educational intervention. In H. C. Quay & J. S. Werry (Eds.), *Psychopathological disorders of childhood* (3rd ed., pp. 583–621). New York: Wiley.

Marriago, K., Fine, S., Moretti, M., & Haley, G. (1986). Relationship between depression and conduct disorder in children and adolescents. *Journal of the American Academy of Child Psychiatry, 25,* 687–691.

Martin, R. (1988). *Assessment of personality and behavior problems.* New York: Guilford.

Matson, J. L., & Ollendick, T. H. (1988). *Enhancing children's social skills: Assessment and training.* Elmsford, NY: Pergamon.

McMahon, R., & Forehand, R. (1988). Conduct disorder. In E. J. Mash & L. G. Terdal (Eds.), *Behavioral assessment of childhood disorders* (2nd ed., pp. 105–153). New York: Guilford.

McMahon, R., Forehand, R., & Griest, D. (1981). Effects of knowledge of social learning principles on enhancing treatment outcome and generalization in a parent training program. *Journal of Consulting and Clinical Psychology, 49,* 526–532.

Moos, R. H. (1974). *Preliminary manual for family, work, and group environment scales.* Palo Alto, CA: Consulting Psychologists.

Moos, R. H., & Moos, B. S. (1984). *Family environment scale manual.* Palo Alto, CA: Consulting Psychologists.

Nickerson, M., Light, R., Blechman, E., & Gandelman, B. (Eds.). (1976, Winter). Three measures of problem solving behavior: A procedural manual. *JSAS Catalog of Selected Documents in Psychology* (Ms. No. 1190).

Ollendick, T., & Hersen, M. (1984). *Child behavior assessment.* New York: Pergamon.

Patterson, G. (1982). *Coercive family process.* Eugene, OR: Castalia.

Patterson, G. (1986). Performance models for antisocial boys. *American Psychologist, 41,* 432–444.

Patterson, G., Reid, J., Jones, R., & Conger, R. (1975). *A social learning approach to family intervention.*

Vol. I: Families with aggressive children. Eugene, OR: Castalia.

Pino, C., Simons, N., & Slawinowski, M. J. (1984). *The Children's Version of the Family Environment Scale Manual.* East Aurora, NY: Slosson Educational Publications.

Prinz, R., Conner, P., & Wilson, C. (1981). Hyperactive and aggressive behaviors in childhood: Intertwined dimensions. *Journal of Abnormal Child Psychology, 9,* 287–295.

Reeves, J. C., Werry, J. S., Elkind, G. S., & Zametkin, A. (1987). Attention deficit, conduct, oppositional, and anxiety disorders in children: II. Clinical characteristics. *Journal of the American Academy of Child and Adolescent Psychiatry, 26*(2), 144–155.

Sayger, T. V., Horne, A. M., Passmore, J. L., & Walker, J. M. (1988). Social learning family therapy with aggressive children: Treatment outcome and maintenance. *Journal of Family Psychology, 1*(3), 261–285.

Siassi, I. (1982). Lithium treatment of impulsive behavior in children. *Journal of Clinical Psychiatry, 43,* 482–484.

Spanier, G. B. (1979). The measurement of marital quality. *Journal of Sex and Marital Therapy, 5,* 288–300.

Spanier, G. B., & Thompson, L. (1982). A confirmatory analysis of the dyadic adjustment scale. *Journal of Marriage and the Family, 44,* 731–738.

Stumphauzer, J. (1973). *Behavior therapy with delinquents.* Springfield, IL: Thomas.

Walker, J., Lahey, B. B., Hynd, G., & Frame, C. (1987). Comparison of specific patterns of antisocial behavior in children with conduct disorder with or without coexisting hyperactivity. *Journal of Consulting and Clinical Psychology, 55,* 910–913.

Werry, J. S., Reeves, J. C., & Elkind, G. S. (1987). Attention deficit, conduct, oppositional, and anxiety disorders in children: A review of research on differentiating characteristics. *Journal of the American Academy of Child and Adolescent Psychiatry, 26*(2), 133–143.

Wilson, J. Q., & Herrnstein, R. J. (1985). *Crime and human nature.* New York: Simon & Schuster.

CHAPTER 7

OPPOSITIONAL DEFIANT DISORDER

Edward R. Christophersen   University of Missouri-Kansas City School of Medicine

Jack W. Finney   Virginia Polytechnic Institute and State University

DESCRIPTION OF DISORDER

Clinical and Associated Features

The development of children includes many optimal behaviors (e.g., speech, language, motor skills) and at times many nonoptimal behaviors (e.g., noncompliance, tantrums, aggression, and other disruptive behaviors). A collection of nonoptimal behavior problems may persist and lead to a diagnosis of oppositional defiant disorder (ODD; American Psychiatric Association, 1987). The diagnosis reflects that the child's disruptive behaviors have exceeded the duration, intensity, and/or severity of these behaviors in children of similar developmental age who are considered to be displaying normal levels.

Children with ODD are frequently identified in the health system and represent a significant proportion of children and adolescents who are receiving mental health services (Finney, Riley, & Cataldo, 1991). ODD, even when identified and treated early, often is associated with, but is not always predictive of, more serious disruptive behavior and psychiatric diagnoses in later phases of development (Baum, 1989; Robins, 1966).

ODD generally begins in the early to middle grade-school years and will have developed by early adolescence; its onset, however, is variable within this age range. As oppositional behavior as a symptom is relatively common in the preschool-age range, especially around the age of 3, care must be taken to distinguish this normal oppositional behavior from a disorder. However, persistence of oppositional behavior for an extended period of time in the preschool-age range may indicate that the disorder is present.

Epidemiology

Epidemiological studies of disruptive behavior disorders generally and ODD specifically are incomplete. Using a number of different measures of children's behavior problems and several different definitions for conduct problems, conduct disorders, juvenile delinquency, ODD, and attention deficit disorder, investigators have reported estimates of prevalence of disruptive behavior ranging from 3.4 to 8.7 percent (Anderson, Williams, McGee, & Silva, 1987; Kashani et al., 1987; Offord, Adler, & Boyle, 1986; Rutter,

Tizard, & Whitmore, 1970). Disruptive behaviors are not only relatively prevalent but they also account for a large portion of children who are referred for mental health services. Improved epidemiological studies that provide information on the prevalence of all disruptive behavior disorders, and studies that provide information on different diagnostic definitions of the disorders (e.g., Lahey et al., 1990) are needed to provide more accurate prevalence estimates.

Etiology

Family, biological and biochemical, and individual psychological factors have been associated with conduct problems in children and adolescents (Quay, 1986b), and all may play a role in the etiology of ODD. While these correlates have been identified in a number of studies, additional evidence for their contribution to the etiology of ODD is needed.

DIFFERENTIAL DIAGNOSIS AND ASSESSMENT

DSM-III-R Categorization

ODD is characterized by hostility, negativistic behavior, and defiant behavior. It includes a pattern of disobedience and negativism, often described as temper tantrums, argumentativeness, and stubbornness (Cantwell, 1989b). The behavior must be chronic (at least 6 months in duration), manifested by violation of minor rules, temper tantrums, asrgumentative and provocative behavior, and stubbornness. However, the disorder is not to be considered secondary to another mental disorder, whether internalizing or externalizing. The *Diagnostic and Statistical Manual, Third Edition Revised* (American Psychiatric Association, 1987) emphasizes a negativistic, hostile, and defiant pattern of behavior. It is below the level of the serious violations of an individual's basic rights that are associated with conduct disorder. Problem behaviors of oppositional defiant disorder, however, are greater than the normal oppositional behavior that is often displayed across

the developmental period, including the opposition of normal children between 18 and 36 months of age and some adolescent rebellion that often occurs during the adolescent years.

Children with oppositional defiant disorder have problems controlling their temper, arguing, and cursing; they appear to be angry, spiteful, resentful, touchy, and easily annoyed; and they may be described by other children as being bullies or mean (Cantwell, 1989b). Oppositional behavior is often setting specific, occurring more often with parents and other familiar adults (e.g., teachers, sitters) with whom the child has frequent contact (Cantwell, 1989b).

Differential Diagnosis

The behavioral features of ODD may be present in a number of children with conduct disorder, a psychotic disorder, or depressive disorder, but each of these diagnoses preempts the diagnosis of ODD. ODD may be present, however, with attention-deficit hyperactivity disorder. Quay (1986a) has suggested that the diagnosis of oppositional disorder is not distinguished in multivariate studies of children. Thus, current clinical uses of this diagnosis are based mostly on the lack of repetitive aggressive patterns of violating others' rights and violating social norms or rules. The diagnosis of conduct disorder is reserved for children whose oppositional, antisocial behavior is severe and persistent. Thus, many children have conduct-problem behaviors. A smaller number will have a time-limited clinical problem, diagnosable but not persistent, at some point in their lives. A smaller number of children will have a distinct conduct disorder that has persisted over time (Cantwell, 1989a).

Assessment Strategies

Behavioral assessment for a child and family has been categorized previously (e.g., Hawkins, 1979; Mash & Terdal, 1988) to include several overlapping functions: (1) determining the problem behaviors for which services are being sought and the directions for further assessments, (2) defining the child's and family's problems and assigning diagnostic labels, (3) formulating a treatment plan based on the conceptualization of the problems, (4) evaluating the effectiveness of treatment and reformulating the plan when progress is not optimal, and (5) evaluating the long-term outcomes of treatment. To implement these assessment functions, clinicians have been advised to use multimethod assessment strategies (Ollendick & Hersen, 1984).

Clinicians gather information in a variety of ways. They interview the child, the parent, and, when appropriate, the child's siblings, teachers, peers, and others who have meaningful contact with the child. Parents and teachers (and older children and adolescents) complete behavioral checklists to provide quantified measures of the child's internalizing and externalizing behavior problems. Direct observations are made, often in an analogue setting, but less often in a home or school setting. Monitoring may be requested of an older child, or parents and teachers may be asked to keep detailed records of child behavior, situational variables associated with problems, and interventions that are in place while the assessment process is completed. It is also important to consider the utility of more traditional standardized intelligence, achievement, and personality tests to assist with identification of other possibly relevant problems and to help formulate a diagnosis. These and other sources of information provide the data with which clinicians formulate a treatment plan for children with ODD.

Interviewing

The assessment process begins with an interview. Interviews may be conducted with the parent or child alone, and subsequently the clinician may wish to interview the family together. Several content areas can be addressed. La Greca (1983) delineates the referral problem, interests, school, peers, family, fears/worries, self-image, moods/feelings, somatic concerns, thought disorder, aspirations, and fantasy for most children, and heterosexual relations, sex, and drug/alcohol use for adolescents. A behavioral interview will also elicit descriptive information from the parent and child about situations of relevance for current behavior problems, apparent antecedents that regularly precede episodes of problem behavior, child (and parent) characteristics that might be important contributors to the problem, and likely consequences that may be maintaining or exacerbating problem behaviors (see Cormier & Cormier, 1985, for a detailed discussion of behavioral interviewing). For children with ODD, the interview process seeks to identify parental child-rearing practices that may be deficient or misguided (Kazdin, 1985; Patterson, 1986). Although interviewing will not provide all needed information, it is the beginning of the assessment process designed to identify both child, parent, and family characteristics that contribute to antisocial behavior (Patterson, 1982).

Behavioral Checklists

Several standardized behavioral checklists or rating scales are available for completion by the parent or teacher of a client, and at least one checklist to be completed by the adolescent client has some promise for the assessment of children with disruptive behavior disorders. A parent may complete the Child Behavior Checklist (CBCL), which provides a range of scores (e.g., internalizing, externalizing, total behavior problems, subscale scores) for children of particular age ranges by sex (Achenbach & Edelbrock, 1983). The Teacher's Report Form and the Youth Self-Report Form of the CBCL provide similar indices of behavior problems (Achenbach & Edelbrock, 1986, 1987). Other behavioral checklists are also available for use with children being evaluated for behavior problems, including the Revised Behavior Problem Checklist (RBPC; Quay & Peterson, 1983) and the Eyberg Child Behavior Inventory (ECBI; Eyberg & Ross, 1978). Furthermore, the Conners Parent Rating Scale and Teacher Rating Scale (Goyette, Conners, & Ulrich, 1978) are often used, particularly when children's problems are suspected to include features of more than one disruptive behavior disorder (e.g., ODD and ADHD) (McMahon & Forehand, 1988).

In many cases, getting assessment input from the child's preschool or school can be beneficial in determining whether the child is oppositional or presents with more serious problems. The Conner's Parent Symptom Questionnaire is standardized down to 2 years of age and the CBCL can be scored for 2- to 3-year-olds, 4- to 5-year-olds, and 6- to 16-year-olds. The Teacher's CBCL is for children 6 years of age and older, but the parent form can often be used with toddlers and preschoolers, particularly those in home daycare. For toddlers and preschoolers, the daycare staff can often be given the same recommendations that are given to the parents.

The Home and School Situations Questionnaires assess how behavior problems may vary across a range of common situations (Barkley & Edelbrock, 1987). These short checklists, completed by a parent or teacher, provide a structured format for learning about behavioral variation across situations. This situational information may suggest which situations are most problematic, or conversely may suggest situational characteristics associated with low rates of problem behaviors.

Behavioral and situational checklists provide a "current" description of parents' perceptions of children's conduct and other behavioral problems, as well as provide a means for repeated assessment during and after treatment. Behavioral checklists, however, do not provide specific and detailed information on dimensions of problem behaviors that may be necessary for developing a treatment formulation. For this information, clinicians often turn to direct observation and self-monitoring.

Direct Observation

Direct observation by the behavioral clinician is almost always conducted in a therapeutic setting. A parent and child are routinely observed during an interview and clinical impressions are used to make decisions about parent and child behaviors that might be changed, for example, to improve communication and the parent-child relationship and/or to reduce conflict and inappropriate parental management styles (Parpal & Maccoby, 1985). Parents may be instructed to make a series of age-appropriate requests of their children and both parent (e.g., rewards, attends, alpha and beta commands) and child behaviors (e.g., compliance, non-compliance, tantrums, aggressive behaviors) are measured (Forehand & McMahon, 1981). Similar parent and child behaviors can be viewed from a coercive family interaction model, which is proposed to develop from early parental mismanagement that escalates into self-perpetuating coercive exchanges (Patterson, 1982). Parents and their older children may be instructed to engage in a problem-solving discussion to allow for observation of communication styles (Foster & Robin, 1988; Robin & Weiss, 1980).

Direct observation in the home and school by the clinician is less common, but structured observation and recording by others is recommended frequently (Forehand & McMahon, 1981). Major dimensions of problem behavior (frequency, duration, intensity, latency) are often specified and data sheets or diaries are prescribed for parents, teachers, and others with regular interaction with children.

Selection of target behaviors for children with ODD and their families may often be made in the absence of empirical validation. This situation is not unique to disruptive behavior disorders, but is common to most areas of behavioral assessment and treatment (Cone, 1980; Hawkins, 1986; Weist, Ollendick, & Finney, 1991). Use of multimethod assessments, and their convergence on common problem behaviors, provides the clinician with indications of problem behaviors that are important targets for change. A range of validation strategies have been proposed by Weist and colleagues (1991), including (1) the selection of behaviors for change based on well-designed assessment and outcome studies of populations similar to the client being served, (2) the use of available normative data against which to compare the child's and family's behavior, and (3) the use of template matching strategies (Cone, 1980; Cone & Hoier, 1986), which consist of the delineation of behavioral targets idiographically matched to the client and situation. Further attention to target selection issues for ODD will identify currently ignored behavior problems and family process issues associated with disorder, as well as establish the validity of the target behaviors and their associated long-term outcomes.

TREATMENT

Evidence for Prescriptive Treatment

Behavior Therapy

Approaches to children's behavior problems (e.g., opposition, noncompliance, tantrums) have been dominated by learning-based treatment and cognitive-behavioral techniques (Kazdin, 1985). A behavioral conceptualization of oppositional defiant disorder views disruptive behaviors as excesses to be decreased (either in frequency, duration, intensity, etc.), and deficient (or absent) adaptive behaviors such as compliance, academic performance, and social skills to be increased in similar dimensions. It has been proposed that early parental mismanagement of children's behavior fails to establish children's compliance, and continued parent demands, child noncompliance, and the child's attempts to avoid continued parent demands and interactions through aggressive exchanges results in a coercive family process (Patterson, 1982). Treatment approaches often differ across developmental periods, with a greater focus on parent training at younger ages and additional attention to the development of interpersonal skills and relationships with others at older ages.

Parent training. Teaching parents improved behavior management techniques is a mainstay of behavior therapy for oppositional children (Patterson, 1982). With young children, parent training often focuses on differential attention for compliance and other desired behaviors, ignoring problem behaviors when possible, and time out for misbehaviors such as noncompliance and tantrums (Christophersen, 1988). Changing parent behaviors that serve as antecedents, such as vague or nagging ways that parents give instructions to their children, and providing structured learning opportunities for techniques of differential attention (The Child's and Parent's Games) provide a curriculum for clinic-based assessment and treatment (Forehand & McMahon, 1981). Other programs use token economy programs to help structure the parents use of reinforcement and response

cost/punishment techniques to change their children's problem behaviors (Christophersen, Barnard, & Barnard, 1981).

There have been several major approaches to parent training for dealing with oppositional behaviors, and these approaches are similar in the procedures that they incorporate. Schaefer and Millman (1982) use a "cookbook" approach, in that they discuss specific behavior problems, give suggestions as to how the problem got started in the first place, and then provide a variety of possible solutions for each problem. Forehand and McMahon (1981) take a similar approach, although they also discuss more general interaction patterns between parent and child. Christophersen (1988) discusses general parent-child interaction, then, in a separate section of the book, provides "cookbook" solutions to common behavior problems. For the most part, these books take the same approach, with minor variations, to educating parents on how to manage their children.

Therapist-directed groups (Rickert et al., 1988) and discussion groups with videotaped modeling of parenting skills can be an effective format for parent training (Webster-Stratton, Kolpacoff, & Hollinsworth, 1988). In addition to clinic-based outpatient services, parent training is often conducted in hospital-based outpatient clinics (Charlop, Parrish, Fenton, & Cataldo, 1987), primary health care clinics (Finney et al., 1991; Kanoy & Schroeder, 1985), and in a small-group continuing education format (Christophersen, Barrish, Barrish, & Christophersen, 1984). Numerous parent training programs and curricula have been developed, and a wide selection of parent training approaches have been summarized (Barkley, 1981; Daniel & Polster, 1984; Schaefer & Briesmeister, 1989).

Several events may lead to more intensive therapeutic approaches. The child matures and engages in an ever-widening range of activities and settings requiring the development of more sophisticated socialization skills (Maccoby & Martin, 1983). One of the major concerns about children with oppositional behavior is that their problems may worsen and their families may become more dysfunctional (Patterson, 1986). Parents may be insular, isolated from appropriate support systems within which to learn and provide appropriate child rearing (Dumas & Wahler, 1983; Wahler, 1980).

Anger control for adolescents. Anger control has also been viewed as an important goal for children and adolescents with conduct and oppositional defiant disorders. Feindler and colleagues (Feindler, 1987; Feindler & Ecton, 1986; Feindler, Ecton, Kingsley, & Dubey, 1986) have developed the Art of Self-Control Program, which uses a self-regulatory, coping-skills approach to teach adolescents to moderate, regulate, and prevent anger and aggression and to use problem-solving strategies to avoid escalation in provoking situations. Feindler's anger-control approach is based on Meichenbaum's (1985) stress inoculation training approach. Structured sessions involve (1) self-monitoring of anger and its associated cognitive, behavioral, and physiological components; (2) relaxation and deep breathing techniques; (3) coping self-statements; (4) self-reinforcement strategies; (5) assertiveness; and (6) problem-solving skills training (Feindler, 1987). Modeling, roleplaying, social reinforcement, and feedback techniques are used to foster anger-control skills. Outcome studies show that anger-control training is effective in producing more appropriate reactions to provocations and reducing arousal and anger behaviors, but additional evaluation of generalization and maintenance is needed to determine the range of outcomes for conduct-disordered and oppositional adolescents.

Barrish and Barrish (1989) have adapted the cognitive behavior modification approach for use by parents. Similar to Feindler's Art of Self-Control program, they recommend a stop-think-act approach to anger control that can be utilized by the parents and by the child. They discuss the importance of substituting "helpful thoughts" for "hurtful thoughts."

Out-of-home treatment. Out-of-home treatment of oppositional behavior is rarely needed, but such treatment may be used as a respite program for parents by removing the child from patterns of interaction that reinforce the oppositional behavior (Cantwell, 1989b). With increasingly tighter monitoring by third-party-payers, children with just oppositional behavior are much less likely to be approved for hospitalization.

Parent training and child-focused cognitive-behavioral treatment can be effective for reducing oppositional defiant disorders. These interventions have limitations. The case has been made for early intervention, regardless of mode or setting of therapy, to prevent the development of more severe conduct problems as the child matures (Patterson, 1982). Controlled evaluation of early intervention for oppositional behaviors is needed to show if, in fact, the association of early externalizing problems to later disruptive behavior disorders and antisocial personality disorders can be reduced.

Pharmacotherapy

Cantwell has stated:

> Pharmacotherapy has not been found effective, in general, for children with oppositional defiant disorder or for children with oppositional defiant disorder combined with or resulting from an underlying conduct disorder. However, children with ADHD with oppositional defiant disorder may benefit from some types of psychopharmacological intervention, including stimulants or tricyclic antidepressants. (1989b, p. 1844)

Cantwell (1989b) also stated that pharmacotherapy should never be used as the sole treatment for a child or adolescent with oppositional defiant disorder or oppositional defiant disorder combined with or resulting from an underlying conduct disorder. However, children with ADHD with oppositional defiant disorder may benefit from some types of psychopharmacological intervention, including stimulants or tricyclic antidepressants. When a drug is prescribed, it should be prescribed only in conjunction with psychological interventions. In the case of children and most adolescents, psychological interventions almost always include parental involvement. The prescription of multiple medications is not indicated for children and adolescents. There is no evidence, in children and adolescents, that the combination of two psychoactive drugs is more effective and safer than a single drug.

Psychoactive drugs are often prescribed to children and adolescents in the hope that the drug will make the patient more amenable to psychological treatments. It has been said that the only lasting effects of pharmacotherapy are due to concurrent psychological treatments. However, very little research has been done in this area.

Alternative Treatments

Family therapy may be of use when the child is enmeshed in a negative family system. However, family therapy, while possibly effective in dealing with a dysfunctional family, has not been investigated specifically for children with ODD. While it is likely that many families of children with ODD may benefit from a family therapy approach, experimental evidence for its effectiveness is needed.

Selecting Optimal Treatment Stratgegies

The decision of which treatment strategy to use with oppositional defiant disorder is simplified by the fact that medication is useful only in cases where the child presents with symptoms in addition to those associated with oppositional defiant disorder, such as ADHD, and the fact that inpatient hospitalization is rarely appropriate with this diagnosis. Thus, the therapist must decide what procedures, in addition to parent training, may be necessary or indicated.

Problems in Carrying Out Interventions

The most commonly encountered problem in dealing with oppositional defiant disorder is noncompliance on the parents' part. As Patterson (1982) has pointed out, some parents get into a coercive cycle where their coercive behavior produces coercive behavior on the child's part which, in turn, leads to further coercive behavior on the parents' part. Breaking this cycle is sometimes difficult. Also, when dealing with oppositional defiant disorder, whether the oppositional behavior

is dealt with directly (e.g., with discipline) or less directly (e.g., with ignoring), there is sometimes an escalation in the child's oppositional behavior prior to a decrease (Drabman & Jarvie, 1977). This initial increase is sometimes a cause for concern for the parents if they have not been prepared for it in advance.

Relapse Prevention

Three strategies for relapse prevention that we use in our office are: (1) in vivo demonstrations of the procedures with the child for the benefit of both the parent and the child, (2) written summaries of our treatment recommendations that are given to parents at the end of each clinic visit (Christophersen, 1988), and (3) a 24-hour treatment hot line for parents who have children currently in treatment.

CASE ILLUSTRATION

David has been followed since birth by a pediatrician. When the mother brought David in for his 2-year well-child visit, his mother told the pediatrician that she was beginning to have some behavior problems with him. The pediatrician assured her that this was probably just the "terrible two's" and recommended that she try to wait it out. By the time David was 3½ years old, his mother had phoned the pediatrician three times with questions about his noncompliant and often obnoxious behaviors. With the third phone call, the pediatrician recommended that the mother make an appointment in Behavioral Pediatrics for an evaluation and recommendations regarding behavior management. When David's mother phoned to schedule her appointment, she was advised that several parent report forms would be mailed to her to be filled out and brought with her for the first appointment. These included a General Intake Form, a Conners Parent Symptom Questionnaire, and a Parent CBCL. When they arrived for their appointment, David's mother was asked for the report forms, which were scored by the receptionist, while she waited briefly for her scheduled appointment.

Case Description

David is a 3½-year-old boy, whose parents complain that he will not do what he is told, who has temper tantrums when he does not get his way, blames others for his mistakes, and gets angry and resentful when he does not get his way. His was the product of a normal, full-term pregnancy and labor and delivery with no remarkable childhood diseases. Both of his parents are in good health and gainfully employed as professionals. The General Intake Form revealed that the problems with David were of greater than 6 months' duration and that none of the family members was under any unusual stress beyond that which stemmed from David's oppositional behavior.

Differential Diagnosis and Assessment

Both the Conners and CBCL suggested that David was a behavior problem. On the Conners, he scored high for behavior problems but within the normal range, for his age, on hyperactivity, learning problems, psychosomatic problems, and nervous/overactive. On the CBCL, he scored high on aggressive, but was within normal limits on somatic complaints, delinquency, depression, and anxiety. By history, David was able to concentrate for at least 30 minutes to one hour, was not unusually distractible, did not have any trouble remaining seated for any length of time, was not unusually noisy in his play, did not talk too much, and could wait his turn in games with his mom or his dad. These symptoms all helped to rule out attention-deficit hyperactivity disorder at this time. Since he was not unusually cruel to people or animals, did not steal or set fires, and respected the rights of others it was also unlikely that he was presenting with a conduct disorder. There also was no history in either family of either ADHD or any personality disorders. It was clear that he met diagnostic criteria for ODD.

During the first office visit, David was observed to misbehave almost continuously, with no real evidence of rule-governed behavior. His mother almost constantly warned him that he was going to get into trouble if he kept up that type of behavior. He opened drawers in the exam room, got out toys, climbed on furniture, and generally did whatever he desired. Neither his mother nor his father ever actually disciplined him during this visit, preferring, instead, to warn and reprimand him repeatedly. His mother commented during the interview, on several occasions, "See, that's the kind of behavior I'm talking about—that's the kind of thing he does all of the time at home." Interestingly, the parents reported that, although the preschool teacher said that David was "all boy," she did not report any remarkable problems with him.

During the history, neither parent reported many activities that they enjoyed with David. Most of their interaction with him consisted of routine home care, errands, and the like. There did not appear to be much quality time with David. The father did report that David "loved to roughhouse, although he didn't know when to stop." It was determined that the father seemed to enjoy playing rough with David, even at times when the mother said that such playing made her nervous and when she asked that they "not to that in the house."

Treatment Selection

After some discussion with his parents, it was decided that both parents needed much more effective child management strategies. David, without any history consistent with ADHD, was not really a candidate for any medication. It was decided, in conjunction with both parents, to work on some behavior management skills at home.

Initially, both parents were instructed in the use of "time in." This was interesting since the therapist began using brief, nonverbal, physical contact with David during the office visit, including a period of 5 to 10 minutes talking to the parents while David played on the floor with some toys, and he appeared to "calm down" readily. He appeared to be very responsive to the brief, physical contact. While playing with David, the therapist pointed out directly, and by way of examples, the importance of refraining from reprimanding and warning David when he misbehaved.

There was a discussion about the futility of trying to change the child's behavior by lecturing and/or reasoning with him. The parents admitted that, although these methods had not worked for them, they did not know what else to do with him. They said that they were a little confused. If David was not behaving like they wanted him to, how would he ever know that he was supposed to change if they didn't tell him. It was explained to the parents that David was simply too young with which to reason. The parents admitted that they had thought this a number of times, particularly when they were trying to reason with him, but they also admitted that they had read a book that recommended that they share their feelings with David and that they let him know how his behavior was affecting his parents.

The therapist explained the need for really high-quality "time in," as well as the need to refrain from any aggressive play with David. The mother appeared relieved that the therapist had addressed the aggressive in-house play. After some further discussion, the appointment was terminated, with a followup appointment scheduled for the next week. The parents were provided with written handouts on the time-in technique, cognitive development as it relates to discipline, and reducing aggressive behavior in the home.

At the second office visit, the parents reported that time in appeared to be working with David and that he was playing more calmly and seemed to be enjoying himself more. They also reported no decrease in his temper tantrums or his demanding behavior. The father did report that he had not played roughly with David all week long. The therapist initiated a discussion about the use of time out for behavior infractions. A lengthy discussion ensued, after which the therapist demonstrated the use of time out with David several times. He was able to quiet down in time out pretty readily, with the therapist distracting them in order to keep them from attending to David's acting out during these brief time outs. At the end of the discussion, the parents were given written handouts on the use of time out with toddlers and scheduled for a return appointment two weeks later. They were also asked to provide the preschool teacher with a copy of the written hand-

outs on time in, cognitive development, and time out.

Treatment Course and Problems in Carrying Out Interventions

The parents reported that they had seen a pretty dramatic improvement in David's behavior after they began to implement the time-out procedures. But they both stated that they found it difficult to completely ignore him when he was supposed to be in time out. They felt that David did not understand that he needed to be quiet in order to get up from time out — so they had been reminding him that he needed to be quiet in time out. This usually resulted in David stating that he "didn't have to go to time out if he didn't want to" and that "they couldn't make him stay in time out." There was further discussion with the parents about the importance of the contrast between time in and time out, and that they were only feeding David's obnoxious behavior each time they talked to him in time out. Indeed, it was pointed out that time out was not being implemented if they were talking to him. They asked, "you mean that we aren't even supposed to talk to him when he acts up during a time out." The therapist reiterated the rules for the use of time out and initiated a discussion about helpful and hurtful self-talking. After some discussion, the parents stated that they thought that they understood better now what time out was all about and that the self-talking discussion could be very beneficial to them. They were given a written handout on parent coping skills, which is primarily a discussion about helpful/hurtful self-talking.

The treatment course was unremarkable. The family returned for their third office appointment and reported that David was much better behaved, that he would now go to time out when he was asked to, that he was self-quieting much better, and that several family friends had even made unsolicited comments about how much better behaved he was. One friend even asked the mother what they were doing differently. The preschool teacher also stated that David seemed to be "calmer now."

Outcome and Termination

After the third office appointment, it was mutually decided that the family did not need to return. A followup appointment was recommended 6 weeks later, with the understanding that the followup appointment would be canceled if David was continuing to behave better. They did, in fact, cancel the followup appointment, telling the receptionist that David was continuing to do very well.

Followup and Maintenance

The outcomes of treatment of psychological problems may be considered limited if children and their parents later seek additional services. However, medical services for acute and chronic illnesses may be needed repeatedly over a number of months or years (Riley, Finney, & Cataldo, 1987), and this repeated use of services is not considered a limitation of the medical treatment. For common behavior problems and more serious disorders, the need for periodic, psychological services should be considered an expected course of events. As the child, parent, and family mature, they may be faced with new situations, novel stressors, and age-specific behavior problems. The necessary changes for a family to accommodate these new developments may be facilitated by additional psychological services. Clinicians may wish to encourage parents to routinely schedule a one-year followup appointment for discussion of parenting strategies useful for their developing child.

SUMMARY

The vast majority of uncomplicated cases of oppositional defiant disorder can be managed in 2 to 3 office visits, provided of course that the parents are able to implement the treatment recommendations and that they do not have any unusual stressors in their lives. Use of office demonstrations and written handouts summarizing the treatment recommendations have significantly improved parental compliance and treatment outcome. This finding is consistent with the literature on medical compliance (Christophersen, Finney, & Friman, 1986).

Early intervention for children's conduct problems is likely to be more effective than later treatment for older adolescents' and adults' antisocial behaviors. At present, there are no studies documenting this assertion. In fact, it appears incredibly difficult, if not impossible, to design such a comparative study.

Oppositional defiant disorder involves a variety of noncompliant, aggressive, and negativistic behaviors that have been assessed with clinical interviews, rating scales, direct observation, and self-report measures. Similar techniques are used with adults, but content of the assessment is consistent with developmental differences between children and adults.

Treatment of children's behavior problems has been approached from parent training as well as child-focused and residential group home perspectives. These treatment approaches produce significant improvements in children's behavior, but children with ODD often are rated as having clinical problems after treatment when compared with nonclinical peers. Disruptive behavior disorders in children and adolescents have received considerably more attention than the treatment of related adult behavior disorders. Pharmacological therapies are of limited effectiveness for children's behavior disorders, and in general are only appropriate when used in conjunction with psychological therapy.

REFERENCES

Achenbach, T. M., & Edelbrock, C. (1983). *Manual for the Child Behavior Checklist and Revised Child Behavior Profile.* Burlington: Department of Psychiatry, University of Vermont.

Achenbach, T. M., & Edelbrock, C. (1986). *Manual for the Teacher's Report Form and Teacher Version of the Child Behavior Profile.* Burlington: Department of Psychiatry, University of Vermont.

Achenbach, T. M., & Edelbrock, C. (1987). *Manual for the Youth Self-Report Profile.* Burlington: Department of Psychiatry, University of Vermont.

American Psychiatric Association. (1987). *Diagnostic and statistical manual of mental disorders* (3rd ed., rev.). Washington, DC: Author.

Anderson, J. C., Williams, S., McGee, R., & Silva, P. A. (1987). DSM-III disorders in preadolescent children: Prevalence in a large sample from the general population. *Archives of General Psychiatry, 44,* 69–76.

Barkley, R. A. (1981). *Hyperactive children: A handbook for diagnosis and treatment.* New York: Guilford.

Barkley, R. A., & Edelbrock, C. (1987). Assessing situational variation in children's problem behaviors: The Home and School Situations Questionnaires. In R. J. Prinz (Ed.), *Advances in behavioral assessment of children and families* (Vol. 3, pp. 157–176). Greenwich, CT: JAI Press.

Barrish, H. H., & Barrish, I. J. (1989). *Managing parental anger* (2nd ed.). Kansas City, MO: Westport Publishers.

Baum, C. G. (1989). Conduct disorders. In T. H. Ollendick & M. Hersen (Eds.), *Handbook of child psychopathology* (2nd ed., pp. 171–196). New York: Plenum.

Cantwell, D. P. (1989a). Conduct disorder. In H. I. Kaplan & B. J. Sadock (Eds.), *Comprehensive textbook of psychiatry* (5th ed., pp. 1821–1828). Baltimore: Williams & Wilkins.

Cantwell, D. P. (1989b). Oppositional defiant disorder. In H. I. Kaplan & B. J. Sadock (Eds.), *Comprehensive textbook of psychiatry* (5th ed., pp. 1842–1845). Baltimore: Williams & Wilkins.

Charlop, M. H., Parrish, J. M., Fenton, L. R., & Cataldo, M. F. (1987). Evaluation of hospital-based outpatient pediatric psychology services. *Journal of Pediatric Psychology, 12,* 485–503.

Christophersen, E. R. (1988). *Little people: Guidelines for commonsense child rearing* (3rd ed.). Kansas City, MO: Westport Publishers.

Christophersen, E. R. (1990). *Beyond discipline: Parenting that lasts a lifetime.* Kansas City, MO: Westport Publishers.

Christophersen, E. R., Barnard, S. R., & Barnard, J. D. (1981). The Family Training Program manual: The home chip system. In R. A. Barkley (Ed.), *Hyperactive children: A handbook for diagnosis and treatment* (Appendix B, pp. 437–448). New York: Guilford.

Christophersen, E. R., Barrish, I. J., Barrish, H. H., & Christophersen, M. R. (1984). Continuing education for parent of infants and toddlers. In R. F. Dangel & R. A. Polster (Eds.), *Parent training: Foundations of research and practice* (pp. 127–143). New York: Guilford.

Christophersen, E. R., Finney, J. W., & Friman, P. C. (1986). Medical compliance in pediatric practice. In N. A. Krasnegor, J. D. Arasteh, & M. F. Cataldo (Eds.), *Child health behavior: A behavioral pediatrics perspective* (pp. 435–452). New York: Wiley.

Cone, J. D. (1980, November). *Template matching procedures for idiographic behavioral assessment.* Paper presented at the meeting of the Association for the Advancement of Behavior Therapy, New York.

Cone, J. D., & Hoier, T. S. (1986). Assessing children: The radical behavioral perspective. In R. J. Prinz (Ed.), *Advances in behavioral assessment of children* (Vol. 2, pp. 1–27). Greenwich, CT: JAI Press.

Cormier, W. H., & Cormier, L. S. (1985). *Interviewing strategies for helpers: Fundamental skills and cognitive behavioral interventions.* Monterey, CA: Brooks/Cole.

Daniel, R. F., & Polster, R. A. (Eds.). (1984). *Parent training: Foundations of research and practice.* New York: Guilford.

Drabman, R. S., & Jarvie, G. (1977). Counselling parents of children with behavior problems: The use of extinction and time-out techniques. *Pediatrics, 59*(1), 78–85.

Dumas, J. E., & Wahler, R. G. (1983). Predictors of treatment outcome in parent training: Mother insularity and socioeconomic disadvantage. *Behavioral Assessment, 5,* 301–313.

Eyberg, S. M., & Ross, A. W. (1978). Assessment of child behavior problems: The validation of a new inventory. *Journal of Clinical Child Psychology, 7,* 113–116.

Feindler, E. L. (1987). Clinical issues and recommendations in adolescent anger-control training. *Journal of Child and Adolescent Psychotherapy, 4,* 267–274.

Feindler, E. L., & Ecton, R. B. (1986). *Adolescent anger control: Cognitive-behavioral techniques.* New York: Pergamon.

Feindler, E. L., Ecton, R. B., Kingsley, D., & Dubey, D. (1986). Group anger control training for institutionalized psychiatric male adolescents. *Behavior Therapy, 17,* 109–123.

Finney, J. W., Riley, A. W., & Cataldo, M. F. (1991). Psychology in primary health care: Effects of brief targeted therapy on children's medical care utilization. *Journal of Pediatric Psychology, 16,* 447–461.

Forehand, R. L., & McMahon, R. J. (1981). *Helping the noncompliant child: A clinician's guide to parent training.* New York: Guilford.

Foster, S. L., & Robin, A. L. (1988). Family conflict and communication in adolescence. In E. J. Mash & L. G. Terdal (Eds.), *Behavioral assessment of childhood disorders* (2nd ed., unabridged, pp. 717–775). New York: Guilford.

Goyette, C. H., Conners, C. K., & Ulrich, R. F. (1978). Normative data on revised Conners Parent and Teacher Rating Scales. *Journal of Abnormal Child Psychology, 6,* 221–236.

Hawkins, R. P. (1979). The functions of assessment: Implications for selection and development of devices for assessing repertoires in clinical, educational, and other settings. *Journal of Applied Behavior Analysis, 12,* 501–516.

Hawkins, R. P. (1986). Selection of target behaviors. In R. O. Nelson & S. C. Hayes (Eds.), *Conceptual foundations of behavioral assessment* (pp. 331–382). New York: Guilford.

Kanoy, K. W., & Schroeder, C. S. (1985). Suggestions to parents about common behavior problems in a pediatric primary care office: Five years of follow-up. *Journal of Pediatric Psychology, 10,* 15–30.

Kashani, J. H., Beck, N. C., Hoeper, E. W., Fallahi, C., Corcoran, C. M., McAllister, J. A., Rosenberg, T. K., & Reid, J. C. (1987). Psychiatric disorders in a community sample of adolescents. *American Journal of Psychiatry, 144,* 584–589.

Kazdin, A. E. (1985). *Treatment of antisocial behavior in children and adolescents.* Homewood, IL: Dorsey.

La Greca, A. M. (1983). Interviewing and behavioral observations. In C. E. Walker & M. C. Roberts (Eds.), *Handbook of clinical child psychology* (pp. 109–131). New York: Wiley.

Lahey, B. B., Loeber, R., Stouthamer-Loeber, M., Christ, M. A. G., Green, S., Russo, M. F., Frick, P. J., & Dulcan, M. (1990). Comparison of DSM-III and DSM-III-R diagnoses for prepubertal children: Changes in prevalence and validity. *Journal of the American Academy of Child and Adolescent Psychiatry, 29,* 620–626.

Maccoby, E. E., & Martin, J. W. (1983). Socialization in the context of the family: Parent-child interaction. In E. M. Hetherington (Ed.), *Handbook of child psychology: Vol. 4. Socialization, personality, and social development* (pp. 236–271). New York: Wiley.

Mash, E. J., & Terdal, L. G. (1988). Behavioral assessment of child and family disturbance. In E. J. Mash & L. G. Terdal (Eds.), *Behavioral assessment of childhood disorders: Selected core disorders* (2nd ed., pp. 3–65). New York: Guilford.

McMahon, R. J., & Forehand, R. (1988). Conduct disorders. In E. J. Mash & L. G. Terdal (Eds.), *Behavioral assessment of childhood disorders: Selected core disorders* (2nd ed., pp. 105–153). New York: Guilford.

Meichenbaum, D. (1985). *Stress inoculation training.* New York: Pergamon.

Offord, D. R., Adler, R. J., & Boyle, M. H. (1986). Prevalence and sociodemographic correlates of conduct disorder. *American Journal of Social Psychiatry, 4,* 272–278.

Ollendick, T. H., & Hersen, M. (Eds.). (1984). *Child behavioral assessment: Principles and procedures.* New York: Pergamon.

Parpal, M., & Maccoby, E. E. (1985). Maternal responsiveness and subsequent child compliance. *Child Development, 56,* 1326–1334.

Patterson, G. R. (1982). *Coercive family process.* Eugene, OR: Castalia.

Patterson, G. R. (1986). Performance models for antisocial boys. *American Psychologist, 41,* 432–444.

Quay, H. C. (1986a). Classification. In H. C. Quay & J. S. Werry (Eds.), *Psychopathological disorders of childhood* (3rd ed., pp. 1–34). New York: Wiley.

Quay, H. C. (1986b). Conduct disorders. In H. C. Quay & J. S. Werry (Eds.), *Psychopathological disorders of childhood* (3rd ed., pp. 35–72). New York: Wiley.

Quay, H. C., & Peterson, D. R. (1983). *Interim manual for the Revised Behavior Problem Checklist.* Unpublished manuscript, University of Miami, Coral Gables.

Rickert, V. I., Sottolano, D. C., Parrish, J. M., Riley, A. W., Hunt, F. M., & Pelco, L. E. (1988). Training parents to be better behavior managers: The need for a competency-based approach. *Behavior Modification, 12,* 475–496.

Riley, A. W., Finney, J. W., & Cataldo, M. F. (1987). Primary-care pediatric consultation. *Newsletter of the Society of Pediatric Psychology, 11,* 7–13.

Robin, A. L., & Weiss, J. G. (1980). Criterion-related validity of behavioral and self-report measures of problem-solving communications skills in distressed and nondistressed parent-adolescent dyads. *Behavioral Assessment, 2,* 339–352.

Robins, L. N. (1966). *Deviant children grown up.* Baltimore: Williams & Wilkins.

Rutter, M., Tizard, J., & Whitmore, K. (Eds.). (1970). *Education, health, and behavior.* London: Longmans.

Schaefer, C. E., & Briesmeister, J. M. (Eds.). (1989). therapists for their children's behavior problems. New York: Wiley.

Schaefer, C. E., & Millman, H. L. (1982). *How to help children with common problems.* New York: New American Library.

Wahler, R. G. (1980). The insular mother: Her problems

in parent-child treatment. *Journal of Applied Behavior Analysis, 13,* 207–220.

Webster-Stratton, C., Kolpacoff, M., & Hollinsworth, T. (1988). Self-administered videotape therapy for families with conduct problem children: Comparison with two cost-effective treatments and a control group. *Journal of Consulting and Clinical Psychology, 56,* 558–566.

Weist, M. D., Ollendick, T. H., & Finney, J. W. (1991). Toward the empirical validation of treatment targets for children. *Clinical Psychology Review, 11,* 515–538.

CHAPTER 8

DEPRESSIVE DISORDERS

Kevin D. Stark   University of Texas at Austin
Margaret Dempsey   University of Texas at Austin
John Christopher   University of Texas at Austin

DESCRIPTION OF DISORDER

Clinical Features

Depression in children and adolescents is a syndrome in which a group of symptoms reliably co-occur (Carlson & Cantwell, 1980). The principal symptom involves mood. However, like adult depression, symptoms for children also extend to the cognitive, motivational, and physical domains (Kovacs & Beck, 1977). The symptoms and associated features for each of these domains will be briefly described. For a more detailed description, the interested reader is referred to Stark (1990a).

Affective Symptoms

The quintessential symptom of depression is dysphoric (sad) mood. However, it is important to recognize that dysphoric mood is a nonspecific symptom common to many childhood disorders. It is the severity and duration of dysphoric mood in a depressive disorder that differentiates it from other disorders. Anger and irritability are common symptoms among depressed children and adolescents (Brumback, Dietz-Schmidt, & Weinberg, 1977), but they are often overlooked because they do not fit common preconceptions about depres-

sion. This is unfortunate both because it leads to the misdiagnosis of many youths who actually are depressed and because this particular symptom has proven during treatment to be one of the most intransigent. Like dysphoric mood, angry and irritable mood vary in both severity and duration.

Another primary affective symptom is anhedonia, or the loss of the pleasure response. Anhedonia appears to be associated with endogenous depression and is one of the symptoms that reliably differentiates depressed youths from children who have other internalizing disorders. Low self-esteem is a very common symptom of depression as well as other disorders of childhood. Over 90 percent of the depressed youths that have participated in our research over the past four years have reported very low self-esteem. Perhaps as a result of low self-esteem, many depressed youths also report feeling worthless. When this symptom is present, we immediately combine individual therapy with either parent training or family therapy.

Cognitive Symptoms

Cognitive symptoms of depression include negative self-evaluations, a sense of hopelessness, and morbid ideation. The youngster's actual thought processes may be sluggish due to impaired concentration and indecisiveness. Most of these symptoms are expressed overtly in a variety of ways in the classroom and other settings. Negative self-evaluations are commonly expressed in the child's verbalizations, such as, "I'm no good at that." Hopelessness also may be expressed verbally in such statements as, "Why bother to try? I can't do it anyway." Morbid ideation is often evident in the youngster's essays, diary entries, and choice of reading materials. Poor concentration is often evident in the child's short attention span and "spaciness." Indecisiveness is present when the youngster is given a choice about what to do, and he or she takes an extraordinarily long time to make a decision, or makes a decision and then regrets it. Excessive guilt is also considered to be a cognitive symptom because it is presumed to reflect the child's attributional style.

Motivational Symptoms

The motivational symptoms of diagnostic significance are suicidal ideation and behavior. Depressed children clearly are at risk for thinking about and committing suicide (Carlson & Cantwell, 1982). A somewhat different approach to assessment and treatment needs to be taken when dealing with the suicidal youth (Stark, 1990). The primary concern immediately becomes ensuring the youngster's safety, and treatment must move much more quickly and always involves a multidisciplinary approach. Although children attempt suicide, this occurs less frequently than among adolescents.

Physical and Vegetative Symptoms

Physical and vegetative symptoms include fatigue, sudden changes in appetite and/or weight, sleep disturbance, and psychomotor retardation and agitation. Fatigue is a very common symptom. The majority of depressed youths experience chronic fatigue and complain of being tired most of the time. Sleep disturbances, especially initial insomnia, are common (Kashani, Barbero, & Bolander, 1981), and early morning awakening is less common but associated with endogenous depression. Disturbances in appetite, extreme changes in weight, and psychomotor disturbances

have been less common among the youths we have studied. However, when they are present, the youngsters typically are more severely depressed. Presence of the physical symptoms are good indicators for the inclusion of pharmacotherapy in the overall treatment program.

Associated Features

In our brief discussion of the associated features, we will include the features that are included in DSM-III-R as well as those that are evident in the literature. A number of associated features fit into the category of affective disturbances, including loss of mirth response, weepiness, self-deprecation, feeling unloved and or misunderstood, self-pity, negativism, uncooperativeness, sulking, a belligerent attitude, and generally increased emotionality.

A few of the associated features could be classified as motivational disturbances. Foremost among these are social withdrawal and decreased academic performance. Social withdrawal occurs with both family members and friends. For instance, depressed youngsters often withdraw to their bedrooms, preferring to listen to music rather than going out to play. Depression's influence on academic performance is unclear, with some studies finding a negative impact (e.g., Hollon, 1970) and others (Stark, Livingston, Laurent, & Cardenas, 1991a) finding minimal impact. While psychomotor disturbances and extreme weight fluctuations are associated with severe disturbances, aches and pain (especially headaches and stomachaches) are quite common (Brumback et al., 1977) physical disturbances that are associated with depression.

A number of other associated physical features are evident in the youngster's appearance, including decreased eye contact, paying less attention to overall appearance, and concerns with health. Prepubertal children may also experience mood-congruent hallucinations (usually only a single voice speaking to the child). Additional associated features include running away, and in adolescence, negativistic and antisocial behavior combined with alcohol or drug use. Among depressed children, Anxiety Disorders of Childhood

(Separation Anxiety Disorder, Overanxious Disorder, and Avoidant Disorder of Childhood or Adolescence) and phobias are common age-specific features.

Epidemiology

The prevalence of depressive disorders in children and adolescents has only been recently researched and conclusions are widely discrepant for a variety of reasons (Lobovits & Handal, 1985). Within the general population, the incidence of depression for children has been estimated in one study to be up to 33 percent (Teuting, Koslow, & Hirschfeld, 1982). However, such a figure appears to refer to the presence of depressive symptoms rather than depressive disorders, as most studies have found significantly lower rates.

For example, in a sample of 3,020 elementary school children, Lefkowitz and Tesiny (1985) found 5.2 percent of the children to be rated by their peers as being depressed and, when actual diagnoses are determined, Anderson, Williams, McGee, and Silva (1989) found rates of 0.5 percent for major depression and 1.7 percent for dysthymic disorder among 641 11-year-olds. Kashani and colleagues have conducted a number of epidemiological studies and found rates of 1.85 percent for major depression and 2.5 percent for dysthymic disorder among 641 9-year-olds (Kashani et al., 1983), and, in a later study of 210 8- and 12-year-olds using the Child Assessment Schedule (Kashani, Orvaschel, Rosenberg, & Reid, 1989), rates of 1.4 percent for major depression (0.7 percent when based on parent reports), 0.4 percent major depression, and 0.6 percent dysthymic disorder among 789 7- to 11-year-olds (Costello et al., 1988), and also rates of 2.7 percent for major depression and .3 percent for dysthymic disorder (McCracken et al., 1986).

Another extensive study by Fleming, Offord, and Boyle (1989) analyzed prevalence rates in 1,156 Canadian children by administering diagnostic checklists to children, their parents, and their teachers. Forming three estimates of the prevalence of major depression according to the level of diagnostic certainty, they found 0.6 per-

cent of preadolescents met the criteria at a high level of certainty, 2.7 percent at a medium level, and 17.5 percent at a low level of diagnostic certainty. Whereas diagnosing depression in preschoolers is particularly difficult, Kashani and Carlson (1987) found 0.9 percent of children in their sample were experiencing major depression. However, in an earlier study of 241 preschoolers, Kashani and Ray (1983) found no evidence of major depression.

Among adolescents, Fleming and colleagues' (1989) previously mentioned study examined 1,230 adolescents and estimated a prevalence rate of 1.8 percent for major depressive disorder at a high level of diagnostic certainty, 7.8 percent at a medium level of diagnostic certainty, and 43.9 percent at a low level of certainty. In another study of 943 15-year-olds, 1.2 percent were found to currently have a major depressive disorder, an additional 1.9 percent had one in the past, and 1.1 percent were experiencing dysthymic disorder (McGee et al., 1990). In an earlier study (McGee & Williams, 1988) of 762 13-year-olds, rates of 0.4 percent for major depression and 1.6 percent dysthymic disorder were found. In a smaller sample of 150 predominantly Caucasian adolescents (Kashani et al., 1990), it was found that 4.7 percent suffered from major depression and 3.3 percent from dysthymic disorder.

In addition to studies that determined diagnoses, a number of investigations have looked at the prevalence of depressive symptoms. In a study of 366 Canadian high school students, 31.4 percent were found to be mildly to clinically depressed, as measured by the Beck Depression Inventory (Ehrenberg, Cox, & Koopman, 1990), while of 103 American high school students, 26 percent scored in the moderate range and 6 percent scored within the severe range of depression on the BDI (Sullivan & Engin, 1986). In a study of 1,270 Australian adolescents, Reynolds and Rob (1988) reported that 9 percent of all adolescents agreed they "felt so down that life has lost its meaning." In a Swedish study of 547 high school students using the BDI, Larsson and Melin (1990) found that 8 percent of the subjects reported moderate levels of depressive symptoms and 2 percent reported severe levels.

Among adolescents, differences in prevalence rates have been found across gender and ethnicity. For instance, black and female students have been found to have higher scores on the Epidemiological Studies Depression Scale (CES-D) than white males (Garrison, Jackson, Marsteller, McKewon, & Addy, 1990). Another study (Emslie, Weinberg, Rush, Adams, & Rintelmann, 1990) found that Hispanic females had the highest scores on depression, as measured by the BDI and the Weinberg Screening Affective Scale (WSAS), while white males had the lowest. The same study also reported rates of clinically significant depressive symptoms of 18.1 percent on the BDI and 13.0 percent on the WSAS among 3,294 high school students. Female high school students in Kenya were also found to report more depressive symptoms than males, as measured by the 20-item Health Opinion Survey (Mitchell & Abbott, 1987). Among children there does not appear to be a gender difference in prevalence rates (Kashani et al., 1983; Lefkowitz & Tesiny, 1985; Lobovits & Handal, 1985), although for adolescents, as for adults, females indicate more depressive features than males (Kandel & Davies, 1982; McDermott et al., 1990; Mezzich & Mezzich, 1979; Reynolds, 1985).

Some studies have examined incidence rates among special populations and found a 50 percent rate among special education adolescents, a 20.9 percent rate among special education children (Mattison, Humphrey, Kales, Hernit, & Finkenbinder, 1986), and a 4 percent rate among speech clinic children (Cantwell & Baker, 1982). Among psychiatric patients, no large-scale studies have been conducted, but smaller-scale studies have found high rates of depression among both child and adolescent psychiatric patients. Among adolescents, Strober, Green, and Carlson (1981) found that 17.8 percent of adolescent psychiatric patients were depressed and Olsen (1961) found that 6.2 percent of the adolescent psychiatric patients were depressed. Studies looking at inpatient children have found percentages of children that were depressed ranged from 26 percent (Asarnow, 1988) to 37 percent (Alessi, 1986) to 58 percent (Carlson & Cantwell, 1980) to 59 percent (Kashani, Husain et al., 1981) and also 59 percent by Petti (1978).

Etiology

What leads to the development of a depressive disorder during childhood? The answer to this question certainly remains speculative at this time. It is likely that there are multiple avenues that all lead to the development of a depressive disorder. For example, a child may have a genetic predisposition toward depression that stems from having a depressed parent. Thus, the youngster is biologically at risk and may be exposed to depressogenic thinking, behavior, and a maladaptive parenting style. A child may come from a family without a history of depressive disorders and live with parents who are not experiencing any diagnoseable psychological disorder, but nonetheless develop a depressive disorder. Stark, Rouse, and Livingston (1991b) hypothesize that a combination of biological, cognitive, behavioral, and familial/environmental variables combine to produce and maintain a depressive disorder. Research into the biological basis of childhood depression has only begun to appear. However, due to the numerous gaps in this research and the many similarities in depression during childhood and later in adult life, we have also drawn upon the adult literature.

The majority of research on possible biological bases of depression has focused on the neurotransmitters thought to be responsible for the disorder. More specifically, this research has been largely guided by the early monoamine hypothesis (Bunney & Garland, 1982; Schildkraut, 1978). This hypothesis states that depression results from low levels of catecholamines (e.g., norepinephrine or dopamine) or low levels of indolamines (e.g., serotonin) (Glassman, 1969).

It was hypothesized that low levels would induce depression whereas high levels would induce mania. Empirical research has looked indirectly at one such catecholeamine by measuring the urinary output of 3-Methoxy-4-hydroxy-phenyl ethylene glycol (MHPG)—the principal metabolite of norepinephrine. Indeed, studies on depressed adults (Sacchetti et al., 1979; Taube, Kirstein, Sweeney, Heninger, & Maas, 1978) and children (McKnew & Cytryn, 1979) have found decreased levels of MHPG. However, the results have been conflicting (Murphy, Cambell, Costa, 1978; Schildkrant, 1978; Zis & Goodwin, 1982).

Using MHPG to indirectly estimate norepinephrine levels has been problematic since factors such as time of day, patient's diet, and level of exercise affect the level of MHPG secreted in adults (Muscettola, Potter, Gordon, & Goodwin, 1981; Wehr, Muscettola, & Goodwin, 1980; Wirz-Justice & Richter,f 1979) and children (Shekim, Javaid, Rutledge, Bylund, & Davis, 1984). Serotonin levels have also been implicated as a correlate of depression. Again, levels of a metabolite, 5-hydroxy-indoleacetic acid (5-HIAA), found in the cerebrospinal fluid, has been measured to estimate levels of serotonin. This metabolite has been found to be lower in depressed adults (Kalin, Risch, & Murphy, 1982; Murphy et al., 1978). However, no definitive support has been found for the monoamine hypotheses.

Other biological correlates found in adult depression have included deficient levels of growth hormone in insulin-induced hypoglycemia (Sachar, Finelstein, & Hellman, 1971). Similar results have been reported for depressed children (Puig-Antich et al., 1984). However, discriminant validity has not yet been demonstrated (Weller, Weller, Fristad, & Preskorn, 1984). Another biological marker found in adult depressives is elevated plasma cortisol levels (Sachar, Asnis, Halbreich, Nathan, & Halper, 1980; Gerner & Wilkins, 1983). Again, comparable findings have been found for children (Poznanski, Carroll, Banegas, Cook, & Grossman, 1982). In addition, theories have included a possible disturbance in the regulation of acetylcholine (Janowsky, El-Yousef, Davis, & Sekerke, 1972; Janowsky, Rish, & Gillin, 1983). This theory is based on the recognized interrelationship between acetylcholine (ACH) and the monoamines (Thase, Frank, & Kupfer, 1985). Again, there is only some indirect evidence in support of this hypothesis. To date, there is no clear-cut, definitive biological basis for depression during childhood.

Given the very influential role of the family in a child's life, it is not surprising that research into the possible psychological basis of depression during childhood has begun to focus on dysfunction within the family. In general, this research has attempted to identify the unique characteristics of families with a depressed child. Kaslow, Rehm, and Siegel (1984) attempted to determine whether there were differences in the perceived family environments of children who reported elevated levels of depressive symptomatology. Children who reported elevated scores on the Children's Depression Inventory (CDI; Kovacs, 1983), relative to controls, reported significantly more general dysfunction in their families. Similarly, Forehand and associates (1988) reported that depressive symptomatology as assessed with the CDI was moderately associated with the number of conflicts the youngsters reported with their parents, and with the degree of negative affect associated with these conflicts.

Asarnow, Carlson, and Guthrie (1987) extended these results by comparing perceived family environments of inpatient children who were diagnosed as suicidal, depressed, or as experiencing some other nonpsychotic psychological disorder. The children completed a portion (Cohesion, Expressiveness, Organization, Conflict, and Control scales) of the Family Environment Scale (FES; Moos & Moos, 1981). Results indicated that there were no significant differences between the perceived family environments of depressed children and children with a variety of nonpsychotic disorders. However, the suicidal children described their families as significantly less cohesive, more conflictual, and less controlled.

Results of one of our own investigations (Stark, Humphrey, Crook, & Lewis, 1990) indicated that depressed youths may experience a unique family environment. Depressed children, relative to controls, rated their families as significantly less cohesive; less involved in activities of a social, recreational, or religious nature; and less democratic in the way that decisions were made within the family. They also reported significantly higher levels of conflict and enmeshment. When compared with anxious children, depressed children reported higher levels of conflict, less involvement in enjoyable activities, and less input into family decisions.

Puig-Antich and associates (1985) studied mothers' perspectives of families with a depressed youth. Mothers with either an endogenously depressed, neurotically depressed, other psychologically disturbed, or normal control child were interviewed regarding communication patterns and relationships in their families. Results indicated that impairment was greatest where there was an endogenously depressed child, followed by a neurotically depressed child, and then the psychological control group. Mothers of all of the disturbed children reported significantly less communication with their child. The affective tone of the mother-child relationship was characterized as cold, hostile, tense, and, at times, rejecting. They also reported subjecting their children to more severe punishment. Impairments in communication and the affective tone of the mother-child relationship were significantly worse among families with a depressed child. Furthermore, these dyads engaged in significantly fewer activities together.

Research from both the biological and family areas are inconclusive and thus far have failed to consider the reciprocal influence of the child's biological and genetic dispositions, family dynamics, the youngster's behavior, and his or her faulty information processing. We believe that all of these systems are involved in the development and expression of depressive disorders.

DIFFERENTIAL DIAGNOSIS AND ASSESSMENT

DSM-III-R Categorization

A good deal of controversy has been evident in the literature regarding the description of, and clinical symptomatology that define, a depressive disorder during childhood. Historically, the very existence of depressive disorders during childhood has been denied on theoretical grounds (Beres, 1966; Bibring, 1953; Mahler, 1961; Rie, 1966), or their existence was accepted but they were presumed to exist as underlying disorders that were expressed through other conditions that "masked" them (Glaser, 1968; Toolan, 1962), or their clinical significance was trivialized (Lefkowitz & Burton, 1978). Another major school of thought was that children experienced depressive disorders in a fashion that was similar to adults, but they experience some symptoms in a developmentally unique way (Brumback et al., 1977; Ling, Oftedal, & Weinberg, 1970; Weinberg, Rutman, Sullivan, Penick, & Dietz, 1973).

More recently, and consistent with the DSM-III-R (American Psychiatric Association [APA], 1987), it has been argued that the essential features of depression are identical between youths and adults (e.g., Kaslow & Rehm, 1983). Consistent with this perspective, Cantwell (1983) has made the distinction between the essential diagnostic criteria versus the age-specific associated features. In essence, he believes tht the core diagnostic criteria are the same across ages, but that there also are some additional symptoms that are unique to the individual's age and developmental stage. These latter symptoms are referred to as *age-specific associated features*.

All of this controversy, along with the recognition that there was a need to develop a psychometrically sound set of criteria for classifying the disorder, led to the development of more than a dozen different sets of diagnostic criteria (Carlson & Garber, 1986). At this time, the most widely accepted diagnostic system is the DSM-III-R. With the growing integration of developmental and clinical psychology, and the mushrooming body of research on childhood depression, changes in the diagnostic criteria that reflect a greater sensitivity to developmental issues may be evident in future versions of this system.

Depressive disorders fall within the general category of Mood Disorders within DSM-III-R. The mood disorders are characterized by a primary disturbance in mood—either excessively elevated, irritable, anhedonic, or depressed mood—that occurs for a specified minimum amount of time. These disorders are grouped into two basic categories: bipolar disorders and depressive disorders. Both disorders are characterized by episodes of depression; however, for a diagnosis of bipolar disorder, a manic episode also has to have occurred. In this chapter, we are concerned with depressive disorders, thus we will outline only the diagnostic criteria for depressive disorders.

Within DSM-III-R, there are 3 diagnostic

categories of depressive disorders: Major Depression, Dysthymic Disorder, and Depressive Disorder Not Otherwise Specified. In addition, within the Adjustment Disorders category, there are two disorders that are characterized by a primary disturbance of mood: Adjustment Disorder with Depressed Mood and Adjustment Disorder with Mixed Emotional Features (see American Psychiatric Association, 1987).

Differential Diagnosis

The road map to differential diagnosis that we describe below is our interpretation and summarization of the DSM-III-R decision tree for the differential diagnosis of mood disturbances. The empirical base for this decision tree is steeped in adult research. While we believe that it can be directly applied to youths, empirical support for this contention does not exist. In general, our understanding of depressive disorders during childhood and adolescence lags far behind that of adulthood. Furthermore, it is not possible at this time to do, for example, the sophisticated subtyping of depression that can be completed with adults and often provides the clinician with useful information about the treatment (both psychological and pharmacological) of the affected individual. For this reason, and some additional reasons noted below, we believe that diagnosing depressive disorders in youths can be complicated, and at times more of an art than a science.

Children remain the primary source of information about their subjective experience of depression, but due to developmental limitations, children often are limited in their ability to identify, distinguish, and describe their affective states and accompanying symptoms. When trying to diagnose a youngster, children seem to have difficulty accurately reporting such-time related information as when the current episode began, how long the symptoms are experienced each day, and how many days a week the symptoms are experienced. Thus, parents are commonly the recommended source for such duration data (Reynolds, 1985). Parents also have limitations as accurate raters of their children's symptoms. Their ability to accurately report their child's symptoms may

be dependent on their own mental health, the type of disorder they are rating, and the nature of the symptoms that they are rating (Kazdin, French, & Unis, 1983a).

If there is evidence to indicate that the youngster is experiencing a mood disorder, the first step in the differential diagnosis process is to determine whether there is an organic basis to this disturbance. If it can be determined that there is, then the youngster would receive a diagnosis of an Organic Mental Disorder, possibly Delirium or Dementia. Deliriums appear to be most likely to occur at the extreme ends of the life cycle, whereas dementias are more commonly associated with the elderly. Nonetheless, either can occur during childhood. For example, a youngster may experience an infection that results in the delirium, or a child may have an accident that involves a head injury and produces a dementia. If there is evidence from historical information, a medical examination, or laboratory tests that indicate a specific organic factor to the disturbance, and the individual displays a clear mood disturbance, then a diagnosis of Organic Mood Syndrome would be appropriate. An exception to this would be a case where the mood disturbance occurs only in the presence of a delirium, then Delirium would be the sole diagnosis.

There is another avenue to the development of an organic base to a mood disturbance that would preclude a diagnosis of depression. It is possible for the mood disturbance to stem from psychoactive substance use, abuse, addiction, or withdrawal. This tends to be of greater concern among adolescents than children, but needs to be considered in youngsters from ages 9 and older. A number of substances that adolescents use have direct toxic effects on the central nervous system that produce organic damage as well as dysphoric mood, including alcohol, amphetamines, barbiturates, cocaine, hallucinogens, opioids, phencyclidine, and steroids. With some substances the dysphoria occurs during use, in others it occurs after prolonged abuse, and in still others it occurs during withdrawal. In addition to these illegal substances, oral contraceptives can cause symptoms of a mood disturbance. A differential diagnosis between Psychoactive Substance-Induced

Organic Mental Disorder and a mood disorder would be based on the presence of physical symptoms, the history of drug use relative to the appearance of the mood disturbance, and/or tests for toxicity (Skodol, 1989).

A number of physical maladies may lead to an organic mental disorder and mood disturbance. These physical illnesses would be coded on Axis IV and include pancreatic carcinoma, thyrotoxicosis, corticoadrenal insufficiency, acquired hypothyroidism, cerebrovascular disease, Cushings' syndrome, Parkinson's disease, and lupus. If the symptoms of the depressive disorder did not occur until after the physical malady developed, then a diagnosis of Organic Mental Disorder Not Otherwise Specified would be approprite.

If the mood disturbance does not appear to be organically based, the next decision point is determining whether the mood disturbance and associated symptoms are part of a depressive disorder or a bipolar disorder. The distinction between the two disorders is the occurrence of a manic or hypomanic episode. Research suggests that bipolar disorder is quite rate among children, but that it is probably underdiagnosed among adolescents (Carlson & Strober, 1979). While it would seem like an easy differential diagnosis to make, it can be complicated when the youngster has a history of recurrent episodes of depression that are broken up by symptom-free periods. In such instances, it is possible that the individual was experiencing a hypomanic episode rather than a symptom-free period, but it is not recognized as such due to the previous depression.

It also is possible, due to mood-congruent memory, for the depressed youngster to simply not remember an episode of mania or hypomania (Skodol, 1989). Attention deficit-hyperactivity disorder (ADHD) commonly co-occurs with depressive disorders among children (Bierdman & Steingard, 1989) and this combination can resemble a bipolar disorder. If the ADHD has already been diagnosed, and was evident before the age of 7, and a depressive disorder is now evident, there is little confusion in making the dual diagnosis. However, when ADHD has not been previously diagnosed, and the evaluator does not have access to reliable historical information, it is possible to confuse cyclothymia with a dual diagnosis. It also is important to note that a diagnosis of a bipolar disorder precludes a diagnosis of ADHD. All of these situations highlight the importance of collecting information from multiple sources, especially reliable information about the onset of various symptoms.

The next step in the differential diagnosis process is determining whether the mood disturbance occurs as part of a psychosis. This differentiation becomes difficult when the youngster is experiencing major depression with psychotic features. At this time, we are unaware of any epidemiological studies with children or adolescents that have reported the frequency of occurrence of major depression with psychotic features. It would seem to be quite rare among children, and only slightly less rare among adolescents. Major depression with psychotic features can be differentiated from a psychotic disorder such as schizoaffective disorder by the duration of the depressive episode relative to the psychotic symptoms. If the psychotic symptoms persist beyond the depressive episode, or if the depressive symptoms were brief relative to the duration of the psychotic symptoms, then a psychotic disorder would be diagnosed.

Assuming that there is no organic base to the disorder or history of mania or psychosis, the next step is to determine whether a syndrome of depression exists, and if so, what type it is? This determination is made based on the number, severity, and duration of depressive symptoms. If a diagnosis of Major Depression is made, then two further differentiations are required. First, it is necessary to determine whether the youngster is experiencing an episode of Major Depression with Melancholia. Melancholia would be diagnosed if there was evidence of psychomotor retardation, anhedonia, early morning awakenings, and a distinct difference in the quality of dysphoric mood. Melancholia, or endogenous depression, has been reported to occur in a similar fashion in adolescents and adults. Secondly, it is necessary to note if there is a seasonal pattern to the disturbance. Rosenthal and colleagues (1986) have reported this pattern among pediatric patients. In addition, it is necessary to specify whether it is a

Single Episode, Recurrent, or Chronic form of major depression.

If the symptoms of major depression are evident, another important differential diagnosis is between major depression and the normal grieving that an individual goes through following a significant loss, such as the death of a parent. In some instances, these depressive symptoms can be severe enough to meet the diagnostic criteria for major depressive disorder. However, if the depressive symptoms represent a normal reaction to the loss, a diagnosis of Uncomplicated Bereavement rather than Major Depression would be appropriate.

The differential diagnosis between Major Depression and Dysthymic Disorder usually is fairly straightforward with children who receive a diagnosis of Major Depression reporting a mood disturbance plus at least four symptoms. In addition, the symptoms are present most of the day, "nearly every day." In contrast, youngsters who receive a diagnosis of Dysthymic Disorder have a mood disturbance plus two additional symptoms that are present most of the day, "more days than not." However, it is important to note that these two diagnostic categories are not homogeneous. There is a great deal of variability with respect to the number and severity of symptoms within each group. Thus, there are grey areas where a youngster with a mild case of major depression may be very similar to a youngster with a more severe case of dysthymic disorder, rendering the differential diagnosis more difficult. Another situation where it may be difficult to differentiate between major depression and dysthymic disorder is when the episode of major depression is in partial remission and has the characteristics of dysthymic disorder. Unless historical information about depressive symptomatology is collected, the child will be misdiagnosed as experiencing a dysthymic disorder.

Major depression and dysthymic disorder are not independent, which can make it difficult to recognize the existence of both disorders. Oftentimes a youngster with a chronic dysthymic disorder will also experience an episode of major depression (Kovacs, Feinberg, Crouse-Novak, Paulauskas, & Finkelstein, 1984). In such cases,

the youngster would receive a dual diagnosis of Major Depression and Dysthymic Disorder. There is another situation where the dual diagnosis would be given, when an episode of major depression is followed by a symptom-free period of at least six months and then the child experiences the onset of a dysthymic disorder.

Children who are experiencing an Adjustment Disorder with Depressed or Mixed Emotional features often report symptoms that are similar to those experienced by youths who are experiencing a depressive disorder. The key difference between a depressive disorder and an adjustment disorder is the identification of a psychosocial stressor that has occurred within the past three months that seems to have triggered the depressive symptoms. In addition to a clearly identified stressor, the youngster may not have been experiencing any previous psychological condition in order to receive a diagnosis of an adjustment disorder. If the depressive symptoms remain for more than six months, and they are severe enough, the youngster's diagnosis would be changed to Major Depression. If they continue for at least a year and meet the criteria for Dysthymic Disorder, then the diagnosis would be changed accordingly.

Depression commonly co-occurs with other disorders during childhood (Puig-Antich, Blau, Marx, Greenhill, & Chambers, 1978), which can make it difficult to determine which one is, or which ones are, present. In addition, when the youngster is experiencing multiple disorders and depression is one of them, it is important to determine whether the depressive disorder is primary or secondary. A number of other childhood disorders, including Attention-Deficit Hyperactivity Disorder, Conduct Disorder, Learning Disabilities, and Anxiety Disorders can lead to demoralization. These, in turn, produce the affective disturbance (Rapoport & Ismond, 1990) and decline in self-esteem that characterize depressive disorders. In such cases, the youngster would receive a dual diagnosis; however, the dysthymia would be considered a secondary disorder.

Depressive disorders and anxiety disorders commonly co-occur and can be difficult to differentiate. This is due to both the overlap in symptomatology (as noted below) and the fact that anxiety disorders are the most difficult group to diagnose reliably (Gittelman, 1986; Prendergast et al., 1988). Many of the symptoms of anxiety are associated symptoms of depressive disorders. For example, the concern about the appropriateness of past behavior and current competence that characterize anxiety disorders are also evident among depressed youngsters due to their poor self-esteem and tendency to experience excessive guilt and negative self-evaluations.

Similarly, depressed youngsters, like anxious children, are extremely self-conscious, and, due to an increase in dependence and indecisiveness, they also have a need for greater reassurance. Some depressed youngsters experience a sense of hopelessness that stems from their negative expectancies for the future. These negative expectations for the future can lead to the worry about the future that characterizes children with Overanxious Disorder. Similar to anxious children, many depressed youths experience somatic complaints. The symptoms with the greatest ability to differentiate depressive and anxiety disorders are anhedonia and suicidal behavior. Since most depressed youngsters are not anhedonic or suicidal, this speaks to the difficulty of making a reliable differential diagnosis.

A dual diagnosis of a depressive disorder and anxiety disorder is possible except in the case where the depressive disorder is primary and the youngster also reports symptoms of Generalized Anxiety Disorder. In this case, the Generalized Anxiety Disorder is ruled out. In addition, Undifferentiated Somatoform Disorder is excluded by a mood disorder if it occurs exclusively during the course of the mood disorder.

With the recent addition to DSM-III-R of irritability as one of the possible primary mood disturbances found among children experiencing major depression, the distinction between Oppositional Defiant Disorder and major depression and dythymic disorder becomes somewhat more difficult. Some children exhibit many of the symptoms of Oppositional Defiant Disorder while they are experiencing an episode of depression. If these symptoms are only evident when the depressive disorder is present, then a dual diagnosis is not warranted. However, if the symptoms are present

at times when the youngster is not depressed, then a dual diagnosis would be appropriate.

Assessment Strategies

There have been a large number of articles (Costello, 1986; Chambers, Puig-Antich, Tabrizi, & Davies, 1982; Faulstich, Carey, Ruggiero, Enyart, & Gresham, 1986; Kazdin, 1981; Kazdin, 1987; Kazdin, 1988a; Kazdin, Colbus, & Rodgers, 1986; Kazdin, French, Unis, & Esveldt-Dawson, 1983a; Kendall, Cantwell, & Kazdin, 1989; Lefkowitz & Tesiny, 1980) and chapters (Cantwell, 1983; Costello, 1981; Kazdin, 1988b; Puig-Antich, Chambers, & Tabrizi, 1983; Rehm, Gordon-Leventon, & Ivens, 1987; Reynolds, 1985) written about the assessment of depression during childhood, and the reader who is interested in a more detailed review of this topic is referred to these articles. Due to the highly subjective nature of depressive disorders, self-report measures have been the most commonly used and widely researched assessment devices for assessing depression in children. The primary procedures have been paper-and-pencil measures and semistructured clinical interviews.

The self-report questionnaires consist of lists of the behavioral, cognitive, affective, physical, and motivational symptoms of depression. Typically, youngsters either rate the frequency of occurrence of each possible symptom on a Likert-type scale (e.g., Child Depression Scale; Reynolds, 1987) or they choose among 3 or 4 items that vary along a dimension of severity the one that best characterizes their phenomenological experience (e.g., Children's Depression Inventory [CDI]; Kovacs, 1983). The emerging consensus is that while such measures have acceptable reliability and convergent validity, they lack adequate discriminant validity (Kazdin, 1981; Kendall et al., 1989; Kerr, Hoier, & Versi, 1987; Petti, 1978; Reynolds, 1984; Weller & Weller, 1985). This lack of discriminant validity may be due to the restrictive range of severity of the symptoms that are assessed (Carey, Faulstich, Gresham, Ruggiero, & Enyart, 1987; Romano & Nelson, 1988). To address this issue, we (Stark, 1990) have developed the Child and Adolescent Depression Inventory, which appears to have superior psychometric properties. Nevertheless, it is our belief that such questionnaires are best viewed as measures of general psychological distress. They are useful as screening tools and as a measure of the severity of distress that the youngster is experiencing.

The clinical interview is the primary assessment tool for evaluating the onset, presence, severity, and duration of depressive symptoms. Due to the difficulties in making a differential diagnosis noted above, it is essential that a psychometrically sound interview be administered by a well-trained clinician. These interviews require training and an understanding of child psychopathology to be administered in a reliable and valid manner.

Our preference from among these interviews is the Schedule for Affective Disorders and Schizophrenia for School-Age Children (Kiddie-SADS or K-SADS; Puig-Antich & Ryan, 1986) because it has demonstrated solid psychometric properties (e.g., Ambrosini, Metz, Prabucki, & Lee, 1989; Apter, Orvaschel, Laseg, Moses, & Tyano, 1989) and diagnostic reliability (Ambrosini et al., 1989; Last & Strauss, 1990; Mitchell, McCauley, Burke, Calderon, & Schlored, 1989). In addition, it assesses a breadth of depressive symptoms as well as the symptoms that comprise most of the other major DSM disorders.

The design of the interview assists the interviewer in the differential diagnosis process. During the unstructured portion of the interview, the interviewer identifies the possible disorders that the child is experiencing and gathers historical data that enable the interviewer to establish possible chronological order of onset of the symptoms. Thus, it is possible to determine whether the depressive disorder appeared before, after, or concurrently with other disorders. In addition to assessing the severity of symptoms over the past week, the severity of symptoms is assessed at the time they were most severe over the previous year, thus enabling the interviewer to make such differential diagnoses as a combination of dysthymic disorder and major depression versus major depression in partial remission. However, it is important to note that for many children below the age of 11 years, the distinction between last week

and the most severe time over the past year becomes blurred.

Another strength of the K-SADS is that the anchors that comprise the rating scale for each symptom are well defined and provide the interviewer with useful information about frequency, duration, and intensity of each manifestation of each symptom. This allows the interviewer to make distinctions between clinical and subclinical manifestations of each symptom. As noted above, it is desirable, and probably crucial, to gather information from the youngster's parents. Another advantage of the K-SADS interview is that with a minimum of changes in the wording of items, a parallel version of the interview can be administered to the youngster's parents. Standard procedure is to interview the parent(s) first and then the child.

In addition to interviewing the youngster's parents, the parents' perceptions of their child can be obtained through behavior rating scales. Such measures commonly assess a number of disorders, including depression. Thus, it is possible to obtain data that might indicate that the child is experiencing multiple disorders, including depression. Both the Personality Inventory for Children (PIC; Wirt, Lachar, Klinedienst, & Seat, 1977) and the Child Behavior Checklist (Achenbach & Edelbrock, 1983) include a depression subscale. The PIC is a 600-item true-false questionnaire that is based on the Minnesota Multiphasic Personality Inventory (MMPI). The depression scale is comprised of 46 items that were judged by clinical psychologists to reflect childhood depression. Test-retest reliability for the depression scale is acceptable (Wirt et al., 1977). In addition, support for the validity of the scale has been reported (Lobovits & Handal, 1985). However, only a modest correlation between parent ratings and child-report measures has been found (Leon, Kendall, & Garber, 1980; Reynolds et al., 1985). Similarly, there is a moderate correspondence between depression ratings on the PIC and DSM-III ratings (Kline, Lachar, & Gdowski, 1988). Achenbach and Edelbrock (1983) reported adequate test-retest reliability for the depression subscale of the Child Behavior Checklist, and parents' ratings have distinguished depressed from nondepressed children (Kazdin & Heidish, 1984; Romano & Nelson, 1988).

In addition to these multidimensional measures, a parent version of the CDI has been developed. The Children's Depression Inventory-Parent Form (CDI-P) is a parallel version of the CDI designed to be completed by parents. Each of 27 symptom items has been reworded so that parents rate their child on the presence and severity of each symptom over the past two weeks. High internal consistency reliability (Kazdin, French, & Unis, 1983b) has been reported. The CDI-P distinuishes depression from other DSM-III disorders (Kazdin et al., 1983a; Kazdin, Sherick, Esveldt-Dawson, & Rancurello, 1985a). Correlations between child and parent forms are high with nonclinic populations (Slotkin, Forehand, Fauber, McCombs, & Long, 1988; Wierzbicki, 1987), but less so with psychiatric inpatients (Kazdin, Esveldt-Dawson, Unis, & Rancurello, 1983c).

In addition to these standardized measures, behavioral observations have also been suggested as part of the assessment of childhood depression (Kazdin, Esveldt-Dawson, Sherick, & Colbus, 1985b; Kazdin et al., 1985a). Such an assessment would entail observing the child's overt behaviors during the interview process as well as during unstructured times for behaviors related to depression.

At present, adult research has demonstrated that specific overt behaviors correlate with depression (e.g. Jones & Pasna, 1979; Williams, Barlow, & Agras, 1972). However, similar studies have only begun with children. Preliminary investigations have tried to define which behaviors are approriate to observe. For instance, when broad catgories were observed (e.g., social activity, solitary behavior, and affect-related expression), low correlations were found between these behaviors and scores on parent measures of depression, and none with child-report measures (Kazdin et al., 1985b). However, when more specific nonverbal behaviors are observed (e.g., eye contact, facial expressiveness), they were correlated with both parent and child reports of depression (Kazdin et al., 1985a). However, these relationships are stronger for girls than boys. Thus, more work is needed in this area in order to better pinpoint the specific behaviors

that should be observed in children of both sexes, and in order to determine the psychometric properties of such assessment devices.

TREATMENT

Evidence for Prescriptive Treatments

Behavior Therapy

To date, surprisingly little treatment outcome research has been completed with depressed youths. Clearly, a need for additional treatment outcome research exists. Perhaps the place to begin this endeavor would be to use single-subject designs so that more clinically realistic and individually tailored interventions can be designed for subjects. Only two empirically evaluated case studies using behavior therapy have been completed. Both of these studies suffer from serious methodological flaws but provide us with some information about the effectiveness of such interventions.

Petti, Bornstein, Delamater, and Conners (1980) used a multimodal intervention with a 10-year-old girl who was experiencing a chronic depressive disorder. The intervention consisted of individual (both psychological and pharmacological), group, and family therapy. Hospital staff completed ratings of the youngster's behavior twice a day as a means of assessing impact of the intervention.

During the initial phase of treatment, the therapeutic relationship was used to enhance self-esteem and help resolve some issues surrounding the patient's parents. She also received remedial education to help overcome academic deficiencies. To help improve interpersonal behavior, she participated in a creative drama group. At the same time, she, along with her family, participated in a creative drama group. At the same time, she, along with her family, participated in family therapy. Since the first phase of the intervention did not have a significant impact, she was placed on imipramine, which produced a marked reduction in overt and subjective manifestations of depression. During the final phase of treatment, she participated in social skills training that produced an increase in eye contact, frequency and duration of smiles, duration of speech, and assertiveness.

In the treatment of a 10-year-old male inpatient, Frame, Matson, Sonis, Fialkov, and Kazdin (1982) evaluated the effectiveness of a skills training program that consisted of instruction, modeling, rehearsal, and feedback. This program was directed toward and led to an improvement in eye contact, volume and amount of speech, facial expressions, and body position.

A few group-comparison treatment outcome studies have been completed. However, it is important to note that they have been completed primarily with moderately depressed school children. It is not clear how these youngsters might differ from their counterparts who have been referred for outpatient or inpatient services. In the first of these studies, Butler, Miezitis, Friedman, and Cole (1980) evaluated the relative effectiveness of a roleplaying treatment, cognitive restructuring, attention placebo, and waiting-list conditions for fifth- and sixth-grade students. Intervention programs were administered in small groups during 10 one-hour weekly meetings. Results indicated that the greatest improvement in the subjective experience of depressive symptoms was reported by subjects in the roleplaying condition. These youngsters were taught social skills, sensitized to their thoughts and feelings as well as those of others, and were taught to generate alternative solutions when facing stressful situations. These skills were acquired through roleplaying followed by feedback, and were applied through homework assignments. Children in the cognitive restructuring procedure were taught the relationship between thoughts and feelings, to identify and change maladaptive thoughts, and listening skills. The investigators noted that the children were not as engaged by this intervention.

Stark, Reynolds, and Kaslow (1987) compared the relative effectiveness of self-control and behavioral treatments to a waiting-list condition. The treatments were conducted in 12 45- to 50-minute group sessions. The self-control treatment was designed to teach the youngsters more adaptive skills for self-monitoring, self-evaluation, attributing the causes of good and bad outcomes, and self-consequating. Skills were applied through homework assignments. The behavioral treatment consisted of education about feelings and interpersonal behavior, and a combination of training in problem-solving skills, self-monitoring of pleasant events, activity scheduling, and social skills training. Once again, the skills were applied through homework assignments. Results of the study indicated that children in both treatments reported a significant reduction in depression as assessed through the CDI and a semistructured clinical interview, and they both reported significantly less depression than children in the waiting-list control condition. Subjects in the latter condition reported a minimum of change. The improvements were clinically significant as well as statistically significant, and were maintained at five-week followup.

Results of this initial study were encouraging and led to a second study with a more seriously impaired sample of children from grades 4 to 7. In this study, an expanded cognitive-behavioral treatment was compared with a traditional counseling condition that emphasized activities that were designed to enhance self-esteem. Participants met in groups of 4 with a pair of graduate student therapists. Groups met for 24 to 26 sessions lasting 45 to 50 minutes over a 3½-month period. Meetings were held twice weekly for eight weeks and once a week thereafter. In addition to group meetings, monthly meetings were held with the youngsters' families.

The cognitive-behavioral treatment included training in self-control skills, social and assertiveness skills, cognitive restructuring, and problem solving. The objective of the family meetings was to get the parents to encourage their children to use their coping skills and to engage in more pleasant activities as a family. In the traditional counseling condition, the group interactions, discussions, and suggestions served as the therapeutic vehicle. In addition, during each session children completed an exercise that either helped them learn more about emotions or enhance self-esteem. Therapists behaved in an empathic and nondirective fashion. The objective of the family sessions was to improve communication and increase the family's involvement in pleasant activities.

Results indicated that both treatments were effective at reducing severity of depressive symptoms as assessed with a self-report measure and the K-SADS interview. However, subjects in the cognitive-behavioral condition reported significantly more improvement on the interview and on a measure of depressive cognitions. Improvements were maintained at seven-month followup.

Two control-group studies have been completed with depressed adolescents. In the first study, Reynolds and Coats (1986) evaluated the relative efficacy of a cognitive-behavioral treatment and a relaxation training condition to a waiting-list control condition. The cognitive-behavioral treatment consisted of a combination of training in self-control and behavioral skills. The relaxation treatment consisted of training in progressive muscle relaxation as a coping skill when confronted with stress. Results indicated that both treatments were effective at reducing depression across a self-report questionnaire and clinical interview. These improvements were maintained at a five-week followup.

In another study with depressed adolescents, Lewinsohn, Clarke, Hops, and Andrews (1990) compared the relative effectiveness of a cognitive-behavioral treatment with and without a parent training component. Adolescent participants met for two hours in groups twice weekly for seven weeks. Parents of some of the adolescents also met in groups for seven weekly two-hour meetings. Parents were taught negotiation and conflict resolution skills during their meetings. Results indicated that adolescents in both treatments improved significantly on self-report and interview measures of depression relative to pretreatment assessment and the waiting-list subjects. There were no significant differences between the two active treatments. Parents who participated in the training, relative to parents whose children were the only participants and to waiting-list control parents, reported significantly fewer behavior problems in their children at posttreatment. At a 24-month followup, subjects in both active treatments reported continued improvement.

Pharmacotherapy

While virtually all the antidepressant and mood stabilizing drugs found useful in the treatment of adults have been tested with children, systematic studies with results that can confidently be applied by child psychiatrists are rare" (Rancurello, 1985, p. 88). The most common drug group for treating depression in children is the tricyclic antidepressants, with impramine, amitriptyline, and nortriptyline being the most popular. The specific mechanisms of action are unclear, but it is thought that tricyclics block the reuptake of norepinephrine and serotonin by the presynaptic terminal (Julien, 1988). Conclusions regarding the effectiveness of the tricyclics is mixed for children. Initial controlled studies indicated no difference between imipramine and placebos. However, when the plasma level of imipramine is controlled for, treatment rates have been high (Puig-Antich & Weston, 1983; Puig-Antich et al., 1987).

The tricyclic antidepressants are increasingly being used with children (Elliott, Popper, & Frazier, 1990). The standard maximum does for imipramine is 5 mg/kg in children. As research on the use of tricyclic antidepressants appeared in the literature, concern about their potential harmful side effects also appeared (Kaslow & Rehm, 1983; Matson, 1989; Rancurello, 1985). It seems as though this period of caution was followed by a period of complacency and increased usage. Recently, renewed concern has been voiced (Popper & Elliot, 1990), as three cases of sudden death have occurred among children taking desipramine, one of the drugs in the imipramine family. Based on available clinical data for these three cases, Popper and Elliott (1990) concluded that the likely cause of these deaths was cardiac arrest, and have outlined a set of guidelines for use of such drugs. Prior to discussing their guidelines, some additional general background information about the use of antidepressants will be presented.

There are two basic approaches to pharmacotherapy. The more conservative approach involves using a single medication, whereas the alternative approach involves poly-medicating. Proponents of the latter approach believe that one medication may potentiate the effectiveness of the other medication. However, to date, there is no research to support one practice over the other.

Although all antidepressants have similar side effects, they vary in the relative severity of each one. The most common side effects of the tricyclics include the following, which would indicate the need to stop taking the medication and possibly the need to seek emergency assistance: high fever, extremes of blood pressure, loss of bladder control, muscle stiffness, seizures, trouble breathing, unusually fast heart beat, unusually pale skin, and unusual sweating. In addition to the aforementioned side effects, the following are cause for concern and prompt medical attention would be indicated: blurred vision, confusion, constipation, decreased sexual ability, difficult urination, drowsiness, eye pain, fainting, hallucination, nervousness, shakiness, trouble sleeping, unusually slow pulse, and vomiting. A number of additional side effects are common and typically do not require medical attention, including dizziness or lightheadedness, drowsiness, dry mouth, headache, increased appetite for sweets, nausea, tiredness, unpleasant taste, and weight gain. Many of these latter side effects subside with time or can be compensated for with minimal effort.

To help ensure safe administration of the group of imipramine drugs, Popper and Elliot (1990) have offered a number of suggestions. Prior to the first dose of imipramine, a cardiac history and electrocardiogram (EKG) should be obtained. A prior history of cardiac disorder would contraindicate the use of the medication. Two or three additional EKGs should be obtained while going through the period of dose adjustment and an EKG should be completed 3 to 4 days after each subsequent increase in dosage. In addition, if any cardiac symptoms reappear, another EKG should be administered. Since imipramine can impact blood pressure and heart rate, both need careful monitoring. If the heart rate reaches 135 beats/minute, the dose should be reduced or the medication should be discontinued. Similar measures should be taken if the systolic pressure reaches 130 mg Hg or diastolic pressure reaches 85 mm Hg. It is also recommended that youngsters who are taking antidepressants avoid extreme physical stress and caffeinated products.

Another potential problem that needs to be addressed with both youngster and parents is the potential difficulties that stem from sudden withdrawal from the medication (Petti & Law, 1981). The child can suffer very serious complications from sudden discontinuation of medication. Unfortunately, it has been our experience that parents will neglect to refill prescriptions as the youngster seems to be doing better, which results in a sudden withdrawal. In addition, parents or the youngster may simply decide to discontinue the medication for a variety of reasons, and this could once again produce very serious medical problems.

Alternative Treatments

A few alternative treatments offer promise for use with depressed youths, but they remain only promising since their contribution has yet to be empirically evaluated. Everly (1989), in his review of the literature on the therapeutic impact of physical exercise on adults, concluded that it can elevate mood, improve self-esteem, and enhance a sense of personal control. Simons, McGowan, Epstein, and Kupfer (1985) have noted that the existing research has suffered from methodological flaws. They are cautiously optimistic about the therapeutic effects of exercise. Distance running or jogging has been the primary form of exercise used and it has been shown to be an effective intervention for moderately depressed adults (Doyne, Chambless, & Beutler, 1983; Griest et al., 1979; McCann & Holmes, 1984). Since physical fitness is a desirable achievement for most youths, especially those in the junior high and high school age ranges, it is possible that a similar positive impact on self-esteem and personal control could be achieved.

However, it is important to note that we believe that exercise should be used as one component in a treatment program and that it can help moderate the impact of depression. In addition to the positive impact noted by Everly, it provides the youngster with a distraction from his or her concerns and in some cases a healthy form of escape from a stressful situation. While regular rigorous physical exercise can become part of the youngster's daily routine, it takes a good deal of planning and support from significant others to make it work. The depressed child's psychomotor, psychosomatic, and motivational disturbances all work against getting into a routine of regular exercise.

An underutilized resource in the treatment of depressed youths is school. School personnel, especially teachers, can be a source of support and encouragement for children. Teachers can be taught through inservices (Downing, 1986) to be sensitive to the needs of depressed youths. For example, they can moderate the homework demands placed on youths and they can encourage them to complete assignments. Teachers can provide youngsters with additional academic help that promotes success, since successful experiences counter the depressed youths' pessimistic and self-denegrating thoughts and beliefs. The additional positive attention and relationship with the teacher can also affect the youngsters' negative sense of self. Furthermore, this relationship and social interchange can help the child acquire appropriate social skills. In some instances, the school counselor (Downing, 1988) or psychologist (Stark, 1990a) can implement a desired intervention on a daily basis in the school or they can monitor the youngsters' completion of therapeutic homework. The P.E. teacher and school nurse can develop, implement, and monitor a physical exercise program. The nurse can also provide the youngster with reassuring information that counters their concern about psychosomatic complaints.

Selecting Optimal Treatment Strategies

The primary strategy employed when selecting the optimal treatment procedure has its roots in the behavioral tradition and involves assessing the youngster to identify (1) behavioral excesses and deficits, (2) deficits in coping skills, and (3) deficits and distortions in thinking. In addition to assessing the child, the youngster's family is assessed to identify unhealthy structural parameters, behaviors, and communications that lead to and maintain maladaptive cognitive structures, maladaptive parenting behaviors, parental psychopathology,

and behaviors of family members that lead to and maintain depressive symptoms. Once these disturbances are identified, relevant treatment procedures are employed. The assessment process may involve the use of formal instruments, but more often uses the clinical interview, observation, and the hypothesis generation and testing process. It is important to emphasize that this is a fluid process that begins during the initial contact and continues throughout treatment.

Problems in Carrying Out Interventions

A variety of problems can occur over the course of treating depressed youths. Some of the difficulties are inherent to the disorder and others are nonspecific to dealing with psychologically disturbed youths. A number of symptoms of depression produce roadblocks to effective treatment. Some of the symptoms affect the therapeutic relationship, others impact the youngsters' involvement in therapy, and some have an adverse affect on motivation (Stark et al., 1991b).

The therapeutic relationship is adversely affected by the youngsters' social withdrawal, which reduces their capacity to become engaged in therapy. Withdrawn youngsters commonly shy away from social interactions, may feel extremely uncomfortable in social situations, and may be deluged by a stream of negative self-evaluations and other automatic thoughts while interacting with the therapist. It also limits the extent to which a collaborative relationship can be established and used over the course of treatment. The youngsters' involvement in therapy and motivation is limited by their sense of hopelessness; they do not perceive that their lives can be changed in a positive way, "so why bother to try." Anhedonic youths find treatment boring and derive little pleasure from the experience. Children who experience fatigue do not have the psychological energy to invest in treatment. The youngsters' difficulties concentrating can make it hard for them to follow the flow of therapy, and their propensity for negatively distorting information may lead them to misunderstand the therapist.

A common difficulty with preadolescents and adolescents, regardless of the disorder, is the establishment of trust within the therapist-client relationship. Until they overcome the fear that what they say will be discussed with their parents, or that friends or someone else might find out what they talk about, they often are reluctant to disclose meaningful and therapeutically crucial information. In addition to the trust issue, for many youths there still is a negative stigma surrounding seeing a psychologist, as they often are forced into it by their parents or school personnel. They may approach therapy with an attitude of "I don't have any problems," or "I'm not the one with the problem, you should be working with my mom — she is the one with the problem."

As is evident from much of existing treatment outcome research, group therapy is a common and useful mode of delivering treatment. However, depressed youths seem to be less capable of benefitting from group therapy due to a number of possibly unique characteristics. Their pessimism and egocentricism contribute to the problem. Pessimism appears to be quite contagious among depressed youths. One group member's pessimism or negativity toward treatment can quickly spread to other group members and undermine treatment. They appear to have difficulty decentering and thus supporting and empathizing with other group members. Consequently, group therapy can rapidly deteriorate into individual therapy delivered in a group, one child at a time. They negatively distort the statements and behaviors of other group members, which can lead to hurt feelings and hostility.

A number of impediments to treatment may arise from within a youngster's family environment. The youngster's family may be destructive to treatment through a variety of pathways. A parent's comments about the expense of treatment may, whether intentional or not, lead to excessive guilt and early termination. An important and influential family member may continue to communicate unhealthy messages to the child about the child, the world, or the future. These messages, such as "You are an unwanted burden," may be communicated verbally or more subtlety through overt behaviors. These messages often form the basis of the youngster's maladaptive belief system. As the therapist tries to help the youngster identify evidence that he or she is a worthwhile individual with positive qualities, a parent may be countering this through derogatory statements about the child.

Another example would be in the case of an adolescent boy who is depressed and has dependent personality disorder. The youngster's parent makes all decisions for him, does the chores that an average youth usually does for himself, and does not allow the youngster to stay home alone. This sends the teenager the message that he cannot do anything on his own and needs someone else to do things for him.

Other destructive behaviors in the family include spousal abuse, physical or sexual abuse of the child, parental substance abuse, and conflict. In addition, a parent's own psychological disturbance can complicate treatment. For example, a child may be confused by the behavior and emotional changes of a parent who is experiencing bipolar disorder. In addition, a youngster may become frightened by the separation that results from the hospitalization of a parent.

Relapse Prevention

Depression is an episodic disorder that is likely to recur (Kovacs et al., 1984). Thus, the development of procedures for preventing future episodes is a clinical imperative. As important as this is, due to the infantile state of treatment outcome research with depressed youths, no research addressing this specific issue is currently available. Thus, we will draw conclusions from existing treatment outcome research, relevant research with depressed adults, and our clinical experience.

The existing treatment outcome research with depressed youths suggests that treatment gains obtained through cognitive-behavioral interventions are maintained for short (e.g., five weeks) as well as long (e.g., 24 months) intervals. In two of these studies (Lewinsohn, Clarke, Hops, & Andrews, 1990; Stark et al., 1987), the authors noted that subjects continued to improve following treatment. While it is possible that, per the design of the interventions, the subjects learned coping skills and continued to apply them to their depressive symptoms, it also is possible that these results are due to the fact that subjects tended to be mildly to moderately depressed. They were not clinical samples. Likewise, it is possible that the duration of the followup period in all but the Lewinsohn study may have been too short to allow for another depressive episode to occur. Furthermore, it is important to note that while enhanced generalization and maintenance of treatment effects was the hope and promise of cognitive behavioral interventions in general (e.g., Meichenbaum, 1977), it has largely not been achieved (e.g., Kendall, 1990). Clearly, additional research is needed before any firm conclusions can be drawn.

As pharmacologic treatments become more widely used with depressed youths, it is important to determine whether youngsters who have benefitted from them remain nondepressed or relapse. Furthermore, what are the relative relapse rates among youths treated pharmacologically, psychologically, or with both? If depressed children and adolescents respond to antidepressant medications in a similar fashion to adults, then results from related research with adults may be informative. In general, studies with depressed adults suggest that fewer relapses occur following cognitive-behavioral therapy as compared with antidepressant medication (Blackburn, Eunson, & Bishop, 1986; Kocacs, 1981; Simons, Murphy, Levine, & Wetzel, 1986). In long-term studies of relapse rates over 6 months (Blackburn, Bishop, Glen, Whalley, & Christie, 1981), one year (Kovacs, Rush, Beck, & Hollon, 1981; Simons et al., 1986), and two years (Blackburn et al., 1986), there were significantly more relapses among subjects treated solely with medication than groups given either cognitive therapy or a combination of both. In fact, based on their results, Blackburn and colleagues (1986) suggested that cognitive therapy may offer long-term protection against depression.

In addition to type of treatment, specific risk factors for relapse have been identified, including a greater number of previous depressive episodes, family history of depression, poor health, higher depression level at onset of treatment, and a younger age at onset. In addition, those patients who continue to exhibit high levels of depressive symptoms at the completion of treatment are also more likely to relapse (Simons et al., 1986). The latter factor is important for therapists to keep in mind as the completion of treatment is nearing.

A number of suggestions for preventing relapses have appeared in the adult literature and may be applicable to depressed youth. Hollon and Garber (1990) noted that clients need to be prepared for termination. This preparation may take the form of rehearsing and roleplaying what to do should depressive symptoms reappear. Gonzales, Lewinsohn, and Clarke (1985) have suggested using booster sessions to produce maintenance of treatment effects. However, Baker and Wilson (1985) found that there was no evidence to support this contention. They found that relapse prevention depended in part on the success of the initial treatment. Freeman, Pretzer, Fleming, and Simon (1990) noted the need to intervene at the schematic level in order to prevent relapses. In addition, they noted the importance of planning ahead with clients to identify strategies for handling situations that might trigger a relapse.

In addition to the suggestions offered in the adult literature, a number of recommendations from the general child treatment literature may prove useful in preventing relapses among depressed youth. Kendall (1990) recommended teaching youths a general problem-solving set. As applied to depressed youths (Stark, 1990a), this would entail teaching children to not only deal with everyday annoyances in one's environment as problems to be solved but also that depressive symptoms are viewed as problems to be solved. The youngsters bring the set of coping skills they have acquired to bare on the problem of, for example, dysphoric mood. Thus, the individuals learn that they are not helpless in the face of depressive symptoms whenever they occur.

While schematic change is the goal of therapy with depressed youths, and Stark (1990a) has emphasized targeting core schemata for change, it is important to highlight the point that the therapist cannot be relied on to do all of the cognitive structures and to apply cognitive restructuring techniques to change maladaptive schemata on their own. In addition, they are taught to identify and restructure the thoughts they are having when they experience a change in mood or other depressive symptoms. Thus, it is crucial to teach depressed youths how to independently identify and restructure their depressive thoughts.

While research and clinical insights have focused some attention on what can be done with the depressed individual to prevent relapses, we believe that focusing only on the depressed child or adolescent is inadequate. Efforts also need to be directed toward modifying the environment, and, in the case of a youth, the most important one to modify is the family. Clinical efforts need to be directed toward changing the behaviors and messages of significant family members that lead to and maintain depressogenic thinking and symptoms. To accomplish this goal, family therapy techniques may need to be incorporated into the treatment regimen. Parents may need to be taught more adaptive parenting skills. In addition to being the targets of change, parents can be taught to help their youngsters to use the cognitive and behavioral coping skills that they have been taught. Finally, in the case of family violence, the therapist could continue to work with social services to ensure that the violence is no longer allowed to occur and that the family receives appropriate treatment.

CASE ILLUSTRATION

Case Description

Jennifer, a 9-year-old fourth-grader, lived with her parents and 13-year-old brother. Both parents were employed in semiprofessional jobs that gave them some visibility within the community. An initial historical interview with her parents revealed an unremarkable past with no apparent physical illnesses that could have led to the apparent depressive disorder, no family stressors, and no problems in school. A family history of depression was noted as both a paternal grandmother and uncle had histories of depression. They had been aware of her psychological problems since she was very young, and had taken her to the family physician when she was 5 years old following statements by Jennifer that she believed that she was overweight and wanted to die. The family physician intervened by telling Jennifer that she "wasn't fat—she just is a big-boned girl" and that she should stop thinking about bad things. In addition, he informed the parents that the problem was solved and would pass. This intervention helped for a couple days, but her generally depressed affect returned and continued at a generally moderate level right up to the time she came in for treatment.

Differential Diagnosis and Assessment

On the K-SADS, her parents reported dysphoric mood without any diurnal fluctuation, frequent temper outbursts, negative self-evaluations, social withdrawal, frequent crying, initial insomnia, excessive guilt, and difficulty in social relationships as she seemed to be too controlling. There was no evidence of an organic basis to the depression, no evidence of substance abuse, and no history of a manic episode. In addition, there was no evidence of another psychological disorder being present. Her parents appeared genuinely concerned about her, reported no marital difficulties, no family problems, no personal history of psychological disturbance, nor any other problems. Jennifer presented as a bright, cheerful, and compliant youngster who stated that she came to therapy because she did not like herself and felt sad much of the time.

While her parents were being interviewed, Jennifer completed the CDI and received a score of 17, which is below the recommended clinical cutoff of 19. A review of specific items indicated mild levels of dysphoria, anhedonia, worry, tearfulness, irritability, social withdrawal, loneliness, and feeling unloved. She also reported feeling ugly and self-hatred. Results of the K-SADS interview paralleled these results, as she reported moderate levels of dysphoria, anger/irritability (primarily directed toward her parents), excessive guilt, low self-esteem (including self-hatred), severe initial insomnia, feeling unloved by her parents, and somatic complaints. She did not report any symptoms that would be indicative of any other disorder. In addition, she did not report diurnal mood variation, a distinctly different dysphoria, nor the vegetative symptoms associate with melancholia or endogenous depression. From the available information, it appeared as though Jennifer was experiencing a chronic dysthymic disorder with possible episodes of major depression superimposed.

Treatment Selection

The first step in developing the intervention plan was to determine the appropriate mode of treatment delivery. Individual therapy, combined with parent training, appeared to be the optimal mode of intervention for the following reasons. Jennifer was bright, insightful, motivated, compliant, anxious to please, and eager to change. Thus, it appeared as if she could identify her depressogenic thinking and that she would follow through on therapeutic homework assignments. No problems in family functioning were reported by either the child or parents, and observations of the family revealed no problems with the exception of some mother-daughter enmeshment. It was believed that the enmeshment could be dealt with through some parent training and counseling of the mother.

Since the parents appeared to be quite healthy, it was decided that they would be taught to help Jennifer apply the cognitive and behavioral coping skills that she would be taught during individual therapy. The parents appeared to set excessively stringent and rigid standards for their daughter's behavior and performance, and they appeared to subtly communicate the message that their acceptance and love was dependent on attainment of parentally set standards. These issues became the focus of parent training. Pharmacotherapy was not initially chosen because Jennifer appeared to be an ideal candidate for a cognitive-behavioral treatment program.

Treatment Course and Problems in Carrying Out Interventions

The initial objectives were to (1) produce some symptom relief; (2) help Jennifer (and the therapist) understand the relationship between her thinking, behavior, and mood; (3) increase frequency and quality of social interaction; and (4) reduce parental pressure to achieve and increase unconditional love and affection from her parents. Over a five-week period, the identification and subsequent scheduling of pleasant activities was used to increase Jennifer's engagement in reinforcing and mood-enhancing activities. In addition, to facilitate this happening, her mother had to learn to give her daughter greater independence, learn developmentally appropriate expectations for how her daughter should spend her leisure time, and reduce pressure on her to practice her artistic skills. Jennifer quickly responded to this intervention, and her parents helped her become more socially active. She reported a reduction in the subjective experience of depressive symptoms, and her parents reported fewer angry outbursts. During the summer, Jennifer visited relatives out of state for a month and attended a two-week camp for artistically talented students.

Upon her return, it was evident that Jennifer was now in the midst of an episode of major depression and, as the new school year had started, it became keenly evident that she was experiencing the associated feature of separation anxiety. An attempt was made to review what had been done in the past to help her successfully cope with her depressive symptoms, and to develop a plan for overcoming the separation anxiety, as it became the most pressing problem since she was creating quite a scene in front of the other students in the morning at school. Furthermore, she was having a difficult time making it through the day without crying or having to visit the nurse. All of this was compounded by a dramatic increase in her level of irritability and a sudden resistance to therapy as she became alternatively quite and angry during sessions.

Nevertheless, a set of coping statements was developed that she employed before leaving home, while in the car on the way to school, when leaving her mother, and while in school. Cognitive restructuring techniques were used to help her recognize that nothing was going to happen to her mother while they were apart and that she was safe at school. In addition, a plan was worked out between her mother and her teachers in which

Jennifer arrived early to school and helped a number of teachers prepare for the day. She really enjoyed this and it provided her with adequate distraction to prevent her from becoming uncontrollably upset.

Her school counselor assisted while she was in school and helped her use her coping statements and provided her with a safe place to go for a few minutes to collect herself when she was becoming overwhelmed with anxiety. This plan led to a moderate reduction in the severity of separation anxiety. She continued to complain of feeling tearful upon departure from her mother in the morning and occasionally during school. She was resistant to efforts to use systematic desensitization. Concurrently, her anger and resistance to therapy increased and both the therapist and school counselor were the targets of uncontrollable fits of anger. She was referred for a psychiatric evaluation and given a prescription for Prozac. Prozac was chosen because it had been used effectively with a relative. It failed to produce an improvement in symptoms, so the prescription was changed to 5 mg of Tofranil to be taken twice daily.

The psychiatrist and psychologist, with informed consent, coordinated their efforts, monitored both Jennifer's and her family's progress, and shared relevant treatment information. Jennifer met weekly (four weeks) then biweekly (twice), and finally monthly with the child psychologist to ensure that the Tofranil was not causing any physical harm. Gradual improvement was noted and the Tofranil seemed to make her more amenable to psychotherapy as the anger and resistance were moderated. In addition, further improvement in separation anxiety was evident, there was a reduction in somatic complaints, and an improvement in sleep was reported.

Through activity scheduling and self-monitoring of engagement of pleasant events, her activity level was greatly increased and she began to make and keep friends both at home and at school. Her school counselor continued to assist with treatment and invited her to join a social skills training group, which she did. This combination was extremely successful as she became very social. Concurrently, the therapist worked with her to systematically identify and restructure maladaptive beliefs about herself, others, and the world.

Through parent training, Jennifer's parents were taught to allow her more freedom and to remove some of the rigid structure that was in place for managing her behavior. As this was occurring, her mood began to decline again, she reported feeling as though her parents did not love her, and her parents reported an increase in acting-out behavior. Subsequently, a core belief was identified: "Parents demonstrate their love by setting very rigid and restrictive rules for their child's behavior," and "If my parents aren't doing this, I must not be lovable and they don't love me." Education and cognitive restructuring were used to combat this belief along with family therapy sessions that were designed to help her parents see how they were communicating this rule to her, and to teach them to, and provide them with practice for, expressing love for their daughter through healthier, more direct, and more conventional means.

In addition, her father's level of engagement in the family was increased. He was assigned the task of being the family disciplinarian since he seemed to set more realistic standards for her behavior, and he was assigned the task of teaching his wife how to express love through words and gestures. Jennifer was assigned the role of being the director of family fun (she suggested enjoyable activities for the whole family). In addition, the parents were given a self-monitoring form parallel to Jennifer's. The parents were instructed to self-monitor and self-record healthy expressions of affection and communications that Jennifer was a valued person. Concurrently, Jennifer was instructed to self-monitor her perception of the occurrence of these positive parental behaviors. At the end of the day, Jennifer and her parents were instructed to compare their self-monitoring forms and talk about discrepancies in perceptions. These tended to be very emotional and powerful meetings. An immediate and lasting improvement was noted in Jennifer's affect and depressive symptoms.

Jennifer continued to improve, become more socially active, and generally happy. She successfully flew by herself to an out-of-state friend's home and had a good time while she was there. She did not feel any separation anxiety.

Outcome and Termination

To help determine the appropriateness of termination, Jennifer completed the CDI. She received a score of 9, which is at the mean for this measure and well below the recommended cutoff score of 19. A review of the individual item ratings indicated that no items were rated at the severe level. This was especially noteworthy since she had experienced an extremely embarrassing event the previous day at school that would have caused her to spiral down into an extreme depression in the past. Termination was a prolonged process as Jennifer had, quite surprisingly (because of the rage that had been directed at the therapist during some sessions), become attached to the therapist. She also verbalized a fear that she would regress if she stopped seeing him. Education and homework assignments were used to change this perception.

In addition, termination was completed over four sessions with progressively longer intervals between sessions (two, three, and then four weeks) to help prove to Jennifer that she could remain healthy without seeing her psychologist. Upon termination, it was decided that she would remain on Tofranil for at least three more months to allow her to finish out the school year. At that time, if she is symptom free, the medication will be discontinued.

Followup and Maintenance

Throughout treatment Jennifer was taught cognitive and behavioral coping skills that she could employ to change her depressogenic thinking and maladaptive behavior. Cognitive restructuring efforts were directed toward her core schemata and she was taught to do it herself. In addition, her parents were taught to help cue her to use such procedures. As it became evident that she was improving rapidly and a strategy was being developed for termination, Jennifer was taught a problem-solving strategy that she could apply to her depressive symptoms and any future occurrence of them. Strategies for employing coping skills to deal with depressive symptoms, both behavioral and cognitive skills, were rehearsed in

hypothetical situations as well as in vivo as the meetings were progressively scaled back to biweekly, every three weeks, and then monthly.

To help counter the depressed youngster's propensity for all or nothing thinking in the face of a setback, Jennifer's parents were instructed to take Jennifer to the store to buy a calendar. Each day that things went satisfactorily and that she felt good, she drew a smiley face on the calendar. During the last few months of treatment, she brought the calendar along and it became evident that she was having one or two "bad" days per month. She was instructed to review the calendar whenever she started to feel like things had not gotten any better or when she started to feel like it was all going to fall apart. This way she could see that it is normal to experience a bad day every now and then and that it was not a sign that it was all going to fall apart.

In addition to the individual work with Jennifer to prepare for termination, the therapist met with the family a few times to assess the maintenance of changes in the family system. The impact of the changes was reviewed with the family and the need to fight the tendency to fall back onto old habits was discussed. Also, the family members agreed to have weekly meetings to discuss how each member was doing with respect to maintaining the positive changes.

SUMMARY

Childhood depression is estimated to be prevalent in approximately 0.5 to 3.0 percent of the general population. Its symptoms, much like in adults, manifest themselves in the child's mood, cognitions, and motivation level, as well as in various physical symptoms. In addition, children exhibit many age-specific associated features such as separation anxiety. Although we can be fairly certain of the symptoms that characterize childhood depression, we are far less certain of how or why the disorder develops. We believe that investigations should be conducted as to the joint contribution of chemical imbalances, family/ environmental variables, cognitive disturbances, and behavioral excesses and deficits.

Childhood depression often co-occurs with

other disorders that can make the diagnostic process difficult as we attempt to rule out competing diagnoses. Thus, in order to be thorough and accurate in our assessment of the child, it is recommended that the examiner use a multimethod multi-informant assessment package that includes self-reports, parental reports, clinical interviews, and behavioral observations. A synthesis of this information would offer the most comprehensive and complete clinical picture.

A review of current treatment outcome studies of depressed children indicates that cognitive-behavioral and pharmacological therapies have been most extensively researched. Although only preliminary, research suggests that cognitive-behavioral therapies appear to produce promising results. Pharmacotherapy also has shown promise, and it may prove maximally effective to combine the two therapies.

Due to the recurrent nature of depressive disorders, relapse prevention is of great concern. In order to effectively achieve a prophylactic effect, our treatment efforts must expand beyond the individual child. That is, as the child learns to modify cognitive distortions and develop new coping skills, the family must be engaged in therapy to modify those behaviors that maintain depressive symptoms.

REFERENCES

Achenbach, T. M., & Edelbrock, C. S. (1983). *Manual for the Child Behavior Checklist and Revised Child Behavior Profile.* Burlington: University of Vermont, Department of Psychiatry.

Alessi, N. E. (1986). *DSM-III diagnosis associated with childhood depressive disorders.* Paper presented at the American Academy of Child Psychiatry, Los Angeles.

Ambrosini, P. J., Metz, C., Prabucki, K., & Lee, L. C. (1989). Videotape reliability of the 3rd revision edition of the K-SADS. *Journal of the American Academy of Child and Adolescent Psychiatry, 28,* 723–728.

American Psychiatric Association. (1987). *Diagnostic and statistical manual of mental disorders* (3rd ed., rev.). Washington, DC: Author.

Anderson, J. C., Williams, S., McGee, R., & Silva, P. (1989). Cognitive and social correlates of DSM-III disorders in preadolescent children. *Journal of the American Academy of Child and Adolescent Psychiatry, 28,* 842–846.

Apter, A., Orvaschel, H., Laseg, M., Moses, T., & Tyano, S. (1989). Psychometric properties of the K-SADS-P in an Israeli adolescent inpatient population. *Journal of the American Academy of Child and Adolescent Psychiatry, 28,* 61–65.

Asarnow, J. R. (1988). Peer status and social competence in child psychiatric inpatients: A comparison of children with depressive, externalizing, and concurrent depressive and externalizing disorders. *Journal of Abnormal Child Psychology, 16,* 151–162.

Asarnow, J. R., Carlson, G. A., & Guthrie, D. (1987). Coping strategies, self-perceptions, hopelessness, and perceived family environments in depressed and suicidal children. *Journal of Consulting and Clinical Psychology, 55,* 361–366.

Baker, A. L., & Wilson, P. H. (1985). Cognitive-behavior therapy for depression: The effects of booster sessions on relapse. *Behavior Therapy, 16,* 335–344.

Beres, D. (1966). Superego and depression. In R. M. Lowenstein, L. M. Newman, M. Scherr, & A. J. Solnit (Eds.), *Psychoanalysis — A general psychology* (pp. 479–498). New York: International University Press.

Bibring, E. (1953). The mechanism of depression. In P. Greenacre (Ed.), *Affective disorders* (pp. 13–48). New York: International University Press.

Biederman, J., & Steingard, R. (1989). Attention-deficit hyperactivity disorder in adolescents. *Psychiatric Annals, 19,* 587–596.

Blackburn, I. M., Bishop, S., Glen, A. I. M., Whalley, L. J., & Christie, J. E. (1981). The efficacy of cognitive therapy in depression: A treatment trial using cognitive therapy and pharmacotherapy, each alone and in combination. *British Journal of Psychiatry, 139,* 181–189.

Blackburn, I. M., Eunson, K. M., & Bishop, S. (1986). A two-year naturalistic follow-up of depressed patients treated with cognitive therapy, pharmacotherapy and a combination of both. *Journal of Affective Disorders, 10,* 67–75.

Brumback, R. A., Dietz-Schmidt, S. G., & Weinberg, W. A. (1977). Depression in children referred to an educational diagnostic center: Diagnosis and treatment and analysis of criteria and literature review. *Diseases of the Nervous System, 38,* 529–535.

Bunney, W. E., Jr., & Garland, B. L. (1982). A second generation catecholamine hypothesis. *Pharmacopsychiatry, 15,* 111–115.

Butler, L., Miezitis, S., Friedman, R., & Cole, E. (1980). The effect of two school-based intervention programs on depressive symptoms in preadolescents. *American Educational Research Journal, 17,* 111–119.

Cantwell, D. (1983). Depression in childhood: Clinical picture and diagnostic criteria. In D. P. Cantwell & G. A. Carlson (Eds.), *Affective disorders in childhood and adolescence: An update* (pp. 3–18). New York: Spectrum.

Cantwell, D. P., & Baker, L. (1982). Depression in children with speech, language, and learning disorders. *Journal of Child Psychiatry, 21,* 51–59.

Carey, M. P., Faulstich, M. E., Gresham, F. M., Ruggiero, L., & Enyart, P. (d1987). Children's Depression Inventory: Construct and discriminant validity across clinical and nonreferred populations. *Journal of Consulting and Clinical Psychology, 55,* 755–761.

Carlson, G. A., & Cantwell, D. P. (1980). Unmasking masked depression in children and adolescents. *American Journal of Psychiatry, 137,* 445–449.

Carlson, G. A., & Cantwell, D. P. (1982). Suicidal behavior and depression in children and adolescents. *Journal of the American Academy of Child Psychiatry, 21,* 361–368.

Carlson, G., & Garber, J. (1986). Developmental issues in the classification of depression in children. In M. Rutter, C. E. Izard, & P. B. Read (Eds.), *Depression in young people: Developmental and clinical perspectives* (pp. 399–434). New York: Guilford.

Carlson, G., & Strober, M. (1979). Affective disorders in adolescence. *Psychiatric Clinics of North America, 2,* 511–526.

Chambers, W. J., Puig-Antich, J., Tabrizi, M. A., & Davies, M. (1982). Psychotic symptoms in prepubertal major depressive disorder. *Archives of General Psychiatry, 39,* 921–927.

Costello, C. G. (1981). Childhood depression. In J. E. Mash & L. G. Terdal (Eds.), *Behavioral assessment of childhood disorders* (pp. 305–346). New York: Guilford.

Costello, E. J. (1986). Assessment and diagnosis of affective-disorders in children. *Journal of Child Psychology and Psychiatry and Allied Disciplines, 27,* 565–574.

Costello, E. J., Edelbrock, C., Burns, B. J., Dulcan, M. K., Brent, D., & Janisszweski, S. (1988). Psychiatric disorders in pediatric primary care-prevalence and risk-factors. *Archives of General Psychiatry, 45,* 1107–1116.

Downing, C. J. (1986). Affirmations: Steps to counter negative, self-fulfilling prophecies. *Elementary School Guidance & Counseling, 20,* 174–179.

Downing, c. J. (1988). Counseling interventions with depressed children. *Elementary School Guidance & Counseling, 21,* 231–240.

Doyne, E. J., Chambless, D. L., & Beutler, L. E. (1983). Aerobic exercise as a treatment for depression in women. *Behavior Therapy, 14,* 434–440.

Ehrenberg, M. F., Cox, D. N., & Koopman, R. F. (1990). The prevalence of depression in high school students. *Adolescence, 25,* 905–912.

Elliott, G. R., Popper, C. W., & Grazier, S. H. (1990). Tricyclic antidepressants: A risk for 6–9 year olds? *Journal of Child and Adolescent Psychopharmacology, 1,* 105–106.

Emslie, G. J., Weinberg, W. A., Rush, A. J., Adams, R. M., & Rintelmann, J. W. (1990). Depressive symptoms by self-report in adolescence: Phase I of the development of a questionnaire for depression by self-report. *Journal of Child Neurology, 5,* 114–121.

Everly, G. S., Jr. (1989). *A clinical guide to the treatment of the human stress response.* New York: Plenum.

Faulstich, M. E., Carey, M. P., Ruggiero, L., Enyart, P., & Gresham, F. M. (1986). Assessment of depression in childhood and adolescence. *American Journal of Psychiatry, 143,* 1024–1027.

Fleming, J. E., Offord, D. R., & Boyle, M. H. (1989). Prevalence of childhood and adolescent depression in the community. *British Journal of Psychiatry, 155,* 647–654.

Forehand, R., Brody, G., Slotkin, J., Fauber, R., McCombs, A., & Long, N. (1988). Young adolescent and maternal depression: Assessment, interrelations, and family predictors. *Journal of Consulting and Clinical Psychology, 56,* 422–426.

Frame, C., Matson, J. L., Sonis, W. A., Fialkov, M. J., & Kazdin, A. E. (1982). Behavioral treatment of depression in a prepubertal child. *Journal of Behavior Therapy and Experimental Psychiatry, 3,* 239–243.

Freeman, A., Pretzer, J., Fleming, B., & Simon, K. M. (1990). *Clinical application of cognitive therapy.* New York: Plenum.

Garrison, C. Z., Jackson, K. L., Marsteller, F., McKewon, R., & Addy, C. (1990). A longitudinal study of depressive symptomatology in young adolescents. *Journal of the American Academy of Adolescent Psychiatry, 29,* 580–585.

Gerner, R. H., & Wilkins, J. N. (1983). CSF cortisol in patients with depression, mania or anorexia nervosa and in normal subjects. *American Journal of Psychiatry, 140,* 92–94.

Gittleman, R. (1986). Assessment of the classroom-behavior of hyperactive children. *Nutrition Reviews, 44,* 137–140.

Glaser, K. (1968). Masked depression in children and adolescents. *Annual Progress in Child Psychiatry and Child Development, 1,* 345–355.

Glassman, A. H. (1969). Indolamines and affective disorders. *Psychomatic Medicine, 31,* 107–114.

Gonzales, L. R., Lewinsohn, P. M., & Clarke, G. N. (1985). Longitudinal follow-up of unipolar depressives: An investigation of predictors of relapse. *Journal of Consulting and Clinical Psychology, 53,* 461–469.

Griest, J. H., Klein, M. H., Eischens, R. R., Faris, J., Gurman, A. S., & Morgan, W. P. (1979). Running as treatment for depression. *Comprehensive Psychiatry, 20,* 41–54.

Hollon, S. D. (1989). Cognitive therapy and pharmacotherapy for depression. *Psychiatric Annals, 20,* 249–258.

Hollon, S. D., & Garber, J. (1990). Cognitive therapy for depression: A social-cognitive perspective. *Personality and Social Psychology Bulletin, 16,* 58–73.

Hollon, T. H. (1970). Poor school performance as a symptom of masked depression children and adolescents. *American Journal of Psychotherapy, 24,* 258–263.

Janowsky, D. S., El-Yousef, M. K., Davis, J. M., & Sekerke, J. (1972). A cholinergic-adrenergic hypothesis of mania and depression. *Lancet, 2,* 632–635.

Janowsky, D. S., Risch, S. C., & Gillin, J. C. (1983). Adrenergic-cholinergic balance and the treatment of affective disorders. *Progress in Neuropsychopharmacology and Biological Psychiatry, 7,* 297–307.

Jones, I. M., & Pasna, M. (1979). Some nonverbal aspects of depression and schizophrenia occurring during the interview. *Journal of Nervous and Mental Disease, 167,* 402–409.

Julien, R. M. (1988). *A primer of drug reaction* (5th ed.). New York: Freeman.

Kalin, N. H., Risch, S. C., & Murphy, D. L. (1982). Involvement of the central serotonergic system in affective illness. *Journal of Clinical Psychopharmacology, 1,* 232–237.

Kandel, D. B., & Davies, M. (1982). Epidemiology of depressive mood in adolescents—An empirical study. *Archives of General Psychiatry, 39,* 1205–1212.

Kashani, J. H., Barbero, G. J., & Bolander, F. D. (1981). Depression in hospitalized pediatric patients. *Journal of the American Academy of Child Psychiatry, 20,* 123–134.

Kashani, J. H., & Carlson, G. A. (1987). Seriously depressed preschoolers. *American Journal of Psychiatry, 144,* 348–350.

Kashani, J. H., Carlson, G. A., Beck, N. C., Hoeper, E. W., Corcoran, McAlister, J. A., Fallahi, C., Rosenberg, T. K., & Reid, J. C. (1990). Depression, depressive symptoms, and depressed mood among a community sample of adolescents. *American Journal of Psychiatry, 144,* 931–934.

Kashani, J. H., Husain, A., Shekim, W. O., Hodges, K. K., Cytryn, L., & McKnew, D. H. (1981). Current perspectives on childhood depression: An overview. *American Journal of Psychiatry, 138,* 143–153.

Kashani, J. H., McGee, R. O., Clarkson, S. E., Anderson, J. C., Walton, L. A., Williams, S., Silva, P. A., Robins, A. J., Cytryn, L., & McKnew, D. H. (1983). Depression in a sample of 9-year-old children. *Archives of General Psychiatry, 140,* 1217–1223.

Kashani, J. H., Orvaschel, H., Rosenberg, T. K., & Reid, J. C. (1989). Psychopathology in a community sample of children and adolescents: A developmental perspective. *Journal of the American Academy of Child and Adolescent Psychiatry, 28,* 701–706.

Kashani, J. H., & Ray, J. S. (1983). Depressive related symptoms among preschool-age children. *Child Psychiatry and Human Development, 13,* 233–238.

Kaslow, N., & Rehm, L. (1983). Childhood depression. In R. J. Morris & T. R. Kratochwill (Eds.), *The practice of child therapy* (pp. 27–51). New York: Pergamon.

Kaslow, N., Rehm, L., & Siegel, A. W. (1984). Social-cognitive and cognitive correlates of depression in children. *Journal of Abnormal Child Psychology, 12,* 605–620.

Kazdin, A. E. (1981). Assessment techniques for childhood depression: A critical appraisal. *Journal of the American Academy of Child Psychiatry, 20,* 358–375.

Kazdin, A. E. (1987). Assessment of childhood depression—Current issues and strategies. *Behavioral Assessment, 9,* 291–319.

Kazdin, A. E. (1988a). The diagnosis of childhood disorders—Assessment issues and strategies. *Behavioral Assessment, 10,* 67–94.

Kazdin, A. E. (1988b). Childhood depression. In J. E. Mash & L. G. Terdal (Eds.), *Behavioral assessment of child disorders* (2nd ed., pp. 157–195). New York: Guilford.

Kazdin, A. E., Colbus, D., & Rodgers, A. (1986).

Assessment of depression and diagnosis of depressive disorders among psychiatrically disturbed children. *Journal of Abnormal Child Psychology, 14,* 499–515.

Kazdin, A. E., Esveldt-Dawson, K., Sherick, R. B., & Colbus, D. (1985b). Assessment of overt behavior and childhood depression among psychiatrically disturbed children. *Journal of Consulting and Clinical Psychology, 53,* 201–210.

Kazdin, A. E., Esveldt-Dawson, K., Unis, A. S., & Rancurello, M. D. (1983c). Child and parent evaluations of depression and aggression in psychiatric in-patient children. *Journal of Abnormal Child Psychology, 11,* 401–413.

Kazdin, A. E., French, N. H., & Unis, A. S. (1983b). Child, mother, and further evaluations of depression in psychiatric in-patient children. *Journal of Abnormal Child Psychology, 11,* 167–180.

Kazdin, A. E., French, N. H., Unis, A. S., & Esveldt-Dawson, K. (1983a). Assessment of childhood depression: Correspondence of child and parent ratings. *Journal of the American Academy of Child Psychiatry, 22,* 157–164.

Kazdin, A. E., & Heidish, I. E. (1984). Convergence of clinically derived diagnoses and parent checklists among inpatient children. *Journal of Abnormal Child Psychology, 12,* 421–426.

Kazdin, A. E., Sherick, R. B., Esveldt-Dawson, K., & Rancurello, M. (1985a). Nonverbal behavior and childhood depression. *Journal of the American Academy of Child Psychiatry, 24,* 303–309.

Kendall, P. C. (1990). Challenges for cognitive strategy training: The case of mental retardation. *American Journal on Mental Retardation, 94,* 365–367.

Kendall, P. C., Cantwell, D. A., & Kazdin, A. E. (1989). Depression in children and adolescents: Assessment issues and recommendations. *Cognitive Therapy and Research, 13,* 109–146.

Kerr, M. M., Hovier, T. S., & Versi, M. (1987). Methodological issues in childhood depression: A review of the literature. *American Journal of Orthopsychiatry, 57,* 193–198.

Kline, R. B., Lachar, D., & Gdowski, C. (1988). Convergence and concurrent validity of DSM-III diagnoses and the personality inventory for children (PIC). *Canadian Journal of Behavioral Science, 20,* 251–264.

Kovacs, M. (1981). Rating scales to assess depression in school-aged children. *Acta Paedopsychiatrica, 46,* 305–315.

Kovacs, M. (1983). *The Children's Depression Inventory: A self-rated depression scale for school-aged youngsters.* Unpublished manuscript, University of Pittsburgh, Pittsburgh, PA.

Kovacs, M., & Beck, A. T. (1977). An empirical clinical approach towards a definition of childhood depression. In J. G. Schulterbrandt & A. Raskin (Eds.), *Depression in childhood: Diagnosis, treatment and conceptual models* (pp. 1–25). New York: Raven Press.

Kovacs, M., Feinberg, T., Crouse-Novak, M., Paulauskas, S., & Finkelstein, R. (1984). Depressive disorders in children: I. A longitudinal prospective study of characteristics and recovery. *Archives of General Psychiatry, 41,* 229–239.

Kovacs, M., Rush, A. J., Beck, A. T., & Hollon, S. D. (1981). Depressed outpatients treated with cognitive therapy or pharmacotherapy. *Archives of General Psychiatry, 38,* 33–39.

Larsson, B., & Melin, L. (1990). Depressive symptoms in Swedish adolescent*s. *Journal of Abnormal Child Psychology, 18,* 91–103.

Last, C. G., & Strauss, C. C. (1990). School referral in anxiety-disordered children and adolescents. *Journal of the American Academy of Child and Adolescent Psychiatry, 29,* 31–35.

Lefkowitz, M. M., & Burton, N. (1978). Childhood depression: A critique of the concept. *Psychological Bulletin, 85,* 716–726.

Lefkowitz, M. M., & Tesiny, E. P. (1980). Assessment of childhood depression. *Journal of Consulting and Clinical Psychology, 48,* 43–50.

Lefkowitz, M. M., & Tesiny, E. P. (1985). Depression in children: Prevalence and correlates. *Journal of Consulting and Clinical Psychology, 53,* 647–656.

Leon, G. R., Kendall, P. C., & Garber, J. (1980). Depression in children: Parent, teacher, and child perspectives. *Journal of Abnormal Child Psychology, 8,* 221–235.

Lewinsohn, P. M., Clarke, G. N., Hops, H., & Andrews, J. (1990). Cognitive-behavioral treatment for depressed adolescents. *Behavior Therapy, 21,* 385–401.

Ling, W., Oftedal, G., & Weinberg, W. (1970). Depressive illness in childhood presenting as severe headache. *American Journal of Diseases of Childhood, 120,* 122–124.

Lobovits, D. A., & Handal, P. J. (1985). Childhood depression: Prevalence using DSM-III criteria and validity of parent and child depression scales. *Journal of Pediatric Psychology, 10,* 45–54.

Mahler, M. S. (1961). On sadness and grief in infancy and childhood. *Psychoanalytic Study of the Child, 16,* 332–354.

Matson, J. L. (1989). *Treating depression in children and adolescents.* New York: Pergamon.

Mattison, R. E., Humphrey, J., Kales, S., Hernit, R., Finkenbinder, R. (1986). Psychiatric background of diagnosis of children evaluated for special class placement. *Journal of Child Psychiatry, 25,* 514–520.

McCann, I. L., & Holmes, D. S. (1984). Influence of aerobic exercise on depression. *Journal of Personality and Social Psychology, 46,* 1142–1147.

McCracken, J., Shekim, W., Kashani, J., Beck, M., Martin, J. Rosenberg, J., & Costello, A. (1986). *The epidemiology of childhood depressive disorders.* Paper presented at the American Academy of Child and Adolescent Psychiatry Meeting, Los Angeles.

McDermott, R. J., Hawkins, W. E., Marty, P. J., Littlefield, E. A., Murray, S., & Williams, T. K. (1990). Health behavior correlated with depression in a sample of high school students. *Journal of School Health, 60,* 414–417.

McGee, R., Feehan, M., Williams, S., Partridge, F., Silva, P. A., & Kelly, J. (1990). DSM-III disorders in a large sample of adolescents. *Journal of the American Academy of Child and Adolescent Psychiatry, 29,* 611–619.

McGee, R., & Williams, S. (1988). A longitudinal study of depression in 9-year-old children. *Journal of the American Academy of Child and Adolescent Psychiatry, 27,* 342–348.

McKnew, D., & Cytryn, L. (1979). Urinary metabolites in chronically depressed children. *Journal of the American Academy of Child Psychiatry, 18,* 608–615.

Meichenbaum, D. (1977). *Cognitive-behavioral modification.* New York: Plenum.

Mezzich, A. C., & Mezzich, J. E. (1979). Symptomatology of depression in adolescence. *Journal of Personality Assessment, 43,* 267–275.

Mitchell, J., McCauley, E., Burke, P., Calderon, R., & Schlored, K. (1989). Psychopathology in parents of depressed children and adolescents. *Journal of the American Academy of Child Psychiatry, 28,* 352–357.

Mitchell, S., & Abbott, S. (1987). Gender and symptoms of depression and anxiety among Kikuyu secondary students in Kenya. *Social Science Medicine, 24,* 303–316.

Moos, R., & Moos, B. (1981). *Manual for the Family Environmental Scale.* Palo Alto, CA: Consulting Psychologists Press.

Murphy, D. L., Campbell, I., & Costa, J. L. (1978). Current status of the indoleamine hypothesis of the affective disorders. In M. A. Lipton, A. DiMascio,

& K. F. Killam (Eds.), *Psychopharmacology: A generation of progress* (pp. 1235–1247). New York: Raven Press.

Muscettola, G., Potter, W. Z., Gordon, E. K., Goodwin, F. K. (1981). Methodological issues in the measurement of urinary MHPG. *Psychiatry Research, 4,* 267–276.

Olsen, T. (1961). Follow-up study of manic-depressive patients whose first attack occurred before the age of 19. *Acta Psychiatry Scandinavia, 162,* 45–51.

Petti, T. A., (1978). Depression in hospitalized child psychiatry patients: Approaches to measuring depression. *Journal of the American Academy of Child Psychiatry, 19,* 690–702.

Petti, T. A., Bornstein, M., Delamater, A., & Conners, C. K. (1980). Evaluation and multimodality treatment of a depressed prepubertal girl. *Journal of the American Academy of Child Psychiatry, 19,* 690–702.

Petti, T. A., & Law, W. (1981). Abrupt cessation of high-dose imipramine treatment in children. *Journal of the American Medical Association, 246,* 768–769.

Popper, C. W., & Elliott, G. R. (1990). Sudden death and tricyclic antidepressants: Clinical considerations for children. *Journal of Child and Adolescent Psychopharmacology, 1,* 125–132.

Poznanski, E. O., Carroll, B. J., Banegas, M. C., Cook, S. C., & Grossman, J. A. (1982). The dexamethasone suppression test in prepubertal depressed children. *American Journal of Psychiatry, 139,* 321–324.

Prendergast, M., Taylor, E., Rapoport, J. L., Bartko, J., Donnelly, M., Zametkin, A., Ahearn, M. B., Dunn, G., & Wieslberg, H. M. (1988). The diagnosis of childhood hyperactivity a United States-UK cross-national study of DSM-III and ICD-9. *Journal of Child Psychology and Psychiatry and Allied Disciplines, 29,* 289–300.

Puig-Antich, J., & Ryan, N. N. (1986). *Schedule for affective disorders and schizophrenia for school-age children.* Unpublished manuscript, Western Psychiatric Institute and Clinic, Pittsburgh, PA.

Puig-Antich, J., Blau, S., Marx, N., Greenhill, L., & Chambers, W. (1978). Prepubertal major depressive disorders: A pilot study. *Journal of the American Academy of Child Psychiatry, 17,* 695–707.

Puig-Antich, J., Chambers, W. J., & Tabrizi, M. A. (1983). The clinical assessment of current depressive episodes in children and adolescents. In D. P. Cantwell & G. A. Carlson (Eds.), *Affective disorders in childhood and adolescence* (pp. 157–179). New York: S.P. Medical & Scientific Books.

Puig-Antich, J., Lukens, E., Davies, M., Goetz, D., Brennan-Quattrock, J., & Todak, G. (1985). Psychosocial functioning in prepubertal major depressive disorders: Interpersonal relationships during the depressive episode. *Archives of General Psychiatry, 42,* 500–507.

Puig-Antich, J., Novacenki, H., Davies, M., Chambers, W., Tabrizi, M., Krawiec, V., Ambrosini, P., & Sachar, E. (1984). Growth hormone secretion in prepubertal children with major depression. 1. Final report in response to insulin-induced hypoglycemia during a depressive episode. *Archives of General Psychiatry, 41,* 455–460.

Puig-Antich, J., & Perel, J., Lupatkin, W., Chambers, W. J., Tabrizi, M. A., King, J., Davies, M., Johnson, R., & Stiller, R. (1987). Imipramine in prepubertal major depressive disorders. *Archives of General Psychiatry, 44,* 81–89.

Puig-Antich, J., & Weston, B. (1983). The diagnosis and treatment of major depressive disorder in childhood. *Annual Review of Medicine, 34,* 231–245.

Rancurello, M. D. (1985). Clinical applications of antidepressant drugs in childhood behavioral and emotional disorders. *Psychiatric Annals, 15,* 88–100.

Rapoport, J. L., & Ismond, D. R. (1990). *DSM-III-R training guide for diagnosis of childhood disorders.* New York: Brunner/Mazel.

Rehm, L. P., Gordon-Leventon, B., & Ivens, C. (1987). Depression. In C. L. Frame & J. L. Matson (Eds.), *Handbook of assessment in childhood pathology* (pp. 341–371). New York: Plenum.

Reynolds, I., & Rob, M. I. (1988). The role of family difficulties in adolescent depression, drug-taking and other problem behavior. *Medical Journal of Australia, 149,* 250–256.

Reynolds, W. M. (1984). Depression in children and adolescents: Phenomenology, evaluation, and treatment. *School Psychology Review, 13,* 171–182.

Reynolds, W. M. (1985). Depression in childhood and adolescence: Diagnosis, assessment, intervention strategies and research. In T. R. Kratochwill (Ed.), *Advances in school psychology* (pp. 133–189). Hillsdale, NJ: Erlbaum.

Reynolds, W. M. (1987). *Child depression scale.* Odessa, FL: Psychological Assessment Resources.

Reynolds, W. M., Anderson, G., & Bartell, N. (1985). Measuring depression in children: A multimethod assessment investigation. *Journal of Abnormal Child Psychology, 13,* 513–526.

Reynolds, W. M., & Coats, K. I. (1986). A comparison of cognitive-behavioral therapy and relaxation training for the treatment of depression in adolescents. *Journal of Consulting and Clinical Psychology, 54,* 653–660.

Rie, H. E. (1966). Depression in childhood: A survey with some pertinent contributions. *Journal of the Academy of Child Psychiatry, 5,* 653–685.

Romano, B. A., & Nelson, R. O. (1988). Discriminant and concurrent validity of measures of children's depression. *Journal of Clinical Child Psychology, 17,* 255–259.

Rosenthal, N., Carpenter, C., James, S., Pany, B., Rogers, S., & Wehr, T. (1986). Seasonal affective disorder in childhood and adolescence. *American Journal of Psychiatry, 143,* 356–358.

Sacchetti, E., Allaria, E., Negri, F., Biondi, P. A., Smeraldi, E., & Cazzullo, C. L. (1979). 3-methoxy-4-hydroxyphenylglycol and primary depression: Clinical and pharmacological considerations. *Biological Psychiatry, 14,* 473–484.

Sachar, E. J., Asnis, G., Halbreich, V., Nathan, R. S., & Halpern, F. (1980). Recent studies in the neuroendocrinology of major depressive disorders. *Psychiatric Clinics of North America, 3,* 313–326.

Sachar, E. J., Finkelstein, J., & Hellman, L. (1971). Growth hormone responses in depressive illness. I. Response to insulin tolerance test. *Archives of General Psychiatry, 25,* 263–269.

Schildkraut, J. J. (1978). Current status of the catecholamine hypothesis of affective disorders. In M. A. Lipton, A. DiMascio, & K. F. Killam (Eds.), *Psychopharmacology: A generation of progress* (pp. 1223–1234). New York: Raven Press.

Shekim, W., Javaid, J., Rutledge, M., Bylund, D., & Davis, J. (1984). Factors affecting urinary excretion of 3-methoxy-4-hydroxyphenylglycol in children and its clinical significance. *Journal of the American Academy of Child Psychiatry, 23,* 343–347.

Simons, A. D., McGowan, C. R., Epstein, L. H., & Kupfer, D. J. (1985). Exercise as a treatment for depression: An update. *Clinical Psychology Review, 5,* 553–568.

Simons, A. D., Murphy, G. E., Levine, J. L., & Wetzel, R. D. (1986). Cognitive therapy and pharmacotherapy for depression. *Archives of General Psychiatry, 43,* 43–48.

Skodol, A. E. (1989). *Problems in differential diagnosis: From DSM-III to DSM-III-R in clinical practice.* Washington, DC: American Psychiatric Press.

Slotkin, J., Forehand, R., Fauber, R., McCombs, & Long, N. (1988). Parent-completed and adolescent-completed CDIs: Relationship to adolescent social and cognitive functioning. *Journal of Abnormal Child Psychology, 16,* 207–217.

Stark, K. D. (1990a). *Childhood depression: School based intervention*. New York: Guilford.

Stark, K. D. (1990b). *Child and Adolescent Depression Inventory: Psychometric evaluation of a measure of depression in youth*. Manuscript submitted for publication.

Stark, K. D., Humphrey, L. L., Crook, K., & Lewis, K. (1990). Perceived family environments of depressed and anxious children. *Journal of Abnormal Child Psychology, 18,* 527–547.

Stark, K. D., Livingston, R., Laurent, J. L., & Cardenas, B. (1991a). *Academic achievement, performance in school, and childhood depression*. Manuscript submitted for publication.

Stark, K. D., Reynolds, W. M., & Kaslow, N. J. (1987). A comparison of the relative efficacy of self-control therapy and a behavioral problem-solving therapy for depression in children. *Journal of Abnormal Child Psychology, 15,* 91–113.

Stark, K. D., Rouse, L. W., & Livingston, R. (1991b). Treatment of depression during childhood and adolescence: Cognitive and behavioral procedures for the individual and family. In P. C. Kendall (Ed.), *Child and adolescent therapy: Cognitive-behavioral procedures* (pp. 165–206). New York: Guilford.

Strober, M., Green, J., & Carlson, G. (1981). Phenomenology and subtypes of major depressive disorder in adolescence. *Journal of Affective Disorders, 3,* 281–290.

Sullivan, W. O., & Engin, A. W. (1986). Adolescent depression—Its prevalence in high school students. *Journal of School Psychology, 24,* 103–109.

Taube, S. L., Kirstein, L. S., Sweeney, D. R., Heninger, G. R., & Maas, J. W. (1978). Urinary 3-methoxy-4-hydroxyphenylglycol and psychiatric diagnosis. *American Journal of Psychiatry, 135,* 78–82.

Teuting, P., Koslow, S. H., & Hirschfeld, R. M. A. (1982). *Special report of depression research* (DHHS Publication No. ADM81-1085, National Institute of Mental Health). Washington, DC: U.S. Government Printing Office.

Thase, M. E., Frank, E., & Kupfer, D. J. (1985). Biological processes in major depression. In E. E. Beckham & W. R. Leber (Eds.), *Handbook of depression: Treatment, assessment and research* (pp. 816–913). Homewood, IL: Dorsey Press.

Toolan, J. M. (1962). Depression in children and adolescents. *American Journal of Orthopsychiatry, 32,* 404–414.

Wehr, T. A., Muscettola, G., & Goodwin, F. K. (1980). Urinary 3-methoxy-4-hydroxyphenylglycol circadian rhythm. Early-timing (phase-advance) in manic-depressives compared with normal subjects. *Archives of General Psychiatry, 37,* 257–263.

Weinberg, W. A., Rutman, J., Sullivan, L., Penick, E. C., & Dietz, S. G. (1973). Depression in children referred to an educational diagnostic center: Diagnosis and treatment. *Journal of Pediatrics, 83,* 1065–1072.

Weller, E. B., & Weller, R. A. (1985). Clinical aspects of childhood depression. *Psychiatric Annals, 15,* 368–374.

Weller, E., Weller, R., Fristad, M., & Preskorn, S. (1984). The dexamethasone suppression test in hospitalized prepubertal depressed children. *American Journal of Psychiatry, 141,* 290–291.

Wierzbicki, M. (1987). A parent form of the Children's Depression Inventory—Reliability and validity in nonclinical populations. *Journal of Clinical Psychology, 43,* 390–397.

Williams, J. G., Barlow, D. H., & Agras, W. S. (1972). Behavioral measurement of severe depression. *Archives of General Psychiatry, 27,* 330–333.

Wirt, R. D., Lachar, D., Klinedienst, J., & Seat, P. D. (1977). *Multidimensional description of child personality: A manual for the Personality Inventory for Children*. Los Angeles: Western Psychological Services.

Wirz-Justice, A., & Richter, R. (1979). Seasonality in biochemical determinations: A source of variance and clue to the temporal incidence of affective illness. *Psychiatry Research, 1,* 53–60.

Zis, A. P., & Goodwin, F. K. (1982). The amine hypothesis. In E. S. Paykel (Ed.), *Handbook of affective disorders* (pp. 175–190). New York: Guilford.

CHAPTER 9

SEPARATION ANXIETY DISORDER

Bruce A. Thyer University of Georgia

Joseph Himle University of Michigan Medical Center

Daniel J. Fischer University of Michigan Medical Center

DESCRIPTION OF DISORDER

The clinical phenomenon labeled separation anxiety disorder (SAD) first made its official appearance in psychiatric nomenclature in 1980, when it was included in the third edition of the *Diagnostic and Statistical Manual of Mental Disorders* (DSM-III, American Psychiatric Association [APA], 1980). The 1980 criteria were revised somewhat in the revision of the DSM-III (DSM-III-R, American Psychiatric Association, 1987), and now provide the following clinical description: Excessive anxiety must have persisted for at least two weeks in a child, centered on fears of being separated from those to whom the child is attached (usually a parent). The onset of this condition must have occurred prior to age 18 years, although the diagnosis may be initially made among adults, providing the history is consistent with an onset prior to age 18.

Virtually all the features associated with SAD can be attributed to this central fear of being apart, either temporarily or permanently, from one's attachment figures (referred to as "parents"

for the remainder of this chapter). Among school-aged children, a refusal to go to school, and the display of behaviors which produce such an outcome, may be a prominent feature. Such behaviors include complaints of illness or other various somatic features, tantrums, paroxysms of apparent terror, fleeing school during the course of the day to return home, and so on. Among younger children, shadowing behavior may be the major feature, wherein the child closely follows the parent about throughout the day or frequently checks on the parent's whereabouts. Quite young children may demand that they be allowed to sleep with their parents. Children with SAD may refuse to participate in other activities that involve separation from parents, including going to Sunday school, camp, overnight stays with friends of relatives, or day excursions with peers.

Clinical Features

The DSM-III-R diagnostic criteria for SAD are reprinted in Table 9–1. It is important to note that

Table 9–1. Diagnostic Criteria for Separation Anxiety Disorders

---

A. Excessive anxiety concerning separation from those to whom the child is attached, as evidenced by at least three of the following:

(1) unrealistic and persistent worry about possible harm befalling major attachment figures or fear that they will leave and not return.

(2) unrealistic and persistent worry than an untoward calamitous event will separate the child from a major attachment figure, e.g., the child will be lost, kidnapped, killed, or be the victim of an accident.

(3) persistent reluctance or refusal to go to school in order to stay with major attachment figures or at home.

(4) persistent reluctance or refusal to go to sleep without being near a major attachment figure or to go to sleep away from home.

(5) persistent avoidance of being alone, including "clinging" to and "shadowing" major attachment figures.

(6) repeated nightmares involving the theme of separation.

(7) complaints of physical symptoms, e.g., headaches, stomachaches, nausea, or vomiting, on many school days or on other occasions with anticipating separation from major attachment figures.

(8) recurrent signs or complaints of excessive distress in anticipation of separation from home or major attachment figures, e.g., temper tantrums or crying, pleading with parents not to leave.

(9) recurrent signs or complaints of excessive distress when separated from home or major attachment figures, e.g., wants to return home, needs to call parents when they are absent or when child is away from home

B. Duration of disturbance of at least two weeks.

C. Onset before the age of 18.

D. Occurrence not exclusively during the course of a Pervasive Developmental Disorder, Schizophrenia, or any other psychotic disorder

---

Source: From *Diagnostic and Statistical Manual of Mental Disorders, Third Edition, Revised)* (pp. 60–61) by the American Psychiatric Association, 1987, Washington, DC: APA. Copyright 1987 by American Psychiatric Association. Reprinted by permission.

the signs and symptoms associated with SAD (listed as potential features 1–9 in Table 9–1) are not in themselves the defining criteria for the diagnosis, *unless* these features are clearly attributable to the primary feature of the condition, the excessive anxiety concerning separation. For example, it is not simply a refusal or reluctance to go to school that makes the case for SAD, it is school refusal *due to* separation fears.

Associated Features

Children and adolescents with SAD may voice concerns over something bad happening to their parents (e.g., accidents or illness), particularly when they are apart from them. Such fears may be amorphous in younger children with SAD but take on more concrete forms of expression among adolescents or older children ("Mom might be robbed while shopping!" or "I'm afraid to go to the store, I might be kidnapped like those kids on the milk carton!"). The DSM-III-R (APA, 1987, p. 59) has contended that a fear of the dark is a common associated feature among children with SAD, but this author is not aware of any research supporting this point. The diagnosis of SAD appears equally frequently among boys and girls, and similar signs and symptoms appear to characterize the expression of the disorder in the two genders (Francis, Last, & Strauss, 1987).

Epidemiology

There do not appear to be any reliable data concerning the nationwide incidence or prevalence of SAD among children and adolescents in the United States (or elsewhere). The recently completed NIMH epidemiological catchment area study (Robins & Regier, 1991) focused exclusively upon adult disorders, not those occurring among the young. There are a number of studies that have tabulated the occurrence of various *symptoms,* such as school refusal, that are associated with the diagnosis of SAD, but in the absence of compelling data derived from the formal DSM-III or DSM-III-R criteria, confident statements regarding the epidemiological characteristics of SAD are unavailable. The DSM-III-R ambiguously claims that "the disorder is apparently not uncommon" (APA, 1987, p. 60).

In one community study of 210 children and adolescents, Kashani and Orvaschel (1990) used structured diagnostic assessments to uncover 27 (13 percent) respondents who appeared to meet the criteria for SAD. The sample of 210 respondents were selected from among the community's population of school children. A completely random sampling procedure was not possible, but strenuous efforts were made to adhere as closely as possible to a random selection process. If replicated, the finding that approximately 13 percent of school-aged children and adolescents meet the criteria for SAD suggests indeed tht the disorder is not "uncommon." It is likely however, that the 13 percent figure is an overestimate. For example, Benjamin, Costello, and Warren (1990) utilized a reliable structured interview protocol to assess the prevalence of anxiety disorders among a sample of 300 children from families enrolling in a health maintenance organization. The one-year percent prevalence for SAD, utilizing both parent and child reports, was 4.1 percent, less than a third of that obtained by Kashani and Orvaschel (1990). This latter figure is quite similar to that obtained by Anderson, Williams, McGee, and Silva (1987) among New Zealand 11-year-olds (3.5 percent prevalency rate). At present, the clinician specializing in children or adolescents can reasonably expect to encounter clients suffering from SAD on a fairly regular basis.

Etiology

At present, empirical research has not isolated one or more clearly compelling and well-supported etiological formulations of separation anxiety disorder. Because separation anxiety is a normal and expected developmental phenomenon both in humans and infrahuman species (cf. Thyer, 1987), its ubiquitousness suggests that it is an evolved adaptive response enhancing the reproductive success. Crying and contact seeking in the absence of the mother may help her locate a lost infant. It is probably not a coincidence that separation anxiety in humans usually appears about the time that infants become more mobile. It is possible that separation anxiety *disorder* represents the failure of a child to make a successful transition of this normal developmental phase, or involves a regression to a prior level of functioning in the face of stressors. There is no good evidence to suggest, however, that SAD involves some unique constellation of psychopathological factors, as opposed to normal developmental processes gone awry.

Thyer and Sowers-Hoag offered the following speculations derived from learning theory:

Children with SAD may have a deficit in their learning history, wherein they have not been exposed to the natural desensitization processes involving the gradual separation from parents (perhaps caused by an overprotective parent?). Alternatively, the child may well have experienced one or more major traumatic separation experiences, such as those hypothesized in the descriptive literature (e.g., parent death or illness, child illness, divorce, upsetting changes of residence). Either set of circumstances could parsimoniously account for the child's dependent behavior and anxiousness in the absence of a parent. . . . A third possibility is that "separation anxiety" represents an operant response. Dependent, clinging behavior and contact seeking could be subtly (or overtly) *positively* reinforced by the mother. If the child is fearful (phobic) of pervasive anxiety-evoking stimuli in his or her environment . . . the reluctance to leave home may involve processes of *negative* reinforcement. The success of anxious behavior on the part of the child in enabling him or her to avoid anxiety-evoking stimuli could be perpetuated by the repeated process of fear reduction. (1988, pp. 214–215)

It has been suggested that childhood SAD represents a precursor to the subsequent adult development of panic disorder or agoraphobia (APA, 1987). A careful review of the evidence pertaining to this hypothesis suggests that such a conclusion is premature, and in fact considerable evidence suggests that it is false (Thyer, in press). The treatment literature, to date, has not reached the stage wherein SAD of differing etiologies is recommended to be treated in a differential manner, although school phobia requires such differential treatment (cf. Thyer & Sowers-Hoag, 1986). Hence the lacunae in etiological understanding does not appear of major clinical import at present.

DIFFERENTIAL DIAGNOSIS AND ASSESSMENT

DSM-III-R Categoization

It seems unlikely that significant changes will be forthcoming in the fourth edition of the DSM with respect to the criteria for SAD. In a preliminary report of the Child Psychiatry Work Group (Shaffer et al., 1989), charged with reviewing and revising the DSM-III-R to prepare criteria for the DSM-IV, the authors noted the following issues are being looked at with respect to SAD:

> whether some index of *impairment* should be included in the diagnostic criteria; . . . the criteria for separation anxiety disorder are being reviewed to ensure that common clinical phenomena like the presence of affective symptoms during periods of separation and a preoccupation and over-concern with death and dying are included; . . . [and] the problem of *criterion overlap* between the different anxiety disorders. For example a child with separation anxiety disorder may dread the departure of a parent. As things stand this fear constitutes a criterion for both separation anxiety disorder and OACD" [overanxious disorder of childhood]. (Schaffer et al., p. 832)

The impression gained is that the DSM-IV will represent more of a "fine-tuning" of the DSM-III-R criteria for SAD rather than a complete overhaul.

Differential Diagnosis

The differential diagnosis of SAD is not usually difficult. Among the more common disorders to be excluded are overanxious disorder (OAD), avoidant disorder of childhood or adolescence, simple or social phobia, obsessive-compulsive disorder (OCD), and panic disorder (with or without agoraphobia). A less common differential diagnosis is posttraumatic stress disorder (PTSD; see Last, Strauss, & Francis, 1987, for one of the few empirical studies in the area of differential diagnosis).

Generally the situational specificity of the child's expressed fears, avoidance behavior, and other signs and symptoms reflective of separation anxiety makes it relatively easy to distinguish SAD from other possible diagnoses. When the child is not faced with an actual or anticipated separation from his or her parent, anxious behavior is virtually absent. With OAD, generalized anxiety may be present irrespective of the parents' presence or absence, and the child's fears are not *centered* on possible periods of separation or of harm befalling the parent.

In avoidant disorder of childhood or adolescence, the anxiety-evoking stimuli are clearly related to social situations involving exposure to unfamiliar people. While this may bear some superficial similarity with aspects of SAD, the absence of a preoccupation with separation from parents again makes this diagnostic possibility easy to exclude.

In some cases of simple or social phobia or OCD, the anxiety-evoking stimuli may be so pervasive in the child's psychosocial environment that the child may act similarly to those with SAD. For example, if the child has a simple phobia of dogs, and free-roaming dogs are common in the neighborhood, then clinging behavior, a reluctance to leave the home for school or to run errands, and so on, may be present. Similarly, the child with a social phobia (e.g., undressing for gym class at school) may display extreme reluctance to leave the home, and may superficially resemble the child with SAD in terms of displaying tantruming, crying, somatic complaints, and so forth, upon being urged to go to school. If a child with OCD is afraid of germ contamination, and views germs as ubiquitous outside the home, then he or she may be similarly reluctant to leave the familiar home environment.

Other children or adolescents with OCD may feel compelled to perform checking or washing rituals, activities that can most conveniently be accomplished in the home, and not at school or in the company of others not familiar with his or her "habits." Such children may also *appear* to be quite uncomfortable apart from the parents, or away from the home, or in the face of anticipated parental separations. However, the central fear is related to obsessions and the opportunity to perform ritualistic behavior, *not* separation from parents.

Recently it has become clear that panic disorder and its sequelae (some simple phobias, agoraphobia) may initially occur among children or adolescents (Ballenger et al., 1989; Last & Strauss, 1989; Moreau, Weissman, & Warner, 1989). A consequence of panic attacks may well take the form of an excessive dependency or clinging behavior on the part of the child, and/or a reluctance to leave the home, to be apart from one's parents, or to be alone. A detailed interview with the child (or perhaps the parents) aimed at carefully elucidating a possible history of spontaneous panic attacks *before* the development of the SAD-like behavior should suffice to determine if the child meets the criteria for panic disorder. If so, such a diagnosis would supersede that of SAD.

Children who meet the DSM-III-R criteria for posttraumatic stress disorder (see Eth & Pynoos, 1985, and Lyons, 1987, for reviews) may display some signs and symptoms that resemble those of SAD (clinging, shadowing, reluctance to leave the home or to go to school, aversion to being apart from parents, etc.). Because PTSD is attributable to clearly identifiable psychosocial stressor (being a victim of violence, war, natural catastrophe, etc.), the diagnosis of PTSD would supersede that of SAD.

Assessment Strategies

Clinical Interview

Generally speaking, a thorough clinical interview conducted by a clinician familiar with the DSM-III-R criteria for the various child and adolescent disorders and adult anxiety disorders criteria remains both the most common and useful clinical assessment strategy. With young children, interviews with the parents may form the primary data source, whereas adolescents may be capable of providing sufficient information to arrive at a correct diagnosis. Collateral interviews with parents and other significant persons in the client's life (e.g., teachers) are usually quite useful.

A number of structured and semistructured clinical interviews have been developed of varying degrees of utility in the assessment of children and adolescents. Among the earliest of these are the Schedule for Affective Disorders and Schizophrenia for School-age Children (Kiddie-SADS; Puig-Antich & Chambers, 1978), the Diagnostic Interview Schedule for Children (DISC; Costello, Edelbrock, Dulcan, Kalas, & Klaric, 1984), and the Interview Schedule for Children (ISC; Kovacs, 1985). The Child Assessment Schedule (CAS) constructed by Hodges and associates (Hodges, Kline, Stern, Cytryn, & McKnew, 1982; Hodges, McKnew, Burbach, & Roebuck, 1987) has two

parallel forms, one for use with children and adolescents and one suitable for interviewing parents about their child. The Diagnostic Interview for Children and Adolescents-Revised (DICA-R; Wellner, Reich, Herjanic, Jung, & Amado, 1987) consists of four differing versions, broken down by the age of the client (versions for children ages 6 to 12 versus adolescents ages 13 to 17), or the respondent (versions for the client versus the parent). The DICA-R provides DSM-III-R diagnoses for both children and adolescents.

Each of the preceding structured interview protocols is not specific to the assessment of anxiety disorders, per se, hence the clinician must wade through a series of potentially irrelevant questions to complete the schedule. Other drawbacks include generally low levels of interrater agreement and of a failure (for some) to provide for specific DSM-III-R diagnoses.

The Anxiety Disorders Interview Schedule for Children (ADIS-C) does provide for arriving at DSM-III-R diagnoses, including ruling out inappropriate ones (Silverman & Nelles, 1988), and includes both child and parent versions. The ADIS-C has good interrater reliability and appears (to this author) to be the most useful and accurate of the structured interview schedules currently available for use in assessing children and adolescents with a presumptive anxiety disorder. At present, however, it seems that structured diagnostic interviews are best utilized in clinical research studies (where journal editorial boards demand evidence of reliability in diagnostic formulations) and in training clinicians or researchers to become familiar with the diagnostic nomenclature used with children and adolescents. The routine use of such interview schedules in clinical practice, once a clinician has become familiar with the DSM-III-R and the subtle nuances of the anxiety disorders as manifested among children and adolescents, does not seem warranted. Silverman (1991) provides an excellent overview of current structured interviews for use in the assessment of anxiety disorders among children.

Self-Report Scales

A number of standardized pencil-and-paper self-report scales have been developed for use in assessing clients with a presumptive anxiety disorder; however, most of these instruments were intended for use with adults (e.g., Beck, Epstein, Brown, & Steer, 1988; Westhuis & Thyer, 1989), not children and adolescents. Normative data for such scales, based on adults, is of dubious value in assessing children. Such adult-oriented scales *may* be useful, particularly with the older adolescent, but the results should be interpreted cautiously.

Two child-oriented anxiety scales are the Fear Survey Schedule for Children (FSSC; Scherer & Nakamura, 1968) and the Children's Manifest Anxiety Scale (CMAS; Mattison, Bagnato, & Brubaker, 1988). The FSSC consists of an 80-item questionnaire listing a variety of potentially phobic stimuli falling into several categories (e.g., school, home, social, animal, etc.). The child rates the degree (none, a little, some, much, very much) to which he or she is afraid of the item in question. Both total and subscale (e.g., fears of school) scores may be obtained. The CMAS consists of items answered by the child respondent on a yes-no basis. A CMAS subscale labeled "worry/oversensitivity" appears to be particularly useful in distinguishing children with an anxiety disorder from those not known to have an anxiety disorder (cf. Mattison et al., 1988). However, Hodges (1990) presents data suggesting that the sensitivity of the CMAS is too low for diagnostic purposes, recommending its use instead as more of a screening instrument and symptom inventory.

It is the author's impression that the use of self-report scales of this nature are best used in an *ipsative* manner, not *normatively*. For example, if normative data suggest that a given score on a particular scale reflects the presence (or absence) of an anxiety disorder, it is important to keep in mind that such cutting scores are valid only when applied to large groups of clients, not the individual child or adolescent sitting in one's consulting room. A pencil-and-paper test can, at best, be used to corroborate clinical impressions and diagnostic assessments, not establish them. These same scales can be very useful when employed in an ipsative manner. This involves comparing a given child's score on a pencil-and-paper test, not with some normative data derived from hundreds of others, but with that given child's previous scores on the same measure. By administering such scales several times prior to beginning treatment, a baseline can be established against which subsequent changes in scale scores can be more usefully interpreted. The author is not aware of any written self-report scales that have been specifically designed for use in assessing separation anxiety disorder alone.

There is no evidence that more generic objective standardized tests such as the Minnesota Multiphasic Personality Inventory (MMPI) or intelligence tests have much to contribute in assessing anxious youth. Similarly, the use of projective tests (Rorschach, Thematic Apperception Test, etc.) is rarely, if ever, valuable in arriving at a DSM-III-R diagnosis or in evaluating the effects of treatment. One projective test designed to measure separation anxiety (but not to provide for a *diagnosis* of separation anxiety (but not to provide for a *diagnosis* of separation anxiety disorder) is the Hansburg separation anxiety test: 12 black and white drawings depicting adolescents in situations related to separation or loss (Hansburg, 1980). The young respondent is asked to describe how the person in the picture is feeling (from a list of 17 defense mechanisms provided, such as rejection or anxiety). Each picture is labeled, describing the situation depicted (e.g., mother is being taken to the hospital). Little empirical research has been conducted on this assessment method. Two factor-analytic investigations have found that the theoretically derived subscales developed by Hansburg were not supported (Kroger, 1986; Kroger & Green, 1990), suggesting that the measure lacks content validity. At present, the available evidence does not suggest the incorporation of the Hansburg separation anxiety test into routine clinical assessment, although further research studies are clearly warranted.

Observational Methods

There do not appear to be any published standardized observational assessment strategies for use in evaluating children or adolescents with (presumptively) separation anxiety disorder, similar to behavioral approach tests developed for assessing simple or social phobics or agoraphobics.

The innovative clinician, however, may wish to employ some form of challenge test to evaluate a child's reactions to brief separations from the parent in the consulting room, or ask the parent to undertake some trial, contrived, separation experiences to evaluate the environmental circumstances that may moderate or exacerbate separation anxiety. For example, it may be clinically useful to empirically determine the buffering influence the presence of an older and trusted sibling has on a younger child's separation anxiety when the parent departs, say at a mall or while visiting friends. The child's reaction to these contrived separations can be carefully observed by the clinician or parent, and discussed in the consulting room to be possibly incorporated into treatment plans.

Marker Variables

For some DSM-III-R disorders, various biological markers have been developed that can aid in diagnosis or in evaluating responses to treatment, such as the dexamethasone suppression test used with severely depressed clients. At present, there does not appear to be any such biological marker for use in assessing clients with separation anxiety disorder. A number of potential *psychosocial* marker variables have been proposed as associated with SAD, such as parental history of adult-onset agoraphobia or of childhood SAD. For example, Last, Hersen, Kazdin, Finkelstein, and Strauss (1987) found that children with SAD tended to be younger or to come from families from a lower socioeconomic strata than children with overanxious disorder. These findings were not replicated in a subsequent study by Pruis and colleagues (1990). As in the case of biological markers, there do not yet appear to be any reliable psychosocial marker variables that serve any diagnostic utility.

TREATMENT

Evidence for Prescriptive Treatments

Behavior Therapy

In a review, Thyer and Sowers-Hoag (1988) found a total of 11 published reports describing the behavioral treatment of children and adolescents with separation anxiety disorder. Of these articles, 6 were case reports, 3 employed single-subject research designs, and 2 utilized group research designs. All of the treatments incorporated elements of exposure therapy, either in real life or in imagination, to desensitize the child to the anxiety-evoking stimulus of the parent's absence. Most often this was done gradually, in an effort to minimize the client's fearful reactions, but several studies applied a more rapid approach which, while engendering considerable anxiety on the part of the child, resulted in a more rapid amelioration of symptoms.

On the positive side, the available behavior studies are quite positive, suggesting that the treatment of SAD is both practical, not usually time consuming or costly, and results in enduring positive behavior change and anxiety reduction. Less optimistically, Thyer and Sowers-Hoag (1988) noted that given the 30-year history of clinical research in providing behavior therapy to children and adolescents experiencing separation anxiety, it is disappointing that a larger and more compelling body of empirical findings has not been forthcoming. Nevertheless, behavioral methods have a greater degree of research support than any other psychosocial approach to the treatment of this significant disorder (see also, Thyer, 1991).

Pharmacotherapy

The only medication described by the American Psychiatric Association's (1989, pp. 416–418) test *Treatments of Psychiatric Disorders* as useful in treating children and adolescents with SAD is the tricyclic antidepressant, imipramine. This recommendation is apparently based on two published studies evaluating the effects of imipramine in the treatment of so-called school phobia (Rabiner & Klein, 1969; Gittelman-Klein & Klein, 1971). The earlier study was an open-label trial, whereas the second involved a placebo-control group, both yielding results that suggested that imipramine was useful in returning children to school. A third study, conducted by Berney and associates (1981) and using a lower average dosage of a different tricyclic compound, did not find the medication to be helpful.

More recently, Bernstein, Garfinkel, and Borchardt (1987; unpublished paper cited by Klein & Last, 1989, p. 79) treated a small sample of school-phobic children with imipramine, and in comparing their response with that of the children treated with a placebo, no significant differences were obtained with respect to promoting a return to school. At present, it is difficult to contend that imipramine is a demonstrably effective treatment for children and adolescents experiencing separation anxiety disorder.

Another category of psychotropic medication that has been tested with children experiencing SAD has been the triazolobenzodiazepine compound alprazolam (trade name Xanax). Klein and Last (1989, p. 80) provided a preliminary report of an uncontrolled study involving 18 youngsters (mean age = 11) with SAD, treated with six weeks of alprazolam (average daily dosage = 1.9 mg). Apparently considerable improvements were obtained. In contrast, use of the benzodiazepine diazepam (trade name Valium) produced disruptive disinhibitory behavioral side effects among children with SAD, leading to a premature termination of the planned study and a discontinuation of the Valium treatment. Well-controlled trials of benzodiazepines await publication, and until such time, their use in treating children and adolescents with SAD should be approached with caution. Long-term use of benzodiazepines with children is not recommended due to the drug's inhibitory effects on growth hormone (cf. Cameron & Thyer, 1985).

It is problematic to extrapolate research on so-called school-phobic children to those experiencing separation anxiety, since research has clearly shown that the two conditions are different disorders (Last, Francis, Hersen, Kazdin, & Strauss, 1987). Furthermore, the term *school phobia* is not a DSM-III or DSM-III-R diagnosis. Rather, *school avoidance* may be the sequelae of a number of conditions or factors. For example, an aversion to school may be secondary to a social phobia or a simple phobia concerning aspects of the school environment, a reflection of true separation anxiety disorder, an operant response inadvertently maintained by parental contingencies, or related to truancy associated with conduct disorder (see Thyer & Sowers-Hoag, 1986, for a review of

potential etiologies of school phobia). Although it is true that most children with SAD display school refusal, it remains unclear what proportion of apparently school-phobic children suffer from SAD.

Alternative Treatments

The American Psychiatric Association's (1989) treatment manual provides separate clinical examples of the use of psychodynamic therapy and of family therapy to treat children experiencing SAD. Unfortunately, the treatment manual, like the DSM-III-R, is not supported by references to empirical research, hence the reader is unable to judge the appropriateness of these recommended treatments. To the author's knowledge, there is no evidence beyond that of clinical anecdote that indicates that either of these two alternative treatments is effective in treating SAD.

Selecting Optimal Treatment Strategies

The impression gained from a comprehensive survey of clinical research on SAD is that behavior therapy is the first choice treatment. Generally, depending on the intensity of treatment and the interventions selected, clinical improvements should be apparent within one month. The failure to find significant improvements within a month would suggest that an alternative behavioral treatment may be warranted. Should efforts using behavioral approaches fail, the addition of tricyclic medication (e.g., imipramine) to behavioral treatment may be useful (for placebo value if nothing else!).

If significant familial dysfunction is present, then educational efforts directed at the parents can be useful (e.g., if the mother or father consistently gives in to the child's tearful demands not to leave them). At all times, clear rationales should be provided to the caregivers since most often they will bear the major responsibility for carrying out treatment plans and for the success or failure of intervention. Marital/familial dysfunction can exist independently of a child's SAD, but if assessment reveals a clear relationship, then therapy directed toward the parent, couple, or family as a whole may be indicated to address SAD indirectly.

Problems in Carrying Out Interventions

The misdiagnosis or incomplete assessment of a child or adolescent who appears to meet the criteria for SAD may be a cause of treatment failure. For example, if a child with apparent SAD has, in reality, experienced sexual abuse at the hands of a neighborhood pedophile while traveling to and from school, and this crucial factor is not uncovered, then the clinician can provide all the behavior therapy, medication, verbal psychotherapy, or family therapy in the world and not achieve a successful outcome. This would be an example of an inaccurate identification of the child's anxiety-evoking stimuli.

Consistency on the part of the parents in carrying out agreed upon treatment plans can also be a frequent source of treatment failure. How many times have we carefully explained treatment programs to parents, had them agree to faithfully carry them out, and then return the following week stating that the program didn't work, only to find out upon detailed inquiry that they had done the exact opposite of what was requested! Similarly, the cooperation of significant others (with respect to SAD) in the child's life is essential. School officials or teachers may be unwilling or unable to cooperate in arranging a graduated schedule to return a child to school, or to put up with a child's (hopefully temporary) being upset in class, after having been dropped off there by mommy as part of a treatment program.

Relapse Prevention

Assuming that a child's SAD has been satisfactorily resolved, the clinician must prepare for the possibility of relapse. A return of SAD is most likely following the child or family's experiencing significant psychosocial stressors or illness. If a child has had an illness during which time he or she received greater than normal solicitude, atten-

tion, and care, upon recovery from the illness one would not be surprised to find a return of SAD-like behavior. This can usually be dealt with by discussion such possibilities with the parents at termination and prompting them to apply the behavioral skills they have learned in treatment once more to the newly dependent child. Similar caveats are in order should a parent experience a severe illness or separation from the child that is traumatic.

Other times of particular vulnerability to relapse include returning to school after an absence due to illness or vacation or the child having spent period of time with another caregiver (aunt, sitter) who reinforces SAD-type behavior. Should the family move, which could involve the child attending a different school, a reemergence of SAD symptoms could occur—something also likely to happen if the child experiences some upsetting events at school or traveling to and from there. Again, prevention involves anticipation on the part of the clinician, and prior instructions and training of the parents on how to deal with such occurrences, should they happen.

CASE ILLUSTRATION

Case Description

Susie is an 11-year-old white girl who presented at the Behavior Disorders Clinic with fear and avoidance of situations in which she would be apart from her mother. Her parents reported that Susie displayed a long-standing fear of such separations since she was a toddler. At the present time, with the exception of school, Susie insists that her mother or father accompany wherever she goes, never leaving her alone. She does not spend any time outside of her home (in the yard or elsewhere in the neighborhood) unless escorted by her mother. She avoids going outside to get the daily mail or to swim in the backyard pool without her mother accompanying her or clearly watching from inside the house.

Rarely does Susie allow her mother to leave her with a babysitter. If the chosen babysitter is especially familiar to her and her mother's absence will be short, Susie may allow her mother to leave her if she has a trusted friend at home as a companion. Susie is involved in many outside activities such as going to movies, playing in the park with friends, 4-H Club, church youth groups, and swimming. However, her mother must transport her and remain to monitor Susie during these activities. If, during these periods, she recognizes that her mother is not within sight, she huddles, terrified, crying, and screaming, waiting for her mother to reappear.

Because of her fears of being separated from her mother, Susie frequently turns down invitations to birthday parties at friends' homes. She does, however, frequently have friends over to her house, and her parents consider her to be quite sociable. Even when accompanied by her mother, she typically clings to her hand for fear of her mother getting lost, injured, or kidnapped. She also reports substantial worry that her mother will be harmed and taken away from her. To ensure her mother's safety, she attempts to restrict her mother's activities, as evidenced by her unwillingness to allow her mother to go grocery shopping or to undertake other activities of a similar nature. She typically requests her father to go instead. At the initial visit to the Behavior Disorders Clinic, Susie refused to be interviewed by the evaluating clinician, crying excessively and clinging to her mother. She demanded that her mother accompany her to the interview room and remain with her throughout the evaluation.

Susie currently attends school regularly and excels academically. Her ability to attend school is enhanced by the fact that her mother has recently obtained a job at the school as a teacher's aide in another classroom. This enables her to provide assistance to her daughter in case she becomes frightened and unable to remain in the classroom. Susie rarely demands leaving the classroom with her mother except when thunderstorms are possible. In fact, her fear in these situations is so exaggerated that the sight of a few dark clouds in an otherwise cloudless blue sky will prompt fear, crying, and demands for her mother to come. After being rescued and taken out of the classroom by her mother, Susie rarely returns immediately after the weather clears. Instead, she remains with her

mother in the school office or, in some cases, leaves school and returns home with her mother for the remainder of the day. Her fear of storms is pervasive across settings, including the home. Although her parents deny that they have similar fears, this appears questionable, as the family has arrangements to have a friend at the local radio station call them prior to public announcements of storm watches and warnings.

Her mother reported first using a babysitter when Susie was approximately 1½ years of age. She was left with the sitter for three and a half hours during which she continually cried. The mother never again attempted to leave her alone with a babysitter until Susie was much older. Susie entered preschool at approximately 3½ years of age. At this time, her parents again noticed that she had problems with excessive anxiety and difficulty being apart from her mother.

She frequently cried at school when her mother left, often refused to go to school, or required her mother to remain with her at school for the day. During this time, conflicts were taking place between her parents and one of her older sisters regarding the sister's association with undesirable company and her wish to leave home. As a result of the daughter's threats to leave home, her parents resorted to slashing the tires of her car, hiding her car keys, and other similar measures to keep her from leaving. Concurrently, another of the sisters married and moved away with her husband to California. During this time, the parents took Susie to see a local psychologist in order to help her with her fears and anxiety difficulties. She was seen in treatment for approximately two years. Although the parents report that this verbal therapy was somewhat beneficial in alleviating Susie's general anxiety level, she continued to have problems being away from her mother, which persist today and prompted referral to the Behavior Disorders Clinic.

Differential Diagnosis and Assessment

It appeared that Susie met the DSM-III-R criteria for separation anxiety disorder. The etiology cannot be clearly determined, however it seems likely that parental overprotectiveness may have inadvertently prevented Susie from experiencing the normal transition out of the separation anxiety phase undergone by most children. It is clear that significant operant elements are serving to maintain her signs and symptoms of SAD. Her parents cater to her demands, and she is clearly the central power-figure in the family, at least in matters concerning separation issues. To the extent that she experiences genuine fear when apart from her mother, Susie's anxiety, weeping, and dependent behaviors are negatively reinforced by the mother's coming to comfort her. To the extent that Susie enjoys all this attention and solicitude, SAD behaviors are positively reinforced. Because this pattern has persisted for a number of years, and her behavior has been reinforced on what is in effect a variable-ratio/variable-interval schedule, SAD behavior is likely to be quite durable and resistant to extinction. It is worth noting in this context that separation anxiety disorder of childhool *can* persist into adulthood (see Butcher, 1983, for an example).

Treatment Selection

Because of the duration and strength of Susie's SAD, and the extensive degree of control she exerted over the family, it was felt that a graduated program involving teaching her to tolerate increasingly longer periods of separation from her mother would be unworkable. Rather, treatment focused on several sessions of parent education, carefully delineating the therapist's formulations of Susie's SAD, how she probably had not been given the opportunity to "outgrow" the separation anxiety phase of development, and that strenuous efforts would be needed to bring about a rapid resolution of her problem and a restoration of the family to normal living, free from Susie's unreasonable demands.

The therapist arranged for several demonstrations of the use of operant extinction in the consulting room with Susie. In one session it was arranged that mother and father were to leave Susie alone in the consulting room with the therapist, stating that they would be back soon. While a videocamera recorded what transpired, the therapist took a matter-of-fact approach to Susie's near hysterics and attempted to engage her in appropriate play and conversation. Whenever Susie paused briefly, the therapist complimented her on calming down, and gave her a potato chip, Susie's preferred snack (it was shortly before lunchtime). After 25 minutes, Susie calmed down and began to engage in appropriate play, after which the therapist knocked on the door and the parents returned to find their daughter calm.

The videotape was reviewed with the parents by the therapist, who commented on his use of a matter-of-fact demeanor, refusal to attend to Susie's SAD behavior, and corresponding reinforcement of appropriate talk and play activities. The results of this trial were quite surprising to the parents, who had predicted that Susie would have maintained her hysterics for several hours, if not forever. These trials were repeated on two more office visits, with Susie calming down in a shorter time period on each trial, serving to illustrate that Susie (1) would not go crazy if left alone, (2) would not be harmed by the experience, and (3) would begin calming down more rapidly if the method were applied consistently.

Arrangements were made for mother to obtain a teacher's aide position in a different school, beginning on a certain date. On that date, the father was to take Susie to school and leave her there, in the care of the teacher. A joint therapist-parent-teacher conference was arranged, wherein it was agreed that if Susie became fearful in class, her behavior was to be ignored unless it became disruptive. If that happened, the teacher would matter-of-factly take Susie to the nurse's office, where she was to remain lying down until she felt ready to return to the classroom. The room was to be free of distractions, and Susie was not allowed any reading materials or permitted to engage the nurse in lengthy conversation. Rather, she was to lie down until she felt better.

At home, the mother was to go about her errands away from the house as necessary. If asked by Susie, the mother was to explain in a matter-of-fact manner that she was leaving to go shopping (or whatever) and that she would be back by _____ (time). If Susie protested, her mother was to simply state, "You are old enough to be by yourself sometimes now," and then leave. Appropriate supervision was, of course, arranged with a trusted babysitter. The babysitter was instructed to take Susie to her room, give her a chance to calm down, leave her there, and not attend to her anxious behavior if Susie became upset. Otherwise, she was to engage Susie in preferred activities during the mother's absence.

Both siblings and parents agreed not to provide Susie with reassurance when she voiced her unrealistic worries ("Mommy will be kidnapped"!) but instead to provide her with praise and other forms of reinforcement when any improvements became apparent.

The preceding treatment program has a number of precedents in the literature. In one series of 50 patients treated in a similar manner by Kennedy (1965), all 50 responded favorably. Patterson and Brodsky (1966) presented a more detailed description of the successful treatment of a single child. Copies of these articles were given to the parents to read and discuss with the therapist for further guidance.

Treatment Course and Problems in Carrying Out Interventions

Formal treatment began on a Monday, the same day that Susie's mother began her new position. It was announced at breakfast that Mom would now be working at another school and that Dad would be taking Susie to school today (siblings took the bus, as usual). Susie immediately began to protest, but both parents matter-of-factly stated that the decision had been made for Mom to take a better job and that Susie was now old enough to attend school without her mother being there. They reminded her of the many days she had gone to school without having to seek out her mother and said that they expected today would be similar. Susie began to weep and continued her protests, but she allowed her father to escort her to the car.

Susie and her father arrived at the classroom a bit before the usual time, so that Susie would not be subjected to entering a crowded classroom while weeping, as indeed she was. Dad saw her seated, sniffling, at her desk, and wished her a good day, stating that he would be by to pick her up at the end of the school day. Other children were entering the room at this point and Susie sat there looking distressed and a bit bewildered.

As school began, Susie went up to the teacher and stated that she wanted to go home and wanted her mommy. The teacher instructed her to return to her seat and begin work like the other kids. Susie complied but a few minutes later returned with similar complaints. As instructed, the teacher took Susie to the school nurse, who was aware of the program and agreed to supervise her until Susie felt rested enough to return to class.

Shortly before lunch, Susie (now quite bored) requested to be allowed to return to class. The nurse escorted her there and Susie joined her class in time to eat. She returned to her classroom and participated without incident for about an hour before returning to the teacher, stating that she wanted to go home. The teacher reminded her that her father would be by to pick her up at the end of the day (in less than two hours), praised her for working so well, and asked her if she would assist her by erasing the blackboards (a favorite task of the children). Susie did so, which took about 10 minutes, again receiving praise from the teacher, and a further task of helping to pass out some assignments. After this, she was instructed to return to her seat and begin her work.

At the end of the school day, the teacher took Susie to the pick-up ramp where Susie's father was waiting. The teacher gave him a brief report, emphasizing Susie's courage and helpfulness, and said that she was confident that Susie would continue to do well. Once in the car with Susie, her father was subjected to tearful recriminations that continued during dinner and also directed toward her mother. Finally, Susie was told that this would have to stop or she could go to her room. Susie left in a pout, claiming that she would never go to school again, that her parents didn't love her, and so on. Later that evening, the parents received the expected phone call from the clinician who discussed the day with them and offered suggestions for dealing with Susie the following day.

The next morning, Mom and Dad got up a bit

earlier than usual, anticipating problems. Susie informed them that she was not going to school today; instead, she would accompany her mother to her new job. The parents presented a united front, informed Susie that she *was* going to school that day, she would not accompany her mother, and that she was to be dressed for breakfast in 15 minutes. They then left the room. Fifteen minutes later they returned to find Susie half dressed and tearful, sullenly refusing to put on any more clothes. In a matter-of-fact manner, without scolding, they began to dress Susie, who protested and finally dressed herself and came downstairs. Breakfast was not pleasant. Susie ate little, continued to protest and weep, and had to be given slight assistance to enter the car with her father.

At school, Susie's dad escorted her to the classroom, kissed her goodbye with encouraging words, and left. The morning of the second day was a repeat of the first, except Susie only remained lying down alone in the nurse's office for a single hour before asking to return to class. The teacher again made efforts to provide Susie with diverting tasks and praised her work.

On the homefront, Susie's mother deliberately began undertaking errands unaccompanied by Susie, who was left in the care of an older sibling. Mom found it difficult to view her daughter's tear-streaked face in the rear-view mirror as she drove off to shop, but continued these solitary errands. One night, both parents arranged an evening out for the two of them, and a babysitter for Susie (older siblings would also be out for the evening). The sitter had been coached on how to handle Susie and the parents left the sitter with a rental videotape Susie had been asking to see. When they returned home, they found Susie in bed, but awake and tearful. The sitter reported no untoward incidents, apart from Susie's initially incessant worrying about her parents' whereabouts and well-being (which the sitter ignored, after offering a single reassurance).

The next few weeks had their ups and downs, but nothing that the parents could not handle by themselves or in consultation with their therapist. One day in school was particularly upsetting. The regular teacher was ill and a substitute teacher replaced her for the day. Unfamiliar with Susie's history and current program, she quickly became extremely concerned when Susie said she wanted to go home and began to cry. The substitute teacher called the school secretary to locate the parents to pick Susie up. After laborious efforts and miscommunicated messages, the father arrived at the school genuinely concerned that his daughter was ill or injured. He did take her home, and the next day presented an exacerbation of Susie's tearful protests and somatic complaints, which had been gradually diminishing. However, by persevering with the program (and a return of the regular teacher to the classroom), the lost ground was quickly regained.

Outcome and Termination

After about three months, Susie was regularly going to school without protest or tears and was allowing her mother to leave the home on errands. The mother's refusal to supervise Susie when she went outside initially led to her staying inside a great deal. But when this became apparent, both parents united in requiring Susie to spend time outside playing. Working in conjunction with one of her girlfriends' parents, they arranged an overnight stay for Susie at this home two houses down the street. After four months, during which time office visits were tapered, the parents agreed with the therapist's suggestion to terminate the case.

Followup and Maintenance

At monthly intervals during the next six months, the therapist called Susie's parents to monitor her progress. Two months after termination, there was an exacerbation of Susie's SAD following her coming down with the flu and staying home from school for four days. However, by continuing the program, the parents were able to deal with this setback within a week. It was very clear that having cooperative, informed, and intelligent parents was what made this outcome successful.

SUMMARY

The condition called separation anxiety disorder remains underresearched both in terms of etiological understanding and in clinical interventions. However, it appears that behavior analysis and therapy approaches have much to offer in the case of such clients. Treatment almost always involves the entire family and is aimed at a restructuring of the inadvertently arranged environmental contingencies that have perpetuated the signs and symptoms of SAD in the identified client. A thorough assessment and accurate diagnosis is essential in correctly treating the condition. The role of medications in treating SAD, including tricyclic antidepressants, is unclear, but recent studies suggest that these compounds are not as effective as was once thought.

REFERENCES

American Psychiatric Association. (1980). *Diagnostic and statistical manual of mental disorders* (3rd ed.). Washington, DC: Author.

American Psychiatric Association. (1987). *Diagnostic and statistical manual of mental disorders* (3rd ed., rev.). Washington, DC: Author.

American Psychiatric Association. (1989). *Treatments of psychiatric disorders* (Vol. 3). Washington, DC: Author.

Anderson, J. C., Williams, S., McGee, R., & Silva, P. A. (1987). DSM-III disorders in preadolescent children. *Archives of General Psychiatry, 44,* 69–76.

Ballenger, J. C., Carek, D. J., Steele, J. J., et al. (1989). Three cases of panic disorder with agoraphobia in children. *American Journal of Psychiatry, 146,* 922–924.

Beck, A. T., Epstein, N., Brown, G., & Steer, R. A. (1988). An inventory for measuring clinical anxiety: Psychometric properties. *Journal of Consulting and Clinical Psychology, 56,* 893–897.

Benjamin, R. S., Costello, E. J., & Warren, M. (1990). Anxiety disorders in a pediatric sample. *Journal of Anxiety Disorders, 4,* 293–316.

Berney, T., Kolvin, I., Bhate, S. R., Garside, R. F., Jeans, J., Kay, B., & Scarth, L. (1981). School phobia: A therapeutic trial of clomipramine and short-term outcome. *British Journal of Psychiatry, 138,* 110–118.

Butcher, P. (1983). The treatment of childhood-rooted separation anxiety in an adult. *Journal of Behavior Therapy and Experimental Psychiatry, 14,* 61–65.

Cameron, O. G., & Thyer, B. A. (1985). Treatment of pavor nocturnus with alprazolam (letter). *Journal of Clinical Psychiatry, 46,* 504.

Costello, A. J., Edelbrock, C., Dulcan, M., Kalas, R., & Klaric, S. H. (1984). *Report on the NIMH Diagnostic Interview Schedule for Children/DISC.* Unpublished manuscript.

Eth, S., & Pynoos, R. S. (Eds.). (1985). *Post-traumatic stress disorder in children.* Washington, DC: American Psychiatric Press.

Francis, G., Last, C. G., & Strauss, C. C. (1987). Expression of separation anxiety disorder: The roles of age and gender. *Child Psychiatry and Human Development, 18,* 82–89.

Gittelman-Klein, R., & Klein, D. F. (1971). Controlled imipramine treatment of school phobia. *Archives of General Psychiatry, 25,* 204–207.

Hansburg, H. G. (1980). *Adolescent separation anxiety: A method for the study of adolescent separation problems* (Vol. 1). New York: Robert Krieger.

Hodges, K. (1990). Depression and anxiety in children: A comparison of self-report questionnaires to clinical interview. *Psychological Assessment, 2,* 376–381.

Hodges, K. K., Kline, J., Stern, J., Cytryn, L., & McKnew, D. (1982). The development of a child assessment schedule for research and clinical use. *Journal of Abnormal Child Psychology, 10,* 173–189.

Hodges, K. K., McKnew, D., Burbach, D. J., & Roebuck, L. (1987). Diagnostic concordance between two structured child interviews, using lay examiners: The Child Assessment Schedule and the Kiddie-SADS. *Journal of the American Academy of Child and Adolescent Psychiatry, 26,* 654–661.

Kashani, J. H., & Orvaschel, H. (1990). A community study of anxiety in children and adolescents. *American Journal of Psychiatry, 147,* 313–318.

Kennedy, W. A. (1965). School phobia: Rapid treatment of fifth cases. *Journal of Abnormal Psychology, 70,* 285–289.

Klein, R. G., & Last, C. G. (1989). *Anxiety disorders in children.* Newbury Park, CA: Sage.

Kovacs, M. (1985). The interview schedule for children. *Psychopharmacology, 21,* 991–994.

Kroger, J. (1986). Factor structure of the Hansburg separation anxiety test. *Journal of Clinical Psychology, 42,* 605–611.

Kroger, J., & Green, K. (1990). Subscale structure and stability of the Hansburg Separation Adolescent

Separation Anxiety Test. *Journal of Clinical Psychology, 46,* 850–856.

Last, C. G., Francis, G., Hersen, M., Kazdin, A. E., & Strauss, C. C. (1987). Separation anxiety and school phobia: A comparison using DSM-III criteria. *American Journal of Psychiatry, 144,* 653–657.

Last, C. G., Hersen, M., Kazdin, A. E., Finkelstein, R., & Strauss, C. C. (1987). Comparison of DSM-III separation anxiety and overanxious disorders: Demographic characteristics and patterns of comorbidity. *Journal of the American Academy of Child and Adolescent Psychiatry, 26,* 527–531.

Last, C. G., & Strauss, C. C. (1989). Panic disorder in children and adolescents. *Journal of Anxiety Disorders, 3,* 87–95.

Last, C. G., Strauss, C. C., & Francis, G. (1987). Comorbidity among childhood anxiety disorders. *Journal of Nervous and Mental Disease, 175,* 726–730.

Lyons, J. A. (1987). Posttraumatic stress disorder in children and adolescents: A review of the literature. *Developmental and Behavioral Pediatrics, 8,* 349–356.

Mattison, R. E., Bagnato, S. J., & Brubaker, B. H. (1988). Diagnostic utility of the Revised Children's Manifest Anxiety Scale in children with DSM-III anxiety disorders. *Journal of Anxiety Disorders, 2,* 147–155.

Moreau, D. L., Weissman, M., & Warner, V. (1989). Panic disorder in children at high risk for depression. *American Journal of Psychiatry, 146,* 1059–1060.

Patterson, G. R., & Brodsky, G. A. (1966). A behavior modification program for a child with multiple problem behaviors. *Journal of Child Psychology and Psychiatry, 7,* 277–295.

Pruis, A., Lahey, B. B., Thyer, B. A., Christ, M. A. G., Loeber, R., & Loeber, M. (1990). Separation anxiety disorder and overanxious disorder: How do they differ? *Phobia Practice and Research Journal, 3*(2), 51–59.

Puig-Antich, J., & Chambers, W. (1978). *The Schedule for Affective Disorders and Schizophrenia for school-aged children.* New York: New York State Psychiatric Institute.

Rabiner, C. J., & Klein, D. F. (1969). Imipramine treatment of school phobia. *Comprehensive Psychiatry, 10,* 387–390.

Robins, L. N., & Regier, D. A. (Eds.). (1991). *Psychiatric disorders in America: The epidemiologic catchment area study.* New York: Free Press.

Scherer, M. W., & Nakamura, C. Y. (1968). A fear survey schedule for children (FSS-FC): A factor analytic comparison with manifest anxiety (CMAS). *Behaviour Research and Therapy, 6,* 173–182.

Shaffer, D., Campbell, M., Cantwell, D., Bradley, S., Carolson, G., Cohen, D., Denckla, M., Frances, A., Garfinkel, B., Klein, R., Pincus, H., Spitzer, R. L., Volkmar, F., & Widiger, T. (1989). Child and adolescent psychiatric disorders in DSM-IV: Issues facing the work group. *Journal of the American Academy of Child and Adolescent Psychiatry, 28,* 830–835.

Silverman, W. K. (1991). Diagnostic reliability of anxiety disorders in children using structured interviews. *Journal of Anxiety Disorders, 5,* 105–124.

Silverman, W. K., & Nelles, W. B. (1988). The anxiety disorders interview schedule for children. *Journal of the American Academy of Child and Adolescent Psychiatry, 27,* 772–778.

Thyer, B. A. (1987). *Treating anxiety disorders: A guide for human service professionals.* Newbury Park, CA: Sage.

Thyer, B. A. (1991). Diagnosis and treatment of child and adolescent anxiety disorders. *Behavior Modification, 15,* 310–325.

Thyer, B. A. (in press). Childhood separation anxiety disorder and adult-onset agoraphobia: A review of the evidence. In C. G. Last (Ed.), *Anxiety across the lifespan.* New York: Springer.

Thyer, B. A., & Sowers-Hoag, K. M. (1986). The etiology of school phobia: A behavioral approach. *School Social Work Journal, 10,* 86–98.

Thyer, B. A., & Sowers-Hoag, K. M. (1988). Behavior therapy for separation anxiety disorder. *Behavior Modification, 12,* 205–233.

Wellner, Z., Reich, W., Herjanic, B., Jung, K. G., & Amado, H. (1987). Reliability, validity, and parent-child agreement studies of the Diagnostic Interview for Children and Adolescents (DICA). *Journal of the American Academy of Child and Adolescent Psychiatry, 26,* 649–653.

Westhuis, D. J., & Thyer, B. A. (1989). Development and validation of the Clinical Anxiety Scale. *Educational and Psychological Measurement, 49,* 153–163.

CHAPTER 10

OVERANXIOUS DISORDER

Philip C. Kendall Temple University
Kimberli R. H. Treadwell Temple University

DESCRIPTION OF DISORDER

Clinical and Associated Features

Overanxious children display a characteristic style of pervasive worry that is not focused on a particular event, situation, or object. In the second edition of *Diagnostic and Statistical Manual of Mental Disorders* (DSM-II; American Psychiatric Association, 1968), overanxious children were clasified within the behavior disorders as having an "overanxious reaction." This reaction included chronic anxiety, excessive fears and self-consciousness, a need to meet the expectations of others, and exaggerated autonomic responses (Jenkins, 1968). These symptoms have remained central to the current diagnosis of Overanxious Disorder (OAD), a term that was introduced into the diagnostic system in 1980 (DSM-III; American Psychiatric Association, 1980). OAD is the most common major anxiety disorder of childhood.

Characteristic concerns of children with OAD include excessive worry about future events—such behaved appropriately or made the correct decision about what to wear. They may display an overconcern about personal competence in athletic, social, or academic domains, the quality of a given performance, or evaluation by others. An extreme need for reassurance is often displayed, sometimes manifested by an inability to complete homework or projects without continuous feedback that they are doing a good job. Marked self-consciousness is also characteristic.

The nature of overanxious children's worries contribute to a picture of pseudomaturity. Their anxieties about needing to meet deadlines, keeping appointments, adhering to rules, and inquiring about the dangers of situations often create this illusion of maturity. Therefore, these children often get along well with adults, such as teachers. As a consequence, children with OAD are often overlooked by parents and teachers as having a disorder, because they are agreeable and do not usually present with behaviorally disruptive behaviors, as would be apparent in attentional difficulties or conduct problems.

Preparation of this chapter was supported in part by a National Institute of Mental Health grant (No. 1 R01 MH44042-01A1) awarded to Philip C. Kendall. We also gratefully acknowledge the assistance of Laura Bross and Bonnie Howard for comments on a draft of this chapter.

In addition, overanxious children often display ailments for which no physical basis can be established. These children are tense much of the time and often have multiple somatic complaints, such as headaches, stomachaches, and fatigue (Strauss, 1988). Generally, anxiety itself has physiological symptoms, typically involving activity in the autonomic nervous system. Physical symptoms that appear to be connected with anxiety include diffuse abdominal pain, enuresis, headaches, muscular tension, sweating, and jittery behavior (Barrios & Hartmann, 1988; Kendall et al., 1991).

On a larger scale, behavioral indices of youth with overanxious disorder involve observable actions. Some children may refuse to attend school, or may complain of somatic discomfort to try to stay out of school, on days of examination or other evaluative performances. At the Child and Adolescent Anxiety Disorders Clinic at Temple University, children with OAD report behavioral symptoms such as avoidance of schoolwork for fear of making errors, frequent visits to the school nurse with various somatic complaints, inability to participate in group sports or activities due to self-doubts about performance, or taking an inordinate amount of time inquiring about upcoming events. Excessive motor habits may be evident, such as nail biting, hair pulling, or hand wringing.

Cognitive features of OAD involve dysfunctional (distorted) thinking processes (Kendall, 1985). For example, children exaggerate (in catastrophic terms) the importance of events or experiences, think that if they cannot succeed at a task in two tries they will never gain competence, and equate minimal errors with total failure. Perfectionistic tendencies are often present, displayed both as unrealistic expectations for performance and as extreme self-criticism. For instance, an OAD child may be disappointed and fear that she will not get into a good college when she receives a grade of 92 percent on a middle-school exam instead of a 100 percent. Parallel to this is an overzealous seeking of approval from adults. These children must often be reassured repeatedly while working on a task, such as a book report, to assure them that they are doing a good job.

Fears of peer evaluation and embarrassment due to poor performance may lead these children to avoid participating in age-appropriate activities, such as social or sporting events. They also may not join groups, like the Girl Scouts, for fear of appearing foolish to others. These children are also liked significantly less by their peers than nondisordered children and are often socially neglected (Strauss, Lahey, Frick, Frame, & Hynd, 1988).

Epidemiology

A 1986 review of the literature noted that the available epidemiological data for pediatric anxiety disorders concerned only anxiety symptoms, not the disorders themselves (Orvaschel & Weissman, 1986). The subjects surveyed across studies were between 3 and 12 years old. From these data, Orvaschel and Weissman concluded that anxiety symptoms were more prevalent in girls than in boys, but that considerable variation occurred depending on the age of the child and the content of symptoms. Studies of 3-year-olds found prevalence rates for abnormal worry to range from 2.6 to 8.0 percent in community samples (Richman, Stevenson, & Graham, 1975; Earls, 1980). Children aged 5 to 8 displayed excessive worry in about 4 percent of the population (Kastrup, 1976). Children up to 12 years in age exhibit between 4 and 33 percent prevalence rates for worrying (Lapouse & Monk, 1958; Abe & Masui, 1981). Naturally, the prevalence of symptoms is not the same as that for a disorder.

A limited amount of research has specifically studied the prevalence rates of OAD. Studies focusing on clinic-referred children have found prevalence rates of OAD as the primary diagnosis to be 14 percent (Silverman & Nelles, 1988). Referrals to an anxiety clinic have found rates of 15 percent (Last, Strauss, & Francis, 1987) and 29 percent (Last, Hersen, Kazdin, Finkelstein, & Strauss, 1987). In our clinic, 86 percent of anxiety-disordered cases have OAD as their primary diagnosis. In pediatric settings, the prevalence for OAD was estimated at 2.0 to 2.8 percent and at 5 percent (Costello et al., 1988; Cantwell & Baker, 1989b). In community samples the prevalence was estimated at 2.8 and 3.6 percent (Anderson,

Williams, McGee, & Silva, 1987; Bowen, Offord, & Boyle, 1990).

Another nonreferred sample of 62 children displayed overanxious concerns at a rate of 10 percent (Bell-Dolan, Last, & Strauss, 1990). It was also reported in this study that one third of the children endorsed overconcern about competence and excessive needs for reassurance—specific diagnostic criteria for OAD. These subclinically anxious children endorsed higher frequencies of anxiety, depression, and loneliness on self-report measures, compared to the nonanxious non-referral children. At 12-month followup, the subclinically anxious children did not develop anxiety disorders, and symptoms actually lessened in frequency on self-report measures. These findings suggest that a wide range of anxiety symptoms are normal in children between the ages of 5 and 8 years and that anxious symptoms do not necessarily lead to anxiety disorders. Further research is warranted to explore the prevalence of anxiety symptoms in nonreferred child populations.

The stability and continuity of anxiety disorders from childhood to adulthood have also been examined. In the review cited above, Orvaschel and Weissman (1986) concluded that childhood anxiety disorders were generally related to adult anxiety disorders, but with little diagnostic specificity. For instance, OAD in childhood may in general be related to adult anxiety disorders, but not specifically to generalized anxiety disorder (GAD) (Cantwell & Baker, 1989a). Others have suggested that direct links between childhood and adult anxiety exist (Rutter, 1985). Due to similar theoretical manifestations, temporal continuity is suggested in overanxiousness, with its childhood manifestation as OAD and its adult variation as GAD.

Findings on differences in the sex ratio of this disorder are inconclusive. Studies thus far have found a higher prevalence of OAD in males compared to females at a ratio of 1.7:1 (Anderson et al., 1987). Males accounted for 63 percent of OAD cases in another clinical study (Cantwell & Baker, 1989b). These findings are inconsistent with the literature studying fears and anxieties in children, which has often indicated that girls display a significantly greater amount of fear than boys do

(Houston, Fox, & Forbes, 1984; Ollendick, Matson, & Helsel, 1985). However, others' findings of no significant gender differences in OAD (e.g., Last, Strauss et al., 1987) are consistent with our experience at our anxiety disorder clinic. Future research will be necessary to examine the nature of these differences. Perhaps specific fears are differentially expressed by children, and the generalized anxiety of OAD is not.

Etiology

Many factors are important in the etiology of disorders, yet few have been studied in OAD. Most research has examined developmental differences in the manifestation of OAD and has left etiology largely unexamined. In literature on adult twin studies, genetic factors for anxiety disorders, such as generalized anxiety disorder, have not been implicated (Torgersen, 1983). Similar research for children, and specifically for OAD, is warranted. Other influences on children's development to be addressed include temperament, early environmental stressors, and parenting practices. This will allow a more complete understanding of the development and manifestation of OAD.

Cognitive concepts such as expectations, attributions, self-statements, problem-solving skills, and schemata are currently receiving research attention. The interrelationships of these factors have been implicated in the development of maladaptive anxiety symptoms and disorders in children and adults (Kendall, 1991). Since behavioral events do not occur in a vacuum, it is important to examine the manner in which children cognitively disambiguate their behavioral experiences. Repetitions of behavioral events and the related cognitive processes will result in some degree of consistency in both behavior and cognition. Upon the accumulation of a history of behavioral events, the child entertains anticipatory cognition (expectancies). If children have early anxiety-producing negative experiences, they may develop distorted cognitive schema, involving anxiety-laden expectations of future behavioral events. The emotional intensity of a behavioral event also influences the importance the child attributes to a self-fulfilled anxious expectation, with events involving higher emotional intensity exerting a more powerful influence on the cognitive schema.

The differences in age among children with separation anxiety disorder (SAD) and OAD suggest that developmental differences in these disorders exist, but there is currently no longitudinal research of OAD. More information on the role of cognitive developmental differences and development of anxiety disorders would prove valuable to mental health professionals. Related information concerning the impact of family factors on childhood anxieties is also unknown. The effects of child-rearing practices, parental anxieties, family structure, and patterns of affective expression in the family on the development of OAD in youth merit future research (see Siqueland, Steinberg, & Kendall, 1991). A developmental perspective will be necessary in research on the etiology of OAD to distinguish normative and maladaptive anxieties in children (Barrios, Hartmann, & Shigetome, 1981).

It is known that children often appear to experience relatively transitory and developmentally appropriate fears and anxieties that are generally not in need of clinical services. These fears are adaptive in the sense that they allow the child to develop information-processing styles and coping strategies to deal with day-to-day living in which anxieties are encountered (Kendall & Ronan, 1990). The fears help the child develop appropriate means to cope with anxiety-related situations. However, what is considered a normative fear for a young child can be inappropriate and maladaptive for an older child. Developmental differences that have been noted in studies of child fears point to the importance of children's age in the manifestation of anxiety.

DIFFERENTIAL DIAGNOSIS AND ASSESSMENT

Cross-sectional research has provided preliminary data in the examination of developmental differences in children with OAD (Strauss, Lease, Last, & Francis, 1988). Significant differences were reported between the overall number of symptoms endorsed per group. Children older than 12 years of age tended to endorse more than five of the total seven symptoms of OAD, when compared to children younger than age 12. Overall, 28 percent of the older group presented all seven criteria for OAD, whereas only 4 percent of the younger group met all seven. Comorbidity patterns also differed significantly by age. Younger children more often received a concurrent diagnosis of separation anxiety disorder or attention deficit disorder, whereas older children more often had a concurrent simple phobia or major depression.

Strauss and colleagues (1988) also found that older children scored significantly higher than the younger ones on the trait and state subscales of the State-Trait Anxiety Inventory-Child Scale (STAIC; Spielberger, 1973), the worry/oversensitivity factor of the Revised Children's Manifest Anxiety Scale (RCMAS; Reynolds (Richmond, 1978), and the Child Depression Inventory (CDI; Saylor, Finch, Spirito, & Bennett, 1984). Compared to normative data for these three instruments, only the older group exhibited elevated anxiety and depression. The younger group was within nondeviant levels for these instruments.

It appears that as children age, the manifestation of OAD changes in regard to the content and quantity of OAD-related symptoms. OAD in children over the age of 12 present with a greater number of overall symptoms and a greater amount of anxiety concerning past events. Comorbidity patterns shift as the children age, from concurrent diagnoses of SAD and ADD to phobias and depression (Brady & Kendall, in press; Last, Hersen et al., 1987). Similar results are also reflected on self-report measures. This increase in reported symptoms appears to be specific to OAD, and not merely a factor of increased age, since findings in SAD often reveal that younger children report more symptomatology than do older children (Francis, Last, & Strauss, 1987).

DSM-III-R Categorization

Overanxious Disorder is categorized under the heading of Anxiety Disorders of Childhood or

Adolescence. OAD is one of the three childhood anxiety disorders, the other two being Separation Anxiety Disorder and Avoidant Disorder of Childhood. Unrealistic or excessive anxiety for a period of six months or longer is the hallmark symptom of Overanxious Disorder. Children must exhibit at least four of seven criteria to achieve clinical status. These criteria involve excessive or unrealistic worry or concerns about future events, the appropriateness of past behavior, or personal competence in one or more areas (athletic, academic, social). Excessive self-consciousness and need for reassurance may also be present. According to DSM-III-R, OAD may be diagnosed in the presence of another Axis I disorder. Differential diagnosis involves determining that anxiety is not related to a psychotic or mood disorder.

Associated features involve somatic complaints for which no physical basis can be established and marked feelings of tension (American Psychiatric Association, 1987). The onset of OAD may be sudden or gradual, and often symptoms are exacerbated by stress. No particular age of onset has been identified. However, several studies have found that the average age of children with OAD who seek therapeutic services centers around 13 years (Last, Hersen et al., 1987). The DSM-III-R also notes that this disorder is more common in the eldest children in small families in upper socioeconomic groups and in families that focus on achievement.

Given the recent emergence of diagnostic categories for child anxiety, there are few published studies of reliability and validity for OAD. Research has focused on DSM-III criteria rather than the 1987 revised edition. Support from case studies attests to the face validity of OAD, although little research addresses this issue (Strauss, 1988). Childhood anxiety is still an evolving domain. A task force is currently examining criteria for childhood anxiety disorders for DSM-IV, to be published December of 1992. Specifically, they are examining whether the degree of impairment of a disorder will be included in diagnostic criteria and whether criteria between anxiety disorders overlap (Shaffer et al., 1989).

Differential Diagnosis

The characteristic anxiety associated with OAD involves excessive or unrealistic worry. The anxiety is not focused solely on situations involving separation from attachment figures, as in SAD, nor is it focused on contact with unfamiliar people, as in avoidant disorder (AD). A jittery restlessness may be exhibited by children with OAD or with attention-deficit hyperactivity disorder, but there is no undue concern about the future in the latter. The anxiety must have lasted for at least six months; if not, adjustment disorder with anxious mood might be considered. Finally, if the anxious symptoms occur due to a psychotic disorder or mood disorder, OAD should not be diagnosed.

Diagnostic Issues

Perhaps due to the relatively brief status of OAD as a diagnostic entity, an examination of the validity and specificity of OAD has been only recently undertaken (Shaffer et al., 1989). Questions regarding OAD's specificity have emerged in the light of overlapping features and comorbidity rates with other childhood disorders (Thyer, Sowers, & Karen, 1988). For instance, several overlapping features exist between OAD and SAD and AD, producing high comorbidity rates between these disorders. In clinic samples, 57 percent of children with a primary diagnosis of OAD received a secondary diagnosis of an anxiety disorder (Last, Hersen et al., 1987). Others report that 36 percent of OAD children received at least one additional anxiety diagnosis, and 18 percent received two or more additional anxiety diagnoses (Last, Strauss, & Francis, 1987). This study also reported that those children diagnosed with SAD were most likely to receive a secondary diagnosis of OAD.

A study specifically addressing the differences between cases of OAD only and OAD with a coexistent diagnosis of SAD found several significant findings (Last, Hersen et al., 1987). Children with OAD alone were significantly older than those with both disorders and were mostly postpubescent children. OAD children were more likely to have a concurrent diagnosis of simple phobia than children with SAD. Children with OAD were also from higher socioeconomic levels than were children with SAD. No significant differences for gender or race (mostly Caucasian) for both groups were reported.

Low to moderate comorbidity rates also exist for OAD and nonanxiety-related diagnoses. Several studies have examined the comorbidity rates of depression with OAD. These rates range from 9 to 33 percent (Last, Strauss et al., 1987; Bowen et al., 1990; Last, Hersen et al., 1987; for review, see Brady & Kendall, in press). Our clinic has found a comorbidity rate of 22 percent for anxiety disorders in general and depression in children. Oppositional disorders are also commonly seen in children with a primary diagnosis of OAD (Last, Strauss et al., 1987).

Assessment Strategies

To assess and diagnose childhood anxiety, several considerations must be taken into account, such as differences in developmental level and normative behavior standards. Children are most often referred for psychological services by a parent or teacher, so the child may not understand why he or she is in treatment. Also, the diagnosis of anxiety in children is continuing to be refined and modified. The comorbidity of childhood anxiety with other disorders has been reported, and an ongoing debate exists concerning whether factor analytic or clinically derived classification systems are more appropriate.

Comprehensive assessment of anxiety has generally been tripartite. Three domains of manifestation are examined: the cognitive, behavioral, and physiological. Clinical interviews, self-report measures, behavioral observation, and physiological recording are strategies that can be employed to elicit expressions of anxiety across these three response categories.

Clinical Interviews

Historically, the clinical interview has been the most common method of assessing children (Greenspan, 1981). Highly structured interviews offer the clinician or researcher the advantage of standardized diagnostic categories according to DSM-III or DSM-III-R criteria. These structured interviews also may be more appropriate for anxious children, who have been shown to respond better to specific rather than open-ended questions (Ollendick & Francis, 1988).

Examples of interview schedules include the Child Assessment Schedule (CAS; Hodges, Kline, Fitch, McKnew, & Cytryn, 1981), the Schedule for the Assessment of Conduct, Hyperactivity, Anxiety, Mood, and Psychoactive Substances (CHAMPS; Mannusa & Klein, 1987), the Diagnostic Interview Schedule for Children (DISC; Costello, Edelbrock, Dulcan, Kalas, & Klaric, 1984), the Diagnostic Interview for Children and Adolescents (DICA; Herjanic & Reich, 1982), the Interview Schedule for Children (ISC; Kovacs, 1983), and the Schedule for Affective Disorders and Schizophrenia for School-Aged Children (K-SADS; Puig-Antich & Chambers, 1978). These interviews have generally low reliability for diagnosing anxiety disorders, which points to the difficulty of assessment of anxiety (Silverman & Nelles, 1988). The Anxiety Disorders Interview Schedule for Children (ADIS-C; Silverman, 1987) has been used in the CAADC at Temple University because it focuses *specifically* on the various anxiety disorders of childhood and adolescence. We have had to employ in-house revisions in order to assess the absence or presence of other conditions such as a depressive condition or an attentional difficulty.

Self-Report Scales

Self-report inventories are widely used strategies for assessing child anxiety in both research and clinical settings. Such measures allow the presence and content of fears and anxieties to be assessed, but alone are not sufficient for assigning specific diagnoses. Several scales are useful in assessing children with OAD. The Revised Children's Manifest Anxiety Scale (RCMAS) is a 37-item scale with dichotomous answers that yields an overall anxiety score and several scaled subscores tapping physiological, cognitive, and behavioral manifestations of anxiety (Reynolds & Richmond, 1978). A lie subscale reflects a child's tendency to respond in a socially desirable manner. Reliability for the measure is estimated at .85, and test-retest reliability is reported to be in the .90s (Reynolds & Paget, 1981). Concurrent validity was also established (Spielberger, 1973).

The State-Trait Anxiety Inventory for Children (STAIC; Spielberger, 1973) is a 40-item measure. Scores are standardized and normative data are available. Internal reliability is reported at .82, with a test-retest reliability of .65. Construct and concurrent validity was reported to be adequate by the authors. The Youth Self-Report (YSR; Achenbach, 1987) measures social competencies in a 17-item format and behavioral problems in a 103-item format. It is a child report measure that serves as a complement to the Child Behavior Checklist (CBCL; Achenbach & Edelbrock, 1983). Symptoms are organized through factor-analytic techniques that divides them into two broad-band factors: internalizing and externalizing disorders. Test-retest reliability for the YSR was .69 for referred adolescents and .81 for nonreferred youth. An advantage to this measure is that child self-reports can be compared to parent and teacher CBCL reports of child functioning. The Social Anxiety Scale for Children (SASC; LaGreca, Dandes, Wick, Shaw, & Stone, 1988) is a factor-analytic divided measure that comprises a Fear of Negative Evaluation Scale (FNE) and a Social Avoidance and Distress (SAD) scale. Moderate internal consistency (alphas .83 and .63 for FNE and SAD, respectively) have been found, and acceptable test-retest reliability (r = .70) has been reported.

The Children's Anxious Self-Statement Questionnaire (CASSQ; Kendall & Ronan, 1989) is a self-report instrument that taps the content of anxious youths' self-statements. The CASSQ has a test-retest reliability of .92 and two factor-analytic scales: negative self-focused attention and positive self-concept and expectations. This measure has shown meaningful discriminant validity. The Coping Questionnaire for children and parents provides data concerning a child's perceived ability to cope with a personally identified anxious situation (Kendall, 1989). Its reliability and validity is currently under investigation.

No behavioral observation system for coding behavior of anxious children is yet available. This is due in part to challenges in observing behavior that are specific to anxiety. Circumstances that are anxiety provoking differ for children, as do behavioral manifestations (Kendall et al., in press; Strauss, 1988). For instance, some children may be fidgety in anxiety-related school incidents, whereas others may have stomachaches when participating in sporting events. Direct observational coding systems merit further research because they could facilitate the identification of antecedents and consequences of anxiety symptoms.

Although physiological manifestations of anxiety have been explored extensively in adults, similar work has not been completed for children (Kendall et al., 1991). The most commonly used techniques are cardiovascular and electrodermal measures (Werry, 1986). However, these techniques lack adequate normative data for children. Idiosyncratic patterns of response during physiological assessment were also noted in children. Furthermore, little correspondence has been found between different physiological responses and subjective or cognitive components of anxiety (Barrios & Hartmann, 1988). Future elaboration of the biological concomitants of anxiety are necessary to establish normative data in children.

TREATMENT

Evidence for Prescriptive Treatments

Based on a review of the treatment outcome research, it is clear that there are precious few controlled empirical reports. There are data to support the beneficial effects of behaviorally oriented programs for anxiety and fears (King, Hamilton, & Ollendick, 1988), psychopharmacological treatments (Lydiard, Roy-Byrne, & Ballenger, 1988), and recent single-subject data supporting positive outcomes for a cognitive-behavioral treatment (Kane & Kendall, 1989). No single treatment has been found to be the most effective for Overanxious Disorder, and thus multiple modes of treatment have been recommended (Cantwell & Baker, 1989a).

Effective *behavioral treatments* have been employed for specific fears and phobias in childhood, modeled after anxiety-reduction approaches in the adult literature (King et al., 1988). No controlled outcome studies exist for generalized anxieties such as OAD. However, effective behavioral procedures for OAD might be developed in a manner similar to phobias, based on the adult literature regarding successful treatment for Generalized Anxiety Disorder (GAD; see Barrios & Shigetomi, 1979).

Most *pharmacotherapy* of anxiety disorders has focused on adults suffering from panic disorder or GAD. The tricyclic antidepressants and monoamine oxidase inhibitor (MAOI) antidepressants have been the standard treatment for panic, and benzodiazepines have been the traditional treatment for GAD (Lydiard et al., 1988). Buspirone is increasingly being used for GAD because it is as, if not more, effective than benzodiazepines and it does not carry the risk of dependence (Murphy, Owen, & Tyrer, 1989).

Various types of psychotropic drugs have been used to treat anxiety in children, including benzodiazepines, general antidepressants, and antipsychotics (Barkley et al., 1990; Gittelman & Kopliewicz, 1986; Simeon & Ferguson, 1985). Benzodiazepines have been used most often for child anxiety. The behavioral effects of these drugs are based on their effects of the central nervous system, such as disinhibition, anticonvulsant effects, reduction of arousal, central muscle relaxation, and potentiation of depressant drugs (Simeon & Ferguson, 1985). Adverse effects include impulsivity and aggression. Despite the widespread use of benzodiazepines, their effectiveness for OAD and the other childhood anxiety disorders has not been supported (Barkley et al., 1990). Anxiolytic efficiency has also not been demonstrated in childhood anxiety disorders, and few controlled studies exist. Buspirone is an alternative pharmacological treatment. A case report supports the use of buspirone for OAD (Kranzler, 1988). Controlled studies are needed to examine the effectiveness of pharmacological treatment, both alone and in adjunct with psychotherapy for OAD.

The preliminary effects of a *cognitive-behavior therapy* (CBT) for anxiety-disordered children ages 9 through 13 are promising. This cognitive-behavioral approach (Kendall, Kane, Howard, & Siqueland, 1989) places greatest emphasis on integrating the modification of cognitive information-processing of interpersonal and social contexts with behavioral practice. The model stresses the learning process and the influence of contingencies in the environment, while validating the centrality of the individual's mediating information processing style in the development and remediation of psychological distress (Kendall, 1985).

It is held that the accumulation of experiences form the cognitive structures through which anxious children filter their current experiences. A dominant structure for anxious children is threat of loss, criticism, or harm. Their information processing style complements this structure, and OAD children view events as fearful, threatening, and uncertain. Expectations associated with fear are triggered as the children attempt to make sense of the world.

Cognitive-behavioral treatment seeks to provide treatment experiences that challenge preexisting anxious structures and to replace those structures with ones that will enable successful coping. Through therapist-guided corrective efforts to modify cognitive processing, the OAD child's dysfunctional schemas are reduced. The therapist shapes attributions about prior behavior and expectations for future behaviors to help the child construct new schemas for coping and solving problems. The goal is for the child to develop a cognitive structure for future events that includes accurate cognitions and adaptive skills.

To the extent that anxious children's inaccurate expectations contribute to their emotional distress, they need performance-based experiences and guidance to correct distorted processing. This results in confidence to proceed toward new situations with a more reasonable set of expectations. Our treatment utilizes in vivo experiences to accommodate this process. The emotional intensity of situations should determine the extent to which a behavioral event influences the child's cognitive structure, therefore therapy includes genuine anxious arousal (in vivo) to be an involving and corrective experience.

It is not the intention of our program to totally

cure anxiety; rather, our goal is to help each child in the successful management of anxious distress (see Kendall, 1989). Some form of anxiety in these children's lives is likely to persist, but if dysfunctional expectations and processing styles are modified, the level of anxiety experienced and the outcome of that experience will change in the direction of adaptive functioning. Many parents report that their OAD children have demonstrated an overanxious style since they were very young, and most children corroborate this description. Therefore, our plan is not to seek an analysis of the *course* or causes of the disorder, but to work to teach youth some adaptive styles of coping and how and when to use them to manage unwanted anxious arousal.

Selecting Optimal Treatment Strategies

Treatment Program

Our 16- to 20-week treatment program for OAD combines cognitive strategies and behavioral procedures (e.g., relaxation, cognitive strategies, problem solving, and imaginal and in vivo exposure) organized into two segments (Kendall et al., 1991; Kendall et al., in press). The first 8 or so sessions are the training segment, during which children learn to identify anxious processing. The second 8 sessions constitute the practice segment during which children begin to use skills acquired in the first 8 sessions in specific situations that are anxiety provoking for the child. The details of these two segments are described below.

Our overall goal is to teach OAD children to recognize their signs of anxious arousal and to let these signs serve as cues for the use of management strategies that minimize the debilitating aspects of anxiety (Meichenbaum, 1977). Specifically, we first teach the child to recognize anxiety, then to learn a variety of skills to cope with this anxiety and reduce its debilitating aspects. We strive to lower the child's level of personal distress and to improve the child's performance on developmental tasks—to create a sense of mastery.

In our program the therapist functions as a coping model as the new skills are introduced and

demonstrated. A therapist might describe a personal anxiety-provoking incident to the child and then describe coping strategies to effectively manage the situation. Then the therapist describes another situation, this time asking the child to help identify possible physical arousals, cognitive beliefs and expectations, and action plans. Throughout the training program, the level of anxiety is gradually increased. "Show That I Can" (STIC) tasks are assigned after each session for the child to complete during the ensuing week to reinforce what was addressed during the session. The therapist introduces a new skill, demonstrates it, then asks the child to roleplay, using a "tag-along" procedure (Ollendick, 1983). The child then roleplays the skill alone.

The Training Segment

Following relationship-building activities, the first 8 sessions address four basic skill areas. First, the child learns about his or her bodily reactions to feelings, especially physical symptoms specific to anxiety. In session 1 the child is encouraged to participate and verbalize feelings and experiences to help himself or herself to become a more expert reporter of personal experience. Children may be given a copy of *The Coping Cat Workbook* (Kendall, 1990) as an at-home supplement to their therapy. The first STIC task introduces the diary format of these tasks, and the child is asked to report a pleasant experience in the ensuing week. Compliance with STIC tasks is encouraged by a reward system. Children receive stickers for completed tasks and earn small rewards, such as markers or a tape, after sessions 4 and 8.

Sessions 2 and 3 further examine the concept of physical reactions to feelings and the discrimination between different types of feelings and theie bodily concomitants. These concepts are first introduced in the abstract, by looking at cartoons and magazines. The focus then moves to noticing emotions in family members and friends. The concept of roleplaying is introduced and the child is invited to participate in roleplaying different emotions. Somatic responses to anxiety are the focus of session 3. The child is asked to record bodily reactions to one pleasant and one anxious experience for the week's STIC task.

Having identified his or her physical symptoms of anxiety, the child is taught to use these symptoms as cues for relaxation. In session 4, children are taught a deep-breathing technique and modified progressive muscle relaxation. The child is given a tape of the relaxation exercise and is encouraged to practice the relaxation exercise every night for a week as the STIC task.

Second, in session 5, the child and therapist focus on recognition and evaluation of "self-talk." Self-talk includes the child's internal dialogue (e.g., expectations) about others and about situations. For the anxious child, the internal dialogues tend to center around unrealistic (catastrophic) appraisals of future events, negative self-evaluations, perfectionistic standards for performance, heightened self-focused attention or concern about what others are thinking, and concerns about failure. Cartoons with empty thought bubbles are used to facilitate awareness of self-statements. Responses to cartoons offer the therapist glimpses of the child's thought processes and degree of flex-

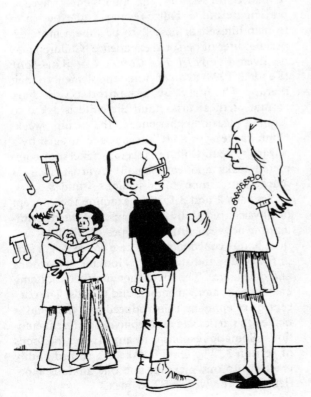

ibility. The impact of personal thoughts over responses in anxiety-provoking situations is addressed as the therapist begins to introduce coping self-talk instead of anxious self-talk. The STIC task involves writing down two anxiety-provoking situations during the week and noting the accompanying self-talk.

Third, beginning around session 6, step-by-step collaborative problem solving is introduced to help modify the anxious self-talk and to develop coping strategies. Feelings, thoughts, and possible coping strategies are examined in a triple-column format, and the child and therapist generate alternative solutions to a variety of difficult situations. The child then evaluates the possibilities and decides on the best personal course of action. As a STIC task, the child is asked to begin to cope with anxious situations by using the triple-column format and to record the results.

Session 7 introduces the fourth skill: self-evaluation and the rewarding of performance. OAD children often have difficulty evaluating themselves fairly and tend to set perfectionistic standards for themselves. The possibility of rewarding one's self for partial success is also introduced, to allow the child to realistically rate and reward himself or herself for the positive features of how he or she handled a situation. This allows the child also to evaluate what things they might do differently in the future, without self-denigration. The child generates a list of possible self-rewards that they receive for outside achievements. These self-rewards are very important for the OAD child, who often relies on outside sources, such as parents or teachers, to provide judgments and a sense of achievement. The child continues this lesson during the week by noting and recording two situations that were problematic and for which the child rated and rewarded the coping method.

The four concepts are summarized by the acronym FEAR—an acronym that facilitates the child's recall of the planned coping strategy. Children are taught to notice whether they are *F*eeling frightened, *E*xpecting bad things to happen, the *A*ttitudes and actions that will help, and *R*esults and rewards for coping. Children and therapist roleplay the use of the FEAR steps and read a pertinent short story. The child is asked to explain the FEAR steps to a parent during the week, which serves as a reminder of the new coping method.

The Practice Segment

The second treatment segment is devoted to the application and practice of the FEAR steps in increasingly anxious situations. Coping modeling, roleplaying, and STIC tasks are still utilized. It is in these next 8 sessions that the child practices using the FEAR steps in anxiety-provoking situations, with the therapist serving as a coach/collaborator. The first few sessions involve imaginal exposure to nonthreatening situations, and then, following initial successful experiences, sessions gradually progress to in vivo exposure to more threatening situations. We encourage children to take risks and to attain new skills. Each child's program is individually tailored to address specific worries. Often data from the Coping Questionnaire are utilized to guide the content of in vivos.

Later, in vivo exposure involves anxious experiences that are at the top of the child's anxiety hierarchy. The child and his or her therapist might go to particular sites, such as the snake pit at the zoo, the local shopping mall, or an age-appropriate social event to observe naturally occurring situations and to help the child to process his or her experiences in a nonanxiety-provoking manner.

STIC tasks for the last 8 sessions involve using the FEAR steps learned from the training segment during out-of-session situations. The child records the successes and the difficulties that are experienced (as in *The Coping Cat Workbook*).

Consolidation of therapeutic gains is presented in the final therapy session, when the child makes a "commercial" about his or her accomplishments, to *SH*ow *O*thers ho*W* (SHOW off). Examples have included a rap video, mini-skits, and cartoons. This commercial is intended to tell others how to cope with fear. That is, it informs the listener, in the child's own words, of what to do to master unwanted anxiety. We tape the commercial and give each child a copy of his or her product to take home. Thus, the child has an opportunity to demonstrate success in a creative task and in his or her management of anxiety.

Problems in Carrying Out Interventions

The generalized problem-solving approach utilized in the FEAR plan can be used to better manage anxiety and anxiety-related problems in daily life. As mentioned previously, we do not purport to cure anxiety but to equip the child with problem-solving capabilities in the context of more adaptive expectations and attributions concerning life experiences. The guiding principle to posttreatment activity is to *practice* these skills. Therapeutic intervention is the first step in a process of realigning maladaptive developmental trajectories to better prepare the child for the inevitable challenges experienced in later adjustment. The child is encouraged to continue to practice the FEAR steps to maintain therapeutic gains.

Relapse Prevention

Several guidelines are helpful in guiding children toward consolidation of treatment-produced gains. The first general guideline for the therapist is to shape and encourage "effort" attributions regarding the management of anxiety. Hard work in therapy is linked to the benefits the child has gained, to encourage the child to reward efforts for partial successes after therapy.

A second guiding principle for posttreatment functioning is introducing the concept of "lapses in efforts," rather than "relapses." Mistakes and partial successes are constructively framed as a vital part of the learning process itself, rather than as evidence of incompetence. Through therapy, the therapist has worked with the child to process errors rationally when they naturally occur. The main goal in relapse prevention is for the child to label and accept setbacks as temporary and then to return to problem solving. Mistakes then do not become excuses to throw in the towel or to confirm anxious thought processes but are construed as learning experiences.

Therapeutic contact after completion of the structured program is another way to maintain goals. The therapist might assure the child that they are still working together and make a phone contact to affirm that message. Regarding any new problems, a refocusing on the FEAR steps is helpful. In some instances, when the child has encountered a particularly difficult situation that has not gone well and/or when a therapeutic contact can prevent a hypothesized setback, we recommend a booster session. A child may experience a particularly negative event, such as death in the family or failing a class. A booster session would involve looking back at the event and systematically reframing it with the use of the FEAR plan. The examination of cognitive and behavioral alternatives and actions, and their consequences, can help the child to better understand the difficult situation in a more adaptive manner. These contacts allow the therapist to assess a child's progress and to remind the child of problem-solving skills and to continue the establishment of a relationship between these skills and real-life problems. Preventive booster sessions are sometimes planned when a future event might create high levels of anxiety, such as entering a new school or an impending divorce. Sessions can be scheduled to help the child cope in a proactive, anticipatory fashion.

CASE ILLUSTRATION

Case Description

The following case illustration* is in general characteristic of overanxious disorder. It is one of four case examples discussed by Kendall and associates (in press). Any identifying information has been changed to protect confidentiality.

Kerry presented as an attractive 11-year-old girl of normal height who was very concerned about her appearance. She was friendly and polite but exhibited nervous mannerisms such as biting her nails and twisting her hair. She lived in an intact nuclear family—her mother worked as a fourth-grade teacher and her father was a certified public accountant. Kerry was the oldest of four siblings. She was particularly close to the youngest sister, and reported normal sibling quarrels with her two brothers. Kerry's mother reported that she and

her daughter had a conflicted relationship. At times Kerry had great difficulty separating from her mother, while at other times Kerry would openly show anger toward her mother.

Kerry's parents admitted to high expectations for their own performances, but denied any open communication of equally high expectations for Kerry's performance. Kerry did quite well academically, usually making grades of A in an accelerated program. However, receiving an occasional B+ upset her; she worried that she consequently would not make the honor roll. It seemed that Kerry was not manifesting anxiety-related symptoms in the classroom, since her teacher was surprised to discover she was receiving treatment for anxiety disorders. Although Kerry was overly concerned about what others thought of her, she appeared to have a fairly normal social life with a group of girlfriends. Kerry's mother contacted the clinic because she was concerned about her daughter's extreme anxiety regarding school. Over the past few weeks, Kerry had started to cry and refused to go to school in the mornings. Despite her daughter's protests, Kerry's mother insisted she go to school, and Kerry managed to comply.

Kerry was experiencing a great deal of anxiety in relation to her studies, and was plagued by fears of failing. She pushed herself very hard to study, and would often stay up late at night or stay indoors on the weekends to complete assignments. At the same time, Kerry complained about being "overworked." Although she was only in the fifth grade, she was concerned about making the grade in high school so she could enter a good college. Indeed, her anxiety about school was so great that she would sometimes experience a vague, overwhelming feeling occasionally accompanied by somatic complaints, such as shaking, headaches, and chills. The intensity of the somatic responses, accompanied by Kerry's inability to clearly describe what specific situation led to the feelings, seemed to indicate panic attacks. However, differential diagnosis did not identify full-blown panic attacks.

Kerry was extremely perfectionistic and self-conscious, yet worried that others might think that she was incompetent and incapable. In fact, her fear concerning grades stemmed from that of

---

*We wish to thank the therapist, Elizabeth Kortlander, for the use of this case material.

being teased if she failed to meet her own standards. In addition, she was very concerned with pleasing others. She felt particularly anxious when faced with choices, fearing that she would hurt others' feelings if she made a wrong choice. For example, she described one occasion when both her brother and a neighbor had asked her to play with them. She so feared being perceived as mean by one or the other that she was unable to make a choice with whom to play. She ran back and forth between the two yards until she became so anxious and overwhelmed by the situation that she had to go inside and lie down on a couch. Fortunately, Kerry was motivated to try to change the patterns that were causing her such great distress.

Differential Diagnosis and Assessment

Kerry's primary diagnosis, based on both the parent and child Anxiety Disorder Interview Schedule (ADIS), was overanxious disorder. In addition, Kerry's interviewer noted a limited number of depressive and obsessive-compulsive features. Her mother's interview produced a secondary diagnosis of separation anxiety and several symptoms of school phobia and depression. Kerry's self-report scores indicated high levels of anxiety (STAIC Trait T-score = 65; RCMAS T-score = 58). Her mother's report on the CBCL also indicated high levels of anxiety (T-score = 72). The specific target behaviors selected for treatment concerned going to school, taking tests, and having to choose particular friends with whom to spend time. Treatment was initiated in the summer, so no information was available from the teacher prior to the beginning of treatment.

Treatment Selection

Kerry was accepted into the Child and Adolescent Anxiety Clinic at Temple University to participate in the cognitive-behavioral treatment program.

Treatment Course and Problems in Carrying Out Interventions

The major focus of therapy for Kerry was on her "need to be perfect" and her attempts to please everyone in order to avoid their disapproval or anger. These issues were evident during the very first sessions of treatment.

It was fairly easy to establish a superficial rapport with Kerry, due to her wish for her therapist to like and approve of her. However, it soon became clear that it would be more difficult to establish a relationship with Kerry in which she could trust the therapist enough to reveal imperfections, worries, and secrets. Thus, while she quickly picked up on the concepts presented to her during session, she had difficulty discussing her own experiences in reference to these concepts. Overcoming Kerry's desire to please and to appear perfect involved the therapist's coping modeling of her own imperfections and finding humor in her own mistakes. The use of humor was gradually extended to include Kerry's imperfections through the use of gentle teasing. The therapist also directly challenged Kerry's expectation of perfection and created ambiguous situations in which the correct answer was not apparent. Kerry's efforts and performance were accepted and praised.

Kerry was quite aware of her somatic responses to anxiety due to her panic-like features. However, her ability to accurately recognize the association between the onset of anxiety and somatic symptoms fluctuated. Lower-level anxiety was indicated by headaches and stomachaches, which Kerry could easily identify. Higher levels of anxiety left her feeling overwhelmed, which Kerry also learned to use as a cue.

Kerry's concerns with perfectionism became evident in her concerns with her STIC tasks. For instance, she would often write several pages about an incident, although she was asked to write only a paragraph. Initially, she was nervous about talking about an event and would ask the therapist to read her written version instead. With encouragement, Kerry progressed to reading it out loud, and eventually recounted the experiences verbally. Kerry learned to let go of the control she initially wanted over how the STIC tasks were presented in therapy and risked doing a "less than perfect" job in presenting the material to the therapist.

While Kerry's extreme physiological reactions to anxiety suggested that relaxation training might be especially beneficial, she actually found learning these skills difficult. She rushed into the exercises with such vigor that she made herself more tense and experienced relaxation-induced anxiety. For example, she reported that in one situation she started to get frightened and tried to relax by tensing and relaxing her hands. She did this to the point of digging her fingernails into the palms of her hands. To help counteract this, Kerry was instructed to begin slowly, taking three deep breaths. In addition, she was reminded that in stressful situations, she was to focus on realizing that her muscles were tense and to concentrate on relaxing them.

The concept of self-talk was difficult for the therapist to address, since Kerry was only partially aware of her cognitions in anxiety-provoking situations. She argued with the therapist's attempts to modify her cognitions in these instances, and was unwilling to consider counterarguments. The therapist chose to ask Kerry to take another's point of view and describe the cognitions. For instance, Kerry was convinced that if she did not receive an A on a report card, she would be teased, regardless of the amount of discussion to the contrary. Eventually she was asked how she would view a friend who did not always get A's. She responded that it would be fine. The therapist then discussed the differences between her response to this situations and her perception of how others would respond to the same situation.

This helped Kerry to shift her focus away from what she thought others were thinking and onto what others were doing. She was often asked to identify behaviors that served as clues to the responses of others. Kerry's extreme fear of looking "stupid" and being laughed at in dance class provided a good example. Kerry was asked to watch for other dancers' mistakes and to notice whether others laughed at the person or were concentrating on their own work. Kerry discovered that everybody made mistakes and nobody seemed to notice, much less laugh.

Another method used to challenge Kerry's cat-astrophic perceptions of situations was to model her behavior in an extreme form so that she could appreciate the humor in the situation. For example, the therapist, with a very straight face, commented that Kerry's tendency to twist her hair would probably make her go bald. Taken off guard, Kerry burst out laughing. She learned to take some teasing and to be able to see the humor in situations, which helped to alleviate her catastrophic expectations.

Problem solving was quite difficult for Kerry to master. She relied heavily on her mother to solve problems for her, and claimed in therapy that she did not know how to cope in imagined situations. In the beginning, the therapist generated possibilities to help Kerry and attempted to thwart her perfectionistic tendencies by including ludicrous possibilities as options. As therapy progressed, the therapist was less willing to generate the alternatives, and they would sometimes sit in silence until Kerry came up with an idea. Interestingly, as Kerry made progress in her problem-solving skills, she had difficulty attributing her solutions to herself. She tended to attribute solutions to the therapist, and consequently did not recognize herself as competent.

Her tendency to view herself as incompetent in light of contrary evidence caused Kerry to be harsh in her self-evaluations and rewards. Though therapy helped Kerry in part to overcome her perfectionistic standards, she found it difficult to completely alter this pattern. She was able to begin being somewhat less self-critical in many areas, but was unable to do so in schoolwork. Not surprisingly, Kerry had a difficult time rewarding herself; as therapy progressed, however, she was able to follow through with rewards such as 30-minute TV study breaks. Positive self-evaluation was particularly difficult because Kerry felt like she was "bragging." She remained fairly dependent on external sources for approval.

Simply being in treatment for her anxiety problems was an in vivo experience for Kerry. She found the process of interacting with the therapist anxiety provoking, as evidenced in her experience of the STIC tasks. Apparently, her fear was that if she was less than perfect, the therapist would become angry at her and reject her for her stupidity.

Early in vivo experiences focused on the issue of perfectionism. One low-level in vivo involved asking Kerry to draw simple pictures with her eyes closed and then asking an unfamiliar person to help her hang these drawings on the wall. Though a relatively simple task, it allowed the therapist to address Kerry's fear of appearing incompetent in the presence of others and her desire to feel in control of situations. Kerry initially divided the sheet of paper in half by drawing a line down the middle. On the side where she was drawing with her eyes open, she wrote "Drawings I am good at" and on the other side where she was to do the drawings with her eyes closed she wrote "Drawings I am bad at." The therapist responded by telling Kerry she had to draw with her eyes closed on the side labeled good, and with her eyes open on the side labeled bad. The therapist used coping modeling (i.e., the therapist drew with her eyes closed) to help Kerry cope with her imperfect drawings and encouraged Kerry to use the FEAR steps to help herself. The drawings Kerry did with her eyes closed were fairly humorous and, via gentle teasing, the therapist was able to help Kerry laugh at them. In this manner, Kerry was helped to understand that teasing and laughter are not always malicious.

A central anxiety-provoking conflict for Kerry consisted of the tension she felt between wanting to have fun and at the same time feeling "guilty" that she was not doing her schoolwork. Throughout sessions, the therapist stressed that it was just as important to have fun as it was to work by focusing on the fun things that Kerry had done during the week. A midlevel in vivo addressed this issue. Kerry was asked to plan an activity on a weekend when she had lots of homework to do. She planned to go to a movie, and the FEAR steps were employed to explore her fears and to help her cope with this situation. The important point was for Kerry to learn through practice that what she feared—failing—would not happen even if she allowed herself to have some fun.

A high-level in vivo experience was developed out of a previous taping task when Kerry had to listen to her own recorded voice. Kerry was asked to play this tape for three graduate-student confederates. Because she thought that people might think she was "weird" for doing this, she problem-solved about how to explain her task. It was determined that she would say that her therapist was asking her to do it, which was in fact the situation, and Kerry seemed comfortable with this explanation. As in the previous taping task, ideas were generated about how to proceed with the taping and how to determine if those listening to her replaying of the tape thought she sounded silly. To encourage independence, the therapist left the room while the tape was replayed, and Kerry reported that this made the task harder. Again, she was able to complete the task, although she felt somewhat anxious about it. The taping task provided Kerry with the opportunity to take the focus off herself and focus more on the responses of others. This was an important theme in her treatment because Kerry was very self-focused and had great difficulty using other sources of information to help her maintain an accurate frame of reference about her experience.

Outcome and Termination

At the end of treatment, Kerry had difficulty separating from the therapist. She had continual problems attributing her gains to herself, insisting that the therapist had the answers for how to cope. Posttreatment results indicated that Kerry, to a great extent, maintained the significant reduction in symptoms that she had reported at midpoint evaluation. She also reported some increase in her ability to cope with going to school and taking tests. Her mother told the interviewer about vast improvement in her daughter, but also noted a few continuing symptoms. Kerry's mother perceived improvement in her daughter's ability to cope, rather than a change in her personality, which she perceived to be anxious in nature.

Though some of Kerry's perfectionism remains and threatens to cause problems in the future, she did learn to question whether she really must be perfect. She was able to develop a more realistic assessment of the level of performance required of her in any particular situation. A big gain for Kerry was to take steps toward mixing work and pleasure, so she did not feel trapped every time she had work to accomplish. Kerry may continue to have dependency problems when problem solving, although it is hoped that her parents will continue to address this issue by encouraging her to independently use her FEAR steps. Kerry told her therapist that she felt she had gained confidence in herself. Also, she developed a capacity to laugh at herself if she looked foolish.

Her gains in laughing at herself were particularly apparent in the taping of her commercial. Kerry spontaneously played around with how to do various things in the situation she had created (such as pretending to go down a flight of stairs by sinking to her knees and becoming melodramatic in her theatrical presentation of what she did when she became anxious). When she and the therapist watched the tape, there was a lot of laughter. Kerry did not seem to need to make this last piece of therapy perfect.

Followup and Maintenance

Several weeks after termination, the therapist received a phone call in which Kerry described several bouts of insomnia accompanied by panic-like symptoms. Accompanying these symptoms were fears of failing school. A booster session was held to help Kerry recognize her own capacity to use the FEAR steps without the aid of the therapist. In a parent meeting, the parents were encouraged to continue to help Kerry in active problem solving. Also, a brief discussion of their own perfectionistic self-expectations may have slowed down the general pace of family life so that they could all better enjoy themselves.

This cognitive-behavioral intervention treatment program has shown preliminary successful outcome in the preduction of childhood anxieties and anxiety disorders. In a multiple baseline trial of four subjects with a primary diagnosis of OAD, posttreatment and 12-month followup assessments indicated reductions in anxiety, as reported by child, parents, and an independent diagnostician (Kane & Kendall, 1989). These changes showed significant improvements from pretreatment assessment, and returned the child to scores within the normal range as expected from normative data.

In a pilot study at our clinic, we completed the treatment of 27 cases of childhood anxiety disorders (Kendall et al., in press). Our research project was a randomized clinical trial, with an eight-week wait-list condition. At posttreatment assessment, self-report measures (RCMAS, STAIC-T, CASSQ, FSSC-R, and CDI) for treated subjects evidenced significant reductions in pathological responses and were within normative ranges. Children's self-rated coping was also found to be significantly higher. Parents' reports on the CBCL and STAIC (parent version) also evidenced significant reductions in reports of anxiety in their children. Diagnoses of OAD based on the ADIS were compared from pretreatment to posttreatment. Using the parents' diagnostic interview data, 60 percent of the treated cases had *no* diagnosis at posttreatment, while 7 percent of the wait-list condition showed such change.

These findings support the use of cognitive-behavioral treatment strategies for OAD. Disordered children, after treatment, were not distinguishable from a nondisturbed reference group, a convincing demonstration of this approach's therapeutic efficacy. For example, in our pilot study, when examining the STAIC-Trait Anxiety scale, and separately, the RCMAS, results indicated that 100 percent of treated deviant cases returned to within nondeviant limits at posttreatment (Kendall et al., in press). Our clinic remains active in the provision of services for anxiety-disordered youth, and we continue to assess and evaluate the outcomes of this program. We are currently examining long-term maintenance of results. Another randomized clinical trial is currently underway, which will continue to contribute to our knowledge of treatment efficacy for overanxious disorder and other childhood anxiety disorders.

SUMMARY

Overanxious disorder is a childhood disorder characterized by a pervasive style of worry not focused on any particular situation, object, or event. Research has begun to examine this diagnostic entity but is still in its infancy. Future evolutions are bound to occur in the forthcoming *Diagnostic and Statistical Manual,* fourth edition, as research explores manifestations of OAD in referred and nonreferred populations. Currently, evidence has begun to accumulate and describe the epidemiology and etiology of OAD. Even less evidence exists for controlled studies of effective therapeutic interventions, although pharmacological and cognitive-behavioral programs are promising. It will be important to continue to develop methods of reliably identifying children with OAD and successful interventions for this disorder.

REFERENCES

Abe, K., & Masui, T. (1981). Age-sex trends of phobic and anxiety symptoms. *British Journal of Psychiatry, 138,* 297–302.

Achenbach, T. M. (1987). *Manual for the Youth Self-Report and Profile.* Burlington: University of Vermont, Department of Psychiatry.

Achenbach, T. M., & Edelbrock, C. (1983). *Manual for the Child Behavior Checklist and Revised Child Behavior Profile.* Burlington: University of Vermont, Department of Psychiatry.

American Psychiatric Association. (1968). *Diagnostic and statistical manual of mental disorders* (2nd ed.). Washington, DC: Author.

American Psychiatric Association. (1980). *Diagnostic and statistical manual of mental disorders* (3rd ed.). Washington, DC: Author.

American Psychiatric Association. (1987). *Diagnostic and statistical manual of mental disorders* (3rd ed., rev.). Washington, DC: Author.

Anderson, J. C., Williams, S., McGee, R., & Silva, P. A. (1987). DSM-III disorders in preadolescent children: Prevalence in a large sample from the general population. *Archives of General Psychiatry, 44,* 69–76.

Barkley, R. A., Barclay, A., Conners, C. K., Gadow, K., Gittelman, R., Sprague, R. L., Swanson, J., & Rapoport, J. (1990). Task force report: The appropriate role of clinical child psychologists in the prescribing of psychoactive medication for children. *Journal of Clinical Child Psychology, 19* (suppl.), 1–38.

Barrios, B. A., & Hartmann, D. P. (1988). Fears and anxieties. In E. J. Mash & L. G. Terdal (Eds.), *Behavioral assessment of childhood disorders* (2nd ed.). New York: Guilford.

Barrios, B. A., Hartmann, D. P., & Shigetome, C. (1981). Fears and anxieties in children. In E. J. Mash

& L. G. Terdal (Eds.), *Behavioral assessment of childhood disorders* (pp. 259–304). New York: Guilford.

Barrios, B. A., & Shigetomi, C. C. (1979). Coping skills training for the management of anxiety: A critical review. *Behavior Therapy, 10,* 491–522.

Bell-Dolan, D. J., Last, C. G., & Strauss, c. C. (1990). Symptoms of anxiety disorders in normal children. *Journal of the American Academy of Child and Adolescent Psychiatry, 29,* 759–765.

Bowen, R. C., Offord, D. R., & Boyle, M. H. (1990). The prevalence of Overanxious Disorder and Separation Anxiety Disorder: Results from the Ontario Child Health Study. *Journal of the American Academy of Child and Adolescent Psychiatry, 29,* 753–758.

Brady, E. U., & Kendall, P. C. (in press). Comorbidity of anxiety and depression in children and adolescents. *Psychological Bulletin.*

Cantwell, D. P., & Baker, L. (1989a). Anxiety disorders. In L. K. G. Hsu & M. Hersen (Eds.), *Recent developments in adolescent psychiatry* (pp. 162–199). New York: Wiley & Sons.

Cantwell, D. P., & Baker, L. (1989b). Stability and natural history of DSM-III childhood disorders. *The Journal of the American Academy of Child and Adolescent Psychiatry, 28,* 691–700.

Costello, E. J., Costello, A. J., Edelbrock, C., Burns, B., Dulcan, M. K., Brent, D., & Janiszewski, S. (1988). Psychiatric disorders in pediatric primary care: Prevalence and risk factors. *Archives of General Psychiatry, 45,* 1107–1116.

Costello, E. J., Edelbrock, L. S., Dulcan, M. K., Kalas, R., & Klaric, S. H. (1984). *Report on the NIMH Diagnostic Interview Schedule for Children (DIS-C).* Washington, DC: National Institute of Mental Health.

Earls, F. (1980). The prevalence of behavior problems in three year old children. A cross-cultural replication. *Archives of General Psychiatry, 37,* 1153–1157.

Francis, G., Last, C. G., & Strauss, C. C. (1987). Expression of separation anxiety disorder: The roles of age and gender. *Child Psychiatry and Human Development, 18,* 82–89.

Gittelman, R., & Kopliewicz, H. S. (1986). Pharmacotherapy of childhood anxiety disorders. In R. Gittelman (Ed.), *Anxiety disorders of childhood.* New York: Guilford.

Greenspan, S. I. (1981). *The clinical interview of the child.* New York: McGraw-Hill.

Herjanic, B., & Reich, W. (1982). Development of a structured psychiatric interview for children:

Agreement between child and parent on individual symptoms. *Journal of Abnormal Child Psychology, 10,* 307–324.

Hodges, K., Kline, J., Fitch, P., McKnew, D., & Cytryn, L. (1981). The Child Assessment Schedule: A diagnostic interview for research and clinical use. *Catalog of Selected Documents in Psychology, 11,* 56.

Houston, B. K., Fox, J. E., & Forbes, L. (1984). Trait anxiety and children's state anxiety, cognitive behaviors, and performance under stress. *Cognitive Therapy and Research, 8,* 631–641.

Jenkins, R. L. (1968). Classification of behavior problems of children. *American Journal of Psychiatry, 125,* 1032–1039.

Kane, M. T., & Kendall, P. C. (1989). Anxiety disorders in children: A multiple-baseline evaluation of a cognitive-behavioral treatment. *Behavior Therapy, 20,* 499–508.

Kastrup, M. (1976). Psychic disorders among pre-school children in a geographically delimited area of Aarhus county, Denmark. *Actra Psychiatrica Scandinavia, 54,* 29–42.

Kendall, P. C. (1985). Toward a cognitive-behavioral model of child psychopathology and a critique of related interventions. *Journal of Abnormal Child Psychology, 13,* 357–372.

Kendall, P. C. (1989). The generalization and maintenance of behavior change: Comments, considerations, and the "no cure" criticism. *Behavior Therapy, 20,* 357–364.

Kendall, P. C. (1989). *The coping questionnaire.* Available from the author, Psychology Department, Temple University, Philadelphia, PA 19122.

Kendall, P. C. (1990). *The coping cat workbook.* Available from the author, Psychology Department, Temple University, Philadelphia, PA 19122.

Kendall, P. C. (1991). Guiding theory for therapy with children and adolescents. In P. C. Kendall (Ed.), *Child and adolescent therapy: Cognitive-behavioral procedures.* New York: Guilford.

Kendall, P. C., Chansky, T. E., Freidman, M., Kim, R., Kortlander, E., Sessa, F. M., & Siqueland, L. (1991). Treating anxiety disorders in children and adolescents. In P. C. Kendall (Ed.), *Child and adolescent therapy: Cognitive-behavioral procedures.* New York: Guilford.

Kendall, P. C., Chansky, T. E., Kane, M. T., Kim, R. S., Kortlander, E., Sessa, F., Ronan, K. R., & Siqueland, L. (in press). *Anxiety disorders in youth: Cognitive-behavioral intervention.* New York: Pergamon.

Kendall, P. C., Howard, B., & Epps, J. (1988). The anxious child: Cognitive-behavioral treatment strategies. *Behavior Modification, 12,* 281–310.

Kendall, P. C., Kane, M. T., Howard, B. L., & Siqueland, L. (1989). *Cognitive-behavioral therapy for anxious children: Treatment manual.* Available from the first author, Psychology Department, Temple University, Philadelphia, PA 19122.

Kendall, P. C., & Ronan, K. R. (1989). *The Children's Anxious Self-Statement Questionnaire (CASSQ).* Available from the first author, Psychology Department, Temple University, Philadelphia, PA 19122.

Kendall, P. C., & Ronan, K. R. (1990). Assessment of children's anxieties, fears, and phobias: Cognitive-behavioral models and methods. In C. R. Reynolds & R. W. Kamphaus (Eds.), *Handbook of psychological and educational assessment of children: Personality, behavior, and context.* New York: Guilford.

King, N. J., Hamilton, D. I., & Ollendick, T. H. (1988). *Children's phobias: A behavioral perspective.* Chichester, England: Wiley.

Klein, R. G., & Last, C. G. (1989). *Anxiety disorders in children.* Newbury Park, CA: Sage.

Kovacs, M. (1983). *The interview schedule for children.* Manuscript submitted for publication.

Kranzler, H. R. (1988). Use of Buspirone in an adolescent with Overanxious Disorder. *Journal of the American Academy of Child and Adolescent Psychiatry, 27,* 789–790.

LaGreca, A. M., Dandes, S. K., Wick, P., Shaw, K., & Stone, W. L. (1988). Development of the Social Anxiety Scale for Children: Reliability and current validity. *Journal of Clinical Child Psychology, 17,* 84–91.

Lapouse, R., & Monk, A. (1958). An epidemiologic study of behavior characteristics in children. *American Journal of Public Health, 48,* 1134–1144.

Last, C. G., Hersen, M., Kazdin, A. E., Finkelstein, R., & Strauss, C. C. (1987). Comparison of DSM-III separation anxiety and overanxious disorders: Demographic characteristics and patterns of comorbidity. *The Journal of the American Academy of Child and Adolescent Psychiatry, 26,* 527–531.

Last, C. G., Strauss, C. C., & Francis, G. (1987). Comorbidity among childhood anxiety disorders. *Journal of Nervous and Mental Disease, 175,* 726–730.

Lydiard, R. B., Roy-Byrne, P. P., & Ballenger, J. C. (1988). Recent advances in the psychopharmacological treatment of anxiety disorders. *Hospital and Community Psychiatry, 39,* 1157–1165.

Mannusa, S., & Klein, R. (1987). *Schedule for the*

Assessment of Conduct, Hyperactivity, Anxiety, Mood, and Psychoactive Substances (CHAMPS). Behavior Disorders Clinic, Long Island Jewish Medical Center, New Hyde Park, NY: Authors.

Meichenbaum, D. (1977). *Cognitive-behavioral modification: An integrative approach.* New York: Plenum.

Murphy, S. M., Owen, R., & Tyrer, P. (1989). Comparative assessment of efficacy and withdrawal symptoms after 6 and 12 weeks' treatment with diazepam or buspirone. *British Journal of Psychiatry, 154,* 529–534.

Ollendick, T. H. (1983). Reliability and validity of the Revised Fear Survey Schedule for Children (FSSC-R). *Behavior Research and Therapy, 21,* 685–692.

Ollendick, T. H., & Francis, G. (1988). Behavioral assessment and treatment of childhood phobias. *Behavior Modification, 12,* 165–204.

Ollendick, T. H., Matson, J. L., & Helsel, W. J. (1985). Fears in children and adolescents: Normative data. *Behaviour Research and Therapy, 23,* 265–267.

Orvaschel, H., & Weissman, M. M. (1986). Epidemiology of anxiety disorders in children: A review. In R. Gittelman (Ed.), *Anxiety disorders of childhood* (pp. 58–72). New York: Guilford.

Puig-Antich, J., & Chambers, W. (1978). *The Schedule for Affective Disorders and Schizophrenia for School-Aged Children (Kiddie-SADS).* New York: New York State Psychiatric Institute.

Reynolds, C. R., & Paget, K. D. (1981). Factor analysis of the Revised Children's Manifest Anxiety Scale for blacks, whites, males, and females with a national normative sample. *Journal of Consulting and Clinical Psychology, 49,* 352–359.

Reynolds, C. R., & Richmond, B. O. (1978). What I think and feel: A revised measure of children's manifest anxiety. *Journal of Abnormal Child Psychology, 6,* 271–280.

Richman, N., Stevenson, J. E., & Graham, P. J. (1975). Prevalence of behavior problems in three-year-old children: Anm epidemiologic study in a London borough. *Journal of Child Psychology and Psychiatry, 16,* 277–287.

Rutter, M. (1985). Psychopathology and development: Links between childhood and adult life. In M. Rutter & L. Hersov (Eds.), *Child and adolescent psychiatry: Modern approaches* (2nd ed., pp. 720–742). Oxford: Blackwell.

Saylor, C. F., Finch, A. J., Spirito, A., & Bennett, B. (1984). The Children's Depression Inventory: A systematic evaluation of psychometric properties. *Journal of Consulting and Clinical Psychology, 52,* 955–967.

Shaffer, D., Campbell, M., Cantwell, D., Bradley, S., Carlson, G., Cohen, D., Denckla, M., Frances, A., Garfinkel, G., Klein, R., Pincus, H., Spitzer, R. L., Volkmar, R., & Widiger, T. (1989). Child and adolescent psychiatric disorders in DSM-IV: Issues facing the work group. *Journal of the American Academy of Child and Adolescent Psychiatry, 28,* 830–850.

Silverman, W. K. (1987). *Anxiety Disorders Interview Schedule for Children.* Unpublished manuscript, available from author, SUNY-Albany.

Silverman, W. K., & Nelles, W. B. (1988). The anxiety disorders interview schedule for children. *Journal of the American Academy of Child and Adolescent Psychiatry, 27,* 772–778.

Simeon, J. G., & Ferguson, H. B. (1985). Recent developments in the use of antidepressant and anxiolytic medications. *Psychiatric Clinics of North America, 8,* 893–907.

Siqueland, L., Steinberg, L., & Kendall, P. C. (1991). *Familial influences on internalizing disorders in childhood and adolescence.* Manuscript submitted for publication, Temple University, Philadelphia, PA 19122.

Spielberger, C. D. (1973). *Preliminary manual for the State-Trait Anxiety Inventory for Children ("How I Feel Questionnaire").* Palo Alto, CA: Consulting Psychologists Press.

Strauss, C. C. (1988). Behavioral assessment and treatment of overanxious disorder in children and adolescents. Special Issue: Behavioral assessment and treatment of childhood anxiety disorders. *Behavior Modification, 12,* 234–251.

Strauss, C. C., Lahey, B. B., Frick, P., Frame, C. L., & Hynd, G. W. (1988). Peer social status of children with anxiety disorders. *Journal of Consulting and Clinical Psychology, 56,* 137–141.

Strauss, C. C., Lease, C. A., Last, C. G., & Francis, G. (1988). Overanxious disorder: An examination of developmental differences. *Journal of Abnormal Child Psychology, 16,* 433–443.

Thyer, B. A., Sowers, H., & Karen, M. (1988). Behavior therapy for separation anxiety disorder. Special Issue: Behavioral assessment and treatment of childhood anxiety disorders. *Behavior Modification, 12,* 205–233.

Torgersen, S. (1983). Genetic factors in anxiety disorders. *Archives of General Psychiatry, 40,* 1085–1089.

Werry, J. S. (1986). Diagnosis and assessment. In R. Gittelman (Ed.), *Anxiety disorders of childhood* (pp. 73–100). New York: Guilford.

CHAPTER 11

PHOBIC DISORDERS

Wendy K. Silverman   Florida International University
Andrew R. Eisen   Fairleigh Dickinson University

DESCRIPTION OF DISORDER

Clinical Features

The Phobic Disorders are comprised of three disorders: Social Phobia, Simple Phobia, and Agoraphobia without History of Panic Disorder (DSM-III-R subset of panic disorder) (American Psychiatric Association, 1987). The clinical feature common to all the phobic disorders is that the child experiences anxiety upon encountering the feared object or event, leading to avoidance of such objects or events. The specific clinical features of each disorder are briefly summarized below.

The primary clinical feature of social phobia involves fear of appraisal by other people accompanied by the fear that one's behavior may result in humiliation or embarrassment. There is also a generalized type in which the individual fears most social situations. Consequently, the individual avoids situations (i.e., social phobic situations) that provoke these fears. In children and adolescents (hereafter referred to as children) frequent types of social phobias include school, public speaking, blushing, crowds, dressing in front of others, and eating or drinking in front of others (Strauss & Last, 1991).

In contrast to children with social phobia, children with simple phobia display marked avoidance that is restricted to specific objects or situations (but not social events). Common phobias observed in childhood include attending school (e.g., a specific object or event, such as a specific teacher, the school bell, etc.; not social), animals, heights, thunder, and darkness.

In Agoraphobia without History of Panic Disorder the avoidance behavior is due to the fear of developing a symptom(s) that could be debilitating or embarrassing. This is accompanied by the fear that one might get "stuck" in a place or situation while have such symptom(s), along with the fear that escape might be difficult or embarrassing. To limit the posibility of this from occurring, the individual restricts travel. Relative to social and simple phobia, agoraphobia is uncommon in children and adolescents. For this reason and also because there is a more extensive literature on social and simple phobias, this chapter will focus on social and simple phobias only.

This chapter was written with the support of grant MH44781-01A1 from the National Institute of Mental Health.

Associated Features

Strauss and Last (1991) conducted a comparative analysis of youngsters diagnosed with either social phobia (SOP; $N = 29$) or simple phobia (SIP; $N = 38$) that provides some interesting information about the associated features of these two disorders. First, 24 percent of the children diagnosed as SOP received this diagnosis only; 39 percent of the children diagnosed as SIP received this diagnosis only. Second, whereas overanxious disorder was the most common additional diagnosis among the SOP group (41 percent; 16 percent for the SIP group), separation anxiety disorder was the most common additional diagnosis among the SIP group (29 percent; 17 percent for the SOP group). Not surprisingly, avoidant disorder was an additional diagnosis in 21 percent of the SOP cases but in only 3 percent of the SIP cases. Finally, while 17 percent of the SOP cases had an additional diagnosis of any affective disorder, this was true for only 5 percent of the SIP cases.

Epidemiology

Since 1987 several community-based epidemiological studies have been reported in the literature. An important methodological advance of these studies over previous research (see Silverman & Nelles,d 1990, for review of previous research) is the employment of diagnostic criteria (DSM-III or DSM-III-R) and structured interview schedules. Anderson, Williams, McGee, and Silva (1987) examined the prevalence of DSM-III disorders in 792 11-year-old children in New Zealand. In terms of the two disorders of interest here, SOP and SIP, the rates were found to be 1.0 and 2.4 percent, respectively. Four years later, at the age of 15, these children were reevaluated (McGee et al., 1990). SIP was the third most common disorder with a prevalence rate of 3.6 percent (although since fear of public speaking was most common, as Beidel [in press] points out, it is unclear why these cases were viewed as SIP rather than SOP). The prevalence rate of SOP was reported as 1.1 percent. In a sample of Puerto Rican children ($N = 777$; 4 to 16 years old), Bird

and colleagues (1988) found that 3.9 percent met criteria for SIP, which decreased to 2.6 percent when a functional impairment criterion was used.

In two cross-sectional studies (ages 8, 12, or 17) (Kashani, Orvaschel, Rosenberg, & Reid, 1989; Kashani & Orvaschel, 1990), SIP had a prevalence rate of 3.3 percent and SOP had a prevalence rate of 1.1 percent. Among an adolescent sample ($N = 150$; 14 to 16 years old), Kashani and Orvaschel (1988) found that 8.7 percent ($N = 13$) of the sample were identified as anxiety disorder cases according to DSM-III criteria and clinically significant functional impairment. Of these 13 cases, 7 met criteria for phobic disorder. A more specific breakdown of these 7 cases (i.e., SIP versus SOP) was not given.

Etiology

Extensive theorizing about but little empirical study on the etiology of SIP in children has occurred; however, for SOP in children, there has been *both* little theorizing and little empirical study. We first briefly summarize what is known about the etiology of SIP, followed by a similar discussion for SOP.

Simple Phobia

With respect to SIP, first, a familial component does appear to exist. In the only family study conducted to date (Fyer et al., 1990), a significantly higher risk (31 percent) was found for SIP among the first-degree relatives ($N = 49$) of SIP probands who had no other anxiety disorder as compared with the first-degree relatives ($N = 119$) of "normal" controls (11 percent). As important as family studies are, they do not allow one to disentangle the genetic influences that contribute to the disorder from the environmental/learning influences (Silverman, Cerny, & Nelles, 1988). And clearly, the impact of environment/learning is considerable (e.g., Marks, 1987; Rachman, 1977).

Several learning-based theories have been proposed to explain the etiology of SIP. (See Silverman & Kearney, in press, for a more detailed account of these theories.) Most influential has been Rachman's theory that proposes three prime pathways for fear acquisition: *conditioning, vicarious exposure,* and transmission through *information and instructions.* Research has supported the existence of these three major pathways in the development of adult subclinical fears and phobias (e.g., Hekmat, 1987; McNally & Steketee, 1985; Murray & Foote, 1979).

Recent evidence corroborates the importance of these pathways in children (Ollendick, King, & Hamilton, in press). Specifically, Ollendick and colleagues administered a questionnaire to assess the pathways for 10 highly prevalent fears (e.g., nuclear war, fire—getting burned, etc.) among a large sample (*N* = 1092) of Australian and American school children (9 to 14 years of age). Vicarious and instructional factors were attributed by a majority of the children as being most influential (56 and 89 percent, respectively), although these indirect sources of fear were often combined with direct conditioning experiences. These findings support the notion that childhood fears are multiply determined and overdetermined (Ollendick, 1979). Like the research conducted with adults, however, this work has the limitation of being based exclusively on subjects' retrospective reports. An additional limitation is that the child participants were drawn from a nonclinical population; whether similar findings would emerge using a clinical sample requires investigation.

In addition to the above pathways, SIP may develop via operant conditioning (i.e., the positive consequences that follow a fearful response [avoidance] may initiate and maintain fearfulness [avoidance]). Thus, a child may display avoidance of a certain stimulus (e.g., a dog); the child's parents who attend to this behavior may inadvertently be positively reinforcing the child's fear response.

The two-factor model (Mowrer, 1939) posits that fear responses to specific stimuli are acquired via classical conditioning but are maintained via operant conditioning (i.e., through the reduction of visceral arousal via avoidance). Problems with the two-factor model have been noted, however (Graziano, DeGiovanni, & Garcia, 1979), and revisions for the model have been proposed (see Barrios & O'Dell, 1989; Silverman & Kearney, in press, for discussions).

Finally, cognitive models have also been developed to explain the development of SIP. In general, these models are based on the assumption that emotional and behavioral problems, including phobias, are due to maladaptive thinking. To overcome one's phobia, therefore, one must succeed in controlling one's faulty cognitions (e.g., "All dogs bite and give rabies") and use more appropriate "self-talk" (e.g., "Actually, most dogs are pretty friendly and a dog has never bitten me before; why should it happen now?").

Social Phobia

As mentioned earlier, relative to SIP, there has been much less theorizing and empirical study conducted on the etiology of SOP. The same pathways described above as being involved in the etiology of SIP (i.e., classical and/or operant conditioning, vicarious exposure, information, and instructions), however, are applicable to SOP. For example, nausea and vomiting during a class presentation in school may perhaps lead to the development of SOP in a youngster via classical conditioning. Alternatively, observing this happen to another child may lead to SOP in the youngster via vicarious exposure.

Although the cognitions of children with SOP have not been examined, interfering cognitive processes appear to exist with adult social phobics (Heimberg, Vermilyea, Dodge, Becker, & Barlow, 1987); and a cognitive model to explain the impairment observed among these individuals has been formulated (Heimberg & Barlow, 1988). The extent to which similar interfering cognitive processes are involved in the etiology of SOP in children warrants further examination.

Although the genetic and family factors involved in the development of SOP have not been examined, such work has been conducted in the area of social anxiety and shyness (see Bruch, 1989, for review). The extent to which similar factors are involved in the development of SOP requires investigation. It may be that shyness, social anxiety, and social phobia represent a continuum; however, each may possess their own set of unique etiological determinants while also sharing a common set of determinants. It is the task of future investigators to determine what these factors are and to understand the process by which they unfold.

DIFFERENTIAL DIAGNOSIS AND ASSESSMENT

DSM-III-R Categorization

The Phobic Disorders (i.e., social phobia, simple phobia, and agoraphobia without history of panic disorder) are all classified under the DSM-III-R category of Anxiety Disorders (or Anxiety and Phobic Neuroses). As noted earlier, agoraphobia without history of panic disorder is subsumed under the Panic Disorder subcategory, which also includes panic disorder, panic disorder with agoraphobia, and panic disorder without agoraphobia.

The DSM-III-R subcategorizations that comprise the Phobic Disorders are the same for both children and adults. Thus, the Phobic Disorders are classified with the other "adult" anxiety disorders (e.g., obsessive compulsive disorder, generalized anxiety disorder, etc.) rather than with the "Anxiety Disorders of Childhood and Adolescence" (i.e., separation anxiety disorder, overanxious disorder, and avoidant disorder). Although our clinical experience has been that the "adult" diagnostic criteria for SIP and SOP may be applied with children, a few caveats are in order. First, some child simple phobics do not understand that their fear is irrational and beyond what might actually occur in reality. Second, for a child to experience anxiety about what others think about him or her (as in SOP), a certain degree of social perspective-taking skills is required. Not all children have necessarily attained such a degree of skill, however.

Differential Diagnosis

Several guidelines provided by DSM-III-R are useful to assist in the differential diagnosis of the Phobic Disorders. First, however, it is important to clarify the difference between SIP and SOP. Although one might view the distinction to be straightforward, this is not necessarily the case.

As mentioned earlier, for example, children with a fear of public speaking in the McGee and associates (1990) study were diagnosed as SIP, although Beidel (in press) questioned why such cases were not diagnosed as SOP. To the extent that these children feared humiliation or embarrassment in a public speaking situation, then SOP would appear to be the more appropriate diagnosis. It is important, therefore, to carefully identify whether the fear elicited in a circumscribed situation (e.g., speaking in class) is concerned primarily with the consequences that might result from public scrutiny in that situation (i.e., humiliation or embarrassment). If affirmative, then SOP is the appropriate diagnosis. If, on the other hand, the fear pertains to the circumscribed situation per se (not a social situation), then SIP is the appropriate diagnosis.

Also important is to ensure that the circumscribed feared stimulus is not a fear of having a panic attack (panic disorder) or having a panic attack in a certain place, such as a shopping mall, and not being able to escape or get help (panic disorder with agoraphobia). One must also carefully determine whether this fear of going certain places is in fact accompanied by clear panic attacks (and not just limited symptom attacks; agoraphobia without history of panic disorder). Overall, however, cases of panic disorder and its variants present rather infrequently in child clinics, and the commonality of these disorders in adolescents is a matter of controversy (see Kearney & Silverman, in press).

The discussion thus far has focused on differential diagnosis within the subcategory of Phobic (and Panic) Disorders. There are other anxiety disorders that frequently require differentiation from the Phobic Disorders. One is obsessive compulsive disorder (OCS). Similar to obsessions, phobias have a repetitive and ruminative quality to them. Obsessions, however, also typically involve repetitive thoughts of violence, dirt, or contamination. Thus, a child with OCD who displays washing rituals would not also be diagnosed as having a SIP of dirt or a SOP of public washrooms.

Another disorder that needs to be distinguished from the Phobic Disorders is posttraumatic stress disorder (PTSD). Just as the phobic stimulus in SIP and SOP must be unrelated to the content of the obsessions of OCD, it must also be unrelated to the trauma of PTSD. Citing an example from Silverman and Nelles (1990), if a child with a previous history of abuse now displays phobic avoidance of stimuli associated with the trauma (e.g., dark-haired, moustached men), fear of dark-haired, moustached men would not be viewed as a separate SIP or SOP. Further, phobic disorders do not involve the more generalized distress observed in PTSD.

The final disorder that is important to differentially diagnose from SOP is avoidant disorder (a subcategory of Anxiety Disorders of Childhood and Adolescence). DSM-III-R's guidelines are that youngsters with either one of these disorders avoid certain social situations and feel anxious with others. Children with SOP, however, display much greater preoccupation and concern over public scrutiny and its consequences (i.e., humiliation and embarrassment) than do children with avoidant disorder. Since few youngsters present with a primary diagnosis of avoidant disorder (see Last, Strauss, & Francis, 1987; Silverman & Nelles, 1988; Silverman & Eisen, in press), however, it has not been possible to empirically confirm this distinction.

Assessment Strategies

It has become common to conceptualize phobias as a complex multichannel/response pattern of behavior, consisting of at least three different but interrelated channels: the cognitive/subjective, the behavioral, and the physiological (Lang, 1968, 1977). For children who present with either SOP or SIP, therefore, a scientist-practitioner would assess each of the three channels in order to determine how the phobia is a "problem" (e.g., negative cognitions, avoidance behavior, sweaty palms, etc.).

To assess the cognitive or subjective domain, one would employ interviewing techniques, questionnaire measures, and self-monitoring procedures. To assess the behavioral domain, naturalistic or analogue observations would be employed. To assess the physiological domain, some type of

psychophysiological recording such as heart rate or skin conductance would be employed. The assessment of multiple sources (e.g., parents, teachers) is also important whenever one works with children with behavior problems, in general, and with phobic problems, specifically (Mash & Terdal, 1989). Specific strategies for assessing the above are now briefly discussed.

The clinical interview is the most prominent assessment instrument used by clinical researchers to assess the subjective/cognitive domain, although it may be used as well to inquire about the other two domains (e.g., "Does your heart beat fast when you see a dog?; "Do you try as hard as you can to stay away from parties?"; etc.). As a way to reduce interrater variability, several structured interviews for children have been developed over the past several years (e.g., the Diagnostic Interview Schedule for Children [DISC], Costello, Edelbrock, Kalas, Dulcan, & Klaric, 1984; the Schedule for Affective Disorders and Schizophrenia for Children [K-SADS], Puig-Antich & Chambers, 1978; The Anxiety Disorders Interview Schedule for Children [ADIS-C], Silverman & Nelles, 1988; etc.).

Most of the existing child interview schedules contain sections that allow for the assessment of SIP and SOP. In our work with the child and parent versions of the ADIS, we have obtained satisfactory kappa coefficients for SIP and SOP (0.84 and 0.73, respectively.) Silverman (1991) concluded in a recent review, however, that due to methodological limitations in the diagnostic reliability studies conducted, there is insufficient evidence to suggest that any one interview clearly provides reliable diagnoses of anxiety disorders in children.

Self-report measures are also widely used methods of assessing the subjective/cognitive domain. Although there is no one scale specifically designed to assess the DSM criteria for SIP and SOP, there are measures available that assess children's fears to specific objects or events (e.g., the Fear Survey Schedule for Children-Revised [FSSC-R], Ollendick, 1983) and in social situations (e.g., the Social Anxiety Scale for Children-Revised [SASC-R], LaGreca & Stone, 1991). There are also social phobic-like items on the

FSSC-R (e.g., "Giving oral reports") and on the Children's Manifest Anxiety Scale-Revised (CMAS-R; Reynolds & Richmond, 1978) (e.g., "I worry what other people will think of me") that might be useful for assessing SOP.

In addition, we recently developed the Childhood Anxiety Sensitivity Index (CASI; Silverman, Fleisig, Rabian, & Peterson, 1991) designed to assess the degree to which bodily signs of anxiety (e.g., heart beating fast, etc.) is frightening to the child. The CASI also contains items that might be useful for the assessment of SOP (e.g., "Other kids can tell when I feel shaky"). In addition, to the extent that a phobic child complains of physiological symptomatology, administering the index might be useful to gauge how much it is the symptomatology per se that is distressing to the child and not merely the phobic stimulus or event.

Despite the apparent appeal—from both a clinical and research perspective—in administering self-report measures, the research support for these measures' construct validity is weak. Rather than measuring anxiety or fear (or depression) per se (e.g., Hodges, 1990; Ollendick & Yule, 1990; Silverman, Jaccard, & Rygh, 1986), these instruments may be measuring "negative affectivity" along the lines of Watson and Clark's (1984) notion. The sensitivity of these measures for diagnostic purposes also appear to be low (Hodges, 1990).

Children's self-ratings of fear and overall distress have also been obtained by investigators using a "Fear Thermometer" (e.g., Melamed, Yurcheson, Fleece, Hutcherson, & Hawes, 1978). The advantages of the Fear Thermometer are that it simplifies the rating task for children and removes some of the variability attributed to language skills when young children respond to questionnaires (Barrios, Hartmann, & Shigetomi, 1981). Melamed and associates (1978) found high temporal stability for the Fear Thermometer and found it to be significantly correlated with the FSSC-R.

An additional way to assess youngsters' cognitive and subjective states is to have them self-monitor their daily avoidance behavior, their degree of fearfulness toward the fear stimulus, and accompanying cognitions. We have found self-monitoring to be useful in our clinical work, and preliminary support for the psychometric properties of children's self-monitoring data has recently been reported by Beidel and her colleagues (Beidel, Neal, Lederer, in press).

To assess the behavioral domain, analogue observation methods (i.e., Behavioral Approach Tasks [BAT]) have been widely used with children with SIP. The BAT represents a test of the child's behavioral limits as it measures the distance the child can approach the fear-provoking object in a natural environment. Unfortunately, the BAT's psychometric properties have not been adequated studied. Further, there are no standardized procedures and instructions that exist in the literature for using BATs with children.

Although behavior observation methods have not been employed with children diagnosed specifically as SOP, they have been used with children who display social anxiety and/or skills deficits (e.g., Esveldt-Dawson, Wisner, Unis, Matson, & Kazdin, 1982; O'Connor, 1969). Research is necessary, however, to determine the extent to which instruments such as these are suitable for assessing SOP in children. Moreover, rather than (or in addition to) rating the child's behavior across standardized situations, it might be useful to observe the child in a laboratory simulation of a personally relevant social phobic situation (e.g., making a classroom presentation, initiating a conversation with a peer, etc.). Such an approach has been found to be useful in the assessment of adult social phobia (Heimberg, Becker, Goldfinger, & Vermilyea, 1985); its utility with child social phobia requires investigation as well.

The final assessment strategy is psychophysiological recording. According to a recent review (see Silverman & Kearney, in press), heart rate appears to be the preferred physiological measure, although further work corroborating this notion is still necessary. In our work with children with SIP, we have found it useful to assess heart rate during the BAT (i.e., during an actual exposure in the phobic situation). Whether a similar approach might be useful with children with SOP (i.e., assess heart rate while the child is exposed to the social phobic situation) also warrants study.

Finally, as indicated at the start of this section,

obtaining information about the child's phobic/avoidance behaviors from additional sources, such as the child's parents, is important in order to obtain a comprehensive and complete picture of the child's problem(s). This is also important given that different sources typically have different perspectives about the child's problem(s) (Achenbach, McConaughy, & Howell, 1987).

With respect to the interview of the parent, most of the existing child-structured interviews have parallel parent versions. These are used to obtain information about the child problem(s) from the parent's perspective, in addition to a diagnosis based on the parent report (as well as a compositive diagnosis — based on combining the child and parent interview data).

Questionnaire measures specifically designed to assess other sources' views about SIP or SOP in children have not been developed. In our research/ clinical activities, therefore, we have modified several of the child self-report measures discussed above (e.g., the FSSC-R, the CMAS-R) to render them appropriate for the parent to complete on the child. We also ask the parent(s) to complete the Child Behavior Checklist (Achenbach & Edelbrock, 1983) on their youngster. There are several subscales that are relevant to SOP (e.g., social withdrawal, and uncommunicative) and to SIP (e.g., schizoid or anxious).

TREATMENT

Evidence for Prescriptive Treatments

Behavior Therapy

There are several problems with the research literature in this area that, consequently, render it difficult to draw any firm conclusions as to "what works best" and, thus, as to what therapists ought to prescribe. The problems with the research include the following: (1) the lack of adequately controlled experimental studies (most of the literature is comprised of either case reports and/or single case studies); (2) the lack of research conducted on clinical samples (most of the work

has been conducted on children with situational fears, such as fears of medical or dental procedures [e.g., Melamed et al., 1978]); (3) the lack of formal diagnostic procedures when clinical samples have been studied; (4) the lack of multi-method-multisource assessment procedures; and (5) the lack of systematic followup procedures.

Despite these difficulties with the research literature, there is one conclusion that can be drawn: The essential element that should be prescribed in any effective behavioral program to reduce phobic symptomatology and avoidance behavior is *exposure*. Exposure plays a major role in the treatment of phobic disorders and is viewed as the treatment of choice by most anxiety researchers (Marks, 1975). (When working with child patients, we would further recommend that the exposure be gradual in nature.) In treating a child with a simple phobia of dogs, therefore, a therapist might prescribe the following exposure exercises — both between and within sessions: (1) seeing pictures of dogs in magazines, (2) going to a pet shop and looking at a dog through the window, (3) going to a pet shop and petting a small puppy that is being held by somebody, (4) petting a larger dog that is on a leash, (5) petting yet a larger dog that is running around loose, and so on. Similarly, a child diagnosed as SOP who primarily avoids social gatherings might be prescribed the following exposure tasks: (1) observing a party on video, (2) actually going to a party, (3) asking a peer a question at the party, (4) engaging in a brief conversation with a peer at the party, and so on.

Although exposure appears to be key to any successful behavioral treatment program for childhood phobic disorders, there is reason to suspect that the effects of exposure may be enhanced through various adjunctive strategies. These strategies include (1) contingency management procedures, (2) modeling, (3) systematic desensitization, and (4) cognitive or self-control procedures.

Briefly, contingency management procedures, based on the principles of operant conditioning, stress the importance of the causal relationship between stimuli and behavior (Morris & Kratochwill, 1983). When employing contingency management procedures with phobic children, external agents of change (parents, teachers, therapists, etc.) rearrange the environment to ensure that the appropriate consequences follow child .approach (e.g., positive reinforcement) and avoidance behavior (e.g., no reinforcement/extinction). The child is also taught to engage in approach behaviors in sequential steps, with each step gradually approximating the desired target behavior (i.e., "shaping" or "successive approximations" [Martin & Pear, 1983]).

Contingency management procedures have been used most frequently to treat "school phobics." Not all school phobics would necessarily receive diagnoses of SIP or SOP, however, and other problems such as separation anxiety disorder might also be primary (e.g., Burke & Silverman, 1987; Last & Strauss, 1990). In addition to school phobia, contingency management procedures have been used successfully to treat children with fears of social situations (Allen, Hart, Buell, Harris, & Wolf, 1964; Jackson & Wallace, 1974), heights (Holmes, 1936), and small animals (Obler & Terwilliger, 1970).

Based on the principles of observational learning, modeling procedures involve the child observing others handle the feared object or situation without fear. As a result, the child learns to be less fearful or anxious. The models observed may be actual or live models, or observed on films/videotapes, or symbolic models. Modeling procedures have been experimentally tested the most extensively (Barrios & O'Dell, 1989), although the focus has been on situational fears (e.g., Melamed & Siegel, 1975). In addition to these situational fears, modeling procedures have been found to be effective in reducing children's fears of small animals (e.g., Bandura & Menlove, 1968; Davis, Rosenthal, & Kelley, 1981; Hill, Liebert, & Mott, 1968), water (Lewis, 1974), heights (Ritter, 1969), and test taking (Mann, 1972).

Formally introduced by Wolpe (1958), systematic desensitization involves the child learning to countercondition his or her learned fear response to some object or situation. Three phases are typically involved: (1) teaching the child an antagonistic response (e.g., relaxation), (2) constructing a fear hierarchy, and (3) pairing the antag-

onistic response to each item on the hierarchy. Some of the types of phobias that have been successfully treated with systematic desensitization include darkness (Kelley, 1976), loud noises (Tasto, 1969; Wish, Hasazi, & Jurgela, 1973), test taking (Laxer, Quarter, Kooman, & Walker, 1969; Mann & Rosenthal, 1969), needles and injections (Ayer, 1973; Rainwater et al., 1988), water (Bentler, 1962; Ultee, Griffioen, & Schellekens, 1982), and heights (Croghan & Musante, 1975).

Finally, self-control/cognitive procedures stress the important contribution of cognitive processes to behavior change with each child directly involved in regulating his or her own behavior. In terms of phobic disorders, the self-control approach focuses on helping children develop specific thinking styles and applying these skills whenever they are confronted with a particular feared stimulus. In our work with phobic (and anxious) children, we use the STOP acronym to teach the child self-control skills where: S stands for "Scared?"; T stands for "Thoughts"; O stands for "Other thoughts or Other things I can do?"; and P stands for "Praise." Self-control/cognitive procedures have been effective in reducing children's nighttime fears (Graziano, Mooney, Huber, & Ignasiak, 1979; Graziano & Mooney, 1980), darkness (Kanfer, Karoly, & Newman, 1975), public speaking (Cradock, Cotler, & Jason, 1978; Fox & Houston, 1981), and bowel movement phobia (Eisen & Silverman, in press).

Although the brief summary just presented of each adjunctive strategy might suggest their utility (either singly or compounded) as a way to enhance the effects of exposure, it is important to keep in mind the methodological limitations of the treatment research, noted earlier. Thus, other than unequivocally recommending exposure, we hesitate to advocate for any *specific* adjunctive strategy in the treatment of phobic disorder at this time until more adequate research on each of these strategies is conducted. In addition, the *relative* effectiveness of these strategies requires study. (Indeed, this is a primary focus of a major research project underway in our research clinic [(i.e., the relative effectiveness of contingency management versus self-control procedures]).

Finally, including the peer group in the design

of a SOP intervention may prove to be yet another useful adjunctive strategy (Dodge, 1989). Although this strategy has not been used with children specifically referred to as "socially anxious" or "socially phobic," it has been found to be beneficial in altering the behaviors of socially incompetent (i.e., rejected) children (Bierman & Furman, 1984). The rationale behind the approach is that rejected children require structured positive experiences with their peer group to modify their peers' negative perceptions of them. They also require skills training to help them attain (and maintain) improved peer acceptance. Given that a subsample of rejected children are likely to be socially anxious and/or phobic (La Greca, Dandes, Wick, Shaw, & Stone, 1988), it would appear that peer group involvement/skills training merits further testing as an adjunctive strategy for SOP treatment.

Pharmacotherapy

Although a spectrum of pharmacological agents (e.g., antidepressants, antihistamines, stimulants, and anxiolytics) has been used in the treatment of anxiety and its disorders in children (see Gittelman & Kopliewicz, 1986, for a review), a paucity of research data is available that examines the therapeutic efficacy of such agents with clearly defined samples of SIP and SOP children. Early reports of anxiolytic administration with "neurotic" children (e.g., Cytryn, Gilbert, & Eisenberg, 1960; Lucas & Pasley, 1969) were methodologically flawed (e.g., mixed samples, diagnostic imprecision) and demonstrated minimal therapeutic value. Although research regarding therapeutic efficacy is strongest in placebo-controlled investigations on antidepressants for school phobia (e.g., Gittelman-Klein & Klein, 1971, 1973, 1980) and obsessive-compulsive disorder (e.g., Flament et al., 1985; Leonard, Swedo, Rapoport, Coffey, & Cheslow, 1988), further work is still necessary in these areas as well.

Given the lack of systematic drug studies with phobic disorder children, it might be informative to briefly examine the efficacy of pharmacological treatments with adults with similar clinical presentation. With respect to SIP in adults, studies conducted have not shown pharmacotherapy (e.g.,

benzodiazepines or beta-blockers) to be of value in isolation (e.g., Bernadt, Silverstone, & Singleton, 1980; Campos, Solyom, & Koelink, 1984) or as a successful adjunct to exposure-based therapy (e.g., Sartory, 1983, Whitehead, Robinson, Blackwell, & Stutz, 1978).

With respect to social phobia in adults, the efficacy of antidepressants (e.g., Klein, Rabkin, Gorman, 1985) and beta-blockers (e.g., Falloon, Llyod, & Harpin, 1981) has been shown to be of marginal therapeutic value. Alternatively, recent evidence has indicated promising results using the monoamine oxidase inhibitor, phenelzine (e.g., Liebowitz, Fyer, Gorman, Campeas, & Levin, 1986; Liebowitz et al., 1988). For example, Liebowitz and colleagues (1988) compared the beta-blocker atenolol with the MAO inhibitor phenelzine in a randomized placebo-controlled design with social phobic patients. After eight weeks of treatment, 64 percent of patients administered phenelzine were classified as treatment responders by blind independent clinicians, compared to 36 percent and 31 percent for patients receiving atenolol and placebo, respectively. In addition, phenelzine responders reported less anxiety in social situations. Since adolescent and adult social phobics experience similar clinical presentation (e.g., Klein & Last, 1989), the evaluation of phenelzine with adolescent social phobics appears warranted.

Alternative Treatments

The literature on alternative treatments for phobic children is also sparse. Psychodynamic/play therapy is the most common approach used. Treatment involves focusing on intrapsychic conflicts with respect to such issues as resistance, interpretation, transference, and countertransference. The play dramatizations are used to help provide indications of inner conflicts.

Although few controlled studies exist (e.g., Miller, Barrett, Hampe, & Noble, 1972), the literature is replete with case reports (e.g., Bornstein, 1949; Finell, 1980; Scharfman, 1978; Sperling, 1967). For example, Bornstein (1949) and Scharfman (1978) each used play dramatizations as a way to provide phobic children with opportunities to reexperience and act out fantasies. In each case, the analyst made interpretations based on the child's play activities, suggesting symbolic themes of projected and displaced emotions (e.g., anger, abandonment, loneliness) to account for the presence of phobic symptoms. According to the authors, through the repetition of play dramatizations in fantasy and reality (e.g., going to school), the children were able to properly direct their displaced emotions, resulting in ego change and, ultimately, diminished phobic symptoms. Although Bornstein (1949) and Scharfman (1978) both provided elaborate intrapsychic explanations to account for symptom resolution, in our view, the mechanism of change remains unclear. Indeed, our interpretation is that anxiety reduction may have resulted as a function of both imaginal (e.g., acting out play situations in session) and in vivo (e.g., enforcing school attendance) exposure elements that were inherent in the treatment.

Selecting Optimal Treatment Strategies

Apparent from our review of the treatment strategies, any treatment approach selected for phobic disorder should include exposure. The question is which additional adjunctive strategies, if any, should also be included in order to: (1) improve the likelihood that the child will expose himself or herself to the feared stimulus and/or (2) enhance the effects of exposure.

Our review of pharmacotherapy indicates rather weak support for its efficacy. Thus, until more convincing evidence appears, we would not be prone to recommend medication to children as an adjunct. This leaves us with play therapy and the other behavioral strategies (i.e., contingency management, modeling, systematic desensitization, and self-control procedures). How would one decide on which of these strategies to include in one's exposure-based intervention? Certainly, the age of the child is an important factor to consider. Indeed, if we were to rank order the various adjunctive strategies by developmental sequence (i.e., the extent to which children are likely to benefit from the approach as a function of increasing age) our ranking would be (1) play, (2) modeling,

(3) contingency management, (4) systematic desensitization, and (5) self-control procedures.

In our view, play is likely to be a useful way to introduce and facilitate exposure in young children whose language skills are still not yet developed. For example, a young dog phobic could use dolls to gradually approach a stuffed animal (e.g., a dog). In addition, the dolls could help the child to express "expected" outcomes (e.g., getting bitten). The child's therapist could then model (using the dolls) alternative scenarios that would promote enhanced coping on the child's part (e.g., petting a very friendly dog). Eventually, the child could apply what was learned in in vivo situations.

With somewhat older children, dolls and the like are probably no longer necessary. Rather, the therapist might serve as a model for the child by approaching the feared stimulus with some initial fear, but then handling the fear and successfully interacting with the stimulus. All along the child is "tagging along" (Ollendick & Cerny, 1981). There are still some children, however, who may require an extra "push" (i.e., incentive) to get them to approach the feared object or event. These children may also have parents who find it difficult to enforce a certain number of weekly exposures on their child. (This may be due, in part, to the Protection Trap, discussed in the next section.) Such families are likely to benefit from the highly structured nature of the contingency management approach. In our contingency management programs, the parent and child are required to sign a written contract each week that states, that "If the child does (a specified exposure task) then (a specified reward is provided by the parent)." This approach appears to be a useful way to actually get the child to approach the feared stimulus while also augmenting parental encouragement and support for the child's efforts.

Clinically, our experience has been that systematic desensitization and self-control/cognitive procedures are most appropriate for older and more verbal children. With respect to systematic desensitization, we occasionally find that young children have a difficult time engaging in the imagery phase of the desensitization procedure. (Some youngsters also have difficulty with the relaxation phase.) It is also difficult to determine whether the children have in fact achieved a vivid and emotionally arousing image—an important ingredient for fear reduction. Therefore, it appears that before selecting systematic desensitization as an adjunct, it is incumbent on the clinician to gauge adequately the child's imagery (and relaxation) capabilities and skills.

Along similar lines, since the self-control approach focuses primarily on modifying the child's thinking about the fear-producing situation or object, our clinical experience has been that children who are able to think of "what is possible" (approximately 12-year-olds and older) tend to benefit more from this cognitive procedure relative to children who can think only of what is "real" (i.e., approximately 8- to 11-year-olds). Preliminary evidence in our clinic also suggests that self-control/cognitive procedures are most efficacious with anxious children who experience a plethora of cognitive symptoms (e.g., worries, negative thoughts, etc.; Eisen & Silverman, in press; Eisen & Silverman, 1991). This, too, tends to be more characteristic of older children than younger children.

Unfortunately, scant attention has been paid in examining how developmental factors differentially influence the effectiveness of self-control procedures (or any of the other adjunctive procedures). Thus, this is a major focus of our own research efforts. In the meantime, it is important for the clinician to be cognizant of the developmental issues just raised in order to select an optimal treatment strategy.

Problems in Carrying Out Interventions

In actual clinical practice, the preceding interventions may not always be implemented as smoothly and easily as one might like. Difficulties come up—with the child, with the parent, and/or with the intervention itself—that interfere with carrying out the intervention. In this section, we review the major issues that we have encountered in our work.

The initial set of issues are actually not specific to child phobia cases but are universal to any

clinical case: (1) child/parent motivation, (2) competing demands, and (3) concomitant emotional problems—either in the parent and/or in the child.

Obviously, without motivation, successfully carrying out any intervention will be an uphill battle. In our work, motivation is assessed at the initial assessment session with the child and parent. We make it clear to clients right from the start that we have no magic wand that will make the child's phobia go away. Rather, the success of the treatment rests primarily with the child and the parent and with their adherence to the program's prescribed steps. Usually our clients understand and accept this notion, and because the phobia is highly interfering with the child's functioning, motivation tends to be high. Indeed, we do not accept clients with low motivation into our treatment program. Like motivation, the extent to which the parent and child can commit to treatment at the present time also requires careful assessment and discussion. To the extent that there are "too many other things going on" (e.g., father just got laid off from work, another child is having major problems in school, etc.), a decision to postpone treatment until "things have settled down" may be in order.

In addition, it is necessary to ensure that the child's phobic disorder is in fact primary and that other coexisting problems (e.g., depression, attention deficit-hyperactivity disorder, etc.) are not more serious and require targeting. Similarly, the presence of severe pathology in the parent also requires careful assessment. If parental pathology does exist, it is necessary to determine whether the pathology will interfere with the parent's ability to be involved in the treatment program and assist in working on the child's phobia problem. A decision might then need to be made to postpone treatment for the child until the parent receives some type of treatment.

Assume, then, that we are working with a motivated child and parent; that the parent is relatively healthy; that phobic disorder is clearly the primary problem area for the child; and, finally, that the parent and child can fully commit to treatment at this time. Given this assumption, what other factors might interfere with carrying out the intervention?

In many cases we have found it difficult to get the child to carry out his or her exposure task prescribed that week (either in the session and/or out). There are several reasons why this might occur. Perhaps the most common reason has to do with inadequacies with the specific exposure task that had been prescribed. One of the first tasks of the therapist at the beginning of the treatment is to develop a fear hierarchy with the child. The steps of the hierarchy comprise the in vivo exercises (i.e., "We will be taking small steps in this program to help you become less afraid of [phobic stimulus]"). If a child has difficulty carrying out the prescribed exercise, it frequently is because the particular step that was assigned that week (i.e., the in vivo exercise) was "too big" for the child.

For example, whereas just a week before the child successfully "petted a small dog in a pet shop," this week the child refuses to do the next step on the hierarchy (i.e., "play with a medium-sized dog in a neighbor's yard"). Careful probing of the child might reveal that his or her refusal to perform this exercise actually has to do with the child not feeling ready for it and that it is "too big a leap," especially in light of the preceding step. In such instances, it is up to the therapist to modify the hierarchy accordingly so that the next task is one that the child feels comfortable in handling (or at least attempting).

Another reason why it might be difficult for the child to carry out his or her prescribed exposure task is because the parent(s) may not be supporting (and may actually be discouraging) the child's efforts to do so. In our work, we call this the Protection Trap. That is, some parents have a difficult time watching their child confront the feared stimulus during the in vivo exercises. (For some, it is because they have the fear themselves.) Such parents are concerned that their child will become too uncomfortable or distressed. Thus, the parents' instincts are to protect their child from these uncomfortable feelings by either not encouraging or by actually discouraging the child's exposure efforts.

We handle the Protection Trap by dealing with it directly with all parents as soon as the exposure phase of treatment begins (i.e., even before any signs of it appear). Thus, we explain to parents that although it is not unusual for some parents to behave in the ways indicated above, we also remind them how countertherapeutic such behavior is as it contradicts the entire premise of our program. That is, rather than supporting and reinforcing the child's approach/exposure, the parents' protective behaviors are actually supporting and reinforcing the child's avoidance. With many parents, our explanation and discussion of the Protection Trap appear to be sufficient. Unfortunately, however, there are always a few parents who, no matter how much we emphasize the "dangers" of engaging in the Protection Trap, disregard our warnings. They still interfere with the child's exposure efforts.

Relapse Prevention

It cannot be assumed that the progress observed in one's clients during treatment will automatically be maintained unless relapse prevention is explicitly programmed and structured into the treatment program. In our work, an entire session is devoted to relapse prevention (Marlatt & Gordon, 1985) and the major ideas behind it are reviewed in yet another. The approach that we use to explain relapse prevention to phobic children is briefly described below.

We begin by reviewing with the child the progress that he or she has made thus far in the program. We reinforce this progress and provide the explicit expectation that progress will continue; there is no reason why it should not, especially if the child continues to practice the skills he or she has learned in treatment (i.e., approach behavior). We also indicate, however, that sometimes, unfortunately, "slips" do occur. This leads us into a discussion with the child about what we mean by "slips" and how they may be handled.

We find it useful to use the analogy of being on a diet, successfully losing weight and then going to a party and eating a piece of cake. We discuss with the child whether this means that the whole diet is "blown." Does it mean that all the weight will come back on? Should the person now continue to overeat because he or she ate this one piece of cake? Even our youngest subjects (age 7) are able to understand that the answer to all of the above questions is negative. Nor is it difficult for them to see the parallel between the diet example and their own experience in overcoming their phobia.

Thus, the children come to understand that although they are presently having "good days," the possibility of having "bad days" exist as well. They should not despair if this occurs; rather, they should recognize such occurrences are not unusual. Relapse happens; the children should know to pick themselves up and remember to continue using the steps they have learned in the program.

It is also crucial that relapse prevention be discussed with the parent(s). Overall, the same ideas indicated above are presented to the parent during the parent session. In addition, an emphasis is placed on the importance of the parent (and the other family members) in genuinely believing that all is not lost in the event of a slip and, more importantly, to communicate this belief to the child.

CASE ILLUSTRATION

Case Description

Joe, a 13-year-old white male, was referred to the Child Phobia and Anxiety Program at Florida International University because he was experiencing anxiety in social situations at school. In addition, despite a desire to socialize with his peers, Joe spent all his free time at home by himself. Joe was also terrified of dogs and remained housebound if a dog was in close proximity in his neighborhood. Although Joe excelled in academics at school, his parents were concerned that he was becoming increasingly socially withdrawn and feared his inadequate social behavior would hinder Joe's development.

Differential Diagnosis and Assessment

Both Joe and his parents were interviewed with the child and parent versions of the Anxiety Disorders Interview Schedule for Children (ADIS-C; Silverman & Nelles, 1988), respectively. Joe also completed several self-report measures, in-cluding the FSSC-R, SASC-R, CMAS-R, and the CASI. In addition, his parents were administered the Child Behavior Checklist (CBCL) and parent versions of the FSSC-R and CMAS-R.

During the child interview, when asked to describe his problem, Joe fidgeted, lacked eye contact, and spoke very softly. He appeared tense and tried his best to calculate how his responses would be interpreted. He repeatedly reassured the interviewer, "I'm not anxious."

The interview with Joe's parents resulted in a more complete picture of Joe's anxiety and overall functioning. For example, Joe's parents stated that he was extremely anxious when interacting with peers at school or outside the home. They reported that he would use them to hide from other students when they picked him up from school. They also stated that they could not remember the last time Joe socialized with a friend at home or elsewhere. In addition, they spoke of how frightened Joe was when he spotted a dog. For instance, if Joe noticed a dog on the other side of his street block (about one fourth mile away), he would run home and lock all the doors in his house as fast as he could. He would stand in the kitchen and tremble until it was clear that the dog was no longer in close proximity. Sometimes he would wait in his house for several hours before deciding to go back outside again.

The interviews yielded DSM-III-R composite diagnoses of social and simple phobias with severity/impairment ratings of 7 and 6 (0–8 scale; 0 = absent, 8 = very severely disabling), respectively. It was apparent that Joe was primarily concerned about the consequences of public scrutiny (i.e., humiliation and embarrassment) in a wide range of social situations (e.g., school and parties). In addition, it was evident that he was afraid of a circumscribed stimulus (e.g., dogs) as well. A history of panic attacks and agoraphobic avoidance was not reported. Although Joe's anxiety-provoking thoughts had a ruminative quality to them, their content was free of harmful intent (e.g., violence) and repetitive rituals were not indicated. Further, neither Joe nor his parents reported any traumatic incidents that may have been associated with the development and maintenance of Joe's simple and social phobias.

On the child self-report measures, the data indicated that Joe scored high on general fearfulness and anxiety and endorsed many social phobic-type items on the questionnaires (e.g., "Meeting someone for the first time" on the FSSC-R; "I am afraid that other kids won't like me" on the SASC-R, etc.). On the parent-completed CBCL, all of Joe's subscales were in the nonclinical range, with the exception of the "schizoid" and "socially withdrawn" subscales.

Since Joe experienced excessive anxiety when interacting with his peers, a personally relevant social phobic simulation was administered with concurrent measurements of self-ratings of fear and heart rate. The simulation involved Joe attempting to engage in a conversation with five adolescents already conversing. During the assessment, Joe's heart rate was found to be elevated during the "performance" phase relative to baseline. Joe was unable to engage in any kind of conversation. Trembling and shaking with fear, he did not make eye contact with his audience. He remained in the simulation for one minute before terminating. Joe rated himself a "five" or "extremely afraid" on the Fear Thermometer's five-point scale.

At the conclusion of this multisource multimethod assessment, Joe was asked to self-monitor his fear (0–8 scale; 0 = none, 8 = very severely disturbing), avoidance behavior, and accompanying cognitions on a daily basis for two weeks with respect to social phobic situations and dogs. His parents were also asked to record daily ratings of their impressions of Joe's anxiety and avoidance behavior as well. The two-week self-monitoring data indicated that Joe reported frequent negative thoughts in social situations (e.g., at school), experienced elevated levels of daily anxiety (mean = 6), and was avoiding every opportunity to socialize with his peers or confront dogs. This was corroborated by parent reports.

Treatment Selection

As indicated earlier, exposure (imaginal and in vivo) appears to be the treatment of choice among anxiety researchers for alleviating phobic symptomatology and avoidance behavior. For this reason, graduated exposure was prescribed as a vital part of Joe's anxiety management program. Because Joe was experiencing a myriad number of worries and negative thoughts concerning social phobic situations and dogs, we also prescribed a self-control/cognitive procedure using the STOP acronym. In addition, because Joe reported some difficulty in performing several of the in vivo exposures due to excessive anxiety, we used participant modeling. Specifically, Joe observed and then "tagged along" with the therapist during both the imaginal and in vivo exposures. This provided him with the opportunity to rehearse and practice the skills learned.

Treatment Course and Problems in Carrying Out Interventions

As just indicated, the intervention was a multicomponent program consisting of graduated exposure, self-control/cognitive therapy, and participant modeling. Joe was first presented with both graded imaginal and in vivo exposures based on his individualized fear hierarchy. Joe's hierarchy contained elements regarding school (e.g., taking tests, physical education, interacting with peers), social events (e.g., parties), and situations involving dogs with different degrees of closeness (e.g., pet shop, neighborhood, within petting distance, etc.). Although Joe successfully completed some of the early in vivo exposures (e.g., taking a test, going to a pet shop), cognitive distortions (e.g., "I will never make friends," "Everyone will laugh at me," "All dogs are vicious," etc.) were keeping him from engaging in exposures of greater difficulty. For this reason, Joe was taught the STOP technique.

Using the STOP technique, Joe was taught to use positive coping self-statements ("The party will be fun," "Most dogs are friendly," "I can handle it if I really try") instead of the negative, maladaptive self-statements that were maintaining his anxiety. The importance of *partial successes* was greatly emphasized to reduce Joe's unrealistic expectations regarding performance activities. In addition, Joe was taught to praise himself (e.g., "I handled myself well at the party") after each exposure regardless of how successful he was in completing the task. Although the STOP technique enhanced both Joe's self-control and coping skills during in session exposures, he was having difficulty applying this technique outside his therapist's office. For this reason, participant modeling was then employed.

As noted earlier, the therapist utilized participant modeling to help Joe successfully and confidently use the STOP technique to decrease his anxiety. Joe was first invited to "tag along" with his therapist in imaginal exposure situations of progressively greater difficulty. Once Joe became skilled with the procedure, he was asked to practice the imaginal roleplay scenes alone. When Joe was ready, he continued to complete the more difficult in vivo exposures. To help promote maintenance and generalization of treatment effects, exposures were conducted at the clinic, at home, and at school. Throughout treatment, Joe's therapist and parents provided encouragement and support for successful use of the coping strategies.

Outcome and Termination

During the course of treatment (10 weeks), Joe was able to gain greater control over his anxiety and successfully progressed through the exposure sessions. The last two weeks of treatment were devoted to discussing the topics of relapse prevention and termination. During these sessions, Joe's therapist explained the concept of "slipping" and discussed strategies to prevent this from occurring (e.g., practice STOP). At the conclusion of treatment, Joe was given a "slipping" handout that carefully outlined steps to take in the event that Joe "slipped" in the future.

During these last two weeks, Joe and his therapist discussed the highlights of the therapy program and his feelings regarding termination. Joe felt sad about leaving therapy, but he was excited in his knowledge that he had become increasingly self-sufficient in confronting his fears and he felt confident he would continue to improve.

Joe's posttreatment data indicated a 70 percent reduction in negative thoughts and an 80 percent increase in positive thoughts (as compared to baseline). His daily anxiety ratings were reduced 50 percent as well. Parental reports were consis –

tent with this. In addition, Joe improved remarkably on several questionnaires (e.g., CASI, SASC-R, FSSC-R) and the parent-completed CBCL indicated the "schizoid" and "socially withdrawn" subscales were within normal limits. More importantly, Joe and his parents reported Joe as being more relaxed at school and at home. Over the course of treatment, Joe attended several social outings and was able to pet familiar dogs of small to medium sizes. His parents expressed great satisfaction in seeing Joe's "social side" beginning to emerge.

Followup and Maintenance

At the conclusion of treatment, Joe continued to practice the STOP technique frequently in a wide variety of phobic situations. At the three-month followup point, his practice was evident since Joe no longer met DSM-III-R criteria for simple phobia of dogs. In fact, Joe and his family were discussing the possibility of getting a small dog in the near future. With respect to Joe's social phobia, he continued to improve but at a slower pace. Joe's parents indicated that even though Joe "slipped" on more than one occasion, he didn't overreact and "bounced back" rather easily. They were pleased that Joe was beginning to problem solve effectively.

At the six-month followup point, Joe proudly showed his therapist pictures of his cocker spaniel. At this time, Joe no longer met DSM-III-R criteria for social phobia. Nevertheless, he still experienced mild anxiety in new social situations (e.g., parties) but both Joe and his parents strongly agreed that Joe's past avoidance behavior was gone. When Joe's therapist asked him if he was still practicing his STOP, Joe replied, "Of course, I'm reminded wherever I go, especially when going for a drive." At 12-month followup, Joe and his parents reported continued improvement.

SUMMARY

In this chapter we have described the exposure-based treatments that appear to be empirically supported and clinically indicated for child and adolescent phobic disorders (i.e., simple and social phobia). As we indicated earlier, however, we hesitate to make any further recommendations about how the effects of exposure may be enhanced via other adjunctive strategies (e.g., contingency management, modeling, etc.) until more adequate data on this issue are adduced.

In addition to the above, etiological factors, prescriptive assessment strategies, and differential diagnosis were discussed. How to go about selecting the optimal intervention was also discussed, as well as the issue of relapse prevention. The case of Joe provided a nice illustration of the above issues.

A chapter summary would not *be* a chapter summary if it did not include the familiar adage "further research is necessary." Thus, adhering to custom, we would like to indicate here that further research on devising and testing prescriptive assessment and treatment strategies for phobic disorders in children is required. However, we would also like to underscore another key point that we hope we have made salient to the reader of this chapter—namely, that despite the fact that further research is necessary, a substantial body of knowledge (based on the research/clinical activities of investigators) *does* exist that indicates that certain things are better to do than *not* to do when it comes to assessing and treating childhood SIP and SOP.

For example, we know that a tripartite assessment strategy is preferable to assessing only one channel or mode; that we are on firmer ground if we obtain information from multiple sources rather than just one source; that structured interviews are more reliable for diagnosing phobic (and anxiety) disorders than are unstructured interviews; and, of course, that whatever treatment strategy one selects, it should include exposure rather than not. Our hope is that this chapter will increase the likelihood that clinicians who work with phobic-disordered youngsters will at least incorporate these basic principles in their assessment and treatment procedures. If our chapter is successful in this way, then a major goal of the present volume will have been attained.

REFERENCES

Achenbach, T. M., & Edelbrock, C. S. (1983). *Manual for the Child Behavior Checklist and Revised Child Behavior Profile.* Burlington: University of Vermont, Department of Psychiatry.

Achenbach, T. R., McConaughy, S. H., & Howell, C. T. (1987). Child/adolescent behavioral and emotional problems: Implications of cross-information corrections for situational specificity. *Psychological Bulletin, 101,* 213–232.

Allen, K., Hart, R., Buell, S., Harris, R., & Wolf, M. (1964). Effects of social reinforcement on isolate behavior of a nursery school child. *Child Development, 35,* 511–518.

American Psychiatric Association. (1987). *Diagnostic and statistical manual of mental disorders* (3rd ed., rev.). Washington, DC: Author.

Anderson, J. C., Williams, S., McGee, R., & Silva, P. A. (1987). DSM-III disorders in preadolescent children. *Archives of General Psychiatry, 44,* 69–76.

Ayer, W. A. (1973). Use of visual imagery in needle phobic children. *Journal of Dentistry for Children, 40,* 41–43.

Bandura, A., & Menlove, F. (1968). Factors determining vicarious extinction of avoidance behavior through symbolic modeling. *Journal of Personality and Social Psychology, 8,* 99–108.

Barrios, B. A., Hartmann, D. P., & Shigetomi, C. (1981). Fears and anxieties in children. In E. J. Mash & L. G. Terdal (Eds.), *Behavioral assessment of childhood disorders* (pp. 259–304). New York: Guilford.

Barrios, B. A., & O'Dell, S. L. (1989). Fears and anxieties. In E. J. Mash & R. A. Barkley (Eds.). *Treatment of childhood disorders* (pp. 167–221). New York: Guilford.

Beidel, D. C. (in press). Social phobia and overanxious disorder in school age children. *Journal of the American Academy of Child and Adolescent Psychiatry.*

Beidel, D. C., Neal, A. M., & Lederer, A. S. (in press). The feasibility and validity of a daily diary for the assessment of anxiety in children. *Behavior Therapy.*

Bentler, P. M. (1962). An infant's phobia treated with reciprocal inhibition therapy. *Journal of Child Psychology and Psychiatry, 3,* 185–189.

Bernadt, M. W., Silverstone, T., & Singelton, W. (1980). Behavioral and subjective effects of beta-adrenergic blockage in phobic subjects. *British Journal of Psychiatry, 137,* 452–457.

Bierman, K., & Furman, W. F. (1984). The effects of social skills training and peer involvement on the social adjustment of preadolescents. *Child Development, 55,* 151–162.

Bird, H. R., Canino, G., Rubio-Stipec, M., Gould, M. S., Ribera, J., Sesman, M., Woodbury, M., Huertas-Goldman, S., Pagan, A., Sanches-Lacay, A., &

Moscoso, M. (1988). Estimates of the prevalence of childhood maladjustment in a community survey in Puerto Rico. *Archives of General Psychiatry, 45,* 1120–1126.

Bornstein, B. (1949). Analyses of a phobic child. *Psychoanalytic Study of the Child, 3–4,* 181–226.

Bruch, M. A. (1989). Familial and developmental antecedents of social phobia: Issues and findings. *Clinical Psychology Review, 9,* 37–47.

Burke, A. E., & Silverman, W. K. (1987). The prescriptive treatment of school refusal. *Clinical Psychology Review, 7,* 353–362.

Campos, P. E., Solyom, L., & Koelink, A. (1984). The effects of timolol maleate on subjective and physiological components of travel air phobia. *Canadian Journal of Psychiatry, 29,* 570–574.

Costello, A. J., Edelbrock, C., Kalas, R., Dulcan, M. K., & Klaric, S. H. (1984). *Development and testing of the NIMH Diagnostic Interview Schedule for Children (DISC) in a clinic population: Final report.* Rockville, MD: Center for Epidemiological Studies.

Cradock, C., Cotler, S., & Jason, L. A. (1978). Primary prevention: Immunization of children for speech anxiety. *Cognitive Therapy and Research, 2,* 389–396.

Croghan, L. M., & Musante, G. J. (1975). The elimination of a boy's high-building phobia by in vivo desensitization and game playing. *Journal of Behavior Therapy and Experimental Psychiatry, 6,* 87–88.

Cytryn, L., Gilbert, A., & Eisenberg, L. (1960). The effectiveness of tranquilizing drugs plus supportive psychotherapy in treating behavior disorders of children: A double-blind study of 80 outpatients. *American Journal of Orthopsychiatry, 30,* 113–129.

Davis, A. F., Rosenthal, T. L., & Kelley, J. E. (1981). Actual fear cues, prompt therapy, and rationale enhanced participant modeling with adolescents. *Behavior Therapy, 12,* 536–542.

Dodge, K. A. (1989). Problems in social relationships. In E. J. Mash & R. A. Barley (Eds.), *Treatment of childhood disorders* (pp. 222–244). New York: Guilford.

Eisen, A. R., & Silverman, W. K. (1991). *Should I relax or change my thoughts? A multiple baseline examination of cognitive therapy, relaxation training and their combination with overanxious children.* Manuscript submitted for publication.

Eisen, A. R., & Silverman, W. K. (in press). Treatment of an adolescent with bowel movement phobia using self-control therapy. *Journal of Behavior Therapy and Experimental Psychiatry.*

Esveldt-Dawson, K., Wisner, K. L., Unis, A. S.,

Matson, J. L., & Kazdin, A. E. (1982). Treatment of phobias in a hospitalized child. *Journal of Behavior Therapy and Experimental Psychiatry, 13,* 77–83.

Falloon, I. R. H., Lloyd, G. G., & Harpin, R. E. (1981). The treatment of social phobia: Real life rehearsal with nonprofessional therapists. *Journal of Nervous and Mental Disease, 169,* 180–184.

Finell, J. (1980). Psychoanalytic play therapy. In G. S. Belkin (Ed.), *Contemporary psychotherapies.* Chicago: Rand McNally.

Flament, M., Rapoport, J. L., Murphy, D., Linnoila, M., Karoum, F., Potter, W., & Ismond, D. (1985). Clomipramine treatment of children with obsessive-compulsive disorder: A double-blind controlled trial. *Archives of General Psychiatry, 42,* 977–986.

Fox, J. E., & Houston, B. K. (1981). Efficacy of self-instructional training for reducing children's anxiety in evaluative situations. *Behaviour Research and Therapy, 19,* 509–515.

Fyer, A. J., Mannuzza, S., Gallops, M. P., Martin, L. Y., Aaronson, C., Gorman, J. M., Liebowitz, M. R., & Klein, D. F. (1990). Familial transmission of simple phobias and fears. *Archives of General Psychiatry, 47,* 252–256.

Gittelman, R., & Kopliewicz, H. S. (1986). Pharmacotherapy of childhood anxiety disorders. In R. Gittelman (Ed.), *Anxiety disorders of childhood.* New York: Guilford.

Gittelman-Klein, R., & Klein, D. F. (1971). Controlled imipramine treatment of school phobia. *Archives of General Psychiatry, 25,* 204–207.

Gittelman-Klein, R., & Klein, D. F. (1973). School phobia: diagnostic considerations in the light of imipramine effects. *Journal of Nervous and Mental Disease, 56,* 199–215.

Gittelman-Klein, R., & Klein, D. F. (1980). Separation anxiety in school refusal and its treatment with drugs. In L. Hersov & I. Berg (Eds.), *Out of school* (pp. 321–341). New York: Wiley.

Graziano, A. M., DeGiovanni, I. S., & Garcia, K. A. (1979). Behavioral treatment of children's fears: A review. *Psychological Bulletin, 86,* 804–830.

Graziano, A. M., & Mooney, K. C. (1980). Family self-control instruction for children's nighttime fear reduction. *Journal of Consulting and Clinical Psychology, 48,* 206–213.

Graziano, A. M., Mooney, K. C., Huber, C., & Ignasiak, D. (1979). Self-control instructions for children's fear-reduction. *Journal of Behavior Therapy and Experimental Psychiatry, 10,* 221–227.

Heimberg, R. G., & Barlow, D. H. (1988). Psychosocial

treatments for social phobia. *Psychosomatics, 29,* 27–37.

Heimberg, R. G., Becker, R. E., Goldfinger, K., & Vermilyea, J. (1985). Treatment of social phobia by exposure, cognitive restructuring and homework assignments. *Journal of Nervous and Mental Disease, 173,* 236–245.

Heimberg, R. G., Vermilyea, J. A., Dodge, C. S., Becker, R. E., & Barlow, D. H. (1987). Attributional style, depression, and anxiety: An evaluation of the specificity of depressive attributions. *Cognitive Therapy and Research, 11,* 537–550.

Hekmat, H. (1987). Origins and development of human fear reactions. *Journal of Anxiety Disorders, 1,* 197–218.

Hill, J. H., Liebert, R. M., & Mott, D. E. W. (1968). Vicarious extinction of avoidance behavior through films: An initial test. *Psychological Reports, 2,* 192.

Hodges, K. (1990). Depression and anxiety in children: A comparison of self-report questionnaires to clinical interview. *Psychological assessment: A Journal of consulting and Clinical Psychology, 2,* 376–381.

Holmes, F. B. (1936). An experimental investigation of a method of overcoming children's fears. *Child Development, 7,* 6–30.

Jackson, D. A., & Wallace, R. F. (1974). The modification and generalization of voice loudness in a fifteen-year-old retarded girl. *Journal of Applied Behavior Analysis, 7,* 461–471.

Kanfer, F. H., Karoly, P., & Newman, A. (1975). Reduction of children's fear of the dark by confidence-related and situational threat-related verbal cues. *Journal of Consulting and Clinical Psychology, 43,* 251–258.

Kashani, J., & Orvaschel, H. (1988). Anxiety disorders in mid-adolescence: A community sample. *American Journal of Psychiatry, 145,* 960–964.

Kashani, J., & Orvaschel, H. (1990). A community study of anxiety in children and adolescents. *American Journal Psychiatry, 147,* 313–318.

Kashani, J., Orvaschel, H., Rosenberg, T. K., & Reid, J. C. (1989). Psychopathology in a community sample of children and adolescents; A developmental perspective. *Journal of the American Academy of Child and Adolescent Psychiatry, 28,* 701–706.

Kearney, C. A., & Silverman, W. K. (in press). Let's not push the "panic button": A cautionary analysis of panic disorder in adolescents. *Clinical Psychology Review.*

Kelley, C. K. (1976). Play desensitization of fear of darkness in preschool children. *Behaviour Research and Therapy, 14,* 79–81.

Klein, D. F., Rabkin, J. G., & Gorman, J. M. (1985). Etiological and pathophysiological inferences from the pharmacological treatment of anxiety. In A. H. Tuma & J. D. Maser (Eds.), *Anxiety and the anxiety disorders.* Hillsdale, NJ: Erlbaum.

Klein, R. G., & Last, C. G. (1989). Anxiety disorders in children. *Developmental Clinical Psychology and Psychiatry, 20,* 76–83.

La Greca, A. M., Dandes, S. K., Wick, P., Shaw, K., & Stone, W. L. (1988). Development of the Social Anxiety Scale for Children: Reliability and concurrent validity. *Journal of Clinical Child Psychology, 17,* 84–91.

La Greca, A. M., & Stone, W. L. (1991). *Social anxiety scale for children-revised: Relationships with peer, teacher, and children's ratings of social and behavioral functioning.* Manuscript submitted for publication.

Lang, P. J. (1968). Fear reduction and fear behavior: Problems in treating a construct. In J. M. Shlien (Ed.), *Research in psychotherapy* (Vol. 13). Washington, DC: APA.

Lang, P. J. (1977). Fear imagery: An information processing analysis. *Behavior Therapy, 8,* 862–886.

Last, C. G., & Strauss, C. G. (1990). School refusal in anxiety-disordered children. *Journal of the American Academy of Child and Adolescent Psychiatry, 29,* 31–35.

Last, C. G., Strauss, C. C., & Francis, G. (1987). Comorbidity among childhood anxiety disorders. *Journal of Nervous and Mental Disease, 175,* 726–730.

Laxer, R. M., Quarter, J., Kooman, A., & Walker, K. (1969). Systematic desensitization and relaxation of high-test-anxious secondary school students. *Journal of Counseling Psychology, 16,* 440–451.

Leonard, H., Swedo, S., Rapoport, J. L., Coffey, M., & Cheslow, D. (1988). Treatment of childhood obsessive-compulsive disorder with clomipramine and desmethylimipramine: A double-blind crossover comparison. *Psychopharmacology Bulletin, 24,* 93–95.

Lewis, S. (1974). A comparison of behavior therapy techniques in the reduction of fearful avoidant behavior. *Behavior Therapy, 5,* 648–655.

Liebowitz, M. R., Fyer, A. J., Gorman, J. M., Campeas, R., & Levin, A. (1986). Phenelzine in social phobia. *Journal of Clinical Psychopharmacology, 6,* 93–98.

Liebowitz, M. R., Gorman, J. M., Fyer, A. J., Campeas, R., Levin, A., Sandberg, D., Hollander, E., Papp, L., & Goetz, D. (1988). Pharmacotherapy of social phobia: A placebo controlled comparison of phenelzine and atenolol. *Journal of Clinical Psychiatry, 49,* 252–257.

Lucas, A. R., & Pasley, F. C. (1969). Psychoactive drugs in the treatment of emotionally disturbed children: Haloperidol and diazepam. *Comprehensive Psychiatry, 10,* 376–386.

Mann, J. (1972). Vicarious desensitization of test anxiety through observation of videotaped treatment. *Journal of Counseling Psychology, 19,* 1–7.

Mann, J., & Rosenthal, T. L. (1969). Vicarious and direct counterconditioning of test anxiety through individual and group desensitization. *Behaviour Research and Therapy, 7,* 359–367.

Marks, I. M. (1975). Behavioral treatments of phobic and obsessive-compulsive disorders: A critical appraisal. In M. Hersen, R. M. Eisler, & P. M. Miller (Eds.), *Progress in behavior modification* (Vol. 1). New York: Academic Press.

Marks, I. M. (1987). *Fears, phobias, and rituals.* New York: Oxford University Press.

Marlatt, G. A., & Gordon, J. (Eds.). (1985). *Relapse prevention: Maintenance strategies in addictive behavior change.* New York: Guilford.

Martin, G., & Pear, J. (1983). *Behavior modification: What it is and how to do it* (2nd ed.). Englewood Cliffs, NJ: Prentice Hall.

Mash, E. J., & Terdal, L. G. (1989). *Behavioral assessment of childhood disorders.* New York: Guilford.

McGee, R., Feehan, M., Williams, S., Partridge, F., Silva, P. A., & Kelly, J. (1990). DSM-III disorders in a large sample of adolescents. *Journal of the American Academy of Child and Adolescent Psychiatry, 29,* 611–619.

McNally, R. J., & Steketee, G. S. (1985). The etiology and maintenance of severe animal phobias. *Behaviour Research and Therapy, 23,* 431–435.

Melamed, B. G., & Siegel, L. J. (1975). Reduction of anxiety in children facing hospitalization and surgery by use of filmed modeling. *Journal of Consulting and Clinical Psychology, 43,* 511–521.

Melamed, B. G., Yurcheson, R., Fleece, E. L., Hutcherson, S., & Hawes, R. (1978). Effects of filmed modeling on the reduction of anxiety-related behaviors in individuals varying in level of previous experience in the stress situation. *Journal of Consulting and Clinical Psychology, 46,* 1357–1367.

Miller, L. C., Barrett, C. L., Hampe, E., & Noble, H. (1972). Comparison of reciprocal inhibition, psychotherapy, and waiting list control for phobic children. *Journal of Abnormal Psychology, 79,* 269–279.

Morris, R. J., & Kratochwill, T. R. (1983). *Treating children's fears and phobias: A behavioral approach.* New York: Pergamon.

Mowrer, O. H. (1939). A stimulus-response analysis of anxiety and its role as a reinforcing agent. *Psychological Review, 46,* 553–565.

Murray, E. J., & Foote, F. (1979). The origins of fear of snakes. *Behaviour Research and Therapy, 17,* 489–493.

Obler, M., & Terwilliger, R. F. (1970). Pilot study on the effectiveness of systematic desensitization with neurologically impaired children with phobic disorders. *Journal of Consulting and Clinical Psychology, 34,* 314–318.

O'Connor, R. D. (1969). Relative efficacy of modeling, shaping, and the combined procedures for modification of social withdrawal. *Journal of Abnormal Psychology, 79,* 327–334.

Ollendick, T. H. (1979). Fear reduction techniques with children. in M. Hersen, R. M. Eisler, & P. M. Miller (Eds.), *Progress in behavior modification* (Vol. 9). New York: Academic Press.

Ollendick, T. H. (1983). Reliability and validity of the Revised Fear Survey Schedule for children (FSSC-R). *Behaviour Research and Therapy, 21,* 685–692.

Ollendick, T. H., & Cerny, J. A. (1981). *Clinical behavior therapy with children.* New York: Plenum.

Ollendick, T. M., King, N. J., & Hamilton (in press). Origins of childhood fears: An evaluation of Rachman's theory of fear acquisition. *Behaviour Research and Therapy.*

Ollendick, T. H., & Yule, W. (1990). Depression in British and American children and its relationship to anxiety and fear. *Journal of Consulting and Clinical Psychology, 58,* 126–129.

Puig-Antich, J., & Chambers, W. (1978). *The schedule for affective disorders and schizophrenia for school-aged children.* New York: New York State Psychiatric Institute.

Rachman, S. J. (1977). The conditioning theory of fear-acquisition: A critical examination. *Behaviour Research and Therapy, 15,* 375–387.

Rainwater, N., Sweet, A. A., Elliott, L., Bowers, M., McNeil, J., & Stump, N. (1988). Systematic desensitization in the treatment of needle phobias for children with diabetes. *Child and Family Behavior Therapy, 10,* 19–31.

Reynolds, C. R., & Richmond, B. O. (1978). What I think and feel: A revised measure of children's manifest anxiety. *Journal of Abnormal Child Psychology, 6,* 271–280.

Ritter, B. (1969). Treatment of acrophobia with

contact desensitization. *Behaviour Research and Therapy, 7,* 41–46.

Sartory, G. (1983). Benzodiazepines and behavioral treatment of phobic anxiety. *Behavioral Psychotherapy, 11,* 204–217.

Scharfman, M. A. (1978). Psychoanalytic treatment. In B. B. Wolman, J. Egan, & A. O. Ross (Eds.), *Handbook of treatment of mental disorders in childhood and adolescence* (pp. 47–69). Engelwood Cliffs, NJ: Prentice Hall.

Silverman, W. K. (1991). Diagnostic reliability of anxiety disorders in children using structured interviews. *Journal of Anxiety Disorders, 5,* 105–124.

Silverman, W. K., Cerny, J. A., & Nelles, W. B. (1988). The familial influence in anxiety disorders; Studies on the offspring of patients with anxiety disorders. In B. B. Lahey & A. E. Kazdin (Eds.), *Advances in Clinical Child Psychology, 11,* 223–248.

Silverman, W. K., & Eisen, A. R. (in press). Age differences in the reliability of parent and child reports of child anxious symptomatology using a structured interview. *Journal of the American Academy of child and Adolescent Psychiatry.*

Silverman, W. K., Fleisig, W., Rabian, B., & Peterson, R. A. (1991). The childhood anxiety sensitivity index. *Journal of Clinical Child Psychology, 20,* 162–168.

Silverman, W. K., Jaccard, J., & Rygh, J. (1986). *A structural analysis of the relationship between child anxiety, fear, and depression.* Unpublished manuscript.

Silverman, W. K., & Kearney, C. A. (in press). Behavioral treatment of childhood anxiety disorders. In V. B. Van Hasselt & M. Hersen (Eds.), *Handbook of behavior therapy and pharmacotherapy for children: A comparative analysis.* Boston: Allyn and Bacon.

Silverman, W. K., & Nelles, W. B. (1988). The Anxiety Disorders Interview Schedule for Children. *Journal of the American Academy of Child and Adolescent Psychiatry, 27,* 772–778.

Silverman, W. K., & Nelles, W. B. (1990). Simple phobia in childhood. In M. Hersen & C. G. Last (Eds.), *Handbook of child and adult psychopathology: A longitudinal perspective.* (pp. 183–196). New York: Pergamon.

Sperling, M. (1967). School phobias—Classification, dynamics and treatment. *Psychoanalytic Study of the Child, 22,* 375–401.

Strauss, C. C., & Last, C. G. (1991). *Phobic disorders in childhood and adolescence.* Unpublished manuscript.

Tasto, D. L. (1969). Systematic desensitization, muscle relaxation and visual imagery in the counterconditioning of a four-year-old phobic child. *Behaviour Research and Therapy, 7,* 409–411.

Ultee, C. A., Griffioen, D., & Schellekens, J. (1982). The effects of 'systematic desensitization in vitro' and 'systematic desensitization *in vivo.*' *Behaviour Research and Therapy, 20,* 61–67.

Watson, D., & Clark, L. A. (1984). Negative affectivity: The disposition to experience aversive emotional states. *Psychological Bulletin, 96,* 465–490.

Whitehead, W. E., Robinson, A., Blackwell, B., & Stutz, R. (1978). Flooding treatment of phobias: Does chronic diazepam increase effectiveness? *Journal of Behavior Therapy and Experimental Psychiatry, 9,* 219–225.

Wish, P. A., Hasazi, J. E., & Jurgela, A. R. (1973). Automated direct deconditioning of a childhood phobia. *Journal of Behavior Therapy and Experimental Psychiatry, 4,* 279–283.

Wolpe, J. (1958). *Psychotherapy by reciprocal inhibition.* Stanford, CA: Stanford University Press.

CHAPTER 12

OBSESSIVE-COMPULSIVE DISORDER

Greta Francis Brown University
Aureen Pinto Brown University

DESCRIPTION OF DISORDER

Clinical Features

Obsessive-Compulsive Disorder (OCD) in children and adolescents is strikingly similar to that in adults. Obsessive thoughts parallel those found for adults and involve worries about physical harm, germs, fear of doing or having done wrong, and thoughts of a violent or sexual nature. The most common compulsions are cleaning, ordering, touching, counting, hoarding, repeating, and checking rituals. Although adolescents and adults may be acutely aware of the abnormality of their symptoms, young children may not recognize the irrationality of their thoughts and behaviors.

Associated Features

Associated psychiatric conditions that have been reported in adults with OCD also have been reported in children and adolescents with OCD. Major depression and anxiety disorders have been reported in approximately one fourth of children who present with OCD (Flament et al., 1988;

Swedo & Rapoport, 1989). Anorexia nervosa and Tourette's Syndrome also have been linked to OCD for both adults and children (Grad, Pelcovitz, Olsen, Matthews, & Grad, 1987; Kasvikis, Tsakiris, Marks, Basough, & Noshirvani, in press). It has been suggested that depression and anxiety may develop in children secondarily in response to the distress associated with interference from OCD symptoms (Swedo & Rapoport, 1989).

Epidemiology

Two studies have investigated the prevalence of OCD in unselected populations of children. Based on 2,000 unselected 10- and 11-year-olds, 0.3 percent were identified as having OCD features (Rutter, Tizard, & Whitmore, 1970). The current prevalence rate of OCD in nonreferred adolescents is approximately 1 percent, as indicated from the findings of an epidemiological study by Flament and associates (1988). These authors hypothesized that the estimate may be low because children with OCD are likely to be secretive and those with severe forms of the disorder might not have completed the assessment. The prevalence of OCD in clinical samples via retrospective chart reviews has ranged from 0.2 percent of outpatients (Hollingsworth, Tanguay, Grossman, & Pabst, 1980) to 1.2 percent of inpatients (Judd, 1965). Although the male to female ratio of OCD in adolescents referred for treatment is fairly equal (Flament et al., 1988), it appears that among referred children, there is a greater preponderance of males with OCD (Despert, 1955; Flament et al., 1985; Hollingsworth et al., 1980; Marks, 1987; Rapoport, 1986; Swedo & Rapoport, 1989).

Obsessive-compulsive disorder generally begins in late adolescence or early adulthood (Rachman, 1985), with 65 percent of patients developing the disorder before age 25 (Rasmussen & Tsuang, 1986), and 80 percent before age 30 (Emmelkamp, 1982). However, cases of childhood OCD also have been reported (e.g., Francis, 1988; Rapoport, 1986; Rapoport et al., 1981). Cases of the disorder have been reported in children as young as 3 years old (Hollingsworth et al., 1980; Judd, 1965). In an NIMH prospective study (Rapoport, 1986), the age of onset of childhood OCD was reported to be between 3 and 14 years. The age of onset for males was 2.5 years earlier, on the average, than that for females. Onset may be sudden or take place over a few months. These findings suggest that while the full syndrome most often emerges in the adolescent to early adulthood period, it can also be present in childhood.

There is little known about the prognosis for OCD in children and adolescents. In a longitudinal study of children with OCD, 68 percent still qualified for the diagnosis of OCD two to five years later, and the majority had concurrent diagnoses (Rapoport, 1986). Deficits in social adjustment and interpersonal relationships have also been reported for adults whose OCD symptoms began in childhood (Hollingsworth et al., 1980). Although these findings suggest a rather gloomy outlook, it has been suggested that approximately half of adolescent OCD cases remit (Warren, 1960).

Etiology

A variety of etiologic theories of OCD have been postulated, including neurological dysfunc-tion, serotonergic deficits, genetic abnormality, psychoanalytic models, learning theory models, and family systems disturbance. Since a review of these theories is beyond the scope of this chapter, the interested reader is referred to Milby and Weber (1991).

DIFFERENTIAL DIAGNOSIS AND ASSESSMENT

DSM-III-R Categorization

According to the DSM-III-R (American Psychiatric Association, 1987), the cardinal features of OCD are recurrent obsessions or compulsions of sufficient severity to cause distress or impairment in functioning, or to be excessively time consuming. Obsessions are persistent thoughts, images, or impulses that, at least initially, are experienced as unwanted, intrusive, and senseless. Attempts are made to ignore, neutralize, or suppress the obsessions. The individual recognizes that the obsessions are a product of his or her mind (e.g., not thought insertion). Compulsions refer to purposeful behaviors that are performed in a stereotyped manner or repeated according to certain rules. While the compulsion is performed as a way to decrease or prevent distress, the activity either is excessive or unrealistic. Typically the person recognizes that the compulsive behavior is problematic; however, this may not be true for very young children or individuals with overvalued ideas.

Differential Diagnosis

Obsessive-compulsive disorder in children and adolescents needs to be differentiated from normal childhood rituals. Many normal youngsters have superstitious beliefs related to eliciting good luck or preventing bad luck. Similarly, children often prefer familiar routines and display developmental rituals, particularly at transition times (Gesell, Ames, & Ilg, 1974). In order to assess the extent to which OCD is a variant of normal developmental rituals, Leonard, Goldberger, Rapoport, Cheslow, and Swedo (1990) evaluated the developmental histories of 38 children with OCD and 22 matched normal controls. The authors reported that OCD children did not differ from normal controls in number or type of superstititious beliefs. However, OCD children did exhibit more persitent developmental rituals.

Anorexia nervosa may be confused with OCD in youth. Although the restrictive eating behaviors of anorectic children may be described as compulsive, these behaviors typically are not viewed by the child as unreasonable or excessive. Similarly, the overconcern among anorectics about weight and body image typically is not perceived as intrusive or senseless. There are times when OCD may properly be diagnosed in youngsters who refuse to maintain their body weight (i.e., when refusal to eat is related to fears of contamination rather than fears of gaining weight).

OCD must be differentiated from Tourette's Syndrome. Although the verbal and motor tics associated with Tourette's are repetitively produced, they are not performed in a purposeful or intentional manner or according to certain rules. Moreover, the repetitive behaviors of OCD typically are more complex than motor or vocal tics.

Some of the characteristics of trichotillomania mirror those of OCD. Youngsters with trichotillomania repeatedly engage in hair pulling, which is associated with a sense of relief or decrease in tension. However, in trichotillomania the repetitive behavior is confined to hair pulling and does not appear in response to obsessive thoughts.

Children with other anxiety disorders often demonstrate ruminative worries. The frequency of such worries may appear similar to what is described in OCD, but their content is related to the specific anxiety disorder. For instance, children with Separation Anxiety Disorder frequently worry excessively about the safety of their parents. Moreover, youngsters with OCD often demonstrate avoidance of feared objects or situations that may appear virtually identical to avoidance associated with phobic disorders. Phobias should not be diagnosed when the avoidance is related to OCD, such as when situations are avoided because of fears of contamination.

Youngsters with psychotic symptoms may exhibit delusional beliefs that appear obsessive in nature. OCD should not be diagnosed when such persistent beliefs are clearly delusional.

Assessment Strategies

A comprehensive assessment of childhood OCD should include information pertaining to the content, frequency, and intensity of obsessions and compulsions; degree of discomfort and avoidance experienced; impairment in functioning; and presence of comorbid conditions. Such an evaluation can best be achieved through the use of a variety of methods and sources of information in combination. Among the different methods available to assess OCD in children and adolescents are clinical interviews, self-report inventories, and direct behavioral observations by the clinician. Parents and teachers also are valuable sources of information toward obtaining a complete clinical picture of the disorder. As with the assessment of any child, a developmental history provides important information.

The Clinical Interview

The clinical interview of the child and family should be geared toward establishing the diagnosis and collecting information pertinent to treatment planning. Of particular importance in the assessment of obsessions is information regarding specific external anxiety cues (tangible objects), internal anxiety cues (thoughts, images, or impulses), and worries about disastrous consequences (Steketee & Foa, 1985). Identifying the source of anxiety is important, as it can aid in the development of treatment plans that involve habituation to the source of anxiety. The functional relationship of each ritual to the anxiety cues and to passive and active avoidance behaviors also should be determined via a behavioral functional analysis. A detailed account of the events surrounding the onset of current symptoms may provide information regarding variables associated with the maintenance of symptoms. Comorbid conditions such as depression and anxiety also need to be assessed, as they may be predictors of treatment success (Basoglu, Lax, Kasvikis, & Marks, 1988; Steketee & Foa, 1985). Additionally, a general history involving information about family and peer relationships, developmental history, and educational progress should be gathered.

The *role of the family* in the assessment of childhood OCD is crucial, as young children might be unable or unwilling to express the nature of their difficulties, and adolescents might be secretive and minimize their fears and behaviors. Interviewing parents may be helpful in gathering descriptive information about symptoms, providing a chronology of events, and reporting information of which children and adolescents may not be aware (e.g., developmental history).

There are several structured and semistructured interviews that are appropriate for use with OCD children and adolescents. These include the Diagnostic Interview for Children and Adolescents-Revised (DICA-R; Herjanic & Campbell, 1977; Welner, Reich, Herjanic, & Campbell, 1987), Diagnostic Interview Schedule for Children (DISC; Costello, Edelbrock, Kalas, Kessler, & Klaric, 1982; Costello, Edelbrock, Dulcan, Kalas, & Klaric, 1984), Schedule for Affective Disorder and Schizophrenia for School-Age Children (K-SADS; Chambers et al., 1985), Interview Schedule for Children (ISC; Kovacs, 1983), Anxiety Disorders Interview Schedule for Children (Kiddie ADIS or ADIS-C; Silverman & Nelles, 1988), and Children's Assessment Schedule (CAS; Hodges, McKnew, Cytryn, Stern, & Kline, 1982).

Although none of these interviews was designed specifically to assess OCD, all of them cover many areas of child psychopathology, including symptoms of OCD, and thereby allow the assessment of comorbidity. Most of the available semistructured, symptom-oriented interviews also allow for behavioral observations during the interview process. An additional advantage of all the interviews named above is that they have parallel forms for children and parents, thereby permitting the collection of information from both children and collaterals.

A cautionary note on the use of structured interviews for OCD is that children may misinterpret questions due to unfamiliarity with unusual behaviors such as obsessions and compulsions (Breslau, 1987). Hence, failure to understand the intent of the question may result in either under

reporting (false negatives) or erroneous reporting of symptoms that are not experienced (false positives). In our clinical experience, it is important to clarify initial questions with examples and concrete descriptions of obsessive thoughts and compulsive behaviors.

Self-Report Measures

The most widely used OCD self-report instruments for children and adolescents are the Children's Yale-Brown Obsessive-Compulsive Scale (CY-BOCS; Goodman et al., 1986) Leyton Obsessional Inventory-Child Version (LOI-CV; Berg, Rapoport, & Flament, 1986), and the Maudsley Obsessive-Compulsive Inventory (MOCI; Hodgson & Rachman, 1977).

The Children's Yale-Brown Obsessive-Compulsive Scale (CY-BOCS; Goodman et al., 1986) has items and format similar to the Yale-Brown Obsessive-Compulsive Scale for Adults (Y-BOCS; Goodman et al., 1989). The CY-BOCS assesses both core and associated symptoms of OCD, along with global severity and improvement. Items are rated on a five-point scale that allows the assessment of response to treatment.

The Leyton Obsessional Inventory-Child Version (LOI-CV; Berg et al., 1986) assesses the presence of persistent thoughts, fear of dirt and/or dangerous objects, cleanliness, order, checking, repetition, and indecision. Positive responses subsequently are assessed for degree of resistance and interference. The *card-sorting method* of administration lends itself to direct behavioral observations of behaviors such as indecision with questions, slowness of task performance, and the need to obsess and/or perform rituals. The LOI-CV reportedly discriminates between adolescent obsessive patients and normal controls; obsessive patients and psychiatric controls differ only on the extent of resistance and interference (Berg et al., 1986). There currently is a 20-item survey version of the LOI-CV that provides age and sex norms for adolescents 13 to 18 years of age (Berg, Whitaker, Davies, Flament, & Rapoport, 1988).

The Maudsley Obsessive-Compulsive Inventory (MOCI; Hodgson & Rachman, 1977) consists of 30 true-false questions. In addition to a general obsessive-compulsive score, the inventory yields five subscales: checking, cleaning, slowness, doubting-conscientiousness, and rumination. It has been reported to have adequate validity and reliability with adults (Rachman & Hodgson, 1980). Clark and Bolton (1985) found that it distinguished between OCD and anxious adolescents on total score and the checking subscale, but not on cleaning, slowness, and doubting subscales. As such, usefulness with adolescents may be limited.

There are several other self-report measures that provide information about anxiety and fears in children. Among these are the Revised Children's Manifest Anxiety Scale (RCMAS; Reynolds & Richmond, 1978), the State-Trait Anxiety Inventory for Children (STAIC; Spielberger, 1973), the Fear Survey Schedule for Children-Revised (FSSC-R; Ollendick, 1983), the Test Anxiety Scale for Children (Sarason, Davidson, Lighthall, Waite, & Ruebush, 1960), and the Social Anxiety Scale for Children (LaGreca, Dandes, Wick, Shaw, & Stone, 1988). These measures can provide useful supplementary information about fears that children with OCD may experience and thus help complete the clinical picture.

Behavioral Observation

Behavioral monitoring of the frequency and duration of ritualistic behaviors, avoidance and exposure tests, and physiological and cognitive indices of anxiety have been used in the assessment of OCD in adults. There are no reports of the systematic use of these measures in children. The interested reader is referred to Turner and Beidel (1988), Foa, Steketee, and Milby (1980), and Marks, Hodgson, and Rachman (1975) for descriptions of the use of these measures with adults.

TREATMENT

Evidence for Prescriptive Treatment

Behavior Therapy

The literature on behavioral treatment of OCD in children and adolescents is limited to a few case reports and single-subject studies that have employed treatment strategies successfully used for adults. Behavioral treatments, especially exposure and response prevention, have emerged as the interventions of choice for adults with OCD, with a 70 percent effectiveness rate (Foa, Steketee, & Ozarow, 1985; Perse, 1988). Although there has not been a systematic investigation of these procedures with children, response prevention, typically used together with other treatment techniques, is the most frequently reported treatment. Other forms of behavioral therapy used with children and adolescents include extinction, positive reinforcement, and thought stopping.

The use of response prevention, combined with in vivo exposure, has been reported by McCarthy and Foa (1988), Zikis (1983), and Apter, Bernhout, and Tyano (1984). McCarthy and Foa (1988) treated a 13-year-old male with excessive fears of causing injury to his family, failing in school, and being teased by peers. His worries were accompanied by compulsive behaviors such as rehearsing homework and repetitive movements. Treatment consisted of 15 outpatient sessions using imaginal and in vivo exposure, together with response prevention over a three-week period, followed by one week of home-based treatment. A reward system also was used in order to increase treatment compliance. Obsessions and compulsions reported were successfully eliminated with no relapse at one-year followup.

Similar success with in vivo exposure and response prevention was reported by Zikis (1983) for an 11-year-old girl who had several rituals and tried to keep her eyes open at night. Rituals were eliminated with two weeks of outpatient treatment applied by the parents. The patient was reported to be symptom free at one-year followup.

In contrast, Apter and colleagues (1984) reported treatment failure following the use of response prevention and in vivo exposure for eight hospitalized adolescents with OCD. Patients were instructed to refrain from performing rituals and to think of something else in place of the obsessional thought. Staff monitoring of the treatment plan was provided only when possible. Given that response prevention was self-imposed, it is possible that treatment failure was related to noncompliance with the regimen.

Of the studies employing primarily response prevention (Allsopp & Verduyn, 1988; Bolton, Collins, & Steinberg, 1983; Clark, Sugrim, & Bolton, 1982; Green, 1980; Mills, Agras, Barlow, & Mills, 1973; Ong & Leng, 1979; Stanley, 1980), the largest study is tht of Bolton and colleagues (1983), which is a review of the records of 15 children admitted to a hospital over a four-year period. The most commonly reported compulsions were checking and cleaning. The general treatment procedure began with outpatient self-imposed response prevention with self-monitoring of symptoms. Concurrently, parents also were taught to use response prevention and to refuse to reinforce rituals.

The success of this procedure was noted to be related to the severity of symptoms and motivation on the part of the adolescent. Following unsuccessful outpatient treatment, inpatient treatment was instituted, with external controls applied by staff to ensure compliance with the treatment. Graded exposure was used for 3 of the 15 inpatients. Additionally, a supportive, therapeutic relationship was provided in most cases. Outcome was assessed by observations on the unit and parental report. Improvement, ranging from complete recovery to "mild" symptoms, was reported in 87 percent of cases after hospitalizations ranging in length from one week to two years.

In another retrospective study, Allsopp and Verduyn (1988) examined the outcome of 26 OCD adolescents approximately 10 years after they had been treated either with outpatient or inpatient treatment. Of these, 14 youngsters were treated with response prevention and family therapy. Seven patients showed complete remission of symptoms at discharge, 9 showed significant improvement, and 2 had little or no change in symptom severity. Of the 20 who participated in the 10-year followup, 10 were symptom free, 6 had significant OCD, and 4 had other psychiatric disorders.

Ong and Leng (1979) employed response prevention to eliminate washing and cleaning rituals in a 13-year-old girl who was prevented from washing by being kept in her room or restrained on her bed. Concurrent treatment was provided by using in vivo modeling, positive reinforcement

of other behaviors, drug treatment, and family interventions. Although improvement was reported, it is not possible to single out the effects of any single procedure. Followup at two years indicated mild relapse, which was responsive to further treatment.

Mills and associates (1973) used response prevention to treat a 15-year-old boy with elaborate morning and evening rituals, including checking and ordering behaviors. Even though only bedtime rituals were targeted for prevention, a concomitant decrease in morning rituals was reported. Rituals stopped within 10 days but returned approximately two months following discharge. At that time, outpatient treatment, consisting of response prevention implemented by the parents, reportedly was successful in reducing rituals.

Extinction procedures have been used to treat childhood OCD (Francis, 1988; Hallam, 1974). Hallam (1974) treated a 15-year-old hospitalized female who had a three-year history of repeatedly asking questions about whether people were spreading rumors or saying unpleasant things about her. The initial phase of treatment, which consisted of refusal to provide reassurance with statements such as, "I can't answer that," reportedly made no impact on the frequency of her reassurance-seeking questions. Subsequently, an extinction procedure was started, during which staff consistently ignored all reassurance-seeking behavior and redirected conversation when asked questions. Halfway through the procedure, a response cost strategy was added. The patient lost one minute of recreation time for each question asked. Although the patient's initial response to extinction included agitation and highly anxious behavior, reassurance seeking was eliminated within three to four weeks. Treatment gains were maintained at 14-month followup. Despite treatment success, the lack of pretreatment baseline data make empirical evaluation of the findings difficult.

The use of extinction to modify reassurance-seeking behavior also has been described by Francis (1988), who used an ABAB single-subject experimental design to collect data during baseline, treatment, and posttreatment phases. The

11-year-old boy was seen on an outpatient basis and treatment was implemented by the parents. He presented with persistent obsessive worries about death and dying, as well as frequent compulsive reassurance-seeking behavior. He frequently voiced fears of dying from various diseases and persistently asked questions such as, "Am I going blind?" "Do you think I will throw up?" and "Am I going to die?" The parents monitored reassurance-seeking questions four times per day. During the eight-day baseline phase, the parents were instructed to respond in their usual way to the child's questions, which consisted of them attempting to reassure him. The eight-day extinction phase involved the parents ignoring all reassurance-seeking questions by looking/turning away and redirecting the conversation.

The therapist maintained frequent phone contact with the family during this phase in order to provide encouragement and support. The return to baseline phase lasted for five days and consisted of a resumption of parental attention to the reassurance-seeking behavior. The onset of this phase occurred spontaneously when the parents began attending to the reassurance-seeking behavior at a time when a number of family members became ill with the flu. Of note, the family illness persisted for another five days following the predetermined end of this phase. The return to extinction phase lasted for 20 days and involved reimplementation of the extinction procedure. A one-month followup assessment was conducted in which the parents monitored the child's behavior for a three-day period.

Results indicated that the extinction procedure was successful in decreasing the frequency of reassurance-seeking behavior to zero within 6 days. During the withdrawal, phase, the child's behavior worsened dramatically, at which time reassurance seeking was occurring at a rate higher than that seen during baseline. Once extinction was reimplemented, the frequency of reassurance-seeking behavior fell to zero within 12 days, and remained at zero for 9 consecutive days and at the one-month followup.

Success with positive reinforcement has been described by Queiroz, Motta, Madi, Sossai, and Boren (1981) in the treatment of two 9-year-olds who hoarded trash and had showering rituals. The therapist educated the patients on appropriate, alternative responses in order to build up a repertoire of adaptive behaviors and allow the compulsive rituals to be phased out. Parents also were trained to give social reinforcements for positive behavior. Both patients were reported to be symptom free at one-year followup.

Positive reinforcement also was reported in the recovery of a 9-year-old male with hand washing and checking rituals. These rituals reportedly stopped following ignoring of the target behaviors and positive reinforcement of appropriate behaviors (Dalton, 1983). Tretment gains were maintained at one-year followup.

Although these behavioral techniques have been used in the treatment of compulsions, the most commonly used technique for obsessive ruminations in youngsters is thought stopping (Campbell, 1973; Ownby, 1983). Campbell (1973) used thought stopping to treat a 12-year-old boy with persistent thoughts about his sister's death. The patient was encouraged to actively engage in the obsessive thought then disrupt it by counting backwards loudly and then thinking of a pleasant scene. Ruminations reportedly decreased by as much as 80 percent within one week of treatment and were eliminated completely at four weeks.

With the exception of two studies (Apter et al., 1984; Clark et al., 1982), there is little information regarding treatment failures in the literature. It is likely that, as with adults (Foa, 1979), treatment failures may be related to comorbid conditions, such as depression, belief that fears are realistic, and poor motivation. In one retrospective study, Allsopp and Verduyn (1988) reported that long-term outcome for treated adolescents was related to a family history of psychiatric illness and lack of response to therapy at initial contact. Information regarding treatment failures is as important to the investigation of effectiveness as are data pertaining to success.

Although the majority of the reports of treatment of childhood OCD describe treatment successes, it is important to keep in mind that there is a need for more systematic research before generalizations about the effectiveness of behavioral treatments can be made. The small number of patients treated in each study, lack of reference to standardized diagnostic criteria, absence of baseline observations, and varying outcome criteria make it difficult to assess treatment effectiveness. Moreover, the use of several different interventions simultaneously makes evaluation of the effectiveness of any single behavioral technique impossible. Furthermore, these studies describe short-term success. Although the longest followup period reported is three years in one study, the average length of followup is one year or less. Given the chronic nature of OCD, demonstration of long-term treatment success is critical.

Pharmacological Treatment

Very little empirical data currently are available attesting to the effectiveness of pharmacological agents in the treatment of OCD in children and adolescents. Clomipramine is the only pharmacological treatment that has been evaluated systematically for youngsters with OCD (Flament et al., 1985; Leonard, Swedo, Rapoport, Coffey, & Cheslow, 1988; Rapoport, Elkins, & Mikkelson, 1980).

Flament and colleagues (1985) conducted a double-blind, crossover design study comparing clomipramine hydrochloride and placebo. Subjects included 19 OCD youngsters between the ages of 10 and 18 years (mean age = 14.5 years) who had experienced significant OCD symptoms for at least one year. The average duration of symptoms was four years. Children with psychosis, mental retardation, or primary affective disorder were excluded from the study. All youngsters but one had a post history of psychiatric treatment for OCD, and one half of the sample had not responded to previous treatment with tricyclic antidepressant medication. The children participated in a one-week baseline monitoring phase followed by 10 weeks of clomipramine or placebo, each of which was administered for five weeks. The mean dose of clomipramine was 141 mg per day. Children and their parents also received supportive psychotherapy. No formal behavior therapy was conducted.

Clomipramine yielded a decrease in obsessional symptoms that was independent of baseline depression levels. However, clomipramine did not produce full recovery of obsessive symptoms. At the end of treatment, 26 percent of youngsters were described as unchanged or only slightly improved, 64 percent of youngsters were described as moderately or much improved, and 10 percent were described as symptom free. There was no change in global measures of depression or anxiety. Unfortunately, the authors provided no information about the kind of compulsive behaviors exhibited by the youngsters, so it is not possible to assess the effect of clomipramine on compulsions.

Leonard and associates (1988) completed a double-blind crossover study comparing clomipramine (CMI) and desmethylimipramine (DMI). Participating in the study were 21 youngsters with OCD between the ages of 8 and 19 years. Subjects had an average symptom duration of 2.7 years, and reportedly were not significantly depressed. Treatment was conducted on an outpatient basis and consisted of a two-week single-blind placebo phase followed by two consecutive five-week trials of CMI or DMI increased to 3 mg/kg. Ongoing assessments of obsessive-compulsive symptomatology, depression, and side effects were gathered. Results indicated that CMI was superior to DMI in alleviating OCD symptoms. These differences were observed by the third week of treatment. DMI produced little or no improvement from baseline, and relapse was apparent within two weeks when DMI followed CMI.

The only other pharmacological agent reported in the literature for the treatment of childhood OCD is fluoxetine. Riddle, Hardin, King, Scahill, and Woolston (1990) described preliminary clinical experience using fluoxetine to treat children and adolescents with OCD. Subjects included five boys and five girls between the ages of 8 and 15 years, six of whom presented with primary Tourette's Syndrome (TS). Four of the OCD/TS youngsters were being treated with other medications concurrently. OCD symptom severity was assessed using the CY-BOCS. Treatment consisted of an open trial of fluoxetine.

Five youngsters were characterized as responders as indicated by "much improved" ratings by their clinician. Each of the responders was on a dose of 20 mg/day and treatment lasted between 4 and 20 weeks. A common adverse side effect, seen in four of the subjects (all but one a non-responder), was behavioral agitation defined by increased motor activity and pressured speech. As the authors readily acknowledge, data in this study must be viewed cautiously, given the lack of a placebo control. The authors reported anecdotically that all five responders have continued on fluoxetine. In fact, they described rapid decompensation in one child whose medication was discontinued temporarily.

Selecting Optimal Treatment Strategies

The current literature suggests that the most effective behavioral treatment for childhood OCD characterized by compulsions with or without obsessions includes exposure and response prevention, coupled with positive reinforcement techniques. For OCD children exhibiting obsessions only, thought stopping would be an appropriate first-line intervention. Clomipramine may also be effective in diminishing obsessive symptoms in youngsters with OCD.

In order to implement such treatments effectively, a number of factors must be considered. The diagnostic assessment should provide information about the presence or absence of compulsions and obsessions in order to develop an appropriate treatment strategy. The degree of distress and impairment must be taken into consideration in order to evaluate whether there is a need for pharmacologic intervention and if such a need is immediate. Furthermore, symptoms may require in vivo or imaginal exposure depending on their content. That is, certain obsessions cannot easily be exposed in vivo, such as those related to aggressive thoughts. Finally, a determination must be made about the parents' ability to implement the treatment aimed at OCD symptoms. Often, parents first require teaching of basic child management techniques.

Problems in Carrying Out Interventions

As with adults who have OCD, it may be difficult to engage a child's participation in treatment. Gaining cooperation and willingness to collaborate with treatment is especially important with children, as the child often is brought in for treatment by parents or guardians and therefore may be resistant, noncompliant, and unmotivated. Explaining the rationale for treatment and encouraging participation in the formulation of plans (e.g., the construction of the hierarchy) with simplicity and clarity lessen fear and apprehension. For both adults and children, initial anxiety regarding assessment and treatment can be alleviated by establishing rapport and providing a supporting therapeutic relationship.

Since motivation and treatment compliance may be lower in children than in adults, procedures that can be directed by the therapist or administered by the parent within the home may be especially helpful. Most behavioral techniques are amenable to application within the home if appropriately modeled, guided, and followed by the therapist.

As with assessment, the inclusion of families in the treatment program is critical for children. A distinguishing feature in the presentation of childhood OCD is the children's tendency to involve parents in rituals or to control the household routine by angry outbursts if family members fail to comply (Bolton et al., 1983). In fact, parents may lack basis child management skills. As such, there is likely to be anger and conflict between the parents over how to manage the child and frustration regarding an inability to control the routines of the household. Moreover, both the child and parent may become anxious and inadvertently contribute to the maintenance of anxiety in the family. Hence, it is important to encourage parents to participate in treatment, learn how to set limits, and break away from overinvolvement in the child's rituals. Although initial attempts to regain control may be met by protest, the ability of the parents to set limits and reestablish appropriate parental control will give them more confidence and the child more security.

It is important to note that treating childhood OCD often is a lengthy and time-consuming process. The therapist may need to implement systematically a variety of interventions over a long period of time in order to achieve symptom relief. The case description below illustrates many of these problems inherent in treating youngsters with OCD.

Relapse Prevention

An important feature of a comprehensive treatment program for both adults and children is the provision of expectations regarding relapse and maintenance strategies to prevent its occurrence. Treatment often must be implemented in a variety of settings in order to promote generalization. In children, a lack of appropriate social skills may become apparent following successful treatment (Bolton et al., 1983), as previous time-consuming behaviors and rules may have resulted in social isolation. Hence, social skills training may be needed for a child to reintegrate effectively into the peer group. Additionally, parents may also need to redirect their own lives so that they no longer revolve solely around the child.

CASE ILLUSTRATION

The following case illustration of a 13-year-old boy with OCD describes typical difficulties encountered in the assessment and treatment of children, as well as the process of selecting and implementing the optimal intervention while being responsive to changing needs during the course of treatment.

Case Description

Jon, a 13-year-old seventh-grader, had been in outpatient treatment for a year before he was referred to us. The referring therapist, who was terminating due to a relocation, reported that Jon engaged in a variety of ritualistic behaviors, including elaborate touching, showering, and bedtime rituals. His symptoms reportedly began soon after his mother was rushed to the hospital for a serious kidney infection, which was treated effectively within a few days. The therapist reported that daily behavioral monitoring of Jon's rituals had been effective in decreasing the symptoms substantially. However, as some behaviors remitted, others appeared in their place.

Differential Diagnosis and Assessment

During initial assessment sessions, we (GF and AP) met with the entire family, consisting of Jon, his parents, both aged 35, and brother Al, aged 11. Jon presented as shy and withdrawn, spoke in monosyllables in a barely audible voice, made no eye contact, and appeared stiff and uncomfortable. The father, a large, burly man, was slow to warm up but, contrary to his appearance, presented as significantly anxious. The mother, a pleasant woman who appeared to be the spokesperson for the family, reported that they had first noticed unusual behaviors when Jon began repeatedly stating the time and talking to his food around age 5.

Subsequently, Jon's parents noted that he was spending a long time in the shower, during which time he stepped back and forth on the mat, showered several times, emptied half the contents of a bottle of shampoo, and winked at the shower head. Jon also arranged his clothes and shoes face down, opened the closed bureau drawers several times, mumbled when he threw his clothes in the laundry hamper, and got into bed in the same way every night. He stepped through doorways with his left foot first and had to touch every doorframe and bannister that he passed. Periodically, he completed a sequence of five steps in the same order. Jon also whistled in short, forced bursts at regular intervals. At mealtime, Jon arranged his food on the plate in a certain way, took a set number of sips each time he got a drink, and always left the same number of pieces of food at the end of a meal. These behaviors were exacerbated when Jon experienced even mild stress. Both parents reported that telling Jon to stop the rituals had been in vain; as Jon became more secretive, they became frustrated about nagging him. Their efforts to have Jon talk to them about his thoughts and feelings also were in vain.

Jon did not demonstrate any compulsions during clinic visits, indicating that he was able to inhibit them in social situations. We attempted to facilitate rapport by having one of us (AP) meet exclusively with him over several weekly sessions, while GF continued to meet with the family. A significant problem that characterized the entire course of treatment was tht it was inordinately difficult to establish any semblance of rapport with Jon. He remained very passive and resisted efforts to ally with him. It was often a struggle just to have him answer "yes" or "no," as he typically shrugged his shoulders to say, "I don't know."

During one session, Jon did provide substantial information about obsessions and compulsions. He stated that he always was afraid that he would fall and be injured or bleed to death, and that his parents would either fall ill or have an accident and die. He believed that the rituals would prevent such "bad luck." He stated that he wanted to stop the rituals but was afraid that his mother would die and it would be his fault. In contrast to his parents, Jon reported only touching and stepping rituals and minimized their frequency. He denied any feelings of sadness, anxiety, or anger.

Jon and his parents were interviewed separately using the Schedule for Affective Disorders and Schizophrenia for School-Aged Children (K-SADS; Chambers et al., 1985), modified by Last (1986) to correspond with DSM-III-R diagnostic criteria for anxiety disorders. Criteria for OCD were met on both parent and child interviews. Although Jon denied all symptoms in other diagnostic categories, his parents endorsed several symptoms of overanxious disorder and separation anxiety disorder, although he did not meet criteria for either diagnosis.

Treatment Selection

The nature of the disorder and treatment options (including behavioral techniques such as response prevention and flooding, medication, and inpatient treatment) were discussed with the family. The initial step was an educative one, in order to keep the parents and Jon informed and allay anxiety resulting from lack of information. The ensuing choice of treatments was based on the nature of specific target behaviors, level of compliance expected from Jon and his parents, and degree of invasiveness of each intervention.

Response prevention, the first treatment option, was initiated by having Jon and his parents monitor compulsions during three time periods (morning, afternoon, and bedtime) over a one-week period. Showering rituals, which were rated the most incapacitating, were targeted during the first week of treatment. Jon's parents were asked to be physically present, take Jon's dirty clothes from him, give him the required amount of shampoo, allot 15 minutes in the shower, hand him clean clothes, and supervise him getting dressed. At the end of each shower, Jon and his parents were instructed to rate his anxiety on 10-point scale. The parents reported that Jon had complied without any resistance or anxiety (rating of zero) and that shower rituals stopped completely. However, they noted that he appeared to be generally more restless and anxious during other times of the day and that touching bannisters and whistling had increased.

Treatment Course and Problems in Carrying Out Interventions

Weeks 1 to 10. As monitoring and response prevention continued successfully with a new target behavior each week, the parents were instructed to encourage Jon to develop independence in changing his own behaviors. It soon became apparent that when response prevention was not implemented, Jon reverted to compulsive behaviors as usual. Additionally, both parents reported that Jon appeared to enjoy their supervision. Further discussion indicated that Jon and his parents had significant difficulty being apart even for short periods, spent all but school time together, and never went anywhere without each other. At this time, a change in the direction of treatment was warranted, as parental attention during response prevention appeared to be providing secondary gain for Jon.

Weeks 11 to 18. Imaginal flooding, directed at obsessional thoughts, was the next treatment of choice. Six hypothetical scenes, based on a hierarchy of Jon's obsessional thoughts (e.g., of injury or death to himself and harm befalling family members), were presented individually during three sessions per week. Anxiety ratings were obtained before, during, and after each presentation of a scene. Ratings and behavioral observations indicated that Jon's initial anxiety was high, but habituation and decreased anxiety was fairly rapid.

Although flooding appeared to be effective in reducing anxiety from fearful thoughts, the parents indicated little improvement in compulsions at home, although Jon reported that he was "much better." The problems that arose at this juncture were unreliable reporting by Jon, including forgetting his weekly monitoring sheet, and failure of treatment gains to generalize outside the clinic. Given the nature of Jon's fears, in vivo flooding was not a viable option.

Subsequently, the parents reported that Jon had been significantly more irritable and oppositional at home and unmotivated to complete school work. They were distressed at their ineffectiveness in disciplining either of their sons, who ignored their repeated requests and "drove them crazy." They admitted that they might have been too lax and overly indulgent in their efforts to be good parents. Their frustration was reflected in discouragement, several canceled appointments, and inconsistency in monitoring.

Weeks 19 to 26. A shift in the focus of treatment was seen as necessary at this time in order to enable the parents to gain control in the home and develop a sense of efficacy, as these factors were interfering with treatment compliance. Child management training was implemented, emphasizing techniques of reinforcement and punishment, and consistency in application. Differences in the parents' approach to discipline emerged at this time, with the mother being more amenable to new ideas and with the father being more skeptical. At this point, it also appeared that the frequency of Jon's rituals had actually decreased, but the parents had failed to acknowledge and reinforce these changes.

Parental anxiety—particularly the father's tendency to catastrophize about Jon's future—resistance to individuation within the family, and reluctance to acknowledge improvement appeared to be relevant to the maintenance of Jon's symptoms. It also emerged that the parents, who in-

itially denied marital problems, did not have a satisfactory relationship apart from that with their children. Jon's mother and father had been divorced when Jon was 5 years old, primarily due to the father's alcoholism, but remarried each other four years later, after the father sought treatment and attained sobriety. He reported that he had been completely abstinent since that time and that he "did it for the kids." Jon had reportedly been upset by the divorce and had received outpatient treatment for a short period. It was evident that Jon's obsessional fears of loss of his parents possibly had been conditioned by the divorce as well as by his mother's sudden kidney infection. These family issues indicated the need for family therapy, as it appeared that Jon's "illness" might have functional value in keeping the family cohesive, thereby limiting opportunities for potential marital discord and/or divorce.

Weeks 27 to 38. Following a few weeks of family therapy, which was considered to be a relatively long-term need, the possibility of medication and inpatient hospitalization was raised. Immediately after, a dramatic improvement was noted in Jon's motivation. He initiated a plan to target selected compulsive behaviors each week and "try not to do them." In a classic case of negative reinforcement, Jon attempted to avoid separation from his parents by abruptly inhibiting compulsive behaviors. Although the parents noted the improvement, they were slow to reinforce the change. After six weeks of steady improvement, whistling was the only ritual that remained unchanged. The decision to hospitalize Jon was dropped and termination of treatment was discussed.

The following week, the parents reported that Jon relapsed into all rituals, making them suspicious that he had been engaging in the compulsions all along but had been successful in hiding them. Jon admitted to the relapse but denied his parents' allegation. There was no identifiable precipitant or stressor related to the relapse. Since 10 months of outpatient treatment had been essentially ineffective, inpatient hospitalization was recommended, much to the distress of the family.

Weeks 39 to 42. During the assessment phase on an adolescent inpatient unit, Jon presented in much the same manner, denying all problem behaviors, being very isolative, and demonstrating great difficulty being separated from his parents. Hourly monitoring by unit staff indicted several touching behaviors and some mealtime rituals that Jon attempted to make "natural," but there were no whistling or stepping rituals.

Recommendations from a comprehensive evaluation included a trial of Clomipramine, coupled with intensive behavioral interventions at the level of milieu, individual therapy, assertiveness training, and family therapy to address issues of parental anxiety, need for individuation within the family, and child management. Within a few days, Jon's withdrawal and passivity began to change and he began to take initiative to earn privileges on the milieu. The parents were encouraged to recognize and reinforce these changes. Only after Jon was able to demonstrate that he could "take care of himself" did the parents develop some confidence in his capabilities and allow him some freedom to express himself.

A trial of Clomipramine was begun with an initial dose of 25 mg twice daily, which was gradually increased to a total daily dosage of 150 mg. Common mild side effects of antidepressant medication were noted, but there were no contraindications.

Jon continued to make steady progress in meeting increased demands for assertiveness and social behavior on the unit. His parents were amazed that he could lead a group meeting and initiate a conversation. Jon began talking spontaneously in a variety of settings, answered questions immediately, and appeared to be much more bright, confident, and pleased with his performance. He also became more comfortable on the unit, engaged with peers, and was significantly less concerned about going home. Jon reported decrease in his fear that his parents would die, and touching behaviors decreased considerably. After a four-week stay, Jon was transitioned back to home and school with increasingly long visits out of the hospital, which were reported to be successful.

Outcome and Termination

Jon was discharged from the hospital. Although it was evident that he was motivated to comply with treatment by his desire to return home quickly, the multifaceted progress he made was dramatic enough to give both him and his parents a renewed perspective on his capabilities. The father, who continued to have the most difficulty being separated from Jon, finally recognized substantial changes in Jon's behavior and acknowledged that he had overprotected him because he was too afraid to allow him to fail. He spontaneously expressed his desire to implement the child management techniques discussed earlier.

Although inpatient treatment was multifaceted, the single most important curative factor during Jon's hospitalization was very likely the in vivo flooding effect of forced separation from his parents, since behavioral improvement began even prior to administration of Clomipramine. During the course of four weeks, Jon was unable to engage in preventive rituals; the fact that his parents remained healthy and free from harm during his absence permitted extinction of his fear of loss.

Followup and Maintenance

The family will continue to attend weekly outpatient sessions in order to monitor treatment gains and transition slowly from the intensity of inpatient treatment. Once gains have been maintained at home, another goal will be to discontinue medication in order to evaluate the need for such treatment. It is hoped that treatment can be terminated within a few months. Jon's mother recently began communicating marital discontent, stating that, in Jon's absence, she and her husband had nothing to talk about and that he was distant and unwilling to be in her company. Accordingly, the next line of attack appears to be in the direction of marital therapy for the parents.

SUMMARY

The purpose of this chapter has been to describe the clinical presentation of OCD in children and adolescents and review evidence for prescriptive treatment of the disorder. A number of promising behavioral and pharmacologic interventions have been studied, although the studies are small in number and most are not methodologically rigorous. Although definitive statements regarding treatment efficacy cannot yet be made, the literature does provide suggestive evicence for a number of interventions. Factors to be considered in selecting treatment options and commonly encountered problems in implementation have been described. A case study has been provided, with the goal of illustrating the often lengthy and complex task of treating children with OCD.

REFERENCES

Allsopp, M., & Verduyn, C. (1988). A follow-up of adolescents with Obsessive-Compulsive Disorder. *British Journal of Psychiatry, 154,* 829–834.

American Psychiatric Association. (1987). *Diagnostic and statistical manual of mental disorders* (3rd ed., rev.). Washington, DC: Author.

Apter, A., Bernhout, E., & Tyano, S. (1984). Severe obsessive compulsive disorder in adolescence: A report of eight cases. *Journal of Adolescence, 7,* 349–358.

Basoglu, M., Lax, T., Kasvikis, Y., & Marks, I. M. (1988). Predictors of improvement in Obsessive-Compulsive Disorder. *Journal of Anxiety Disorders, 2,* 299–317.

Berg, C. J., Rapoport, J. L., & Flament, M. (1986). The Leyton Obsessional Inventory—Child Version. *Journal of the American Academy of Child Psychiatry, 25,* 84–91.

Berg, C. J., Whitaker, A., Davies, M., Flament, M. F., & Rapoport, J. L. (1988). The survey form of the Leyton Obsessional Inventory—Child Version: Norms from an epidemiological study. *Journal of the American Academy of child and Adolescent Psychiatry, 27,* 759–763.

Bolton, D., Collins, S., & Steinberg, D. (1983). The treatment of obsessive-compulsive disorder in adolescence: A report of fifteen cases. *British Journal of Psychiatry, 142,* 456–464.

Breslau, N. (1987). Inquiring about the bizarre: False positives in Diagnostic Interview Schedule for Children (DISC) ascertainment of obsessions, compulsions, and psychotic symptoms. *Journal of the American Academy of Child and Adolescent Psychiatry, 26,* 639–644.

Campbell, L. M. (1973). A variation of thought-stopping in a twelve-year-old boy: A case report. *Journal of Behavior Therapy and Experimental Psychiatry, 4,* 69–70.

Chambers, W. J., Puig-Antich, J., Hirsch, M., Paez, P., Ambrosini, P. J., Tabrizi, M. A., & Davies, M. (1985). The assessment of affective disorders in children and adolescents by semistructured interviews: Test-retest reliability of the K-SADS-P. *Archives of General Psychiatry, 42,* 696–702.

Clark, D. A., & Bolton, D. (1985). An investigation of two self-report measures of obsessional phenomena in obsessive-compulsive adolescents: Research note. *Journal of Child Psychology and Psychiatry, 26,* 429–437.

Clark, D. A., Sugrim, I., & Bolton, D. (1982). Primary obsessional slowness: A nursing programme with a 13-year-old male adolescent. *Behaviour Research and Therapy, 20,* 289–292.

Costello, A. J., Edelbrock, C., Dulcan, M. K., Kalas, R., & Klaric, S. H. (1984). *Development and testing of the NIMH Diagnostic Interview Schedule for Children (DISC) in a clinic population: Final report.* Rockville, MD: Center for Epidemiological Studies, NIMH.

Costello, A. J., Edelbrock, C., Kalas, R., Kessler, M. D., & Klaric, S. H. (1982). *The NIMH Diagnostic Interview Schedule for Children (DISC).* Unpublished interview schedule, Department of Psychiatry, University of Pittsburgh.

Dalton, P. (1983). Family treatment of an obsessive compulsive child: A case report. *Family Process, 22,* 99–108.

Despert, L. (1955). Differential diagnosis between obsessive-compulsive neurosis and schizophrenia in children. In P. H. Hoch & J. Zubin (Eds.), *Psychopathology of childhood* (pp. 240–253). New York: Grune & Stratton.

Emmelkamp, P. M. G. (1982). *Phobic and obsessive-compulsive disorders: Theory, research, and practice.* New York: Plenum.

Flament, M. F., Rapoport, J. L., Berg, C. J., Sceery, W., Kilts, C., Mellstrom, B., & Linnoila, M. (1985). Clomipramine treatment of childhood obsessive-compulsive disorder. *Archives of General Psychiatry, 42,* 977–983.

Flament, M. F., Whitaker, A., Rapoport, J. L., Davies, M., Berg, C. Z., Kalikow, K., Sceery, W., & Shaffer, D. (1988). Obsessive-compulsive disorder in adolescence: An epidemiological study. *Journal of the American Academy of Child and Adolescent Psychiatry, 27,* 764–771.

Foa, E. B. (1979). Failures in treating obsessive-compulsives. *Behaviour Research and Therapy, 17,* 169–176.

Foa, E. B., Steketee, G., & Milby, J. B. (1980). Differential effects of exposure and response prevention in obsessive compulsive washers. *Journal of Consulting and Clinical Psychology, 48,* 71–79.

Foa, E. B., Steketee, G. S., & Ozarow, B. J. (1985). Behavior therapy with obsessive-compulsives: From theory to treatment. In M. Mavissakalian, S. M. Turner, & L. Michelson (Eds.), *Obsessive-compulsive disorder: Psychological and pharmacological treatment* (pp. 49–129). New York: Plenum.

Francis, G. (1988). Childhood obsessive-compulsive disorder: Extinction of compulsive reassurance-seeking. *Journal of Anxiety Disorders, 2,* 361–366.

Gesell, A., Ames, L. B., & Ilg, F. L. (1974). *Infant and child in the culture today.* New York: Harper and Row.

Goodman, W. K., Price, L. H., Rasmussen, S. A., Mazure, C., Fleischmann, R. L., Hill, C. L., Heninger, G. R., & Charney, D. S. (1989). The Yale-Brown Obsessive Compulsive Scale, I: Development, Use, and Reliability. *Archives of General Psychiatry, 46,* 1006–1011.

Goodman, W. K., Rasmussen, S. A., Price, L. H., Mazure, C., Rapoport, J. L., Heninger, G. R., & Charney, D. S. (1986). *Children's Yale-Brown Obsessive-Compulsive Scale (CY-BOCS).* Unpublished scale.

Grad, L. R., Pelcovitz, D., Olsen, M., Matthews, M., & Grad, W. (1987). Obsessive-compulsive symptomatology in children with Tourette's syndrome. *Journal of the American Academy of Child Psychiatry, 26,* 69–73.

Green, D. (1980). A behavioral approach to the treatment of obsessional rituals: An adolescent case study. *Journal of Adolescence, 3,* 297–306.

Hallam, R. S. (1974). Extinction of ruminations: A case study. *Behavior Therapy, 5,* 565–568.

Herjanic, B., & Campbell, W. (1977). Differentiating psychiatrically disturbed children on the basis of a structured psychiatric interview. *Journal of Abnormal Child Psychology, 5,* 127–135.

Hodges, K., McKnew, D., Cytryn, L., Stern, L., & Kline, J. (1982). The Child Assessment Schedule (CAS) Diagnostic Interviews: A report of reliability and validity. *Journal of the American Academy of Child Psychiatry, 21,* 468–473.

Hodgson, R. J., & Rachman, S. (1977). Obsessive compulsive complaints. *Behavior Research and Therapy, 15,* 389–395.

Hollingsworth, C. E., Tanguay, P. E., Grossman, L., & Pabst, P. (1980). Long-term outcome of obsessive-compulsive disorder in childhood. *Journal of the Academy of Child and Adolescent Psychiatry, 19,* 134–144.

Judd, L. L. (1965). Obsessive compulsive neurosis in children. *Archives of General Psychiatry, 25,* 298–304.

Kasvikis, Y., Tsakiris, F., Marks, I., Basough, M., & Noshirvani, N. (in press). Women with obsessive compulsive disorder frequently report a past history of anorexia nervosa. *International Journal of Eating Disorders.*

Kovacs, M. (1983). *The Interview Schedule for Children (ISC): Interrater and parent-child agreement.* Unpublished manuscript, University of Pittsburgh School of Medicine, Pittsburgh, PA.

LaGreca, A. M., Dandes, S. K., Wick, P., Shaw, K., & Stone, W. L. (1988). Development of the social anxiety scale for children: Reliability and concurrent validity. *Journal of Clinical Child Psychology, 17,* 84–91.

Last, C. G. (1986). *Modification of the K-SADS for use with anxiety-disordered populations.* Unpublished manuscript, University of Pittsburgh School of Medicine, Pittsburgh, PA.

Leonard, H. L., Goldberger, E. L., Rapoport, J. L., Cheslow, D. L., & Swedo, S. E. (1990). Childhood rituals: Normal development or obsessive-compulsive symptoms? *Journal of the American Academy of Child and Adolescent Psychiatry, 29,* 17–23.

Leonard, H. L., Swedo, S. E., Rapoport, J. L., Coffey, M. L., & Cheslow, D. L. (1988). Treatment of childhood obsessive-compulsive disorder with clomipramine and desmethylimipramine: A double blind crossover comparison. *Psychopharmacological Bulletin, 24,* 93–95.

Marks, I. M. (1987). *Fears, phobias and rituals.* New York: Oxford Press.

Marks, I. M., Hodgson, R. J., & Rachman, S. (1975). Treatment of chronic obsessive compulsive neurosis by in vivo exposure: A 2 year follow-up and issues in treatment. *British Journal of Psychiatry, 127,* 349–364.

McCarthy, P. R., & Foa, E. D. (1988). Obsessive-compulsive disorder. In M. Hersen & C. G. Last (Eds.), *Child behavior therapy casebook.* New York: Plenum.

Milby, J. B., & Weber, A. (1991). Obsessive-compulsive

disorder. In T. R. Kratochwill & R. J. Morris (Eds.), *The practice of child therapy.* New York: Pergamon.

Mills, H. L., Agras, W. S., Barlow, D. H., & Mills, J. R. (1973). Compulsive rituals treated by response prevention: An experimental analysis. *Archives of General Psychiatry, 28,* 524–529.

Ollendick, T. H. (1983). Reliability and validity of the Revised Fear Survey Schedule for Children (FSSC-R). *Behaviour Research and Therapy, 21,* 685–692.

Ong, S. B. Y., & Leng, Y. K. (1979). The treatment of an obsessive compulsive girl in the context of Malaysian Chinese culture. *Australian New Zealand Journal of Psychiatry, 13,* 255–259.

Ownby, R. L. (1983). A cognitive behavioral intervention for compulsive handwashing with a thirteen-year-old boy. *Psychology in the Schools, 20,* 219–222.

Perse, T. (1988). Obsessive-Compulsive Disorder: A treatment review. *Journal of Clinical Psychiatry, 49,* 48–55.

Queiroz, L., Motta, M., Madi, M., Sossai, D., & Boren, J. J. (1981). A functional analysis of obsessive-compulsive problems with related therapeutic procedures. *Behaviour Research and Therapy, 18,* 377–388.

Rachman, S. J. (1985). An overview of clinical and research issues in obsessive-compulsive disorders. In M. Mavissakalian, S. M. Turner, & L. Michelson (Eds.), *Obsessive-compulsive disorders: Psychological and pharmacological treatment* (pp. 1–47). New York: Plenum.

Rachman, S. J., & Hodgson, R. J. (1980). *Obsessions and compulsions.* Englewood Cliffs, NJ: Prentice Hall.

Rapoport, J. L. (1986). Childhood obsessive-compulsive disorder. *Journal of Child Psychology and Psychiatry, 27,* 289–295.

Rapoport, J., Elkins, R., Langer, D. H., Sceery, W., Buchsbaum, M. S., Gillin, J. C., Murphy, D. L., Zahn, T. P., Lake, R., Ludlow, C., & Mendelson, W. (1981). Childhood obsessive-compulsive disorder. *American Journal of Psychiatry, 138,* 1545–1554.

Rapoport, J., Elins, R., & Mikkelson, E. (1980). Clinical controlled trial of chlorimipramine in adolescents with obsessive-compulsive disorder. *Psychopharmacological Bulletin, 16,* 61–63.

Rasmussen, S. A., & Tsuang, M. T. (1986). Epidemiology and clinical features of obsessive-compulsive disorder. In M. A. Jenike, L. Baer, & W. E. Minichiello (Eds.), *Obsessive-compulsive disorders: Theory and management* (pp. 23–44). Littleton, MA: PSG Publishing.

Reynolds, C. R., & Richmond, B. O. (1978). "What I Think and Feel": A revised measure of children's manifest anxiety. *Journal of Abnormal Child Psychology, 6,* 271–280.

Riddle, M. A., Hardin, M. T., King, R., Scahill, L., & Woolston, J. L. (1990). Fluoxetine treatment of children and adolescents with Tourette's and Obsessive compulsive Disorders: Preliminary clinical experience. *Journal of the American Academy of Child and Adolescent Psychiatry, 29,* 45–48.

Rutter, M., Tizard, J., & Whitmore, K. (1970). *Education, health, and behavior.* London: Longmans.

Sarason, S. B., Davidson, K. S., Lighthall, F. F., Waite, R. R., & Ruebush, B. K. (1960). *Anxiety and elementary school children.* New York: Wiley.

Silverman, W. K., & Nelles, W. B. (1988). The Anxiety Disorders Interview Schedule for Children. *Journal of the American Academy of Child and Adolescent Psychiatry, 27,* 772–778.

Spielberger, C. D. (1973). *Manual for the State-Trait Anxiety Inventory for Children.* Palo Alto, CA: Consulting Psychologists Press.

Stanley, L. (1980). Treatment of ritualistic behavior in an eight-year-old girl by response prevention: A case report. *Journal of Child Psychology and Psychiatry, 21,* 85–90.

Steketee, G., & Foa, E. B. (1985). Obsessive-Compulsive Disorder. In D. H. Barlow (Ed.), *Clinical handbook of psychological disorders* (pp. 69–144). New York: Guilford.

Swedo, S. E., & Rapoport, J. L. (1989). Phenomenology and differential diagnosis of Obsessive-Compulsive Disorder in children and adolescents. In J. L. Rapoport (Ed.), *Obsessive-Compulsive Disorder in children and adolescents* (pp. 13–32). Washington, DC: American Psychiatric Press.

Turner, S. M., & Beidel, D. C. (1988). *Treating obsessive-compulsive disorders.* New York: Pergamon.

Warren, W. (1960). Some relationships between psychiatry and children and adults. *Journal of Mental Science, 106,* 815–826.

Welner, A., Reich, T., Herjanic, B., & Campbell, W. (1987). Reliability, validity and parent-child agreement studies of the Diagnostic Interview for Children and Adolescents. *Journal of the American Academy of Child Psychiatry, 26,* 649–653.

Zikis, P. (1983). Treatment of an 11-year-old obsessive compulsive ritualizer and Tiqueur girl with in vivo exposure and response prevention. *Behavioral Psychotherapy, 11,* 75–81.

CHAPTER 13

ANOREXIA AND BULIMIA NERVOSA

Theodore E. Weltzin   University of Pittsburgh

Jeannie Starzynski   University of Pittsburgh

Regina Santelli   University of Pittsburgh

Walter H. Kaye   University of Pittsburgh

The term *eating disorders* really refers to a number of subgroups of disorders. The boundaries between subgroups and the terminology used to differentiate these subgroups has been in flux. Nevertheless, considerable literature (Beaumont, George, & Smart, 1976; Casper, Eckert, Halmi, Goldberg, & Davis, 1980; Garfinkel, Moldofsky, & Garner, 1980; Garner, Garfinkel, & O'Shaughnessy, 1985; Halmi & Falk, 1982; Herzog & Copeland, 1985; Strober, Salkin, Burroughs, & Morrell, 1982) suggests that certain factors distinguish subgroups of eating disordered patients. These factors include the amount of weight loss, the type of pathological eating behavior, and certain additional psychopathological characteristics.

The best known eating disorder is anorexia nervosa whose most distinguishing characteristic is severe emaciation. Two types of consummatory behavior are seen in anorexia nervosa. Restrictor or fasting anorexics (who fit the DSM-III-R [American Psychiatric Association (APA), 1987] criteria for anorexia nervosa [AN]) lose weight by pure dieting. Bulimic anorexics (who qualify for a DSM-III-R diagnosis of both anorexia nervosa and bulimia nervosa [AN-BN]) also lose weight but have a periodic disinhibition of restraint and engage in bingeing and purging. Compared with restrictors (AN), the bulimic subgroup (AN-BN) has been characterized as displaying significantly more evidence of premorbid behavioral instability, a higher incidence of premorbid and familial obesity, a greater susceptibility to depression, and a higher incidence of behaviors suggestive of impulse disorders (Beaumont et al., 1976; Casper et al., 1980; Garfinkel et al., 1980 ; Garner et al., 1985; Halmi & Falk, 1982; Herzog & Copeland, 1985; Strober et al., 1982).

The third eating disorder is normal weight bulimia (or bulimia nervosa using DSM-III-R criteria). This disorder is at least 10 times more prevalent than anorexia nervosa (Halmi, Falk, & Schwartz, 1981; Pope, Hudson, & Yurgelun-Todd, 1984; Stangler & Printz, 1980). These patients periodically binge and purge, usually by vomiting, but never become emaciated. That is, they maintain a body weight above 85 percent of average body weight (Garner et al., 1985). Normal-weight bulimics resemble bulimic anorexics in terms of impulsivity and a predisposition to obesity (Garner et al., 1985).

DESCRIPTION OF DISORDERS

Clinical Features

Bulimia Nervosa

Bulimia is defined as the rapid ingestion of large amounts of food that is often of high caloric value. The eating is usually inconspicuous and is terminated by sleep, social interruption, abdominal pain, or self-induced purging. Bulimics purge themselves through vomiting, laxatives, or diuretics. Periods of binge eating are often interspersed with fasting and dieting, and weight fluctuations are commonly seen. Bulimic individuals are often aware that they have an abnormal eating pattern and yet are unable to alter it voluntarily.

Bulimia can occur in underweight patients with anorexia nervosa but is much more commonly found in those of normal weight or the obese. We use the terms *normal-weight bulimia* or *bulimic disorder* to describe nonanorexic patients with the symptoms of binge eating described above. The typical duration of the illness prior to treatment is reported to be at least five years (Fairburn & Cooper, 1982).

Anorexia Nervosa

Anorexia nervosa is characterized by a refusal to maintain body weight over a minimal normal weight, a fear of weight gain or becoming fat even though underweight, a disturbance of body image, and amenorrhea, which is the loss of three consecutive menses (APA, 1987). This disorder occurs in one of 250 females during adolescence and the male-to-female ratio is approximately 1:20. The etiology of the illness is unknown, but predisposing factors have been thought to include psychodynamic, social, learning, family, and biological factors. Some evidence indicates success in treating anorexia nervosa with psychotherapy, family therapy, behavior modification, and drug treatments. However, over the long term, most patients do poorly despite treatment. Perhaps overly optimistic claims of success may be due to inadequate followup of patients after treatment (Vandereycken & Pierloot, 1983) or inadequate assessment of placebo response rate (Hsu, 1980; Schwartz & Thompson, 1981).

Associated Features

Anorexia Nervosa

Studies of comorbidity of affective disorders in anorexia nervosa have examined the presence of concomitant psychopathology during the acute phase of the illness and following short- and long-term recovery. The widely varying estimates reflect differential methodological and diagnostic procedures across studies. It has been estimated that 21 to 91 percent of anorexic patients have depressive symptoms when they are underweight and malnourished (Eckert, Goldberg, Halmi, Casper, & Davis, 1982; Hendren, 1983; Morgan & Russell, 1975; Stonehill & Crisp, 1977; Theander, 1970). Interpretation of these findings must consider that the effects of starvation on behavior (Keys, 1950; Strober & Katz, 1988) seem to be similar to the depressive disorders. This high rate of depressive patients with anorexia may be due, in part, to malnutrition. The presence of depressive symptomatology has also been examined in patients with anorexia nervosa after short- and long-term weight recovery. With duration of followup ranging up to 4.9 years, an estimated 15 to 58 percent of patients continued to exhibit depressive symptom disturbance after weight recovery.

The high prevalence of depressive symptoms in anorexics mentioned above has generated trials of antidepressant medications. However, antidepressants have been found at best to be only partially effective. These medications include amitriptyline (Biederman, Herzog, Rivinus, & Ferber, 1985; Halmi, Eckert, & LaDu, 1986), clomipramine (Crisp, Lacey, & Crutchfield, 1987; Lacey & Crisp, 1980), and lithium (Gross et al., 1981). There have been a few family epidemiology studies of the coaggregation of eating and affective disorders. Strober and colleagues (1990), in a large and well-controlled family-epidemiologic study, found an increased prevalence of affective disorders (mainly unipolar) depression among relatives of only the anorexic probands who were themselves depressed. Biederman and colleagues (1985) had similar findings. In contrast, Gershon and others (1984) found equally high rates of affective disorder among relatives of depressed and nondepressed anorexic probands.

The focus on the possible relationship of depression to anorexia nervosa has tended to obscure investigations of other psychopathology in this illness. In fact, patients with anorexia nervosa also have a high prevalence of obsessive-compulsive symptoms or disorders (Cantwell, Sturzenberger, & Burroughs, 1977; Hsu, Crisp, & Harding, 1970; Rowland, 1970; Hudson, Pope, Jonas, & Yurgelun-Todd, 1983a; Rothenberg, 1988). Strober (1980) described the anorexic personality as being markedly obsessional in character makeup, introverted, self-denying, prone to self-abasement with limited spontaneity, overly formalistic, and stereotyped in thinking despite being industrious. Importantly, he noted that these characteristics were ingrained and not related to weight in that they remained present after short-term weight restoration.

Casper (1990) reported that women recovered from restricting anorexia nervosa for 8 to 10 years continued to rate higher on risk avoidance, displayed greater restraint in emotional expression and initiative, and showed greater conformance to authority than age-matched controls, and had a greater degree of self- and impulse-control than their sisters. Finally, several investigators have noted (Kasvikis, Tsakiris, & Marks, Basoglu, & Noshirvani, 1986; T. Insel, personal communication) that adult women with obsessive-compulsive disorder (OCD) have an increased likelihood of a history of anorexia nervosa. Together, these data suggest that some anorexic patients may have more in common with OCD patients than their depressive counterparts.

Bulimia Nervosa

A number of studies have found a high incidence of concurrent depressed mood in patients with bulimia nervosa &Gwirtsman, Roy-Byrne, Yager, & Gerner, 1983; Hatsukami, Eckert, Mitchell, & Pyle, 1984; Herzog, 1982; Hudson, Laffer, & Pope, 1982; Hudson et al., 1983b; Pope, Hudson, Jonas, & Yurgelon-Todd, 1983). In addition, family studies reveal a high prevalence of affective disorders in the relatives of patients with bulimia nervosa. For example, Kassett and colleagues (1986) found that first-degree relatives of bulimia nervosa probands had higher rates of major affective disorders than first-degree relatives of control subjects. Such findings have led investigators to hypothesize that eating disorders are a variant of major affective disorders (Hudson et al., 1983b).

The high incidence of depressive symptoms in bulimic patients has prompted trials of antidepressant medication. Placebo-controlled, double-blind trials of desipramine (Blouin, Blouin, & Perez, 1988; Hughes, Wells, Cunningham, & Illstrupp, 1986), isocarboxazid (Kennedy, Piran, & Garfinkel, 1986), amitriptyline (Mitchell, & Groat, 1984), imipramine (Pope et al., 1983), phenelzine (Walsh, Stewart, & Roose, 1984), and fluoxetine (Freeman, Morris, Cheshire, Casper, & Davis, 1988) show that these medications reduce binge eating and purging behavior and/or improve depressive symptoms. Two important points should be made. First, though these medications improve eating behavior, the majority of patients treated with antidepressants continue to exhibit bulimic behavior. Second, antidepressants are associated with improvement of bulimic symptoms in subjects that are not depressed. In summary, data from antidepressant treatment trials suggest some common biological mechanisms between bulimia nervosa and depression, but it cannot be concluded that bulimia nervosa is a subtype of depressive illness.

Recently investigators have focused on the relationship of other psychopathology in bulimia nervosa. Laessle, Wittchen, Fichter, and Pirke (1989) found that 70 percent of BN patients had a lifetime diagnosis of anxiety disorders, a figure *greater* than the lifetime prevalence (56 percent) of depression. Hudson, Pope, Jonas, Yurgelun-Todd, and Frankenburg (1987) found that BN patients had a 43 percent lifetime prevalence of anxiety disorders in comparison to a 67 percent prevalence of depression. Studies of bulimia nervosa patients have shown a high incidence of alcohol abuse or dependency with a range of between 16 and 49 percent (Beary, Lacey, & Meery, 1986; Bulik, 1987; Hudson et al., 1983b; Hudson et al., 1987; Laessle et al., 1989). For example, Mitchell and colleagues (1985), in a study of 275 bulimic women, found that 23 percent acknowledged a history of alcohol abuse and that 18 percent reported a prior history of treatment for chemical dependency. A high prevalence (between 33 and 83 percent) of women with bulimia nervosa have at least one close relative with alcoholism (Bulik, 1987; Herzog, 1982; trober et al., 1982; Leon, Carroll, Chernyk, & Finn, 1985; Mitchell, Hatsukami, Pyle, & Eckert, 1988; Pyle, Mitchell, & Eckert, 1981). Family epidemiology studies have also found a higher incidence of substance abuse in relatives of patients with bulimia nervosa than in matched controls (Hudson et al., 1987; Kassett et al., 1986).

Overview

At best, it remains controversial as to whether eating disorders and major depression share a common diathesis. Critical examination of clinical phenomenology, family history, antidepressant response, biological correlates, course and outcome, and epidemiology yields *limited* support for this hypothesis (Rothenberg, 1988; Strober & Katz, 1988; Swift, Andrews, & Barklage, 1986). In fact, there is considerable evidence suggesting that eating disorders share some relationship with other disorders. That is, anorexia nervosa may have some relationship to obsessive and compulsive behavior and bulimia nervosa may have share some commonality with anxiety disorders or alcoholism and substance abuse.

Epidemiology

Bulimia Nervosa

Relative to anorexia nervosa, bulimic disorder is more common. Studies in the United States, England, and Japan report the lifetime prevalence of bulimia nervosa in women to be as high as 19.6 percent, whereas in men the disease is much more rare (Halmi et al., 1981; Pope et al., 1984; Pyle, Mitchell, Eckert et al., 1983). In college popula-

tions, surveys place the prevalence of this disorder at 4 to 13 percent (Johnson & Larson, 1982) with a distribution of 87 percent females and 13 percent males (Halmi et al., 1981). As pointed out by Fairburn and Beslin (1990), this high prevalence may be due to overly inclusive criteria for identifying effected individuals. Using strict criteria, the prevalence is more likely to be closer to 1 percent in young adult and adolescent females.

Anorexia Nervosa

A recent study by Lucas, Beard, O'Fallon, and Kurland (1988) found the prevalence of anorexia nervosa in the United States as calculated in residents of Rochester, Minnesota (adjusted for age and sex to the 1970 U.S. white population) to be 113.1 per 100,0900, or 0.1 percent. This broke down into a prevalence of 0.2 percent for females and 0.017 percent for males. The age- and sex-adjusted incidence rates were the highest (7.3 per 100,000 person years) in females between the ages of 15 and 19. In addition, this study found no increase in the occurrence of disorder with time.

A study conducted in Switzerland on the incidence of anorexia nervosa in the canton of Zurich betweend 1956 and 1975 (Willi & Grossman, 1983) found that there was a significant increase in the incidence over time going from 0.38/100,000 to 1.12/100,000 in the total population, and from 3.98/100,000 to 19.84/100,000 in females between the ages of 12 and 25.

Etiology

Anorexia Nervosa

Current theories of the etiology of anorexia include family dysfunction, environmental pressures to maintain low weight, and biological disturbances (Strober & Humphrey, 1987). Theories of the familial contribution to the etiology include dysfunctional interactional patterns that include enmeshment, rigidity, overprotectiveness, and faulty conflict resolution (Minuchin & Fishman, 1981). Also, an increased prevalence of anorexia nervosa has been reported in the siblings (Theander, 1970) and parents (Crisp, Hsu, Harding, & Hartshorn, 1980) of anorexics.

Although environmental factors most likely

play an important role in the etiology of eating disorders, the mechanism by which this occurs is unclear. Hsu (1990) hypothesized that societal pressures to be thin, coupled with a trend in developed countries to have more abundant food sources, set the stage for the development of eating disorders. Thus, dieting, in those susceptible to developing eating disorders, becomes the initiation of the problem.

As previously noted, there has been controversy as to whether or not anorexia nervosa and major depressive disorders share a common diathesis. However, critical examination of clinical phenomenology, family history, antidepressant response, biological correlates, course and outcome, and epidemiology yield limited support for this hypothesis (Strober & Katz, 1988; Rothenberg, 1988; Swift et al., 1986).

5-HT and anorexia nervosa. Considerable data in animals and humans implicate brain serotonin systems in the modulation of appetite, mood, personality, and neuroendocrine function. Thus, a brain serotoninergic dysfunction could contribute to many aspects of the anorexia nervosa symptom complex.

Considerable evidence shows that brain serotoninergic pathways are inhibitory of appetite (Blundell, 1984; Leibowitz & Shor-Posner, 1986; Wurtman & Wurtman, 1979). Theoretically, food restriction and weight loss could be caused by increased serotonin activity. As noted above, anorexia patients are rigid, ritualistic, perfectionistic, and meticulous. A number of studies have found that low levels of CSF 5-HIAA are associated with impulsive, suicidal, and aggressive behavior (Asbert, Traskman, & Thoren, 1976; Brown, Goodwin, Ballenger, Goyer, & Major, 1979; Linnoila et al., 1983; van Praag, 1983). Thus, higher levels of CSF 5-HIAA in long-term weight-restored anorexics are of interest since these patients tend to be the opposite of impulsive and aggressive patients.

It has also been reported (Kaye, Ebert, Gwirtsman, & Weiss, 1984; Kaye, Gwirtsman, George, & Ebert, 1991) that long-term weight restored anorexics had elevated concentrations of CSF 5-HIAA. Furthermore, after probenecid infusion,

weight-recovered nonbulimic anorexics had higher levels of CSF 5-HIAA than did bulimic anorexics.

Taken together, these data suggest that increased serotonin activity could contribute to certain attributes found in both restrictor and bulimic anorexics, including obsessional and overly inhibited characteristics, as well as the pursuit of thinness. Alternatively, it is possible that restrictor and bulimic anorexics exist along a continuum, with restrictors having relatively greater serotonin activity than do bulimic anorexics, as evidenced by the fact that bulimic anorexics have cyclical and episodic behavioral patterns manifested by swings from impulsivity to compulsivity.

OCD and anorexia nervosa. At least three lines of evidence suggest that anorexia nervosa may be related to obsessive-compulsive disorder (OCD) and/or anxiety disorders. First, it has been well recognized that anorexics have a high prevalence of obsessive-compulsive symptoms or disorders, (Cantwell et al., 1977; Hsu et al., 1970; Hudson et al., 1983a; Rowland, 1970; Strober, 1980) as well as other anxiety disorders (Toner, Garfinkel, & Garner, 1986). Rothenberg (1988) reviewed 11 investigations of comorbidity in anorexia nervosa. He found obsessive-compulsive symptoms to be the second msot frequent symptoms (after depression), with an incidence of between 11 and 83 percent during an acute episode of anorexia nervosa or after weight restoration.

Second, two investigators have noted (Kasvikis et al., 1986; T. Insel, personal communication) that adult women with OCD have an increased incidence of prior anorexia nervosa. Third, anorexics have disturbances of serotoninergic (Kaye et al., 1991) activity that persist after long-term weight recovery. A disturbance of this neurotransmitter system has also been implicated in OCD (Traskman, Asberg, & Bertilsson, 1981; Zohar & Insel, 1987).

The possibility of a relationship between anorexia nervosa and OCD raises the question of how anorexic patients respond to a serotonin-specific medication. In fact, some evidence shows that medications affecting the serotonin system have some efficacy in anorexia nervosa. Crisp and colleagues (1987) administered clomipramine, a serotonin reuptake blocker, to anorexics engaged in a program of refeeding and weight gain and found it to be associated with increased appetite, hunger, and caloric consumption during the early stages of treatment. Halmi and others (1986) found that restrictor anorexics had a better response than bulimic anorexics to cyprohepta-dine, a serotonin antagonist. One study (Kaye, Weltzin, Hsu, & Bulik, 1991) treated 31 anorex-ics with an open trial of fluoxetine, a serotonin reuptake blocker that is effective in the treatment of OCD. Response was good in 11 and partial in another 16 anorexics, as measured by the fact that all of these anorexics were able to maintain a weight of > 85 percent ABW (average body weight for height) in 10 ± 7 months as outpa-tients. Additionally, there were improvements in eating behavior, mood, and obsessional symp-toms. In this preliminary investigation, it was also found that restrictors responded significantly bet-ter than bulimic/purging anorexics to a medica-tion with serotonin properties.

Bulimia Nervosa

The reason for the increase in incidence of BN in the past decade is not certain. One possible ex-planation is based on the hypothesis that BN is related to substance abuse, particularly alcohol. BN may serve as a more socially acceptable means, in our current social and cultural climate, of cer-tain women (who have a vulnerability to develop-ing alcohol abuse or dependence) who obtain the same short-term gratification that is found in substance abuse (Kaye et al., 1985; Bulik, 1987).

A number of points of evidence (Vandereycken, 1990) suggest a link between BN and substance abuse. Bulimic patients show an addiction-like behavior (craving, preoccupation with obtaining the substance, loss of control, adverse social and medical consequences, ambivalence toward treat-ment, risk of relapse) Bulik, 1987; Hatsukami et al., 1984; Mitchell et al., 1988), and they often tend to abuse alcohol or drugs. Several authors have noted that bingeing behavior produces a brief reduction in stress and tension that is similar to an intoxication-like state (Abraham & Beaumont, 1982; Johnson & Larson, 1982; Kaye et al., 1986; Strober, 1984). A higher-than-expected prevalence

of substance abuse is reported in relatives of bulimic patients when compared with controls. Studies in humans suggest that the pathophysiol-ogy of bulimia nervosa involves alterations of cer-tain central nervous system neurotransmitter sys-tems, such as opioid and monoamine systems (Jonas & Gold, 1986; Kaye, Ballenger et al., 1990; Kaye, Gwirtsman et al., 1990), which have been implicated in addictive, affective, and anxiety disorders.

Therapeutic strategies for bulimia have been in-spired by existing treatments for addictions, al-though little empirical evidence exists to support this concept. For example, some treatment op-tions—such as the self-help group, Overeaters Anonymous, based on the fundamental premises of Alcoholics Anonymous—have gained in popularity.

DIFFERENTIAL DIAGNOSIS AND ASSESSMENT

DSM-III-R Categorization

The DSM-III-R (APA, 1987) stipulates four criteria to obtain a diagnosis of anorexia nervosa. These include not maintaining weight over a min-imal normal level for age and height (defined as a body weight of 15 percent below expected levels); a fear of gaining weight or becoming fat despite low weight levels; a distorted body image about one's weight, size, or shape; and in women, amenorrhea (an absence of at least three con-secutive menstrual cycles). Bulimia nervosa is diagnosed using five criteria. These consist of repeated episodes of binge eating; feelings of not being in control over eating behavior while binge-ing; engaging in methods to prevent weight gain (e.g., self-induced vomiting, laxative or diuretic abuse, strict dieting or fasting, intense exercising); at least two binge-eating episodes per week over the previous three months; and excessive and per-sistent concern with weight and body shape.

Differential Diagnosis

Unusual eating patterns are symptomatic of several illnesses and psychiatric disorders although in these instances diagnoses of anorexia nervosa or bulimia nervosa are unwarranted. For example, anorexic behavior is seen in patients suffering from tumors, tuberculosis, hypothalamic disease, rigilan enteritis, interior pituitary insufficiencies, Addison's disease, hyperthyroidism, and diabetes mellitus (Garfinkel & Garner, 1982). Also, decreased eating and weight loss is sometimes found in major depression, schizophrenia, hysteria, and obsessive-compulsive disorder. Illnesses associated with bulimic behavior include epileptic-equivalent seizures, CNS tumors, Kluver-Bucy-like syndromes, Kleine-Levin syndrome, and gastrointestinal dysfunction. Bingeing and vomiting are also seen in schizophrenia, psychogentic vomiting, and anxiety disorders (Kaplan & Saddock, 1985).

Assessment Strategies

The assessment of eating disorders involves a comprehensive evaluation that includes medical and psychological evaluations. The need to make sure that abnormal eating behavior does not lead to potentially life-threatening medical problems cannot be overemphasized. Disease-specific mortality rates in anorexia range between 5 and 20 percent, and bulimia nervosa is also associated with potentially life-threatening sequelae. For additional information on assessment, Johnson, Stuckey, Lewis, and Schwartz (1982) detailed a comprehensive approach to the psychological assessment of eating disorders. Mitchell (Mitchell, 1984; Mitchell, Scim, Colon, & Pomeroy, 1987) and Hsu (1990) discuss medical complications and medical evaluations of bulimia and anorexia, respectively.

Assessment of Eating Disorder Symptoms

The initial evaluation should include a complete history of weight, eating behavior, psychological functioning (including perceptions of weight and shape, depression, and anxiety), a complete medical history and examination, and family and developmental history.

Body weight. It is particularly important to document weight at the time of initiation of puberty and at the time of the onset of abnormal eating behavior. For the adolescent, yearly weights, confirmed by pediatric records if possible, should be obtained. For the adult patient, weights at specific time points, including puberty, graduation from high school and college, marriage, and child birth, should be investigated. Also, episodes of significant fluctuations in weight should be obtained.

Dieting. Frequently a history of dieting precedes or coincides with the development of eating disorder symptoms. Therefore, a record of when dieting first began and the regularity of dieting is helpful.

Caloric intake. A careful history of daily caloric intake is important. This should include the number of meals a day, the types of food eaten, and any periods of overeating. We have found that bulimics may not differ from healthy controls by the number of meals they eat; rather, they tend to eat bigger meals in the afternoon and evening. They also tend to eat a higher percentage of snack foods (Weltzin, Hsu, Pollice, & Kaye, 1991).

Menstrual and sexual history. Because menstrual dysfunction occurs in 100 percent of patients with anorexia and approximately 50 percent of normal-weight bulimics, it is important to determine periods of time during which amenorrhea or oligomenorrhea occur. This can serve to support reported periods of recovery or to confirm a more chronic course suggested by long-standing menstrual dysfunction.

Impulsive and destructive sexual behavior is noted in a subgroup of eating disordered patients. This can be an indication of significant impulse control problems or alert the clinician to consider an additional diagnosis of bipolar affective disorder.

Sexual abuse is commonly reported in patients with eating disorders. Thus, it is important to include this in a detailed history, as it may have an impact on patient self-esteem and, if not taken into account, negatively affect treatment response.

Mental state. A complete mental status examination should be done to document any significant affective, anxiety, psychotic, suicidal, or impulse control problems. An adequate assessment of the patients' insight into their problems, judgment, and motivation for change should be conducted, as this can influence subsequent treatment decisions.

It should be determined if the patient meets additional diagnostic criteria especially for depression, anxiety disorders, and substance abuse disorders, as these occur more frequently in eating disorder patients than the general population and can influence treatment decisions.

Social and developmental history. A comprehensive assessment should gather information concerning learning disabilities, interpersonal difficulties, coping skills, and peer relationships.

Previous treatment. The types and extent of previous treatments should be ascertained, including psychotherapeutic approach, family therapy, medication trials, and previous inpatient treatment. Also, any medical treatment for medical complications of eating disorders should be documented, including hypotension, bradycardia, dizziness or blackouts, electrolyte disturbance, or suicide attempts.

Family history. Constructing a family genogram, including any significant physical or medical problems, is an essential component of a comprehensive assessment. Special attention should be given to parental opinions concerning weight, eating, and exercise. Also, it is not uncommon for a family crisis to coincide with the onset of an eating disorder or a worsening of symptoms. The use of the genogram has been demonstrated to be a helpful assessment tool in that it puts into picture form the family constellation of medical and psychiatric illnesses over several generations (McGoldrick, 1985).

Medical history and physical exam. A full physical exam, including neurological assessment and laboratory testing, should be done with underweight anorexics and actively bulimic pa-

tients. Laboratory testing should include complete blood counts, serum electrolytes, serum amylase, liver and kidney function tests, and an electrocardiogram. EEG, CAT, and MRI procedures should be reserved for those patients with suspected neurological illnesses.

TREATMENT

The primary focus of treatment for anorexia nervosa and bulimia nervosa should first be the correction of physiological sequelae of abnormal nutrition and the reversal of the psychological problems associated with these two disorders. Generally speaking, current evidence as to the treatment of both of these disorders should involve a comprehensive treatment approach that involves nutritional therapy, psychotherapeutic treatment, a cognitive-behavioral focus, family interventions, and pharmacotherapy. Below we will present pertinent data that support this contention.

Evidence for Prescriptive Treatments

Anorexia Nervosa

Currently, no single effective treatment for anorexia nervosa has been identified that is supported by rigorous scientific treatment efficacy studies. However, data support the use of a combination of nutritional restoration, behavioral reinforcement of normal eating behavior, cognitive restructuring of "anorexic thinking," and medications with antiobsessional characteristics in the treatment of anorexia nervosa.

Nutritional therapy. Malnourished anorexics have numerous hormonal and neurotransmitter disturbances, including decreased LH and FSH secretion, hypercortisol secretion, and disturbances of opioid, norepinephrine, and serotonin metabolism (Ploog & Pirke, 1987). Although many of these abnormalities return to normal with weight restoration, some, including CSF norepinephrine level and 5-HIAA, remain abnormal in anorexics (Kaye et al., 1984; Kaye et al., 1991).

We know that abnormalities of CSF, serotonin, and norepinephrine metabolism have been linked to other disorders of mood and behavior, including obsessive and impulsive behavior, depression, and anxiety. Therefore, it is possible that nutritionally induced changes in these neurochemicals could inhibit response to treatment, specifically psychological treatments. Conversely, by improving psychological functioning, nutritional recovery and weight gain may increase the effectiveness of specific psychological interventions.

Psychotherapeutic treatment. Behavioral approaches are effective in the weight-gain stage of anorexia treatment (Agras, Dorian, Kirkley, Arnow, & Bachman, 1987). They have been shown to decrease the length of inpatient treatment and increase the rate of weight gain (Agras et al., 1987). However, a strict behavioral program may be no better than more lenient approaches (Touyz, Beumont, Glaun, Phillips, & Cowie, 1984; Nusbaum & Drever, 1990), and in fact may increase the likelihood of patient engaging in purging behavior (Bossert, Schnabel, Krieg, & Berger, 1988).

The effectiveness of individual psychotherapy in anorexia nervosa has been sparse. However, Russell, Checkley, Feldman, and Eisler (1988) reported on the effects of individual versus family therapy in 57 anorexics. They found that in anorexics under the age of 18, patients treated with family therapy had a better outcome than those treated with individual therapy, whereas in the older anorexics the opposite was true. Other controlled trials employing social skills training (Pillay & Crisp, 1981), psychoanalytic therapy (Sohlberg, Rosmark, Norring, & Holmgren, 1987), and cognitive-behavioral treatment were inconclusive (Channon, de Silva, Hemsley, & Perkins, 1989). In spite of this, the importance of incorporating social skills training into treatment should not be overlooked, as themes of loneliness and troubled relationships typically emerge in psychotherapy.

In fact, most current psychotherapeutic interventions in anorexia are based on theoretical models proposed by major investigators in the field based on their clinical experience (Garfinkel & Garner, 1982; Minuchin, Rosman, & Baker, 1987). These areas of focus include those of the development of autonomy, competence, self-control, and the need for parental unity and consistency in dealing with illness-related conflicts.

Pharmacotherapy. A wide variety of psychoactive medications are reported to be beneficial in open trials. Uncontrolled studies have shown efficacy of chlorpromazine (Crisp, Fenton, & Scotton, 1968), L-dopa (Johanson & Knorr, 1977), phenoxybenzamine (Redmond, Swann, & Heninger, 1976), diphenylhydantoin (Green & Rau, 1974), amitriptyline (Biederman et al., 1985), stimulants (Wulliemier, Rossel, & Sinclair, 1975), and naloxone (Moore, Mills, & Forster, 1981). None of these observations has been confirmed under double-blind, controlled conditions.

Recent literature describes a high incidence of mood disorders in anorexics (Cantwell et al., 1977) and their families (Hudson et al., 1987). Several antidepressants have been investigated, including amitriptyline (Beiderman et al., 1985; Moore, 1977; Needlemen & Waber, 1977), clomipramine (Lacey & Crisp, 1980), and lithium (Gross et al., 1981). None of these medications appears to significantly improve mood when compared with placebos. Some partial effects were noted for weight gain, improved attitude, and weight maintenance following discharge, but benefits were relatively minor. Thus, the efficacy of antidepressants in anorexia remains unknown and worthy of further study.

In contrast to claims from open trials, results from double-blind trials do not find a "magic bullet" drug that provides a significant remission of the anorexic symptom complex. Double-blind studies report limited success in treatment of specific problems, such as improving the rate of weight gain during refeeding, disturbed attitudes toward food and body image, depression, or gastrointestinal discomfort.

Two neuroleptics, pimozide (Vandereycken & Pierlott, 1982) and sulpiride (Vandereycken & Van den Broucke, 1984), have been investigated in anorexia because neuroleptics have been considered the drugs of choice (Dally & Sargent, 1960) when brain dopamine pathways may be disturbed

(Barry & Klawans, 1976). Both drugs had limited success in accelerating weight gain or altering anorectic attitudes in some patients for part of the study, but overall drug effect was marginal. These studies do not support the use of pimozide or sulpiride in the routine treatment of anorexia nervosa. Whether other neuroleptics are useful remains unknown.

Cyproheptadine, a drug that is thought to act on the serotoninergic and histaminergic systems, may have beneficial effects on weight gain, mood, and attitude in some patients. Data in comparison to trials of amitriptyline or placebo found cyproheptadine to significantly improve weight gain in restrictor anorectics when compared with bulimic anorectics (Halmi et al., 1986). This is intriguing since bulimic anorectics have reduced central serotonin relative to restrictors (Kaye et al., 1984). These data suggest that cyproheptadine may be modestly helpful in the restrictor subgroup of anorectics and tricyclic antidepressants should be considered in bulimic anorectics when medication is needed.

Gwirtsman, Guze, Yager, and Gainsley (1990) reported that 6 chronic, refractory anorexic patients gained weight during an open trial of fluoxetine. In addition, fluoxetine administration was associated with a reduction in depression and a decrease of obsessive thoughts about food and ritualistic preoccupations. In one case report (Ferguson, 1987), a patient with chronic anorexia and bulimia had improvements in mood and a reduction in pathological eating after three weeks of fluoxetine treatment. In another case report (Wilcox, 1987), a patient with chronic anorexia used up to 120 mg a day of fluoxetine because this dose both improved mood and also helped suppress her appetite so that she was able to lose weight. Crisp and others (1987) found that clomipramine was associated with increased appetite, hunger, and caloric consumption when administered to anorexics during the early stages of refeeding and weight restoration. Serotonin reuptake blockers have been reported to be useful in the treatment of body-dysmorphic disorder (Hollander, Liebowitz, & Winchel, 1989), which has symptoms that overlap in some areas with anorexia nervosa and OCD.

Fluoxetine is a highly specific serotonin reuptake inhibitor (Wong, Hornig, Bymaster et al., 1974). Recent data suggest that anorexics studied after long-term weight restoration and recovery have a disturbance of central nervous system serotoninergic activity (Kaye et al., 1984). Such a defect is possibly trait related and could contribute to a number of symptoms in anorexia nervosa, including obsessionality, anxiety, depression, and pathological feeding behavior.

An open trial of fluoxetine in 31 patients with anorexia nervosa after weight restoration (Kaye et al., 1991), 29 of 31 patients (94 patients) maintained a body weight above the anorexic range in an outpatient setting. This is particularly impressive when considering that these subjects had been at a low of 69 ± 8 percent ABW in their life, had started fluoxetine at 89 ± 6 percent ABW, and were 97 ± 13 percent ABW while on fluoxetine.

The explanation for the apparent efficacy of fluoxetine in this study is not certain. Fluoxetine, particularly in good-response anorexics, had a global effect. That is, administration of fluoxetine was associated with reduced OCD-like symptoms, anorexic core symptoms, anxiety, and depression. Thus, its actions may be related to amelioration of one or more of these symptoms (Benfield, Heel, & Lewis, 1986). Fluoxetine seems to be particularly effective in improving the ability of many of the pure restrictor anorexics to maintain a healthy weight. In contrast, most of the bulimic/purger anorexics had some resumption of pathological eating despite fluoxetine administration.

Many questions remain unanswered. First, it is not certain what dosage of fluoxetine is most therapeutic. All subjects were started on 20 mg a day for three weeks, with an increase in dose dependent on response. Second, it is not known how long anorexics need to be maintained on fluoxetine. Several patients have continued to do well after fluoxetine was stopped. Third, it is not clear whether or not it matters if anorexics are started on fluoxetine when underweight or after weight recovery. Finally, it should be noted that some anorexics had increased dysphoria during the first week of fluoxetine administration, a phenomenon noted in the clomipramine treatment of

OCD (Zohar, Inel, & Zohar-Kadouch, 1988). These symptoms were transient and usually disappeared by the tenth day of treatment.

In summary, although these preliminary results are encouraging, it should be emphasized that only a few patients had a dramatic response with a large reduction in symptoms. It should be cautioned that the apparent response to an open trial of fluoxetine is not a recommendation for its use in this disorder, but its use may be warranted in those patients who are chronically ill and who have suffered multiple relapses despite previous treatment. Rather, this study supports the need for a double-blind placebo-controlled trial to determine whether or not fluoxetine is beneficial as a treatment for anorexia nervosa.

Bulimia Nervosa

The treatment of bulimia, a disorder at least 10 times more prevalent than anorexia nervosa (Stangler & Printz, 1980; Halmi et al., 1981; Pope et al., 1984), is different from anorexia nervosa in several ways (see Herzog & Copeland, 1985).

Nutritional. Most importantly, bulimia nervosa patients do not become emaciated and they maintain a body weight above 85 percent ABW (Garner et al., 1985; Fairburn & Cooper, 1982). Nutritional therapy focuses on replacing abnormal or bulimic behaviors with normal eating behavior, which should include regularly scheduled meals without restricting any particular food groups. Dieting should be discouraged during the initial phases of recovery as food restriction may intensify appetite and increase the likelihood of binge eating. Caloric requirements for weight maintenance (approximately 25 kcal/kg/day) in bulimia are lower than that for anorexia and noneating disorder females (Weltzin, Fernstrom, Hansen, & McConaha, 1991).

Psychotherapy. At this point, the state of the art in treatment of eating disorders involves cognitive-behavioral psychotherapy (Garner, Gairburn, & Davis, 1987). Techniques of self-monitoring, identifying, and restructuring dysfunctional thinking patterns concerning weight, food, self-image, relationships, problem solving, stress reduction and management, time management, and assertiveness training are all areas that need to be addressed in typical bulimic patients. Additionally, bulimic patients have trouble modulating their reactions, behaviors, and the like. Helping them to strike an appropriate balance in multiple areas of their lives may be a general therapeutic theme. With this approach, improvement and reduction in binge eating averages approximately 70 percent (Oesterhed, McKenna, & Gould, 1987).

Family involvement. Family treatment in relation to bulimia is less well explored than in anorexia. This is most likely due to the older age of onset and the fact that many patients no longer reside with their family of origin (Hall, 1987; Vandereycken, 1987). We feel family involvement is important because many family members have become frustrated, angry, and hopeless due to the chronic course of their loved one's illness. The oversecretiveness of the bulimia disrupts the sense of trust within the family and the patient is therefore often met with emotional disapproval (Hall, 1987). Parents typically feel guilty but powerless. The stress of the illness often creates negative change in the family, resulting in emotional distance, withdrawal, and denial. The high rate of sexual abuse and incest found by some authors may certainly contribute to this phenomenology (Oppenheimer, Howells, & Palmer, 1984).

Schwartz, Barrett, and Saba (1984) added to Minuchin's (1978) psychometric description of the anorexic family to better capture the dynamic picture of the bulimic family. In addition to overprotectiveness, conflict avoidance, rigidity, and enmeshment, additional factors are isolation, conscientiousness of appearance, and a special importance placed on food and its meaning (Minuchin, Rosman, & Baker, 1978; Schwartz et al., 1984). It should be emphasized, however, that although many families have some or even all of these characteristics, many have only a few or none. Thus, each family needs to be assessed individually and an eclectic approach seems most helpful with regard to treatment.

The stages of treatment for the bulimic family are: (1) motivating the family for differentiation, (2) guiding the differentiation, (3) targeting the symptoms, and (4) teaching the patient and family about relapse prevention and preparing them realistically for the continued recovery process (Vanderlinden & Vandereycken, 1988). consolidating change is the ultimate goal and a multidimensional approach best serves this program.

The primary therapeutic tasks of working with families is to (1) establish a good working alliance; (2) avoid collusion with denial of reality with regard to the severity of the illness; (3) avoid an authoritarian power stance and involve family and patient in the decision-making process; (4) resist overidentification with parts of the system (i.e., beware of counter transference issues); (5) restore normal eating patterns; (6) restore more positive family interactions; (7) successfully emancipate the patient; and (8) establish a support network for both family and patient as needed (Vanderlinden & Vandereycken, 1988).

Treatment planning should be geared to the goals of reestablishing normal weight and eating patterns as well as the maintenance of these goals. It is important that goals be concrete and achievable, as this will help to minimize patient's and family's sense of importance.

The need to empower the family and patient through education about the illness and the treatment must be underscored. Knowledge is power, and it enables family and patient to feel part of the team. It is always easier to work with the system than against it, and involvement tends to diminish resistance. It is also important for the therapist to evaluate the treatment on an ongoing basis. Making use of fellow professionals for supervision and guidance is an essential component toward improving the clinical care of these families.

Pharmacotherapy. Most double-blind, placebo-controlled trials of tricyclic antidepressants, including imipramine (Agras et al., 1987; Pope et al., 1983), desipramine (Hughes et al., 1986), and amitryptaline (Mitchell & Groat, 1984), when used at adequate dosages, demonstrate that an active drug is significantly better than a placebo in reducing bingeing and vomiting behavior. Additionally, all studies that reported a significant drug-related reduction in frequency of bingeing also reported

an improvement in affective symptoms. Some groups found a correlation between change in binge frequency and mood improvement, whereas other investigators did not. Several studies (Hughes et al., 1986; Walsh et al., 1988) have shown that nondepressed bulimics have similar antibulimic responses to antidepressants. It is worth mentioning that open trials of tricyclic antidepressants have been reported (Brotman, Herzog, & Woods, 1984; Pope et al., 1984) and, in general, the findings are similar to controlled trials.

Studies examining the efficacy of monoamine oxidase inhibitors (MAOIs) in bulimia (Kennedy et al., 1986; Walsh et al., 1988) report improvement in bulimic symptoms similar to that with tricyclic antidepressants (TCAs). In an open trial, Roy-Byrne, Gwirtsman, Edelstein, Yager, and Gerner (1983) reported that only one of eight patients responded favorably to tranylcypromine a dosages of 30 mg or more. All authors recommend careful clinical evaluation of each patient with whom MAOI therapy is initiated, as many bulimic subjects exhibit impulsive behavior patterns and might have great difficulty with adherence to the low tyramine diet necessary for these treatments.

Fluoxitane, a new antidepressant with potent serotonin reuptake blockade characteristics, decreased bulimic symptoms in a severe anorectic patient (Ferguson, 1987) and, in double-blind, placebo-controlled studies, decreased bulimic behavior (Enas, Pope, & Levine, 1989; Freeman et al., 1988).

Trazadone, in a double-blind, placebo-controlled trial (Pope, Keck, McElroy, & Hudson, 1988) was found to significantly improve bulimic symptoms when compared with controls, and was well tolerated by the subjects. Other studies have shown moderate benefit (Pope et al., 1984) or, in one trial of three patients, a worsening of symptoms using trazadone (Wold, 1983). Reports of lithium being effective in anorexic subjects with bulimic symptoms (Gross et al., 1981) have suggested that it may also be beneficial in bulimia. In a trial in 14 normal-weight bulimic subjects, lithium was found to reduce bulimic behavior by 75 to 100 percent in 12 of the subjects (Hsu, 1984). The efficacy of mianserin, another antidepressant, remains undetermined (Sabine, Yonace, Farrington, Barratt, & Wakeling, 1983).

Selecting Optimal Treatment Strategies

Anorexia Nervosa

The treatment of anorexia can generally be divided into two stages. The first is refeeding and weight restoration. The second is maintenance of weight after weight gain in an outpatient setting. It is debatable whether medications are of much use during weight restoration. Our experience is that most anorexia nervosa patients will gain weight with a well-designed nutritional program. There is no "magic bullet" for the treatment of the core symptoms of anorexia nervosa. That is, there is no pharmacological agent that seems to affect the obsessional pursuit of thinness and fear of being fat. Pharmacological treatment may be directed at accessory symptoms, such as anxiety or depression, using appropriate medications.

Few studies have concentrated on helping anorexics maintain weight after weight restoration. This is an important phase of treatment, because only about 50 to 70 percent of anorexics are able to maintain a relatively normal weight after restoration of weight. It is common to see these severely ill patients gain weight in an inpatient tretment unit but rapidly lose weight after discharge. Few studies have assessed whether medications improve mood and attitude or stabilize weight in the long term. These severely ill patients are problematic candidates for drug studies because of medical complications and limited cooperation. They are, however, the group that probably has the majority of the morbidity and mortality associated with anorexia nervosa and more aggressive and innovative pharmacologic approaches are warranted in these chronically ill patients.

Much remains to be learned. In contrast to some other major psychiatric illnesses, current pharmacologic treatment options have limited benefit in patients with anorexia nervosa. However, we suspect that this will soon change for several reasons. First, we are beginning to recognize distinctions between subgroups of anorexics (e.g., bulimics versus restrictor, or good versus bad prognosis patients) and it appears that some groups respond differently to different medications, allowing for more selective treatments that will hopefully lead to better results. Second, much progress has been made in understanding which neuroendocrine and neurotransmitter systems are disturbed in anorexia nervosa. Recent data suggest that there may be trait-related alterations in serotonin (Kaye et al., 1984) and norepinephrine (Kaye et al., 1985) pathways in anorexia nervosa, two systems implicated in the regulation of appetite, weight, and mood. These research findings lead to cautious optimism that we are on the edge of a new era in understanding and treating this disease.

Bulimia Nervosa

Recent data suggest that the initial treatment of choice for bulimia nervosa involves a structured program that utilizes cognitive-behavioral, educational, and nutritional interventions in either a group or individual setting (Mitchell, Pyle, & Eckert, 1990; Fairburn, Kir, O'Connor, & Cooper, 1986). For patients resistant to this approach, the use of antidepressant medications can help to decrease the frequency of binge eating and purging. When outpatient treatment is unable to decrease severe bulimic behavior that is associated with severe medical instability or disabling depression, anxiety, or impulsive behavior, then a period of inpatient treatment should be implemented.

Problems in Carrying Out Interventions

Poor outcome in anorexia nervosa is associated with longer duration of illness, lower minimum weight, premorbid personality and social difficulties, disturbed relationship with family, and previous treatment (Hsu, 1990).

Clinically, the major obstacle to the treatment of anorexia is the intense denial of malnutrition and weight loss as a problem. Even patients who are able to see that they are underweight cannot tolerate the fears of weight gain and becoming "obese." Frequently, anorexics "bargain" with their family that they will not lose weight if they are not made to gain weight. This may lead to the family supporting the patient's noncompliance with a weight gain program. This should be dealt with in terms of improved education as to the unreality of the patient's ability to follow through with such a promise. Families in this situation should be encouraged to have the patient routinely monitored in terms of weight and electrolyte status to avoid catastrophic medical complications if, in fact, they are unable to maintain their weight. This monitoring should be done by the professionals involved so as to avoid setting up a chronic power struggle within the family. When therapists do not wish to weigh the patient themselves, they should then collaborate closely with a medical professional who will keep close track of the patient, as these data play a critical role in case management. Families frequently go through a phase of "wanting to believe" the anorexics' intentions, and it is only after they have gone through repeated disappointments that they are able to set limits in terms of necessary weight gain.

In anorexics who remain significantly underweight, our experience suggests that patients who are less than 80 to 85 percent of ABW do not respond as well to "talk therapies" or medication. In the case of psychotherapy, the cognitive rigidity and inability to spend significant time focusing on thoughts that are not related to food and weight interfere with work in psychotherapy. We have found that during weight gain, more frequent sessions that are of short duration and primarily supportive can set the foundation for therapeutic alliance or bonding. The focus may be a casual exploration of possible interests and/or goals not directly related to food, weight, and appearance, which can point toward future psychotherapeutic work. If the patient is unable to present any such themes, simply taking a respectful interest in the patient over and above the eating disorder can set the stage for future work on relationships and self-esteem, since isolation and loneliness are frequently present. In terms of medication response, it is also possible that some of the neurobiological sequelae of malnutrition decrease the effect of medication in these patients.

In bulimia, indicators of poor prognosis include duration of illness, positive family history of alcoholism and depression (Hsu & Holder, 1986), and higher frequency of binge eating and vomiting (Mitchell, Soll, Eckert, Pyle, & Hatsukami, 1989). A prior history of anorexia nervosa is *not* associated with poor prognosis (Lacey, 1983).

Psychotherapeutically, difficulties may arise in individual sessions with bulimics if there is a history of troubled relationships, impulsivity, and/or intense feelings of guilt and shame. Due to this, mutually respective relationships should be the goal, with realistic expectations being clearly defined. Patients need to be educated about the differences between guilt and shame and why keeping these feelings hidden are harmful. They need to be gently encouraged to reveal painful feelings and incidents. Self-destructive and/or deceptive behaviors that lead to authentic guilt need to be confronted respectfully but honestly, with a vision toward understanding and changing such behaviors.

Relapse Prevention

The concept of relapse prevention in eating disorders involves three main components. First, it must be assumed that there will be continued eating disorder symptoms, either continuously or intermittently during recovery. Patients should assume that they will have continued fears of eating and gaining weight and that they will have periods of time when they hve urges to restrict, binge eat, use laxatives or diet pills, or exercise. Second, given the inevitability of continued eating disorder symptoms, specific planning should be done to determine, in advance, what the patients will do if slips or eating disorder symptoms occur. This should include finding out the location of support groups, identifying peers and family members that can lend support, seeing continued psychotherapy as important, and having clear meal planning. Third, these plans need to be individualized and implemented. Recovery from anorexia and bulimia must be an active process in which patients continuously work at maintaining recovery.

It must be emphasized to patients that taking action is critical to recovery. Frequently, fears, low self-esteem, and long-standing isolation make it very difficult for patients to risk new behaviors. For this reason, relapse prevention strategies are more helpful if they are discussed openly with the individual and tailored to their unique situations and capabilities.

CASE ILLUSTRATION: ANOREXIA NERVOSA

Case Description

Sarah was a 15-year-old female, the oldest of a family of three children, who all lived at home with their mother and father. Sarah was in good health, did very well in school, and was reported by the family to be a "perfectionistic" child who worked hard in school and did not get into trouble.

At the age of 13, Sarah reported to be increasingly worried about her weight, which had increased about 10 pounds over the last six months. This was also a time when she was going through puberty and had begun menstruating. She reported that she began dieting because she did not want to become overweight and because "kids were teasing me at school about my weight." Her dieting consisted of eating low-calorie foods and she also started to run two to three miles a day and bought an aerobics tape that she used at home alone once a day.

Because of these techniques, she lost about five pounds over a one-month period. With this weight loss, she reported feeling a sense of control and accomplishment. It became easier for her to skip meals, usually breakfast and lunch. Sarah also began spending an increasing amount of time either studying or exercising. At this point, she became increasingly self-critical. She would ruminate that she could not make friends because she was not interesting and had nothing to offer. She believed that she was not smart, and she would become extremely upset if she did not make the highest score in class on a test.

She became more irritable with her family and isolated from her friends. She would not eat with her family, and would spend most of her time in her room where she would argue with her younger sisters and parents. This escalated to the point where her family began to become relieved when she was in her room because she was so disruptive with other family members. They believed that she must be going through an adolescent phase, and hoped things would be back to normal soon.

Sarah's parents began to be concerned about her weight as she began to look "a little too thin" and they could hear her exercising in the middle of the night in her room.

One day Sarah's mother received a call from the school counselor who reported that they believed that Sarah had an "eating disorder." Her parents then had her seen by a therapist (recommended by the family physician) who diagnosed her as "anorexic."

The therapist began to meet with Sarah on a weekly basis, weighing her prior to each session. Sarah was noted to be quite depressed and angry with her parents. She minimized their concerns about weight, stating that "my parents think I have a problem with my weight, but I don't." At home, her parents began watching her eating, insisting that she eat with the family. After meals she would go to the bathroom and they could hear her vomiting. At the same time, her weight began to decrease, she continued to exercise two to four hours a week, and she did not contact her friends.

Her therapist met with the parents and reported that Sarah's weight had continued to decrease. The patient was evaluated by the family physician and was found to have a normal exam except for mildly decreased thyroid function tests, amenorrhea, and parotid swelling. She weighed 85 pounds and had mildly decreased pulse and blood pressure.

Differential Diagnosis and Assessment

Sarah was subsequently admitted to the hospital and found to weigh 80 pounds. She was five feet tall and therefore weighed 75 percent ABW. She had normal electrolyte blood counts, but had mildly decreased thyroid hormone levels and was bradycardic. On physical exam she was noted to have dry skin, prominent definition of her skeletal structure, and increased fine hair on her face and arms.

In addition to physical and neurological exams, she had a psychiatric evaluation, nutritional assessment, and family history assessment. She was started on 1,200 kcal a day of meals (35 kcal/kg) and was observed during and one hour after all meals and in the bathroom at all times.

Initial psychiatric evaluation characterized Sarah as a young thin female who made poor eye contact. She was alert and oriented. Formal memory and intellectual testing were normal. She was extremely fidgety and restless during the interview. She reported feeling fat and having a desire to lose weight. She reported a fear of weight gain and panic whenever she would eat because of fearing of "blowing up like a balloon." She reported that she spent 99 percent of her day worrying about weight and food. She at times felt that applying hand lotion or body lotion would cause her to gain weight. She reported exercising two to four hours a day and would do a very structured exercise routine that included 100 each of sit-ups, jumping jacks, deep knee bends, and pushups. Sarah would time herself, always trying to decrease the amount of time it would take her to complete her exercise routine. She was extremely fearful of eating meats, stating she had become a vegetarian over the last year and that she was "allergic to sugar." She repeatedly asked if she would have to gain weight in the hospital, and commented that all of the other patients were much thinner than her.

Sarah reported a persistent sadness that was centered around feeling like she was a failure if she gained weight. She also believed that the only way she would feel better would be if she could diet more and not gain weight. She reported less interest in hobbies that did not relate to dieting or exercising, was not interested in seeing friends, and had difficulty sleeping characterized by going to bed and waking up at 5 A.M. and not being able to fall back asleep.

She also reported persistent worrying about minor matters usually related to weight and food, but also many important items such as what col-

lege to attend and if she will attain the success she desires.

On further questioning, Sarah also reported a preoccupation with doing things perfectly. This caused her to spend much more time on homework because she would end up recopying the same assignment three or four times to make sure it looked perfect. She also reported spending two to three hours a day cleaning at home, and would compulsively organize her room so that her books and clothing would be arranged according to size or color. She reported that if things were not clean and organized, she would not stop thinking about it until she put them in order or cleaned them. She also reported that she did not like other members of the household to clean because it was not up to her standards.

Treatment Selection, Treatment Course, and Problems in Carrying Out Interventions

The initial treatment focus was on nutritional rehabilitation and weight gain. Sarah was required to eat 100 percent of a 1,200 kcal diet and when she was able to accomplish this her calories were gradually increased 250 to 300 kcal every three to four days. Over the first 3 weeks of hospitalization, she gained very little weight. However, when her calories were increased to 50 to 60 kcal/kg/day she began to gain 1 to 2 kg a week. After 10 weeks of hospitalization, she attained her target weight of 102 pounds, or 95 percent of ABW. Her calories were increased to 4,000 kcal a day in the week prior to attaining her target weight to be able to maintain weight gain. After attaining her target weight, her calories were decreased over the course of 1 week to a 2,400 kcal a day for weight maintenance. Sarah then began to self-select in the hospital cafeteria, had meals out of the hospital with staff, and received passes to go home with her parents prior to discharge. She would report persistent urges to restrict her intake and lose weight while on pass but was able to maintain her weight between 100 and 104 pounds.

The primary treatment during the hospital was cognitive-behavior therapy. Its main focus was behaviorally reinforcing healthy eating patterns, as opposed to eating disordered behavior and identifying pathological thinking patterns that would initiate or perpetuate anorexic behaviors. Thought restructuring techniques were used to help Sarah connect positive results with maintaining a healthy body weight and not engage in anorexic behavior under stress. This was done by using a variety of group exercising and a structured treatment manual that Sarah would work on throughout the course of her hospitalization. Taped meal sessions with family and therapist were helpful in exploring dynamics around eating. The simple experience of eating together in a structured setting was anxiety reducing for both patient and family. These tapes were reviewed later to discuss family observations, feelings, and thoughts regarding the exercise. Specific eating tasks were scheduled with staff, such as eating a feared food during the later phases of treatment. Therapeutic meal passes were also scheduled with the family prior to discharge. All of these activities provided experience and information necessary for more complete discharge planning.

In addition, individual therapy was used to identify specific stressful life events and situations that contributed to Sarah's low self-esteem. A move by the family from another city became a focus of treatment. Themes around the loss of friends where she previously lived, guilt feelings about how she avoided saying goodbye to them, and anger at her parents about having to move were addressed. This resulted in Sarah renewing some relationships, which she found to be rewarding and helpful in transitioning to her new home.

During the course of a family evaluation, two major items appeared that needed to be addressed to facilitate Sarah's recovery. First, her mother, who was moderately obese, reported herself to be very fearful that Sarah would become "fat like me." As a result, she reported encouraging Sarah to diet and exercise when her eating disorder began. She would also frequently ask how much Sarah weighed and reward her if her clothes size decreased. She also reported being chronically depressed and felt that she was unattractive to her husband and that her life was going nowhere. Sarah's father, on the other hand, was somewhat

successful in his job in middle management. However, the family reported significant compulsive behavior at home in terms of cleaning and organization. The father reported that he had some problems with completing projects on time at work and he felt that this had recently kept him from a promotion to a more senior level.

With this information, the focus of family therapy was to identify the parents' individual problems and facilitate their working on these. The mother had reported that she had previously attended Overeaters Anonymous and had found this to be quite helpful before they moved. She began attending groups at their new home and reported that this was helping her to control her weight, and she also reported an increase in self-esteem. The father was referred to a psychiatrist and was diagnosed at having obsessive-compulsive disorder and subsequently responded well to an antiobsessional medication.

Outcome and Termination

After discharge, Sarah was referred back to the therapist who treated her prior to admission. We notified the therapist as to interventions that we felt worked in the hospital and made treatment recommendation for outpatient therapy. These included a contract concerning weight maintenance that the patient and family signed stating that if Sarah's weight dropped below 95 pounds, she would be rehospitalized. We recommended that Sarah be followed by a psychiatrist for monitoring of fluoxetine treatment and psychotherapy focusing on themes that were dealt with in cognitive, individual, and family therapy. We also remained available for consultation concerning treatment issues that would arise in outpatient therapy.

Followup and Maintenance

Followup at one year after discharge found that Sarah was maintaining her weight slightly above her target range and was weighing between 105 and 110 pounds. She was able to maintain a regular meal schedule and exercise only one hour a day. She did not return to participating in track but was still involved in the school newspaper and had a boyfriend. Her grades continued to be excellent and she was in the process of planning for college. Themes in individual therapy continued to center around rejection sensitivity with a tendency to have an increase in eating disorder symptoms. However, she learned how to identify this pattern and was doing good work in individual therapy examining possible contributing factors to this problem.

Sarah's mother reported that she was happier, involved in volunteer work, and spending much more time out of the house; Sarah's father was less obsessional and his work was going well. The parents were also able to improve their parenting skills and discuss concerns and proposed interventions with one another before attempting to implement this. This provided more consistency and less opportunity for conflicts over management to develop. The diminished stress and conflict over the illness allowed the parents to focus on their individual problems, which improved their marital communications as well.

Case Summary

This is a typical case history of a restrictor anorexic. The hallmarks of this case include prominent obsessional and perfectionistic traits that increase as weight decreases. Also, when stress increases, patients typically spend more time involved in anorexic behavior and studying. It is also not uncommon to have compulsive behaviors such as cleaning and organizing in these patients and for them to maintain good school or work performance in the setting of poor nutritional low weight.

Denial and resistance to treatment occur in the majority of these patients. Whether patients can see they have anorexia and need to gain weight or do not feel they have a problem, all are extremely fearful of weight gain and typically cannot eat unless in a highly structured setting. If a short-term outpatient treatment does not noticeably improve eating and if the weight of patients is less than 80 percent of ABW, we recommend that inpatient weight gain be initiated. A weight increase of at least to 80 percent ABW should be obtained

before outpatient treatment is attempted. In highly resistent patients, weight gain to 95 percent of ABW followed by a period of weight maintenance should be carried out in a hospital or partial hospitalization setting.

Family intervention initially focused on educating the parents about anorexia nervosa and the process of recovery. Setting firm limits around eating and weight gain were encouraged and frequent phone contact by the psychiatrist and family therapist served to support the parents in this process. The need for continued treatment following discharge was emphasized. Parents and patient were also realistically prepared for recovery (typically having progression, setbacks, and plateaus). Many families and patients hope to be "cured," which can set up a situation in which they will feel devastated, frustrated, angry, and hopeless if realistic expectations regarding recovery process are a part of the hospitalization experience. As Sarah began to improve, the parents began to identify marital issues that were contributing to increase stress at home and agreed to a trial of couples therapy to address these.

Although fluoxetine is not FDA approved in the treatment of anorexia nervosa, Sarah was treated with 40 mg a day, initiated when she reached her target weight. She reported that with the medication she was less anxious about her weight and had less of an urge to clean and organize. Her parents and treatment team found her to be less rigid and more flexible on the medication.

CASE ILLUSTRATION: NORMAL-WEIGHT BULIMIA

Case Description

Lori was a 23-year-old single, white woman employed as a salesclerk for a retail store. Her weight at evaluation was 117 pounds with a high weight in the past of 160 pounds and a low weight of 110 pounds. Her height was 5'4". She recounted always having had a "problem" with weight. At age 13, she went on a restrictive diet for three weeks and lost 10 pounds, but subsequently she gained all of the weight back.

Lori read about purging techniques (e.g., vomiting and laxatives) in popular magazines, but her first personal experience with vomiting occurred at age 18. Following a large Mexican meal, she developed an upset stomach and subsequently vomited. Vomiting alleviated her feeling of fullness, decreased her dread of putting on weight, and introduced her to a practice that would allow her to eat as much as she wanted without gaining weight.

At first, the practice of purging was uncomfortable, but within several months it became a way of life. Food became her "friend"—a way to quell anger and reduce depression and anxiety. Prior to binge eating she often felt lonely, empty, and depressed, and had thoughts of failure. During the binge she escaped from her world of immediate cares to a dulled, inner-directed state. As the binge progressed she experienced feelings of fullness, fatness, and loss of control. Tension built and then fell precipitously following the purge. What originally had been a "friend" over time became an uncontrollable habit. Consuming a loaf of bread, a half gallon of ice cream, a plate of spaghetti, and a bowl of cereal several times a day was expensive, time consuming, and isolating, and often took priority over socializing with friends or going to work. In addition, she had difficulty controlling her alcohol intake and she reported frequent periods of drunkenness.

Lori had a very troubled childhood. On the surface her parents were successful and respected in the community. However, her mother was an alcoholic who had frequent episodes of depression and was often unavailable emotionally for the patient. Her father's behavior was unpredictable, ranging from extreme passivity to displays of frightening rage. Lori was frequently in the middle of family disputes and felt responsible for maintaining peace between her parents. Her parents had high expectations of Lori and never seemed satisfied with her accomplishments.

Differential Diagnosis and Assessment

On mental status exam, Lori was attractive, extroverted, and friendly. She described chronic feelings of depression accompanied by intermittent periods of disrupted sleep, crying spells, and suicidal thoughts. Her affect was bright and appeared incongruent with her stated depressed mood. She spoke of guilt and shame concerning the binge eating and vomiting. She had difficulty verbalizing emotion and would often state that everything was "fine." Physical examination and pertinent laboratory data revealed no physical cause for her vomiting.

Lori reported that at the age of 21 she first decided that she wanted to stop bingeing and vomiting. Typically, she would be able to abstain, with great effort, for a couple of days, but when even a minor stressor would arise, she would resume her binge-purge behavior at the same rate or worse then before. She began lying to friends and family about her eating and would steal food and borrow money from friends and family to binge eat.

At age 23, Lori was referred to a private therapist after a suicide attempt precipitated by a period of heavy bingeing. She was seen weekly and initially was able to decrease her frequency of bingeing and purging. However, when unable to stop bingeing, she began feeling guilty and lied to the therapist, telling her she had stopped so as not to disappoint her. As a result of increasing guilt and frustration, she eventually was unable to continue with this therapist and left treatment precipitously. She tried other treatments, which included an overeaters support group and a behavioral day treatment program, both of which she felt helped her to stop her bingeing initially. In all situations it was only with a great deal of effort that she could keep going for up to a couple of weeks at a time, but she always resumed bingeing and would subsequently feel guilty and stop treatment. Her self-esteem plummeted and depression intensified with feelings of sadness, guilt, hopelessness, and helplessness.

Treatment Selection, Treatment Course, and Problems in Carrying Out Interventions

On initial evaluation at our program, which included routine psychiatric and physical examinations, Lori was bingeing one to three times a day and had a Hamilton score of 23. She was entered into a structured cognitive-behavioral program that focused on methods to control binge eating and learning better methods of solving problems. She was started on desipramine 10 mg a day, which was increased to 150 mg a day over the next two weeks. She reported feeling generally hopeful and was bingeing less but only with a lot of effort. A tricyclic antidepressant level was obtained, which was 98 ng/ml; her does was increased up to 250 mg a day, which gave her a level of 198 ng/ml. Over the next two weeks she decreased her binge frequency to one to two binges a week and felt more hopeful that she could have more control over eating. She also felt less depressed, as her Hamilton-Depression Rating Scale (HAM-D) score decreased to less than ten. At this point she was able to recognize certain stressors that precipitated the urge to binge and was referred to a psychotherapist.

Outcome and Termination, Followup and Maintenance

At one-year followup, Lori was bingeing one to two times a month and felt less depressed and more in control of her life. A trial off of desipramine led to an increase in bingeing, which she could not tolerate. The desipramine was reinstituted with good results. Her weight at one-year followup was 122 pounds. She felt this was too high, but tolerated her mild discomfort, as she was afraid she would binge more frequently if she tried to lose weight.

Case Summary

This is a typical case of bulimia nervosa. The age of onset is typically later than in anorexia because bulimics are aware that their eating is abnormal and they are more likely to conceal their behavior from their family. Depressive symptoms, emotional lability, and low self-esteem are frequent in this disorder and can lead to problems in interpersonal functioning, school performance, and self-destructive behavior, including suicide. Lying and shoplifting are common in bulimia, which can decrease the effectiveness of therapy and be quite frustrating for peer and family members.

Histories of sexual abuse and disruptive home lives, which serve to increase feelings of low self-esteem, are present in this case and common in bulimia. These are frequent themes in individual and family therapies and need to be addressed if present. The failure to identify and address these issues may result in decreased effectiveness of treatment.

For the majority of bulimics, recovery is a long experience. Short-term goals should include maintaining medical and psychological stability so that patients are able to work effectively in outpatient therapy. Goals in outpatient therapy should be to decrease binge-purge behavior to the point of abstinence. However, many patients continue to have episodic urges to binge eat and/or restrict, especially under periods of stress. Antidepressants typically decrease these urges and improve mood and emotional stability. However, only rarely do they lead to abstinence. For this reason, antidepressants should be used adjunctively in the setting of ongoing psychotherapy.

SUMMARY

In summary, anorexia nervosa and bulimia nervosa represent two eating disorders that can occur either separately or together. The hallmarks of these disorders are weight loss associated with an intense fear of weight gain, and episodic binge eating associated with self-induced vomiting or other purging behaviors and a fear of weight gain, respectively. Medical complications, cognitive distortions, depressive and anxiety symptoms, and substance abuse are common and need to be comprehensively assessed in eating disorder patients. Treatment interventions should be multifaceted and involve nutritional rehabilitation, cognitive restructuring, behavioral reinforcement of non-eating disorder behavior, and individual, family, and pharmacological therapy. With a comprehensive approach, a majority of patients should improve. However, even at this point roughly a third of anorexics and bulimics remain significantly impaired by these illnesses.

REFERENCES

Abraham, S. F., & Beumont, P. J. V. (1982). How patients describe bulimia or binge eating. *Psychological Medicine, 12,* 625–635.

Agras, W. D., Dorian, B., Kirkley, B. G., Arnow, B., & Bachman, J. (1987). Imipramine in the treatment of bulimia: A double-blind controlled study. *International Journal of Eating Disorders, 6,* 29–38.

American Psychiatric Association. (1987). *Diagnostic and statistical manual of mental disorders* (3rd ed., rev.). Washington, DC: Author.

Asbert, M., Traskman, L., & Thoren, P. (1976). 5-HIAA in the cerebrospinal fluid: A biochemical suicide predictor? *Archives of General Psychiatry, 33,* 1193–1197.

Barry, V. C., & Klawans, H. L. (1976). On the role of dopamine in the pathophysiology of anorexia nervosa. *Journal of Neural Transmission, 38,* 107–122.

Beary, M. D., Lacey, J. H., & Merry, J. (1986). Alcoholism and eating disorders in women of fertile age. *British Journal of Addiction, 81,* 685–689.

Beaumont, P. J. V., George, G. C. W., & Smart, D. E. (1976). 'Dieters' and 'vomiters' in anorexia nervosa. *Psychological Medicine, 6,* 617–622.

Benfield, P., Heel, R. C., & Lewis, S. P. (1986). Fluoxetine: A review of its pharmacodynamic and pharmacolinetic properties, and therapeutic efficacy in depressive illness. *Drugs, 32,* 481–508.

Biederman, J., Herzog, D. B., Rivinus, T. M., & Ferber, M. A. (1985). Amitryptyline in the treatment of anorexia nervosa: A double-blind study, placebo-controlled study. *Journal of Clinical Psycopharmacology, 5,* 10–15.

Blouin, A. G., Blouin, J. H., Perez, E. I. et al. (1988). Treatment of bulimia with fenfluramine and desipramine. *J Clin Psychopharmacol, 8,* 261–9.

Blundell, J. E. (1984). Serotonin and appetite. *Neuropharmacology, 23,* 1537–1551.

Bossert, S., Schnabel, E., Krieg, J. C., & Berger, M. (1988). Modifications and problems of behavioral inpatient management of anorexia nervosa: A "patient suited" approach? *Acta Psychiatrica Scan, 77,* 105–110.

Brotman, A. W., Herzog, D. B., & Woods, S. W. (1984). Antidepressant treatment of bulimia: The relationship between bingeing and depressive symptomatology. *Journal of Clinical Psychiatry, 45,* 7–9.

Brown, G. L., Goodwin, F. K., Ballenger, J. C., Goyer, P. F., & Major, L. F. (1979). Aggression in humans correlates with cerebrospinal fluid amine metabolites. *Psychiatric Research, 1,* 131–139.

Bulik, C. M. (1987). Drug and alcohol abuse by bulimic women and their families. *American Journal of Psychiatry, 144,* 1604–1606.

Cantwell, D. P., Sturzenburger, S., & Burroughs, J. (1977). Anorexia nervosa. An affective disorder? *Archives of General Psychiatry, 34,* 1087–1093.

Casper, R. C. (1990). Personality features of women with good outcome from restrictive anorexics. *Psychosom Med, 52,* 156–170.

Casper, R. C., Eckert, E. D., Halmi, K. A., Goldberg, S. C., & Davis, J. M. (1980). Bulimia: Its incidence and clinical importance in patients with anorexia nervosa. *Archives of General Psychiatry, 37,* 1030–1035.

Channon, S., de Silva, P., Hemsley, D., & Perkins, R. (1989). A controlled trial of cognitive-behavioral therapy and behavioral treatment of anorexia nervosa. *Behavior Research and Therapy, 27,* 529–535.

Crisp, A. H., Fenton, G. W., & Scotton, L. (1968). A controlled study of the EEG in anorexia nervosa. *British Journal of Psychiatry, 114,* 1149–1160.

Crisp, A. H., Hsu, L. K. G., Harding, B., & Hartshorn, J. (1980). Clinical feature of anorexia nervosa. *Journal of Psychosomatic Research, 24,* 179–191.

Crisp, A. H., Lacey, J. H., & Crutchfield, M. (1987). Clomipramine and 'drive' in people with anorexia nervosa. *British Journal of Psychiatry, 150,* 355–358.

Dally, P. J., & Sargent, W. (1960). A new treatment of anorexia nervosa. *British Medical Journal, 1,* 1770–1773.

Eckert, E. D., Goldberg, S. C., Halmi, K. A., Casper, R. C., & Davis, J. M. (1982). Depression in anorexia nervosa. *Psychological Medicine, 12,* 115–122.

Enas, G., Pope, H., & Levine, L. (1989, May). *Fluoxetine in bulimia nervosa.* New Research #386, presented at the 142 Annual Meeting of the American Psychiatric Association, San Francisco, CA.

Fairburn, C. G., & Beslin, S. J. (1990). Studies of the epidemiology of bulimia nervosa. *American Journal of Psychiatry, 147,* 410–408.

Fairburn, C. G., & Cooper, J. P. (1982). Self induced vomiting and bulimia nervosa: An undetected problem. *British Medical Journal of Clinical Research, 284,* 1153–1155.

Fairburn, C. G., Kir, J., O'Connor, M., & Cooper, R. G. (1986). A comparison of two psychological treatments for bulimia nervosa. *Behaviour Research and Therapy, 24,* 629–643.

Ferguson, J. M. (1987). Treatment of an anorexia nervosa patient with fluoxetine. *American Journal of Psychiatry, 144,* 1239 (letter).

Freeman, C. P., Morris, J. E., Cheshire, K. E., Casper, R. C., & Davis, J. M. (1988, April). A double-blind controlled trial of fluoxetine vs placebo for bulimia nervosa. Abstract: Second International Conference on Eating Disorders, New York City.

Garfinkel, P. E., & Garner, D. M. (1982). *Anorexia nervosa: A multidimensional perspective.* New York: Brunner/Mazel.

Garfinkel, P. E., Moldofsky, H., & Garner, D. M. (1980). The heterogeneity of anorexia nervosa. *Archives of General Psychiatry, 37,* 1036–1040.

Garner, D. M., Fairburn, C., & Davis, R. (1987). Cognitive-behavioral treatment of bulimia nervosa: A critical appraisal. *Behavior Modification, 4,* 398–431.

Garner, D. M., Garfinkel, P. E., & O'Shaughnessy, M. (1985). The validity of the distinction between bulimia with and without anorexia nervosa. *American Journal of Psychiatry, 142,* 581–587.

Gershon, E. S., Schreiber, J. L., Hamovit, J. R., Dibble, E. D., Kaye, W. H., Nurnberger, J., Anderson, A., & Ebert, M. H. (1984). Clinical findings in patients with anorexia nervosa and affective illness in their relatives. *American Journal of Psychiatry, 141,* 1419–1422.

Green, R. S., & Rau, J. J. (1974). Treatment of compulsive eating disturbances with anticonvulsant medication. *American Journal of Psychiatry, 131,* 428–432.

Gross, H. A., Ebert, M. H., Faden, V. B., Goldberg, S. C., Nee, L. E., & Kaye, W. H. (1981). The use of diphenylhydantoin in compulsive eating disorders: Further studies. In R. A. Vigersky (Ed.). *Anorexia nervosa* (pp. 377–385). New York: Raven Press.

Gwirtsman, H. E., Guze, B. H., Yager, J., & Gainsley, B. (1990). Fluoxetine treatment of anorexia nervosa: An open clinical trial. *Journal of Clinical Psychiatry, 51,* 378–382.

Gwirtsman, H. E., Roy-Byrne, P., Yager, J., & Gerner, R. H. (1983). Neuroendocrine abnormalities in bulimia. *American Journal of Psychiatry, 140,* 550–563.

Hall, A. (1987). The patient and the family. In P. J. V. Beaumont, E. P. Burrows, & D. C. Casper (Eds.), *Handbook of eating disorders. Part 1: Anorexia and bulimia* (pp. 189–200). The Netherlands: Elsevier.

Halmi, K. A., Eckert, E. D., & LaDu, T. J. (1986). Anorexia nervosa: Treatment efficacy of cyproheptadine and amitriptyline. *Archives of General Psychiatry, 43,* 177–181.

Halmi, K. A., & Falk, J. R. (1982). Anorexia nervosa: A study of outcome discrimination in exclusive dieters and bulimics. *Journal of the American Academy of Child Psychiatry, 21,* 369–375.

Halmi, K. A., Falk, J. R., & Schwartz, E. (1981). Binge-eating and vomiting: A survey of a college population. *Psychological Medicine, 11,* 697–706.

Hatsukami, D. K., Eckert, E. D., Mitchell, J. E., & Pyle, R. L. (1984). Affective disorder and substance abuse among women with bulimia. *Psychological Medicine, 14,* 701–704.

Hendren, R. L. (1983). Depression in anorexia nervosa. *Journal of the American Academy of Child Psychiatry, 22,* 59–62.

Herzog, D. B. (1982). Bulimia in the adolescent. *American Journal of Disorders in Children, 136,* 985–989.

Herzog, D. B., & Copeland, P. M. (1985). Eating disorders. *New England Journal of Medicine, 313,* 295–303.

Hollander, E., Liebowitz, M. R., & Winchel, R. (1989). Treatment of body-dysmorphic disorder with serotonin reuptake blockers. *American Journal of Psychiatry, 146,* 768–770.

Hsu, L. K. G. (1980). Outcome of anorexia nervosa: A review of the literature (1954–1978). *Archives of General Psychiatry, 37,* 1041–1046.

Hsu, L. K. G. (1984). Treatment of bulimia with lithium. *American Journal of Psychiatry, 141,* 1260–1262.

Hsu, L. K. G. (1990). *Eating disorders.* New York: Guilford.

Hsu, L. K. G., Crisp, A. H., & Harding, B. (1970). Outcome of anorexia nervosa. *Lancet, 1,* 61–65.

Hsu, L. K. G., & Holder, D. (1986). Bulimia nervosa. Treatment and long-term outcome. *Psychological Medicine, 16,* 65–70.

Hudson, J. I., Laffer, P. S., & Pope, H. G. (1982). Bulimia related to affective disorder by family history and response to the dexamethasone suppression test. *American Journal of Psychiatry, 5,* 685–687.

Hudson, J. I., Pope, H. G., Jonas, J. M., & Yurgelun-Todd, D. (1983a). Family history study of anorexia nervosa and bulimia. *British Journal of Psychiatry, 142,* 133–138.

Hudson, J. I., Pope, H. G., Jonas, J. M., & Yurgelun-Todd, D. (1983b). Phenomenologic relationship of eating disorders to major affective disorder. *Psychiatric Research, 9,* 345–354.

Hudson, J. I., Pope, H. G., Jonas, J. M., Yurgelun-Todd, D., & Frankenburg, F. R. (1987). A controlled family history study of bulimia. *Psychological Medicine, 17,* 883–890.

Hughes, P. L., Wells, L. A., Cunningham, C. J., & Ilstrupp, D. M. (1986). Treating bulimia with desipramine: A double-blind, placebo-controlled study. *Archives of General Psychiatry, 43,* 182–186.

Johanson, A. J., & Knorr, N. J. (1977). L-Dopa as treatment for anorexia nervosa. In R. A. Vigersky (Ed.), *Anorexia nervosa* (pp. 363–372). New York: Raven Press.

Johnson, C., & Larson, R. (1982). Bulimia: An analysis of moods and behavior. *Psychosomatic Medicine, 44,* 341–351.

Johnson, C., Stuckey, M. K., Lewis, L. D., & Schwartz, D. M. (1982). Bulimia: A descriptive study survey on 316 cases. *International Journal of Eating Disorders, 2,* 3–16.

Jonas, J. M., & Gold, M. S. (1986). Naltrexone reverses bulimic symptoms. *Lancet, 1,* 807.

Kaplan, H. I., & Sadock, B. J. (1985). *Comprehensive textbook of psychiatry* (4th ed.). Baltimore: Williams and Wilkins.

Kassett, J. A., Gershon, E. S., Maxwell, M. E., Guroff, J. J., Kazuba, D. M., Smith, A. L., Brandt, H. A., & Jimerson, D. C. (1986). Psychiatric disorders in the first-degree relatives of probands with bulimia nervosa. *American Journal of Psychiatry, 11,* 1468–1471.

Kasvikis, Y. G., Tsakiris, F., Marks, I. M., Basoglu, M., & Noshirvani, H. F. (1986). Past history of anorexia nervosa in women with obsessive-compulsive disorder. *International Journal of Eating Disorders, 37,* 1281–1285.

Kaye, W. H., Ballenger, J. C., Lydiard, B., Stuart, G. W., Laraia, M. T., O'Neil, P., Fossey, M., Stevens, V., Lesser, S., & Hsu, L. K. G. (1990). CSF monoamine levels in normal-weight bulimia: Evidence for abnormal noradrenergic activity. *American Journal of Psychiatry, 147,* 225–229.

Kaye, W. H., Ebert, M. H., Gwirtsman, H. E., & Weiss, S. R. (1984). Differences in brain serotonergic metabolism between nonbulimic and bulimic patients with anorexia nervosa. *American Journal of Psychiatry, 141,* 1598–1601.

Kaye, W. H., Gwirtsman, H. E., George, D. T., & Ebert, M. H. (1991). Altered serotonin activity in anorexia nervosa after long-term weight restoration: Does elevated CSF 5-HIAA correlate with rigid and obsessive behavior? *Archives of General Psychiatry, 48,* 556–562.

Kaye, W. H., Gwirtsman, H. E., George, D. T., Jimerson, D. C., Ebert, M. H., & Lake, C. R. (1986, May). *Disturbances in noradrenergic systems in normal weight bulimia: Sympathetic activation with bingeing, reduced noradrenergic activity after a month of abstinence from bingeing.* Presented at the 139th Annual Meeting of the American Psychiatric Association, Washington, DC.

Kaye, W. H., Gwirtsman, H., George, D. T., Jimerson, D. C., Ebert, M. H., & Lake, C. R. (1990). Disturbances of noradrenergic systems in normal-weight bulimia: Relationship to diet and menses. *Biological Psychiatry, 27,* 4–21.

Kaye, W. H., Gwirtsman, H. E., Lake, C. R., Siever, L. J., Jimerson, D. C., Ebert, M. H., & Murphy, D. L. (1985). Disturbances of norepinephrine metabolism and alpha2 adrenergic receptor activity in anorexia nervosa: Relationship to nutritional state. *Psychopharmacology Bulletin, 21,* 419–423.

Kaye, W. H., Weltzin, T. E., Hsu, L. K. G., & Bulik, C. (1991). An open trial of fluoxetine in patients with anorexia nervosa. *Journal of Clinical Psychiatry, 52,* 464–471.

Kennedy, S., Piran, N., & Garfinkel, P. E. (1986). Isocarboxazide in the treatment of bulimia. *American Journal of Psychiatry, 143,* 1495–1496.

Keys, A. (1950). *The biology of human starvation.* Minneapolis: University of Minnesota Press.

Lacey, J. H. (1983). Bulimia nervosa, binge eating, and psychogenic vomiting: A controlled treatment study and long term outcome. *British Medical Journal, 286,* 1609–1613.

Lacey, J. H., & Crisp, A. H. (1980). Hunger, food intake, and weight: The impact of clomipramine on a refeeding anorexia nervosa population. *Postgraduate Medical Journal, 56,* 79–85.

Laessle, R. G., Wittchen, H. U., Fichter, M. M., & Pirke, K. M. (1989). The significance of subgroups of bulimia and anorexia nervosa: Lifetime frequency of psychiatric disorders. *International Journal of Eating Disorders, 8,* 569–574.

Leibowitz, S. F., & Shor-Posner, G. (1986). Brain serotonin and eating behavior. *Appetite, 7,* 1–14.

Leon, G. R., Carroll, K., Chernyk, B., & Finn, S. (1985). Binge eating and associated habit patterns within college students and identified bulimic populations. *International Journal of Eating Disorders, 4,* 43–57.

Linnoila, M., Virkkunen, M., Scheinin, M., Nuutila, A., Rimon, R., & Goodwin, F. K. (1983). Low cerebrospinal fluid 5-HIAA concentration differentiates impulsive from non-impulsive violent behavior. *Life Sciences, 33,* 2609–2614.

Lucas, A. R., Beard, C. M., O'Fallon, W. M., & Kurland, L. T. (1988). Anorexia nervosa in Rochester, Minnesota: A 45-year study. *Mayo Clinical Proceedings, 63,* 433–442.

McGoldrick, M. (1985). *Genograms in family assessment.* New York: Norton Press.

Minuchin, S., & Fishman, H. C. (1981). *Family therapy techniques*. Cambridge, MA: Harvard University Press.

Minuchin, S., Rosman, B. L., & Baker, L. (1978). *Psychosomatic families: Anorexia nervosa in context*. Cambridge, MA: Harvard University Press.

Mitchell, J. E., (1984). Medical complications of anorexia and bulimia nervosa. *Psychiatric Medicine, 1*, 229–255.

Mitchell, J. E., & Groat, R. (1984). A placebo-controlled double-blind trial of amitriptyline in bulimia. *Journal of Clinical Psychopharmacology, 4*, 186–193.

Mitchell, J. E., Hatsukami, D., Eckert, E. D., & Pyle, R. L. (1985). Characteristics of 275 patients with bulimia. *Journal of Clinical Psychopharmacology, 142*, 482–485.

Mitchell, J. E., Hatsukami, D., Pyle, R., & Eckert, E. D. (1988). Bulimia with and without a family history of drug abuse. *Addictive Behaviors, 13*, 245–251.

Mitchell, J. E., Pyle, R. L., & Eckert, E. D. (1990). A comparison study of antidepressants and structured intensive group psychotherapy in the treatment of bulimia nervosa. *Archives of General Psychiatry, 47*, 149–157.

Mitchell, J. E., Scim, H. D., Colon, E., & Pomeroy, C. (1987). Medical complications and medical management of bulimia. *Annals of Internal Medicine, 107*, 71–76.

Mitchell, J. E., Soll, E., Eckert, E. D., Pyle, R. L., & Hatsukami, D. (1989). The changing population of bulimia nervosa patients in an eating disorders program. *Hospital and Community Psychiatry, 40*, 1188–1189.

Moore, D. C. (1977). Amitriptyline therapy in anorexia nervosa. *American Journal of Psychiatry, 134*, 1303–1304.

Moore, R., Mills, I. H., & Forster, A. (1981). Naloxone in the treatment of anorexia nervosa: Effect on weight gain and lipolysis. *Journal of the Royal Society of Medicine, 74*, 129–131.

Morgan, H., & Russell, G. F. M. (1975). Value of family background and clinical features as predictors of long-term outcome in anorexia nervosa: Four-year follow-up study of 41 patients. *Psychological Medicine, 5*, 355–371.

Needlemen, H. L., & Waber, D. (1977). The use of amitriptyline in anorexia nervosa. In R. A. Vigersky (Ed.), *Anorexia nervosa* (pp. 357–362). New York: Raven Press.

Nusbaum, D. (1990). Inpatient survey of nursing care measures of inpatient treatment of patients with anorexia nervosa. *Mental Health Nursing, 11*, 175–184.

Oesterhed, J. D., McKenna, M. S., & Gould, N. B. (1987). Group psychotherapy of bulimia: A critical review. *International Journal of Group Psychotherapy, 37*, 163–184.

Oppenheimer, R., Howells, K., & Palmer, R. L. (1984). *Adverse sexual experiences and victimization in the histories of patients with clinical eating disorders.* Paper presented at the International Conference on Anorexia Nervosa and Related Disorders, Swansea, United Kingdom.

Pillay, M., & Crisp, A. H. (1981). The impact of social skills training within an established inpatient treatment program for anorexia nervosa. *British Journal of Psychiatry, 139*, 533–539.

Ploog, D. W., & Pirke, K. M. (1987). Psychobiology of anorexia nervosa. *Psychological Medicine, 17*, 843–859.

Pope, H. G., Hudson, J. I., Jonas, J. M., & Yurgelon-Todd, D. (1983). Bulimia treated with imipramine: A placebo-controlled double-blind study. *American Journal of Psychiatry, 140*, 554–558.

Pope, H. G., Hudson, J. I., & Yurgelun-Todd, D. (1984). Anorexia nervosa and bulimia among 300 suburban women shoppers. *American Journal of Psychiatry, 141*, 292–294.

Pope, H. G., keck, P. E., McElroy, S. L., & Hudson, J. I. (1988). A placebo-controlled study of trazadone in bulimia nervosa. *Journal of Clinical Psychopharmacology, 9*, 254–259.

Pyle, R. L., Mitchell, J. E., & Eckert, E. D. (1981). Bulimia: A report of 34 cases. *Journal of Clinical Psychiatry, 42*, 60–64.

Pyle, R. L., Mitchell, J. E., Eckert, ED. et al. (1983). The incidence of bulimia in freshmen college students. *Int J Eat Dis, 2*, 75–85.

Redmond, D. E., Swann, A., & Heninger, G. T. (1976). Phenoxybenzamine in anorexia nervosa. *Lancet, 2*, 397.

Rothenberg, A. (1988). Differential diagnosis of anorexia nervosa and depressive illness: A review of 11 studies. *Comprehensive Psychiatry, 29*, 427–432.

Rowland, C., Jr. (1970). Anorexia nervosa: A survey of the literature and review of 30 cases. *International Journal of Clinical Psychiatry, 7*, 37–137.

Roy-Byrne, P., Gwirtsman, H. E., Edelstein, C. K., Yager, J., & Gerner, R. H. (1983). Response to "The Psychiatrist as Mind Sweeper": Eating disorders and antidepressants. *Journal of Clinical Psychopharmacology, 3*, 60–61.

Russell, G. F. M., Checkley, S. A., Feldman, J., &

Eisler, I. (1988). A controlled trial of d-fenfluramine in bulimia nervosa. *Clinical Neuropharmacology, 1,* S146–S159.

Sabine, E. J., Yonace, A., Farrington, A. J., Barratt, K. H., & Wakeling, A. (1983). Bulimia nervosa: A placebo-controlled, double-blind therapeutic trial of mianseren. *British Journal of Clinical Pharmacology, 15,* 195s–20s.

Schwartz, D. M., Barrett, M. J., & Saba, G. (1984). Family therapy for bulimia nervosa. In D. M. Garner & P. E. Garfinkel (Eds.), *Handbook of psychotherapy for anorexia nervosa and bulimia* (pp. 280–307). New York: Guilford.

Schwartz, D. M., & Thompson, M. G. (1981). Do anorectics get well? Current research and future needs. *American Journal of Psychiatry, 138,* 319–323.

Schwartz, S., Rosmark, B., Norring, C., & Holmgren, S. (1987). Two year outcome in anorexia nervosa/bulimia: A controlled study of an eating control program combined with psychoanalytically oriented psychotherapy. *International Journal of Eating Disorders, 6,* 243–256.

Sohlberg, S., Rosmark, B., Norring, C., & Holmgren, S. (1987). Two year outcome in anorexia nervosa/bulimia: A controlled study of an eating control program combined with psychoanalytically oriented psychotherapy. *International Journal of Eating Disorders, 6,* 243–256.

Stangler, R. S., & Printz, A. M. (1980). DSM-III psychiatric diagnosis in a university population. *American Journal of Psychiatry, 137,* 937.

Stonehill, E., & Crisp, A. H. (1977). Psychoneurotic characteristics of patients with anorexia nervosa before and after treatment and at follow-up 4–7 years later. *Journal of Psychosomatic Research, 21,* 187–193.

Strober, M. (1980). Personality and symptomatological features in young, nonchronic anorexia nervosa patients. *Journal of Psychosomatic Research, 24,* 353–359.

Strober, M. (1984). Stressful events associated with bulimia and anorexia nervosa: Empirical findings and theoretical speculations. *International Journal of Eating Disorders, 3,* 3–16.

Strober, M., & Humphrey, L. L. (1987). Familial contributions to the technology and course of anorexia nervosa and bulimia. *Journal Consulting Clinical Psychology, 55,* 654–659.

Strober, M., & Katz, J. L. (1988). Depression in the eating disorders: A review and analysis of descriptive, family, and biological findings. In D. M. Garner

& P. E. Garfinkel (Eds.), *Diagnostic issues in anorexia nervosa and bulimia nervosa.* New York: Brunner/Mazel.

Strober, M., Lampert, C., Morrell, W., Burroughs, J., & Jacobs, C. (1990). A controlled family study of anorexia nervosa: Evidence of familial aggregation and lack of shared transmission with affective disorders. *International Journal of Eating Disorders, 9,* 239–253.

Strober, M., Salkin, B., Burroughs, J., & Morrell, W. (1982). Validity of the bulimia-restrictor criteria in anorexia nervosa. *Journal of Nervous Mental Disease, 170,* 345–351.

Swift, W. J., Andrews, D., & Barklage, N. E. (1986). The relationship between affective disorder and eating disorders: A review of the literature. *American Journal of Psychiatry, 143,* 290–299.

Theander, S. (1970). Anorexia nervosa: A psychiatric investigation of 94 female patients. *Acta Psychiatrica Scandinavia Supplement, 214,* 1–194.

Toner, B. B., Garfinkel, P. E., & Garner, D. M. (1986). Long term follow-up of anorexia nervosa. *Psychosomatic Medicine, 48,* 520–529.

Touyz, S. W., Beumont, P. J. V., Glaun, D., Phillips, T., & Crowie, I. (1984). A comparison of lenient and strict operant conditioning programmes in refeeding patients with anorexia nervosa. *British Journal of Psychiatry, 144,* 517–520.

Traskman, L., Asberg, M., & Bertilsson, L. (1981). Monoamine metabolites in CSF and suicidal behavior. *Archives of General Psychiatry, 38,* 631–636.

Vandereycken, W. (1987). The management of patients with anorexia nervosa and bulimia nervosa—Basic principles and general guidelines. In E. P. Burrows & D. C. Casper (Eds.), *Handbook of eating disorders. Part 1: Anorexia and bulimia,* (pp. 235–254). The Netherlands: Elsevier.

Vandereycken, W. (1990). The addiction model in eating disorders: Some critical remarks and a selected bibliography. *International Journal of Eating Disorders, 9,* 95–102.

Vandereycken, W., & Pierloot, R. (1982). Pimozide combined with behavior therapy in the short term treatment of anorexia nervosa: A double blind controlled crossover study. *Acta Psychiatrica Scandinavia, 66,* 445–450.

Vandereycken, W., & Pierloot, R. (1983). Long-term outcome in anorexia nervosa: The problem of patient selection and follow-up duration. *International Journal of Eating Disorders, 2,* 237–242.

Vandereycken, W., & Van den Broucke, S. (1984). Anorexia nervosa in males: A comparative study of

107 cases reported in the literature (1970 to 1980). *Acta Psychiatrica Scandinavia, 70,* 447–454.

Vanderlinden, J., & Vandereycken, W. (1988). Family therapy in bulimia nervosa. In D. Hardoff, & E. Chigier (Eds.), *Eating disorders in adolescents and young adults* (pp. 325–334). London: Freund.

van Praag, H. M. (1983). CSF 5-HIAA and suicide in non-depressed schizophrenics. *Lancet, 2,* 977–978.

Walsh, B. T., Gladis, M., Roose, S. P., Stewart, J. W., Stetner, F., & Glassman, A. H. (1988). Phenelzine vs placebo in 50 patients with bulimia. *Archives of General Psychiatry, 45,* 471–475.

Walsh, B. T., Stewart, J. W., & Roose, S. P. (1984). Treatment of bulimia with phenelzine: A double-blind, placebo controlled study. *Archives of General Psychiatry, 41,* 1105–1109.

Weltzin, T. E., Fernstrom, M. H., Hansen, D., McConaha, C., & Kaye, W. H. (1991). Abnormal caloric requirements for weight maintenance in patients with anorexia and bulimia nervosa. *American Journal of Psychiatry, 148,* 1675–1682.

Weltzin, T. E., Hsu, L. K. G., Pollice, C., & Kaye, W. H. (1991). Feeding patterns of bulimia nervosa. *Biological Psychiatry, 30,* 1093–1110.

Wilcox, J. A. (1987). Abuse of fluoxetine by a patient with anorexia nervosa [letter]. *American Journal of Psychiatry, 144,* 1100.

Willi, J., & Grossman, S. (1983). Epidemiology of anorexia nervosa in a defined region of switzerland. *American Journal of Psychiatry, 140,* 564–567.

Wold, P. (1983). Trazodone in the treatment of bulimia. *Journal of Clinical Psychiatry, 44,* 275–276.

Wong, D. T., Hornig, J. S., Bymaster, F. P. et al. (1974). A selective inhibitor of serotonin uptake: Lilly 110140 3)(p-trifluoromethylphenoxy)-N-methyl-3-phenylpropylamine. *Life Sciences, 15,* 471–479.

Wulliemier, F., Rossel, F., & Sinclair, K. (1975). La therapie comportementale de l'anorexia nerveuse. *Journal of Psychosomatic Research, 19,* 267–272.

Wurtman, J. J., & Wurtman, R. J. (1979). Drugs that enhance central serotoninergic transmission diminish elective carbohydrate consumption by rats. *Life Science, 24,* 895–903.

Zohar, J., & Insel, T. R. (1987). Obsessive-compulsive disorder: Psychobiological approaches to diagnosis, treatment, and pathophysiology. *Biological Psychiatry, 22,* 667–687.

Zohar, J., Insel, T. R., & Zohar-Kadouch, R. C. (1988). Serotonergic responsivity in obsessive-compulsive disorder. *Archives of General Psychiatry, 45,* 167–172.

CHAPTER 14

GENDER-IDENTITY DISORDERS

John Money   Johns Hopkins University and Hospital
Gregory K. Lehne   Johns Hopkins University and Hospital

DESCRIPTION OF DISORDER

Clinical Features

Gender identity is the private experience of gender role, and *gender role* is the public manifestation of gender identity. Both are like two sides of the same coin and constitute the unity of gender-identity/role (G-I/R). Gender identity is the sameness, unity, and persistence of one's individuality as male, female, or androgynous, in greater or lesser degree, especially as it is experienced in self-awareness and behavior. Gender role is everything that a person says and does to indicate to others or to the self the degree that one is either male or female or androgynous. It includes but is not restricted to sexual and erotic arousal and response, which should not be excluded from the definition.

Gender transposition is the switching or crossing over of attributes, expectancies, or stereotypes of gender-identity/role from masculine to feminine, or vice versa, either serially or simultaneously, temporarily or persistently, and in greater or lesser degree. From the viewpoint of subjective experience, the name given to gender transposition is *gender dysphoria*. A gender-identity disorder is one in which the G-I/R develops or changes so as to be discordant with the signs of the natal sex, with ensuing severe and morbid repercussions that are incompatible with personal well-being.

The pathognomonic feature of a gender-identity disorder, whether in the juvenile years or later, is that the person with the disorder has a sex-transmutational fixation—that is to say a fixed idea *(idée fixe)* of being able to metamorphose into a member of the other sex. This fixation is a disorder of the body image. It is not a delusion of having been born a member of the other sex. The actuality of the natal sex is not refuted, only repudiated. Older patients, translating a nineteenth-century maxim of K. H. Ulrichs ("anima muliebris virili corpore inclusa"), describe themselves as having "a woman's mind trapped in a man's body" (and vice versa for females). They are pragmatic about requiring professional intervention for sex transformation, whereas the logic of young children is of magical transformation by enchantment or divine intervention. In the fantasy logic of very young childhood, changing sex is of the same order as other fairy-tale transmutations, not to mention the mystique of the body changes of puberty. Occasional dressing up and play-acting the role of the other sex does not constitute the body-image transmutation of a gender-identity disorder.

Associated Features

Even very young children with a gender-identity disorder make explicit statements about becoming a member of the other sex. Various associated features may be collectively construed as impersonation or mimesis (gynemimesis in males; andromimesis in females) of the role of the other sex. These children play dress-up and, if clothing is not available, improve cross-dressing styles with fancy paper, towels, scarves, ribbons, and accessories. Unless provided with clothes in the style they demand, they veto various activities, including going to school or on family outings. They become accomplished in using cross-sexed body language, gestures, vocabulary, and speech patterns. Their recreational and vocational-rehearsal play are cross-sexed, and they shun playing with members of their natal sex who, in turn, shun them.

Boys with a gender-identity disorder have a history of not fighting for rank in the dominance hierarchy of boyhood, and of being failures in sports, whereas the contrary applies to girls. Among age-mates, boys are cruelly stigmatized and sometimes victimized for being sissies. Girls also may be stigmatized, although being like a boy is less stigmatizing for girls than "sissyness" is for boys. Despite being stigmatized, the boys are likely to be good students and high academic and vocational achievers, whereas the girls are more likely to be fractious and to be at risk for underachievement. Careers are likely to be cross-sex stereotypic, except that the sex-stereotyping of modern careers is no longer hard and fast.

In both boys and girls with a diagnosis of gender-identity disorder, there is no special likelihood of an additional diagnosis. However, incidents associated with or precipitated by the primary disorder may require crisis intervention. Prepubertally, there is no apparent likelihood of untoward sexual behavior. Postpubertally, sexual delinquency may occur in some cases—so may other delinquencies in the triad of lying, thieving, and sexing, though not predictably or invariably so.

Epidemiology

There are no epidemiological statistics. There is undoubtedly a strong sampling bias in the selection of childhood cases referred for professional attention, in favor of the indigent with accompanying school problems and of the socioeconomically privileged classes. There may also be a sampling bias that accounts for the referral of more boys than girls. If not, then according to available statistics, the sex ratio is disproportionate, with four or more boys to each girl with the syndrome.

Etiology

In experimental animal sexology, the method of creating a gender identity disorder is to manipulate the level of sex hormone reaching the brain of the fetus from the maternal blood stream. It must be done precisely at the critical period after the genital anatomy has differentiated but before the brain has become sexually dimorphic. Masculinization of the brain of the female fetus is accomplished by implanting a pellet of the testosterone under the skin of the mother. Demasculinization of the brain of the male fetus is more complex, as implantation of an estrogen or progestin pellet is likely to induce abortion of the fetus. Surgical castration of the fetus is effective but technically challenging.

An experimentally masculinized female subsequently "impersonates" a male in mating and is accepted as a male by other males and females of the species (and vice versa for a demasculinized male). This experiment is most effectively demonstrated in the four-legged, subprimte species. In sheep, it has been recorded on film (Short & Clark, undated). In the primate species, the prenatal hormonal history is only the first part of the story. The second part is postnatal, and it belongs not to hormones but to social learning and experience.

The possibility of a prenatal, hormonal brain determinant of gender-identity disorder in human beings cannot be dismissed, even though attempts to find it have so far been unsuccessful. It is quite possible that sex steroid plays only a precursor role in a multivariate cascade of determinants that, in sequence, differentiate gender identity, or its disorder, in the brain. During the postnatal period, gender coding becomes, in large part, contingent on stimulus input through the senses, cognitional assimilations, and conceptual learning.

The two antipodean principles of gender coding are identification and complementation. The well-recognized principle of *identification* pertains to the coding of one's own gender schema concordant with the example of others whose natal sex is the same as one's own. Conversely, the less-recognized principle of *complementation* pertains to the coding of one's own gender schema as being not concordant with but reciprocal to the example of others whose natal sex differs from one's own. Identification and complementation models are not only parents but also age-mates and others, including those who, especially in adolescence, are by popular acclaim idols of hero worship.

In the brain, the developmental outcome of the processes of identification and complementation is represented as two gender-coded schemas. One is coded as mine and the other as thine. The constancy of both schemas is established early in the development of most but not all children. In children who develop a gender-identity disorder, the two schemas become cross-coded.

No consistently occurring antecedents of gender identity disorder have yet been discovered. On the basis of retrospective studies of adult transsexual patients, Stoller (1968) postulated a blissful antecedent state of extensive and excessive closeness with the mother during infancy, but the postulate has not been supported statistically. There has also been no statistical support for such a simplistic idea that the mother always wanted a girl instead of a boy (or vice versa). There is no verification of the outdated dogma that gender-identity disorder is caught by social contagion from contact with homosexual or bisexual people, including possibly a parent. No body of evidence has emerged to suggest an elevated incidence of sexual child abuse.

In some cases it can be documented by family photographs that a child, more often a boy than a girl, becomes entranced with cross-dressing when as young as age 3 or 4. By age 6 or 7, the fixation on personal sex transmutation may already be well established, so that gender-identity disorder is diagnosable. Whether or not the occurrence of the disorder is randomly distributed is not known. The likelihood of an antecedent predisposition or

vulnerability factor should not be disregarded lightly. Such a factor might be a propensity for roleplaying. In one followup study of gender-identity disorder in boys (Green & Money, 1966), the prevalence of theatrical play and dramatic improvisation was higher than one would expect by chance, thus suggesting a special talent for switching roles. Some children with gender-identity disorder are able to demonstrate alternately a feminine and a masculine role—the phenomenon of two names, two wardrobes, and two personalities, which may continue into adulthood (Money, 1976). In other children, such bipotentiality resolves into monopotentiality. The pragmatic issue then becomes one not of the cause but the permanence of the effect—that is, of mutability and immutability, regardless of etiology.

DIFFERENTIAL DIAGNOSIS AND ASSESSMENT

DSM-III-R Categorization

Gender-Identity Disorders

302.60   Gender-Identity Disorder of Childhood

302.50   Transsexualism

302.85   Gender-Identity Disorder of Adolescence or Adulthood, Nontranssexual Type (GIDAANT)

Note: The number 302.85 is used twice. Whereas it is claimed that in the vast majority of cases the onset of gender-identity disorder can be traced back to childhood, it is also allowed that an adult may report that the first signs appeared in adulthood. Nonetheless, such a case is illogically categorized in DSM-III-R as one of the disorders usually first evident in infancy, childhood, or adolescence.

Differential Diagnosis

Gender-Role Nonconformity

Boys and girls whose masculinity or femininity, respectively, does not conform to societally established gender stereotypes are stigmatized by adults and peers alike. Boys who are not aggressively assertive, competitive, and staunch when challenged risk being labeled effeminate or sissy, especially if they also show interest in work or play stereotyped as feminine. Girls who are aggressively assertive, competitive, and staunch when challenged, and who are more interested in boys' than girls' stereotypic work and play are, by contrast, not labeled masculinate or virilistic, but more tolerantly as tomboys. In popular usage, the predicted outcome of effeminacy, but not of tomboyism, is a homosexual orientation. In actuality the outcome in either case may be an orientation that is heterosexual, homosexual, or bisexual, with no fixation on a transmutation of sex, no evidence of body-image pathology, and no diagnosis of gender-identity disorder. Homosexuality (as well as bisexuality), per se, is not classified as a sickness or disease or disorder.

Hermaphroditic and Related Disorders

Whereas the different variables of sex are usually all concordant with one another and with the gender identity, in cases of birth defect of the sex organs this is not necessarily so. Thus, it is possible, as in the syndrome of congenital virilizing adrenal hyperplasia (CVAH), for a male rearing and a masculine gender identity to be associated with external male genitalia on the one hand, and female internal genitalia, ovaries, and female (46,XX) chromosomal karyotype on the other. Correspondingly, it is possible, as in the androgen-insensitivity syndrome (AIS) for a female rearing and a feminine gender identity to be associated with female external genitalia on the one hand, and imperfect male internal genitalia, testicles, and a male (46,XY) chromosomal karyotype on the other. These and similar congenital discrepancies are dealt with in detail in the fourth edition of the Wilkins textbook of pediatric endocrinology (Blizzard, Kappy, & Migeon, 1993) and in Money (1968, 1988). The discrepancy between feminine (tomboyish) gender identity and male natal sex may occur also in cases of total ablatio penis secondary to a circumcision accident, if the child is reared as a female with appropriate genital reconstructive surgery.

The fact that gender identity may differentiate discordantly with other variables of sex is of significance neonatally in cases of birth defect of the genitalia when the sex of rearing is being decided so as to be compatible with copulatory function in maturity. It is again of significance later in childhood, when to disregard the gender identity and to impose an enforced change of sex according to the criterion of the chromosomes or the gonads would be malpractice. In addition, it may assume legal significance, as when a sex-chromosome test is used to disqualify a person with, say, a CVAH or AIS diagnosis from sports competition, or to deprive the person of legal rights (e.g., the right of marriage).

In the annals of hermaphroditism, there are some cases — namely those in which the gender identity is discrepant with the sex of civil status — that warrant a secondary diagnosis of gender-identity disorder and a surgical, hormonal, and social reassignment of sex.

Transsexualism

Etymologically, *transsexualism* means crossing sex. It is used as the name for a syndrome and as a synonym for sex reassignment — the treatment procedure. Transsexualism represents the extreme degree of fixation on sex transmutation and metamorphosis of the body to agree with the body image.

The fixation on sex transmutation evolves to become full blown in adolescence (or subsequently). Typically it is not associated with any other diagnosis. However, in rare cases it may be a complication of clinical epilepsy, multiple personality, messianic paranoia (as in the Schreber case made famous by Freud), and paraphilia (e.g., apotemnophilia, in which the primary fixation is on being an amputee). It may be associated with a chromosomal anomaly, in particular the 47,XXY (Klinefelter) syndrome, and the 47,XYY (supernumerary Y) syndrome, but no etiological relationship has been established. Transsexualism may be confused with the skoptic syndrome (Money, 1988), in which the transmutational body-image fixation is not on changing sex but on castration so as to become a eunuch.

Transvestism and Tranvestophilia

Etymologically transvestism means cross-dressing, irrespective of the occasion, function, duration, regularity, or sexuoerotical component. Transvestism, per se, is not a syndrome. The syndrome is *transvestophilia,* one of the paraphilias, also known as *fetishistic transvestism.* It occurs perhaps exclusively in men. It is classified as a paraphilia insofar as the cross-sexed wearing of garments, accompanied by transsexual body imagery, is a contingency of sexuoerotical arousal and attainment of orgasm. Onset of transvestophilia is retrospectively dated to peripuberty or later, although fascination with female clothing may be retrospectively dated to an earlier age. Prospective followup of boys with a diagnosis of childhood gender-identity disorder and a history of childhood cross-dressing has shown, however, that the long-term outcome is not predictably tranvestophilia nor transsexualism (Money & Russo, 1979; Green, 1986). Instead, it is a homosexual gender identity and orientation, in some cases after a failed adolescent attempt at heterosexual dating.

In adolescence and adulthood, transvestophilia is episodic in occurrence. The longer the period of not being cross-dressed, the greater the degree of stress and anxiety, which, in turn, increases the frequency of cross-dressing. Tranvestophilia may continue indefinitely to be episodic or, in midlife or later, may emerge full time into transsexualism. In an unknown proportion of cases in adolescence and subsequently, transvestophilia is combined with asphyxiophilia, the paraphilia of self-strangulation, which may lead to accidental autoerotic death (Boglioli, Taff, Stephens, & Money, 1991; Money, Wainwright, & Hingsburger, 1991).

Gynemimetic or Andromimetic Syndrome

The syndrome of gynemimesis is the lady with a penis syndrome (Money & Lamacz, 1984). Correspondingly, the syndrome of andromimesis is the man with a vulva syndrome. Both syndromes may be regarded as a *forme fruste* of transsexualism. In both syndromes, there is a sex-transmutational body-image fixation. In gynemimesis, it involves taking female hormones, estrogen and progestin (possibly obtained illicitly), for breast growth and other feminizing or partial demasculinizing effects. It may also involve cosmetic plastic surgery, but not genital reconstructive surgery. Correspondingly, in andromimesis, testosterone is taken for its masculinizing effects. Surgical intervention involves mastectomy, hysterectomy, and oophorectomy. If masculinizing genital reconstructive surgery were more technically satisfactory than is presently possible, it would be more in demand.

Gynemimetics and andromimetics dress, live, and work full time in the cross-sexed role, often exaggerating the stereotypes. On the criterion of their natal sex, the large majority are homosexual in orientation. For many gynemimetics, the acme of achievement is to pass as a prostitute. In some bars where they work, their customers are gynemimetophiles—that is, men who are erotically attracted to ladies with a penis.

Like transsexuals, gynemimetics and andromimetics are, with the knowledge of hindsight, likely to say that they knew themselves to be different ever since childhood, even though the difference may not have been readily apparent to others until around the time of puberty. In adolescence they enter a phase of identifying themselves as homosexual, cross-dressing whenever possible, and finally living full time in the cross-dressed role.

Gynemimesis and andromimesis have been identified as occurring worldwide and transculturally, though they may be unknown in some small tribal cultures. The sex ratio appears always to be heavily weighted in favor of gynemimesis, though the final verdict is not in. In some societies neither gynemimesis nor andromimesis is considered a disorder—for example, in most Native American tribal societies (Williams, 1986). Instead, these societies traditionally have a societal niche for gynemimetics and andromimetics. In India, gynemimetics, known as *hijras,* are accommodated as a minority subculture—part caste and part religious cult (Money & Lamacz, 1984; Nanda, 1990).

Assessment Strategies

The statistical chances that the findings from a complete physical and laboratory examination will be noncontributory are extremely high. Nonetheless, there is much wisdom in obtaining such a workup not only as a safeguard against error but also to dispel the popular and professional notion that anything so exotic as gender-identity disorder must be the product of a genetic, hormonal, or other biological anomaly. A complete workup, by showing what are not sufficient causes of gender-identity disorder, will also lead more directly in the future to the discovery of what are the causes. The same principles apply to the use of routinely used psychological tests and procedures (to obtain an IQ, for example), none of which has been designed specifically for the assessment of gender identity, disordered or otherwise. Questionnaires and checklists for the assessment of masculinity, femininity, or androgyny are few in number, mostly unpublished, and designed for screening surveys. They are not acceptable for clinical diagnosis; their percentage of false negatives and false positives is too high.

To obtain information about a gender-identity disorder and its history, one needs an assessment schedule or systematic schedule of inquiry, of which an example is provided in Money and Primrose (1969). Such a schedule allows each evaluation to follow its own logical sequence while ensuring that no topics are overlooked. On each topic, the inquiry never begins as an interrogatory, but as fully open-ended interview, completely nonjudgmental in vocabulary and idiom (see Money, 1986, Chapter 8). The ideal is to conduct an inquiry separately with the patient and each parent or other accompanying person, and, if professional personnel are available, concurrently, so that the respondents do not have an opportunity to coach one another regarding what transpired. By the very nature of the disorder, there is always the possibility of collusion among the participants of what is, in the final analysis, a family dream.

Not all information regarding the family drama may be disclosable forthrightly, but only if it is fictionalized in the manner legitimated by clinical psychological projective techniques—which may be narrative, graphic, or, especially in young children, ludic (toy play). Great contradictions may be revealed. Thus, a quietly docile but linguistically noncommunicative young boy under

evaluation for effeminacy may, when away from his parents, explode into an orgy of mayhem, murder, crashing, and destruction when playing with flexible toy people, animals, guns, trucks, and buildings.

For all parties, the child included, the guarantee of confidentiality is imperative. That does not preclude prior agreements about information that can be shared in a conference of interviewers and respondents together, at the conclusion of the evaluations.

TREATMENT

Evidence for Prescriptive Treatments

Behavior Therapy

Claims made on behalf of the efficacy of behavior therapy in the treatment of gender-identity disorder are based on the operant-conditioning formula of the stimulus/response bond which, unlike the ethological formula, does not contain the chronological constraint of a critical or sensitive period. The ethological formula has not two but three constituents: stimulus/critical period/response. If the timing is either premature or postmature, stimulus/response bonding does not occur, whereas during the critical period not only does it occur but it also becomes long lasting or immutable. Gender identity differentiates from its early bipotential phase and becomes immutably monopotential, concordantly with the natal sex in the majority of people but discordantly in cases of gender-identity disorder. In some instances of discordance, bipotentiality remains only partially unresolved into monopotentiality, more so in younger than older patients. These are the patients who may appear to respond to therapeutic intervention, at least temporarily. There have been no studies of the comparative efficacy of behavior therapy versus other therapies. Accurate comparisons may, in fact, be unattainable, as there are too many variables that cannot, for ethical and legal reasons, be manipulated.

Pharmacotherapy

Neither before nor after puberty are the levels of sex hormones circulating in the blood stream responsible for or correlated with gender-identity disorder. Correspondingly, administration of exogenous sex hormone does not change gender identity from masculine to feminine or vice versa; nor does it change orientation from homosexual to heterosexual or vice versa; nor does it change bisexual to monosexual. The same applies to nonhormonal medications.

Medications that are not hormones may be used for the treatment of concomitant symptoms or syndromes, however. There are no statistics on concomitant diagnoses with respect to their prevalence, type, or range in those with a primary diagnosis of gender-identity disorder. Concomitant disorders are likely to be overlooked more often in prepubertal than postpubertal cases of gender-identity disorder. Those disorders amenable to pharmacologic treatment are depression, suicidal despondency, phobia, and anxiety or panic attacks. Though confirmation studies still need to be done, there is preliminary evidence that, in cases of transvestophilia, when the anxiolytic, buspirone hydrochloride (Buspar) is taken for the relief of anxiety, the fixation on cross dressing may also be relieved, with at least partial remission (Federoff, 1988).

Whereas hormonal therapy is not effective in changing gender identity to agree with natal sex, it is effective in changing at least some of the secondary sexual characteristics of the natal sex so that they match the gender identity of the sex-reassigned transsexual. Hormonal reassignment is a component of the two-year, real-life test (Money & Ambinder, 1978). The other is social reassignment. Both precede those procedures of surgical reassignment that are nonreversible.

For female-to-male hormonal reassignment, the recommended androgen is testosterone enanthate. It is given intramuscularly, 200–400 mg/month, or 100–200 mg/biweekly, the dosage being adapted to height and weight. This treatment induces changes typical of masculinizing puberty: more oily skin, possible acne, voice deepening, and the growth of facial and body hair. Apart from the possibility of irregular breakthrough bleeding,

it suppresses menstrual cyclicity and menstruation. It may enlarge the clitoris, though not sufficiently to permit its surgical reconstruction as a penis. It may increase the intensity of orgasms without altering their occurrence as either single or multiple. Testosterone treatment does not alter the dimensions of the feminized bone structure, and it brings about little if any reduction of breast size. By contrast, it reduces subcutaneous fat padding, promotes muscular development, and, in later life, may bring about shedding of head hair and baldness. As a replacement hormone, it is taken without time limit.

In the case of male-to-female sex reassignment, hormonal reassignment may very well begin not with an estrogenic, feminizing hormone but with a progestinic, demasculinizing hormone—for example, Depo-Provera (medoxyprogesterone acetate), 200 mg/wk, taken by intramuscular injection, the exact dosage adjusted according to height and weight.

While it is being used, though not subsequently, Depo-Provera has a suppressant effect on the secretion of testosterone, the masculinizing hormone, from the testicles, which themselves become smaller and azoospermic. Secretion of ejaculatory fluid from the prostate gland diminishes or ceases, and erection wanes or defaults. Muscular mass decreases. Subcutaneous fat increases, and the skin becomes less oily and less prone to acne. There is no demasculinizing effect on the bone structure, nor on the vocal cords and pitch of the voice, and little, if any, on hirsutism of the face and body. Balding of the head hair, if begun, is arrested.

Whereas progestinic hormones typically demasculinize but do not feminize, estrogenic hormones do both. Thus, to grow breasts, both hormones are combined in the treatment of male-to-female transsexualism. After gonadectomy, the maintenance combination dosage coincides with the hormonal dosage of various brands of the combined form of the birth control pill—for example, Lo-Ovral (Wyeth), which contains a maintenance daily dosage of estrogen (ethinyl estradiol, 0.03 mg) and progestin (norgestrel, 0.3 mg). Alternatively, in Loestrin (Parke Davis) the two hormones are, respectively, ethinyl estradiol,

20.0 mcg, and norethindrone acetate, 1.0 mg. After sex-reassignment surgery, sex-hormone replacement therapy is essential to prevent osteoporosis and other hormonal deficiency reactions.

In some cases of hermaphroditism and related disorders, hormonal replacement therapy in accordance with the gender identity is timed so as to prevent the spontaneous onset or progression of incongruous pubertal masculinization or feminization of the body. The completeness of masculinization or femininization achieved when treatment is begun before onset of puberty is much superior to that when treatment is begun after puberty.

Prepubertal sex-hormonal reassignment is not a prescribed procedure in the treatment of childhood gender-identity disorder, insofar as there are no diagnostic signs by which to make a prognosis of transsexualism in adolescence or adulthood. In adolescence, even if the prognosis is not disputed, sex-hormonal treatment is generally withheld, in view of the perils of malpractice charges, until after age 18. In some cases of male-to-female gender-identity disorder, delay of treatment is contraindicated (Money & Lamacz, 1984), insofar as an antiandrogen may have a beneficial effect on calming unruly and delinquent behavior by way of its direct action on brain cells. In a study of male monkeys, Rees, Bonsall, and Michael (1986) showed that Depo-Provera is absorbed by sex-regulating brain cells of the anterior hypothalamus within 15 minutes after an intramuscular injection.

Alternative Treatments

Correctional therapy. Before gender-identity disorder was given a place in clinical nosology, its status was that of a sin, a vice, or a crime. The treatment policy was disciplinary and correctional. This policy is still encountered, as when parents, teachers, and others resort to chastisement, humiliation, and punishment of juveniles whose behavior is symptomatic of a gender-identity disorder. In the case of boyhood effeminacy, there are some who recommend the strict regimentation of a military school. Others seek religious help by way of conversion, confession, prayer, penance,

and even exorcism. In the case of adolescent gender-identity disorder, and in a jurisdiction where cross-dressing and homosexual acts are criminal offenses, there is a risk of probation or punitive detention in the guise of treatment.

Proponents of the different forms of correction do not follow the statistical methodology of probability sampling or of having a control group. Their correctional claims of success are anecdotal and can be accounted for in terms of self-selection volunteer bias, variations in the natural history of the syndrome, and lack of long-term outcome statistics. There are some individuals in whom a partial or temporary remission of symptoms can be expected as a sequel to any form of intervention or simply to the passage of time.

Conjugate counseling. In some, if not all, cases of juvenile gender-identity disorder, there is evidence that, behind the veil of social propriety, the parents' marital and sexuoerotical history is one of adversarial feuding and abusiveness. The child, it transpires, represents the index case in a yoked network of sexological and related disorders in other members of the household or kinship. For these others, also, therapeutic intervention may be indicated. The network may be traceable through three or more generations.

The yoking together of disorders behind a veil of normalcy, with the child presented up front as proband, is not uncommon in pediatric practice. Munchausen's syndrome by proxy (Money, 1986; Money, Annecillo, & Hutchison, 1985) is a particularly challenging example. So also is the syndrome of psychosocial (child abuse) dwarfism (Money & Annecillo, 1987). The challenge is to be able to unveil the existence of the veiled disorders without so offending and antagonizing the parents that they become lost to followup.

The parents of a child with a gender-identity disorder do not come into the clinic complaining of a sexuoerotical problem of their own, and they do not expect to be confronted with questions that they construe as an assault on privacy. Nonetheless they are entitled, by law, not to have information withheld from them. Part of this information is that it is common, in cases of juvenile gender-identity disorder, for parents to have a serious degree of sexuoerotical incompatibility. The more it can be resolved, the greater is the likelihood of a remission of the child's gender-identity disorder. Those parents who do take the step of self-disclosure then require counseling of their own, in solo sessions sometimes, in couple sessions at other times, and on some occasions in sessions with the child.

There is a formula to explain the mystery of the parent-child yoking effect (Money, 1984), although prevalence of its applicability remains unascertained. The formula is that parental incompatibility threatens to sever the child's pairbond with the parent who may depart. Then ensues a flip-flop reversal of development identification and complementation of which the sequel is a collusional father-son or mother-daughter alliance. In the epistemology of infantile ideation and imagery, the son becomes a sex-transmuted understudy for the role of the father's mythical boy-wife, and the daughter of the mother's mythical girl-husband. The boy, identifying with his mother, substitutes for her in enticing his father not to leave home. Correspondingly, the girl, identifying with her father, substitutes for him in enticing her mother not to leave. These formulations do not need to be put into words to be useful in counseling.

Residential relocation.   Whereas in cases of child abuse and neglect it is common to relocate a child in a benign domicile, in the case of juvenile gender-identity disorder a change of domicile cannot be legally enforced. There are cases, however, when the tribulations in the home of origin reach such a peak of intensity that domiciliary relocation of the child is indicated—a time-limited "rest cure" at the home of a relative or friend may be arranged.

Support groups.   There are no regional or national support groups for children with gender-identity disorders. By contrast, there are many cross-gender support groups organized by adult transvestites and transsexuals. Nationally and internationally, there is an extensive network of well-organized support groups and political-action groups for gay men and lesbians. For parents there is a very effective national support group—the Federation of Parents and Friends of Lesbians and Gays.

Selecting Optimal Treatment Strategies

In view of the limited number of alternative strategies, selection is on the basis mostly on the availability of a counselor or therapist with at least some training and experience in gender-identity disorder, and preferably in general sexology as well, irrespective of adherence to a particular therapeutic doctrine. Therapeutic doctrine is considered, however, in the case of adolescents and older applicants for sex reassignment. On the basis of medical morals, psychotherapists and counselors are divided into those who do and those who do not make referrals for hormonal and surgical sex reassignment. It is in violation of a patient's rights not to inform that patient of one's sex-reassignment referral policy.

It may also be a violation of a patient's rights if that patient is not informed of the practitioner's policy and preparedness about medications for secondary or associated symptoms, and for making referrals, as indicated.

When the primary strategy is for psychotherapy or counseling, then there may be some shifts of focus—for example, to a pedagogical strategy for the transmission of explicit knowledge of reproduction, sexuality, and HIV transmission; or to a group, roleplaying strategy for assertiveness and social skills training, both in addition to counseling about management and lifestyle rehabilitation for the gender-identity status.

Problems in Carrying Out Interventions

The great naivete of contemporary health care lies in the assumption of compliancy. It is more on target to assume noncompliancy as the basic rule, in both children and parents. At the basis of the high prevalence of noncompliancy is the principle of inexistence—namely, that which is no longer recalled no longer exists.

In the expectation of compliancy, it is easy for the practitioner to take for granted the performance of everyday clinical procedures, oblivious to the fact that they are subjectively experienced and construed as noxious and abusive. The practitioner is then open to a malpractice charge, albeit false, of nosocomial abuse or, more damaging, nosocomial sexual abuse. Psychological procedures, including those of imposed behavior therapy, are not excluded from false charges of nosocomial abuse. Behavior therapy may be construed as a form of tyranny, and a form of being punished or deprived for having an identity the way it is, manifesting itself in the way it does. The tyranny is magnified if it is applied only in the clinic or at school, whereas at home the parents drift into noncompliancy.

The Hippocratic teaching is to do no harm. In the present state of knowledge of juvenile gender-identity disorder, rather than to do harm in carrying out interventions, it is preferable to take an observant and supportive therapeutic role, and to intervene with help when a crisis arises. In addition to being Hippocratically correct, this may also be the currently "politically-correct" thing to do, for there are already adherents of the social constructionist theory who maintain that gender-identity disorders are not disorders at all, and, like a homosexual orientation, need no treatment.

In the litigious climate of present-day health care, among the problems in carrying out interventions one does well never to overlook the possibility of accusations of sexual abuse, either true or false. Thus, it is wise never to be the only occupant of a suite or area when conducting an evaluation or counseling session. Inquiry into sexuo-erotical ideation and imagery may be misconstrued as signifying an illicit invitation, hence the precaution of interviewing with a student or trainee as auditor. Another precaution is to obtain from the patient and/or parents a signed contract of informed consent to undergo the proposed procedures of evaluation and treatment.

The greatest impediment to effective interventions is their cost—the cost of long-term followup, which is imperative, and the cost of having a long-term coordinator to ensure that no stone is left unturned and that the case does not become lost to followup.

Relapse Prevention

All things considered, the function of treatment in gender-identity disorder is not to remediate or cure but rather to ameliorate and rehabilitate. Thus, the concept of relapse, in the sense of becoming worse again after having improved, does not apply to gender-identity disorder, per se. Instead of relapse, the more pertinent term might be *deterioration*. Prevention of the deterioration of health and well-being, applying the general principles of health care and health maintenance, is the long-term ideal.

CASE ILLUSTRATION

Case Description

Stephen was referred for evaluation by the school pupil personnel worker. He had been a good student, with no noted problems, until two years ago when his school grades deteriorated, and he was frequently truant. His outlandish dress and provocative behavior at school was disruptive, in a way that suggested a gender identity conflict.

Stephen was a slender, tall, black male who looked young for his 15 years. There was no evidence of facial hair, and his voice was in a middle range, which did not distinctively connote either gender. Inflectionally and gesturally, however, his mannerisms were exaggeratedly feminine. He would flail his arms away from his body, with limp-wristed gestures, purse his lips, roll his eyes, throw back his head waving his longish hair, and utter supercilious or "campy" remarks. He insisted that the examiner call him Stephanie. He wore some eye makeup, and had clear nail polish on his nails, which varied in length. His clothing was unisex—baggy shirts/blouses with full, pleated pants and pumps. He smelled as if he had just doused himself with a flowery feminine toilet water.

He said that he wanted to be a woman but that nobody understood him and would let him be. He was angry at everybody for not accepting him. He also had periods of severe depression, which he hid from others, and was evasive when asked about suicidal thoughts. He said that he had always felt this way, even as a young child. He had tried to hide it, but it did not work anymore because his femininity was so strong. He was teased and threatened at school. His only friends were a few girls with whom he spent some time. He said that his only sexual experiences were being forced to perform oral sex on some boys who hassled him, and this had occurred in the boys' bathroom at school. He denied any masturbation, claiming this would be homosexual. His whole style of presentation seemed to be intended to shock the evaluator and elicit rejection.

Stephen's mother provided more information about his background history. She had worked for years as a teacher's aide in a daycare center. Her husband had worked for the post office until his sudden death from a stroke when Stephen was 11 years old. Her husband was also a Baptist minister of a small storefront congregation. Family values and sex roles were traditional. The couple had one other child, a girl born before Stephen, who died from sudden crib death.

His mother said that Stephen had always been a quiet, good boy. He did what he was supposed to do and never got in trouble. He was small and did not play with the other neighborhood boys, whom she described as tough bullies. He always had an interest in girls and girls' things. From age 6, she remembered he would help her fix and set her hair. He frequently drew pictures of women in different types of fancy clothing and elaborate hairstyles. He used to dance around the house, miming the songs of black female vocalists like Dianna Ross. He was very creative. He even made some of his own clothes and a few outfits for her, although his taste was much more extreme than her traditional style. She was relieved that he had avoided getting into drugs and drinking like the other neighborhood boys. She was concerned that he had started doing so poorly in school, which she thought was because the other children did not accept him. He had always been truthful with her, but now she was not certain if he was telling lies, although she had no specific examples.

Differential Diagnosis and Assessment

The differential diagnosis was between gender-identity disorder of adolescence, nontranssexual type; or transsexualism; or gender-identity disorder NOS, associated with confusion about homosexual orientation. Transvestic fetishism was ruled out by his self-report denying any masturbation or sexual arousal associated with cross-dressing, although he was not necessarily considered a reliable informant.

Physical examination showed that Stephen was a healthy adolescent, with typically developed male genitalia. His pubertal development, Tanner Stage 5, was consistent with his age. No genital or anal lesions, abrasions, or scars were noted. There was no evidence from blood tests or swabs of sexually transmitted diseases or other diseases, and the HIV test that he consented to was negative.

Because Stephen was seen in a research center, we were able to conduct additional medical tests that might not be routinely feasible to perform in other settings. The karotype was typical 46,XY. The endocrinological evaluation was within normal limits for an adolescent, with no laboratory results suggesting abnormal levels of testosterone or estrogen. This ruled out hermaphroditic syndromes, as well as the possibility that he was illicitly taking "sex hormones." Wrist X-ray showed fusion of the epiphyses, indicating that his statural growth was virtually complete. This information would be useful if hormonal treatment were to be considered. Assessment of fertility was not performed.

Although it is possible to use penile phlethsymography to investigate what sexual stimuli are sexually arousing, we did not consider this. Sexual arousal is difficult to assess reliably in an adolescent. It would not actually contribute information useful for the differential diagnosis for a gender-identity disorder, since many different sexual orientations can coexist with gender identity disorders.

In working with adolescents, the clinician's task is not to tell the adolescent what his or her sexual orientation is but rather to assist the adolescent in determining what type of viable lifestyle can be developed that would include sexual fulfillment. Thus, defining sexual orientation is part of the patient's task, not part of the differential diagnosis of the clinician. When DSM-III-R asks for specification of sexual orientation, this is informational only and based on the patient's self-report—it is not strictly diagnostic information. For the differential diagnosis to be further ascertained, developmentally appropriate experience in the "real-life test" would be necessary.

Treatment Selection

The treatment selected was individual psychotherapy. The therapeutic approach was that of the "real-life test" (Money & Ambinder, 1978). Although our private prognostic hunches were that he was more likely to be homosexual than transsexual, this approach was chosen to help Stephen reach his own definitive conclusion about what would suit him. Since he did not talk about the past, there was little to be accomplished with traditional insight-oriented therapies. His behavior was too defiant and oppositional to even consider the use of behavior therapy. Hormonal treatment would have been premature for this adolescent. Family therapy, with his mother involved, might have been considered if he were much younger, but it is not effective with an adolescent where the issues of gender become so closely intertwined with social and sexual behavior.

Stephen was informed that we would be willing to support him in a trial of living as a female, including eventual referral for administration of hormones when he was 18 years old, if he followed the treatment protocol and was convinced that he was ready to try hormones. We also informed him that if his sexual urges were too strong for him to control, we would be willing to refer him for treatment with Depo-Provera. Issues of confidentiality and social responsibility were also discussed, with a signed agreement of understanding and the written consent of his mother.

Stephen was provided with educational information, including sex education. He was also given rehabilitative support in exploring the different options that were available to help him

develop a lifestyle with which he could cope. He was encouraged to participate in group activities—in this case, free community-based discussion groups instead of costly professionally led therapy groups.

The therapist acted as a case manager. One joint session was held with Stephen and his mother together to explain the situation and proposed plan of rehabilitative treatment. Another conference as well as various phone calls and letters, was held with school personnel.

Treatment Course and Problems in Carrying Out Interventions

It was difficult to develop a therapeutic relationship with Stephen. For the first few sessions, his mother brought him to the appointments and then he came alone. He frequently missed sessions or would reschedule them on brief notice. While there were many pertinent issues in his past history, he remained interested only in discussing the present.

Our approach to therapy was to listen nonjudgmentally, to provide him with sex education and information, and occasionally to share stories in the form of parables about other teenagers who had some experiences similar to his own. Instead of trying to hold him to a regular schedule, we allowed him to schedule the sessions. This reduced the problem of missed appointments, and we were also able to see him for longer appointments if he requested. Instead of discouraging his feminization, we told him that he could come looking as much like a woman as he wanted, and we could even work with him to improve his feminine appearance if he desired.

He adamantly denied being homosexual or being sexually active. We heard from a building security officer that Stephen had sexually solicited him in the men's room, but no further action was taken because the officer was aware he was our patient. We did not confront Stephen with this information, but we did become more proactive in talking about safe sex and condom use. We helped him find out information about a variety of community-based groups, ranging from a transsexual support group to the gay teens discussion group. Although he considered his own presentation as a woman to be better than most of the transsexual support group members, he found the gay teen group more closely related to his interests.

He then admitted that he had been engaged in street hustling dressed as a woman, but that he could do better as a guy. He opened up about sexuality, now admitting that he had not been forced into sex with males at school, but had in fact solicited it. Unfortunately, but not unexpectedly, his behavior had become widely known at his school. He had adopted an angry, rejecting "bitch" approach to try to handle the situation, and still found it almost intolerable to go to school.

School personnel began repeatedly calling our offices, questioning the value of Stephen's treatment with us because his school behavior was getting worse (their code words meaning more feminine and sexually taunting) and he might soon be expelled for excessive truancy. Stephen understood that the school and his mother were getting more upset. He also believed that we were keeping his confidentiality instead of working as covert agents for social conventionality.

Stephen was aware that some of his behavior was illegal. We had informed him of the legal limits of confidentiality in our state, and what type of information we would have to report to authorities if he told us. Whether his behavior skirted the reporting laws, or the extent to which he censored what he told us, could not be determined. Fortunately, we were never in a position where we thought the law required us to report him as a victim of sexual abuse or as a sexual abuser.

We encouraged him to show us his fashion drawings (he had many notebooks full) and some of the clothes he had made. We listened nonjudgmentally as he described his difficulties with school, neither blaming him nor the others but trying to understand the perspectives of all parties. We helped him find out about a different high school program that dealt in fashion design. He began to tone down his social outrageousness and cooperate more at school after he set a goal of transferring into the fashion design program. Although the program had very competitive entrance requirements, he was able to transfer into it and was soon very successful. He developed his own, "far-out" style of dress, which was avante garde but not necessarily feminine.

Outcome and Termination

In the new school program, Stephen ceased to dress in women's clothing and stopped street hustling. He now defined himself as gay, and was able to describe articulately the many difficulties facing gay teenagers. We met with him and his mother, and she became able to accept and support her son as gay. He had a group of male and female friends. Most of his male friends were gay and included some young adult black males who were successful in different aspects of the fashion industry. Through these connections, he obtained a part-time sales job in a retail women's store.

Followup and Maintenance

We considered this to be a successful outcome to therapy. In the course of seeing him about 20 times over three years, after the initial history taking we never did have a chance to further discuss his personal history background. We continue to be available to him, as requested. We would not be surprised to hear from him in the future—perhaps with relationship problems or less likely on the issue of sex change. Our hope is that the risk of homicide, suicide, or AIDS has been reduced as a function of treatment.

SUMMARY

Gender-identity disorders involve transposition or discordancy between the natal sex and the private experience of gender role and the public manifestation of gender identity, to an extent that is incompatible with personal well-being. Individuals with these disorders may make explicit statements about becoming a member of the other sex. In some cases the outcome is transsexualism and sex reassignment in adulthood. Transvestism and gynemimetic syndromes are conditions where there is less than a total transposition of gender identity. In other cases, there may be gender-role nonconformity or homosexuality as an outcome without psychopathology.

Assessment can occur only over a period of

time, utilizing information from a variety of sources. There is no biological marker, test battery, or brief interview protocol for assessment. The "real-life diagnostic test" follows the patient in trying out various aspects of gender roles in attempts to be rehabilitated in a gender identity/role that is psychologically viable.

Treatment may include hormonal and surgical reassignment and social rehabilitation. For children and adolescents, treatment more typically involves individual therapy, sometimes with family or conjugate therapy, without pharmacotherapy. Behavioral and correctional therapies are not known to be effective. Difficulties with patient compliance and possible conflicts with social norms and laws make treatment challenging to manage.

REFERENCES

Blizzard, R. M., Kappy, M. S., & Migeon, C. J. (Eds.). (1993). *Wilkins' diagnosis and treatment of endocrine disorders in childhood and adolescence* (4th ed., rev.). Springfield, IL: Thomas.

Boglioli, L. R., Taff, M. L., Stephens, P. J., & Money, J. (1991). A case of autoerotic asphyxia associated with multiplex paraphilia. *American Journal of Forensic Medicine and Pathology, 12,* 64–73.

Federoff, J. P. (1989). Buspirone hydrochloride in the treatment of transvestic fetishism. *Journal of Clinical Psychiatry, 49,* 408–409.

Green, R. (1986). *"The sissy boy syndrome" and the development of homosexuality.* New Haven, CT: Yale University Press.

Green, R., & Money, J. (1966). Stage-acting, role-taking, and effeminate impersonation during boyhood. *Archives of General Psychiatry, 15,* 535–538.

Money, J. (1968). *Sex errors of the body: Dilemmas, education, counselling.* Baltimore: Johns Hopkins University Press.

Money, J. (1976). Two names, two wardrobes, two personalities. *British Journal of Sexual Medicine, 3,* 18–22.

Money, J. (1984). Gender transposition theory and homosexual genesis. *Journal of Sex and Marital Therapy, 10,* 75–82.

Money, J. (1986). Munchausen's syndrome by proxy: Update. *Journal of Pediatric Psychology, 11,* 583–584.

Money, J. (1986). *Venuses penuses: Sexology, sexosophy, and exigency theory.* Buffalo, NY: Prometheus Books.

Money, J. (1988). *Gay, straight, and in-between: The sexology of erotic orientation.* New York: Oxford University Press.

Money, J. (1988). The skoptic syndrome: Castration and genital self-mutilation as an example of sexual body-image pathology. *Journal of Psychology and Human Sexuality, 1,* 113–128.

Money, J., & Ambinder, D. (1978). Two-year, real-life diagnostic test: Rehabilitation versus cure. In J. P. Brady & H. K. H. Brodie (Eds.), *Controversy in psychiatry* (pp. 833–845). Philadelphia: Saunders.

Money, J., & Annecillo, C. (1987). Crucial period effect in psychoendocrinology: Two syndromes, abuse dwarfism and female (CVAH) hermaphroditism. In M. H. Bornstein (Ed.), *Sensitive periods in development: Interdisciplinary perspectives* (pp. 145–158). Hillsdale, NJ: Erlbaum.

Money, J., Annecillo, C., & Hutchison, J. W. (1985). Forensic and family psychiatry in abuse dwarfism: Munchausen's syndrome by proxy, atonement, and addiction to abuse. *Journal of Sex and Marital Therapy, 11,* 30–40.

Money, J., & Lamacz, M. (1984). Gynemimesis and gynemimetophilia: Individual and cross-cultural manifestations of a gender coping strategy hitherto unnamed. *Comprehensive Psychiatry, 25,* 392–340.

Money, J., & Primrose, C. (1969). Sexual dimorphism in the psychology of male transsexuals. In R. Green & J. Money (Eds.), *Transsexualism and sex reassignment* (pp. 115–131). Baltimore: Johns Hopkins Press.

Money, J., & Russo, A. J. (1979). Homosexual outcome of discordant gender-identity/role in childhood: Longitudinal follow-up. *Journal of Pediatric Psychology, 4,* 29–41.

Money, J., Wainwright, G., & Hingsburger, D. (1991). *The breathless orgasm: A lovemap biography of asphyxiophilia.* Buffalo, NY: Prometheus Books.

Nanda, S. (1990). *Neither man nor woman: The Hijras of India.* Belmont, CA: Wadsworth.

Rees, H. D., Bonsall, R. W., & Michael, R. P. (1986). Preoptic and hypothalamic neurons accumulate [^{3}H]medoxyprogesterone acetate in male cynomolgus monkeys. *Life Sciences, 39,* 1353–1359.

Short, R. V., & Clarke, I. J. (Undated). *Masculinization of the female sheep.* Distributed by MRC Reproductive Biology Unit, 2 Forrest Road, Edinburgh, EHI 2QW, United Kingdom.

Stoller, R. J. (1968). *Sex and gender: On the development of masculinity and femininity.* New York: Science House.

Williams, W. L. (1986). *The spirit in the flesh.* Boston: Beacon Press.

CHAPTER 15

SUBSTANCE USE DISORDERS

Stephanie S. Rude   University of Texas at Austin
John J. Horan   Arizona State University

DESCRIPTION OF DISORDER

Clinical and Associated Features

According to the media, our nation's youth are being swept by an epidemic of drug abuse. Private hospitals encourage parents to watch their adolescents for signs of drug abuse and to respond to warning signs by seeking medical treatment. Even governmental officials voice alarm; and the United States has invested millions of dollars on a "war on drugs."

What is the actual nature and proportion of this problem? It is sometimes difficult to discern amidst the hoopla. First of all, the "drug abuse as epidemic" metaphor obscures the fact that drug use does not appear to be on the rise among either adult or youth populations; in fact, since 1980 there have been some indications of a trend toward modest decreases in the incidence of drug use.

Second, the distinction between *drug use* and *drug abuse* is too often obscured. However desirable it might be that adolescents abstain from *all* drug use, some experimentation appears to be normative and in most cases is not associated with lasting ill effects. Baumrind's (1990) 20-year longitudinal study demonstrated that a very small proportion of those who engage in experimental drug use subsequently become abusers or even regular users. Equating use with abuse is likely to cloud theoretical understanding of substance abuse and interfere with clinical interventions.

As Newcomb and Bentler (1989) pointed out, abuse should probably be viewed as a multidimensional problem. Among the factors to be considered in defining substance abuse are the context of consumption (e.g., use while driving), the toxicity of the substance (e.g., substances such as crack cocaine carry greater dangers regardless of context), individual reaction or sensitivity to the drug (drugs taken at very young ages are more likely to interfere with physical and psychological developmental tasks), and the presence of dependence (e.g., needing the substance to get through the day, experiencing withdrawal effects).

In making these points, it is not our intention to trivialize the problem of youthful substance abuse. The small proportion of youths who regularly use drugs translates into thousands of youths nationwide. And the impact of drug abuse upon the lives of these youths and their families can be profoundly negative and lasting. Most tragic, the consequences of substance abuse are sometimes lethal. This is particularly true of two of the most widely abused drugs in the United States: alcohol and tobacco. Automobile accidents are a leading cause of death among youths in the 15- to 24-year age category and alcohol use is frequently implicated. One study using 1980 data estimated that 37 percent of 15- to 24-year-old drivers in fatal motor vehicle accidents were legally intoxicated (Lowman, 1983). The effects of cigarette smoking, though delayed, are no less deadly; cigarette smoking is the foremost preventable cause of death in the nation (Califano, 1979).

Epidemiology

The most widely used and abused drugs among adolescents are tobacco and alcohol (see Newcomb & Bentler, 1989). Some 92 percent of high school seniors have consumed alcohol at least once in their lives; 66 percent have done so during the previous month. Slightly more than a third acknowledge at least one episode of heavy drinking, and 5 percent report drinking alcohol on a daily basis. About one fifth of seniors reported daily smoking of cigarettes.

A substantial number of adolescents experiment with illegal drugs but a smaller proportion report using these drugs on a regular basis. Data on high school seniors, updated yearly by Johnston and his associates (Johnston, Bachman, & O'Malley, 1989), reveal that students commonly experiment with drugs (47.2 percent have tried marijuana and 12.1 percent cocaine) but that the number of students currently involved with these substances on a monthly or daily basis is substantially smaller (2.7 percent for marijuana and 0.2 percent for cocaine).

On a national level, drug use among adolescents and, indeed, among the general population, has not increased and, for many classes of drugs, has shown some evidence of decline since 1980. The exception during this period was cocaine use, but beginning in 1987, use of cocaine appears to have leveled off if not declined slightly.

Etiology

Despite a huge literature on the correlates of substance abuse, definitive statements about etiology are not warranted. A few well-controlled cross-sectional designs (e.g., Block, Block, & Keys, 1988) and longitudinal studies (e.g., Baumrind, 1990; Shedler & Block, 1990) that relate drug use to personal-social variables measured prior to and independently of drug use provide a reasonable foundation for inferences, although these cannot fully establish causality.

Family and/or Parenting Correlates

A wide variety of family variables appear to contribute to substance abuse among children and adolescents. These include favorable attitudes or actual use of drugs by parents (Harford & Grant, 1986; Newcomb, Chou, Bentler, & Huba, 1988), and less direct influences such as the absence of perceived parental support, excessive permissiveness, chaotic living conditions, family disruption through divorce or separation, and inconsistent parenting styles (Block et al., 1988). It appears that disruption within the family may be less important when strong mutual attachments exist between parents and children (Hawkins, Lishner, Catalono, & Howard, 1986). Moreover, Baumrind (1990) indicated that the presence of such attachments along with coherent and consistent parenting styles are "protective" against substance abuse.

Longitudinal data such as that reported by Shedler and Block (1990) provide convincing evidence for the etiological importance of parenting variables. Shedler and Block found that preschool-aged children who later used drugs on a regular basis had mothers who were rated by clinicians as more "cold, unresponsive, and underprotective . . . [as giving] their children little encouragement, while . . . pressuring and [appearing to be] overly interested in their children's 'performance'" (p. 621) than were mothers of children who later only experimented with drugs.

Peer Group

In correlational studies, peer group variables are among the most consistent predictors of substance use (e.g., Newcomb et al., 1988). In addition, peer group influences have been experimentally demonstrated on alcohol consumption

(Dericco & Garlington, 1977) and in the formation of expressed drug attitudes (Stone & Shute, 1977). There appear to be "drug-specific" peer subcultures that engage in, for example, alcohol or marijuana, and eschew the use of other substitutes (Spieger & Harford, 1987). Peer groups most likely exert an influence through modeling and social reinforcement processes (Harford & Grant, 1986).

Personality Variables

The notion that there is a unitary "addictive personality" is controversial and is rejected by many researchers. There *is* support for the less stringent claim that a variety of personality variables indicating poor adjustment distinguish drug abusers from nonabusers. These include unconventionality or nonconformity with adult societal expectations (Baumrind, 1990), sensation seeking and low self-esteem (Hawkins et al., 1986), and depressed mood (Kashini, Keller, Solomon, Reid, & Mazzola, 1985).

Shedler and Block (1990) observed clear differences between their group of *frequent users* of drugs and *experimenters,* with the former group appearing to be "relatively maladjusted as children." Frequent users had more difficulty forming good relationships and were insecure and anxious. Importantly, these clinical ratings were made early in childhood and were independent of later assessments of drug use.

Biological Factors

Family, twin, and adoption studies have shown a definite familial nature to the development of alcoholism, but the relative influence of genetic and environmental factors has not been established. A recent report by Blum and colleagues (1990) offers evidence for the existence of a biological marker for the development of alcoholism. However, many studies suggest a lack of evidence for the existence of biological factors in alcoholism. The lack of consistency may be due to numerous conceptual and methodological flaws that plague this literature. For example, these include inaccurate determination of zygosity, inadequate diagnostic criteria, inappropriate samples, and poor operational definitions of environmental factors (see Murray, Clifford, & Gurling, 1983, for a review).

DIFFERENTIAL DIAGNOSIS AND ASSESSMENT

DSM-III-R Categorization

The DSM-III-R divides substance use disorder into two categories: psychoactive substance dependence and psychoactive substance abuse. Dependence is defined by patterns of use that suggest lack of volitional control (e.g., using the substance more than intended) and a prominant but negative impact on the individual's life (e.g., interfering with performing obligations, withdrawal from other activities). A diagnosis of psychoactive substance dependence is made when some symptoms of the disturbance have persisted for at least one month or have occurred repeatedly over a longer period of time (as in binge drinking).

Psychoactive substance abuse is diagnosed when the full criteria for dependence are not met but a maladaptive pattern of use is indicated by either continued use despite awareness that a persistent problem (occupational, social, psychological, or physical) is caused or exacerbated by use of the substance, or by recurrent use in situations when use is physically hazardous (e.g., drunk driving).

Abuse and dependence often involve several substances. When criteria are met for more than one drug, the DSM-III-R calls for multiple diagnoses. The polysubstance dependency diagnosis is used only when there is ongoing use of multiple categories of psychoactive substance, no single psychoactive substance predominates, and the dependency criteria *are not* met for any specific substance but only for the group of substances.

Differential Diagnosis

Formal psychological assessments are not appropriate until at least 10 to 14 days after detoxification. However, some preliminary medical treatments and decisions may need to be made prior to this point. For example, patients who are currently under the influence of or withdrawing from several substances—notably alcohol, amphetamines, cocaine, opoids, or sedatives—present potentially serious medical problems that require monitoring and intervention by a physician.

One reason to delay formal assessment is that the acute and residual effects of several substances can be difficult to distinguish from certain other psychological disorders. For example, hallucinogens or chronic use of amphetamines or cocaine may produce symptoms that are similar to those associated with psychotic disorders. in some but not all cases, toxicological analyses can aid in identifying acute drug effects.

Drug use may accompany depressive or anxiety disorders as well as personality disorders. Conduct disorder and, later in life, antisocial personality disorder are particularly likely to be accompanied by substance use. Hence, substance-abusing adolescents should be carefully evaluated for other psychological conditions such as the above once the effects of substance abuse have subsided.

Assessment Strategies

There are two broad goals of assessment in the treatment of drug-abusing adolescents. First, the clinician needs to know about the substance use itself—what substances have been consumed in what quantities and with what frequencies? It is also helpful to determine circumstances associated with consumption, the nature of impairment, if any, and the degree to which the client perceives the presence of a problem. This information is relevant to determining whether or not the substance use is problematic, how great a problem it represents, whether it warrants treatment, and what sorts of treatment might be appropriate.

Second, in order to further inform treatment plans, the clinician will need to assess factors that seem to be involved in maintaining substance abuse and those that might help encourage positive alternative behaviors. Here, we believe that it is important to focus assessment on empirically based mediators of substance abuse (e.g., family environment, interpersonal skills, self-acceptance) that are potentially modifiable by treatment. This

will involve taking account of the resources, both personal and environmental, on which an intervention can be built.

Tarter (1990) recently proposed a system of assessment for use in clinical decision making about adolescent substance users in which initial screening assesses a broad range of domains and guides decisions about more in-depth assessment. Although Tarter's proposed system was more comprehensive than what will typically be required, clinicians may find it useful to adopt components of this approach.

An initial step in assessment involves collecting broad-based information relevant to the two goals mentioned previously—determining the nature and pattern of the substance use itself and identifying areas of functioning that may play a role either in maintaining substance use behavior or in an intervention. For this purpose, Tarter developed the Drug Use Screening Inventory (DUSI), a self-administered questionnaire that inquires about substance use *and* about functioning in nine other domains, each chosen for etiological relevance to substance abuse treatment: Behavior Patterns, Health Status, Psychiatric Disorder, Social and Personal Competence, Family Interactions, School Adjustment, Work Skills and Orientation, Peer Relationships, and Recreation.

Several of these domains particularly warrant the clinician's attention, and thus the DUSI may be supplemented with other devices. For example, the clinician should strive to gain as thorough an understanding of the pattern of substance abuse as possible. This information can be gained through an interview or from self-report scales, such as used by Johnston and his colleagues (e.g., Johnston et al., 1989) in their annual national surveys. Alternatively, the Michigan Alcohol Screening Test (MAST; Selzer, 1971) is a rapid and inexpensive device for assessing alcohol-related problems. Likewise, the Alcohol Use Inventory (AUI; Horn, Wanberg, & Foster, 1983) has received some acclaim as a multivariate, differential-diagnostic instrument.

Evidence from a variety of sources suggests the importance of assessment in three other areas: family interactions, personal decision-making ability, and social skills. The family should be be regarded not only as a possible influence maintaining adolescent substance abuse behavior but also as a potential resource that can be mobilized in treatment. In particular, it may be useful to determine whether the parents are effectively monitoring the youth's behavior and are applying contingencies consistently.

The adolescent's personal decision-making skills have been implicated in the etiology of substance abuse and have been taught as components of successful programs for preventing substance abuse. Finally, social skills and peer relationships are among the most important dimensions to assess. Peer relationship variables are consistent predictors of substance abuse. And social skills training, a means for making a positive impact on the peer variables that are implicated in substance abuse, is probably the best documented intervention for reducing future drug use.

Because substance abuse is likely to co-occur with other psychological disturbances, it is recommended that a structured diagnostic interview be part of the assessment process. The Kiddie-Schedule for Affective Disorders and Schizophrenia (K-SADS; Puig-Antich & Chambers, 1978) is widely used for this purpose and has the advantages of flexibility (in providing for tailoring of the degree of probing into various areas) and the availability of parent and child forms for assessing consensus.

TREATMENT

Evidence for Prescriptive Treatment

The literature on the prevention and treatment of substance use contains a diverse array of philosophies and procedures. However, several reviews (e.g., Davidge & Forman, 1988; Horan & Harrison, 1981) have pointed out that, despite the profusion of programs, relatively few are theoretically coherent; even fewer have been evaluated using standard experimental procedures.

Behavior Therapy

Information-based interventions are consistent with the behavioral practice of providing indi-

viduals with the knowledge necessary to evaluate the consequences of their actions. Nevertheless, empirical studies of information-based approaches suggest a disappointing impact on subsequent drug use behavior (Bangert-Drowns, 1988; Horan & Harrison, 1981). It should be noted, however, that most studies on which impact has been evaluated have been methodologically inadequate. Moreover, the approach has perhaps not been given a fair test, since many of the information-based programs that have been evaluated have been replete with credibility-damaging misinformation.

Several studies have provided support for assertion training programs in reducing subsequent drug use in adolescent and preadolescent students. A study by Horan and Williams (1982) exemplifies an intervention approach that weds prescriptive and preventive strategies. Horan and Williams identified 72 nonassertive junior high students (presumably at greater risk of succumbing to peer pressure to use drugs) and randomly assigned them to assertion training or to placebo discussions on peer pressure, or to no treatment. Assertion training employed modeling and guided practice and focused on developing students' competence for saying no in both drug-related and nondrug-related situations with peers. In addition to showing highly significant gains on behavioral and psychometric measures of assertiveness and decreased willingness to use alcohol and marijuana at posttest compared with the control groups, experimental subjects continued to display higher levels of assertiveness, and most importantly, less actual drug use at a three-year followup.

Botvin and colleagues (e.g., Botvin, Baker, Renick, Filazzola, & Botvin, 1984; Botvin, Renick, & Baker, 1983) developed and tested a 20-session cognitive-behavioral life-skills curriculum. The curriculum includes material concerning the consequences of substance use, decision making, resisting social influences to engage in substance use, interpersonal skills, and assertiveness (Botvin, Baker, Dusenburg, Tortu, & Botvin, 1990). In the 1984 large-scale implementation of their program involving 1,311 junior high students from 10 schools, significant effects were produced by carefully selected and closely supervised older peers from the tenth and eleventh grades. Whereas a teacher-led version of their program produced significant effects with students in the 1983 study, it failed to do so in the 1984 evaluation. The authors suggested that the problem may have been due to "implementation failure" on the part of the teachers. They successfully attended to this problem in a more recent large-scale field test involving 4,466 students and two methods of teacher training (Botvin et al., 1990).

The classic comprehensive behavioral approach to addictions treatment (e.g., Miller & Eisler, 1977) includes three objectives: (1) decrease the immediate reinforcing properties of drugs through, for example, aversion therapies and medications such as methadone; (2) teach alternative behaviors; and (3) rearrange the environment so that reinforcement occurs for being "off" drugs. Marlatt's model (e.g., Marlatt & Donovan, 1981) also implies the need for problem-solving skills and cognitive restructuring. The latter is employed to challenge erroneous beliefs about the effects of drugs.

Two case studies report success in using contingency contracting to reduce polydrug abuse (Frederiksen, Jenkins, & Carr, 1976) and alcohol and marijuana abuse (Cook & Petersen, 1985). Unfortunately, controlled research on the effectiveness of specific treatment programs for young addicts is rare. The only controlled experimental evaluation of a behavioral treatment for substance abuse that we are aware of was conducted by Smith (1983), who evaluated a school-based group treatment for adolescent marijuana abusers. The eight-session group program included drug information, problem-solving skills training, interpersonal skills training, and self-monitoring of marijuana use. Compared with the control students, the 10 adolescents who were randomly assigned to the experimental program showed fewer school absences, higher grade point averages, fewer friends using marijuana, and less self-reported abuse of marijuana.

Other approaches to addictions treatment include self-help derivatives of Alcoholics Anonymous. Although behavior principles are rarely if ever articulated in these literatures, they are nevertheless discernible:

A behavioral analysis shows that these groups provide a potently reinforcing group atmosphere which does not tolerate drug or alcohol abuse. New, more adaptive patterns of behavior are encouraged and reinforced through group approval and increased status within the group. Drinking buddies and addicted friends are replaced with more appropriate role models exhibiting complete abstinence. The fact that the "helping agents" were once abusers of drugs or alcohol and therefore represent successful coping models may foster imitation of their behavior and enhance their reinforcing value. (Miller & Eisler, 1977, p. 392)

Pharmacotherapy

The use of pharmacological agents as adjuncts to the treatment of adolescent substance use disorders is not without controversy. A conservative approach to the use of pharmacological agents with children and adolescents seems warranted because of possible unanticipated effects of drugs on growth and development. In addition, there is potential irony in treating drug abuse with yet more drugs, and the implicit message to the client should be taken into account when the use of pharmacological agents is being considered. Having made these qualifications, the use of pharmacological aids to treatment may be indicated in some specific situations. In particular, pharmacotherapy may be necessary to prevent dangerous withdrawal reactions to certain substances as discussed previously under Assessment Strategies. In addition, pharmacotherapy *may* be indicated if the substance abuse is intractable because of a strong physical dependency, as may be the case in addiction to heroine, alcohol, or nicotine.

Two classes of drugs are most often used in treating substance abuse: *Antagonists* block the reinforcing efect of drugs by inhibiting neurotransmission; *agonists* mimic the substance being abused at the neurotransmitter level, creating reinforcing effects similar to those of the abused drug or at least preventing aversive withdrawal effects (Carlson, 1988).

Pharmacological adjuncts are typically specific to the type of substance that is being abused; and within a given abuse category, different pharmacological agents may be used for different purposes. For example, chlordiazepozide purportedly prevents alcohol withdrawal symptoms, whereas antabuse produces nausea if followed by alcohol ingestion. With heroin addicts, methadone is frequently used (Schuster, 1986). Other pharmacological adjuncts to the treatment of opiate addiction includes naltrexone — an antagonist that purportedly inhibits the reinforcing properties of opiates — and buprenorphine, a mixed agonist-antagonist that is said to prevent withdrawal and simultaneously block the opiate's reinforcing properties.

Nicotine gum seems to be an effective adjunct to smoking treatment programs (Lam, Sze, Sacks, & Chalmers, 1987). However, data supporting its use as an adjunct to simple medical advice are less convincing (Russell, Merriman, Stapleton, & Taylor, 1983).

Alternative Treatments

Family interaction variables have received strong support as precursors to adolescent substance abuse (e.g., Block et al., 1988). Two approaches to family-level intervention merit discussion due to their relatively wide implementation and the fact that some controlled outcome research on these approaches exists. These are behavioral family therapy and family systems theory approaches.

Although a variety of treatment strategies are included under the rubric of *behavioral family therapy,* all have several features in common. First, they emphasize the need to define specific target behaviors and specify observable indices of improvement. Second, they employ direct observation (in session or in the home or school) and functional analyses to identify the antecedent and consequent events that maintain target behaviors. Third, they focus on teaching skills that are intended to promote independence from therapeutic assistance and thereby further the maintenance and generalization of treatment benefits.

Behavioral family therapy is also likely to employ training in communication and problem-solving skills and contingency contracting; these procedures have successfully improved family harmony and child behavior (e.g., Frederiksen et al., 1976). A good deal of behavioral skills training is also directed toward parents since they have control or potential control over many of the contingencies that affect their children's behavior.

The problem of keeping individuals in therapy and promoting regular attendance is particularly difficult in family therapy. Patterson, Reid, Jones, and Conger (1975) suggested checking in with the family by telephone several times per week. Other family therapists have suggested making home visits, which are phased out gradually, providing small fee incentives for therapeutic compliance, and using reinforcement for improved session attendance and homework compliance.

Family systems theorists propose that adolescent problems can best be understood and treated by attending to the characteristics of the family. Many of the concepts and treatment strategies employed by family systems therapists are similar to or at least compatible with behavior therapy approaches but not all have not been articulated in behavior therapy. For example, systems theorists pay attention to the process by which the therapist gains access to and influence within the family system. This is important since a low proportion of families who make initial contact actually enter therapy. The family systems therapist may attempt to "join" with the family in order to create a therapeutic alliance and a commitment to treatment. Strategies for doing so include (cf. Stanton, Todd, and associates, 1982) contacting the family within three days of having obtained permission, delivering a nonblaming message to each family member, and presenting the rationale for family treatment in such a way that refusal seems tantamount to endorsing the drug abuser's continued addiction (Bry, 1988). Szapocznik and colleagues (1988) obtained an engagement rate of 93 percent (compared with 42 percent in the control group) by using such strategies.

Once the family has been brought into treatment, the therapist directs them to interact during the session so that it is possible to "discover recurring behavioral sequences, alliances, unspoken family rules, etc., that are maintaining the status quo" (Bry, 1988, p. 41). Dysfunctional system/behavior relationships are then addressed through a variety of additional strategies such as reframing and paradoxical instructions. Reframing (cf. cognitive restructuring) involves explaining a characteristic interaction pattern in a new, more positive way that is compatible with the family's value system. For example, a father's criticism of his adolescent son's drinking behavior might be reframed by the therapist as an expression of concern and an attempt, albeit ineffective, to protect the son. The objective of the interpretation is to alter the interaction sequence by altering the meaning interpretations made by the participants. Theoretically, this will disrupt the son's characteristic interpretation of his father's behavior as signaling disrespect and hostility and will help the father to realize the ineffectiveness of his characteristic behavior while commending his goal of protecting his son.

Paradoxical instruction typically involves prescribing of symptoms. For example, a mother and adolescent daughter who engage in frequent heated arguments might be instructed to make a point of avoiding any consideration of the other's perspective whatsoever. The therapist might stress to both that it is essential that neither be distracted by the slightest attention to understanding the other's feelings or views. Purposefully engaging in symptomatic behavior theoretically strips it of its former function and allows individuals to experience control over it. Kolko and Milan (1983) found that the addition of reframing and paradoxical instruction to a modified token economy intervention reduced previously intractable drug use, school failure, and absenteeism problems.

Once the problematic family system has been destabilized, techniques may be used to restructure the system in more adaptive ways. For example, boundaries within the family may be clarified by establishing rules regarding communication (e.g., allowing family members to express views without interruption) and privacy (e.g., negotiating rights to privacy that the adolescent has or can earn) (Bry, 1988; Stanton et al., 1982).

Although controlled evaluations of family systems therapy are rare, Stanton and colleagues (1982) reported that three different intensities of family intervention, including a relatively weak weekly family trip to the movies, all resulted in less drug use in the identified patient than a traditional individual treatment. An additional treatment effect was a higher percentage of days employed or in school.

Selecting Optimal Treatment Strategies

Despite the need for research on the matching of adolescent substance abusers to appropriate treatments, few studies have provided us with empirically based guidelines. Simpson and Selles (1982) found no interactions between client variables and treatment settings. However, Vaglum and Fossheim (1980) reported that abusers of particular drugs responded differentially to various forms of treatment. Family therapy, followed by individual psychotherapy, was most strongly correlated with reductions in psychedelic drug use, whereas confrontive milieu therapy was negatively correlated with outcome. Conversely, confrontive milieu therapy was strongly correlated with favorable outcomes for opiate and central nervous system stimulant users, followed by family therapy and individual psychotherapy. However, this pattern of results does not lend itself to straightforward interpretation, and since this was a quasi-experimental design, firm conclusions should await replication.

In the absence of evidence supporting the prescriptive value of particular treatments based on client profiles, we must combine what we know about factors that underlie substance abuse problems with what we know about how to produce specific types of behavior change. Accordingly, we propose several questions to guide decisions about treatment.

What Should Be the Treatment Foci?

We suggest that this question be addressed through an assessment scheme that is broad based but that gives particular attention to etiologically important variables, such as family interactions and social skills. The clinician should look for contingencies that may be altered to maintain desired drug-free behaviors. Adolescent drug use may provide negative reinforcement, as when it allows the adolescent to escape unpleasant circumstances (e.g., conflictual family relationships). Alternatively, drug use may provide positive reinforcements, ranging from drug-induced euphoria, to status among peers, to parental concern and attention (as when drug abuse functions as a cry for help). In addition, deficient information about drugs or deficient skills (e.g., assertiveness, decision making) for declining their use may leave an adolescent vulnerable to succumbing to the rewards that may be offered by substance use. These factors can be addressed by the psychosocial skills interventions discussed previously (e.g., assertiveness and decision-making skills training) and by interventions to improve family functioning.

Should the Family Be Brought into Treatment?

It is important to evaluate the role of family interactions in maintaining substance use and in supporting treatment. The etiological role of family variables in adolescent substance abuse is well supported by research. Even in cases where the family seems not to play an important etiological role in the substance abuse, it is likely to be an important source of contingencies and may be mobilized in a treatment plan.

Is Group Therapy Warranted?

In addition to offering the possibility for greater cost effectiveness, group treatment offers particular treatment advantages (cf. Cook & Petersen, 1985). Groups may provide adolescents with relevant peer coping models, with powerful social reinforcements for decreased drug use, and with the opportunity to test perceptions and to experiment with new behaviors in a relatively safe environment.

What Treatment Setting Is Most Appropriate?

There is a lack of consensus about the relative effectiveness of inpatient as compared with outpatient treatment. Detoxification from certain substances, including heavy and chronic alcohol abuse, may require hospitalization because of the importance of medical treatment at this stage. In addition, Cook and Petersen (1985) have noted:

> Residential treatment may be necessary for the client who requires a structured environment because he or she tends to act out, lacks adequate internal controls, or requires a brief period of separation from his or her usual environment. By contrast, a youth with a relatively intact family and other supportive relationships may be more suitable for outpatient care. (p 82)

Problems in Carrying Out Interventions

In addition to the obstacles that are likely to be faced in carrying out any psychological intervention, several problems are especially likely to arise in the treatment of substance abuse. First, adolescents who are brought in for treatment (by parents or the courts) will not always recognize their substance use as problematic. In such cases, an important and early treatment goal may be to change the client's perceptions toward greater awareness of the problems and dangers of their substance abuse. Interventions that make use of peer feedback and support may be useful toward this end.

Obtaining accurate self-reports of substance use from the adolescent may be a formidable challenge. Honest reporting during the initial assessment phase may be facilitated by assurances that details of prior use will not be shared unnecessarily with parents or other authorities. However, this is a thorny area in which the clinician is advised to proceed carefully and with ample forethought. In some situations, withholding information from parents is illegal and/or unethical. This is particularly so when the youth's behavior poses an imminent threat to his or her well-being. In other situations, assurances of confidentiality may simply be clinically inadvisable. The therapist must be careful to avoid the perception by the child that the two are colluding to keep the parents in the dark. In the context of family therapy, such a confidentiality arrangement can be at odds with what is often an important goal—that of strengthening parental monitoring and authority. In most cases it will be important for the clinician to corroborate the adolescent's self-reports with parent and teacher reports of behavior.

Finally, one of the most formidable challenges to effective treatment occurs when the adolescent's family is severely dysfunctional and is unresponsive or unavailable to treatment. In such cases the best strategy may be to try to bring the youth's behavior under the control of a nondrug-abusing peer group. This may be accomplished by involving the youth in an outpatient treatment group that uses the social influence and support of the peer group to facilitate prosocial behavior and abstinence from drugs.

Relapse Prevention

Modification of the environment in which the client operates is important for relapse prevention. This can include helping the adolescent to avoid association with drug-abusing friends and modifying interactions within the family so that the family helps to maintain changes in substance use behavior. Another strategy likely to be useful in preventing relapse is to phase out treatment contact and to include followup booster sessions. Booster sessions, in which the skills focused on during therapy are reviewed and polished, have been established as helpful in the maintenance of a variety of behavior changes (e.g., McDonald & Budd, 1983).

CASE ILLUSTRATION

Case Description

Dirk is a 14-year-old Caucasian male from a middle class-family. His mother contacted the therapist in response to Dirk having been picked up by the police for driving under the influence of alcohol and without a license. For a few months prior to this incident, his parents reported having suspected drug abuse and were concerned that he had fallen in with a bad crowd. They noted that over the past year he had grown sullen and withdrawn at home and, although he had previously been an average student, he had failed two classes during the previous term.

Differential Diagnosis and Assessment

Assessment was conducted during an initial interview in which the therapist met with Dirk and his parents, separately and together, and also during a two-hour session in which Dirk completed written inventories.

During the first meeting, the therapist solicited the perceptions of each family member as to what the problem was and what factors contributed to it. Examples of how discipline and disagreements were handled were sought, and interactions between family members during the interview were observed. The separate meeting with the parents was used to assess whether or not the parents functioned well enough as a couple to be able to work together effectively as parents.

In the initial meeting, the therapist noted several features of the family interaction. Dirk was passive, withdrawn, and sullen. Dirk's father, although seeming to be well intentioned and genuinely concerned about Dirk's welfare, came across in a blustering, authoritarian manner. For example, he commented that he thought Dirk should be "locked up" in an inpatient program but that, at the insistence of his wife, he was willing to "try this" first. Dirk's mother seemed to be working to avoid conflict between Dirk and his father.

During the second session, Dirk completed the Drug Use Screening Inventory (DUSI). The therapist went over his responses with him, tentatively identifying several problem areas, and then conducted a diagnostic interview. Dirk's pattern of substance abuse consisted primarily of episodes of heavy alcohol consumption. He reported 2 to 3 incidents per month, occurring over the past 5 to 6 months, in which he had become intoxicated from a large quantity of hard liquor; on two occasions he had passed out. This drinking was always in the company of the same two friends — boys one to two years older than himself. However, on a recent occasion he had become intoxicated while alone. This last episode seemed to have occurred in response to an argument with his father. Dirk had also smoked marijuana on several occasions and had used inhalants twice. Dirk did not meet diagnostic criteria for any Axis I or Axis II disorders other than alcohol abuse. However, the therapist noted subclinical levels of depression and social anxiety.

Although some experimentation with alcohol is a normative (albeit often risky) event among adolescents, Dirk's pattern of use was a concern because he seemed to exercise so little control over his drinking. He drank very heavily and showed a lack of prudence regarding where and when he drank (e.g., driving while intoxicated). His experimentation with inhalants was also a source of concern because inhalants can cause neurological damage.

Treatment Selection

Once the therapist had formulated tentative recommendations for the focus of the treatment, these recommendations were put before the family and fleshed out in a series of discussions. A detailed contract was negotiated among the family members in order to structure and provide incentives for changes in the behavior of each party.

Four major targets for intervention were identified. First, the therapist noted that Dirk seemed to lack information about the effects of various substances. For example, he was unaware of dangers associated with inhalant use. Hence, the provision of information about drug effect was selected as one component of the treatment.

A second intervention target was Dirk's passive behavior. He went along with what others suggested to him much of the time. When Dirk did make a decision on his own, it was often made fairly impulsively and with little reflection. The components of treatment selected to address these deficits were training in personal decision making and assertiveness to help him recognize his right to exercise control over his own behavior and develop the skills to do so.

A third intervention target was Dirk's tendency to defy his parents in indirect ways. The therapist hypothesized that the noncompliant behavior exhibited by Dirk, which ranged from failing to follow through with chores to abusing drugs, were reinforced by making Dirk feel autonomous and adult-like. Hence, a treatment goal was to teach

Dirk more effective strategies for asserting his autonomy and receiving respect. The decision-making and assertion training treatment components discussed above were expanded to include this target. In addition, communications training with Dirk and his family was planned. This training would teach Dirk to express his desires for autonomy more directly and would encourage his parents to accept and reinforce appropriate expressions of autonomy.

Finally, a fourth target was Dirk's shyness and anxiety in dealing with his peers. His anxiety seemed to make him more eager to win approval by joining in substance use. The expanded assertion training component also included skills for developing friendships.

Contingency Contracting with the Family

The contract included a set of rules that restricted Dirk's activities and thereby limited his opportunity to engage in drug use. It also provided incentives for his participation in the treatment program. The rules were initially fairly restrictive, providing Dirk with little freedom and requiring him to keep his parents closely apprised of his whereabouts. This was seen as appropriate because Dirk had not demonstrated an ability to manage his behavior responsibly. However, a number of steps were built into the contract through which Dirk could earn increased freedom by demonstrating his ability to handle it effectively. Other rewards for desired behaviors were built into the contract as well. An emphasis was placed on rewards that involved interaction between Dirk and his parents, particularly his father with whom he had not spent much time previously. For example, one reward involved attending a basketball game with his father.

Drug Information

Because Dirk had shown a lack of awareness of the consequences of various drugs, the therapist assigned information for him to read and discuss. In the spirit of encouraging a skeptical, empirical attitude, the therapist encouraged him to seek independent verification of this information.

Problem-Solving Training

The goals of this training were to improve Dirk's actual skills in problem solving and decision making, which seemed to be deficient, and to help him become aware of his ability to exercise control over his life. Several individual sessions were spent instructing Dirk in the use of a structured problem-solving/decision-making model (a variation of the approach outlined by D'Zurilla and Goldfried [1971]), and practicing its application, with an emphasis on drug use situations.

Social-Skills Training

The goals of this training were to help Dirk act on his decisions (e.g., decisions to not use drugs) in the face of peer pressure and to help him interact more comfortably and more frequently with peers. Both were areas in which Dirk showed deficiencies. The treatment of choice was a social skills training group with other adolescents. The advantage of this format was that it would give Dirk a chance to practice behaviors and get feedback from peers. In the absence of such a group, the therapist engaged Dirk in roleplays of assertiveness situations and in friendship-building exchanges and assigned between-sessions practice.

Communication Skills Training

A primary goal of this training was to develop more rewarding interactions within the family. The rationale was that family disharmony contributed to Dirk's drug-abusing behavior in two ways. First, it seemed to function as an antecedent condition for his using drugs to express his anger and independence. Second, it impaired his parents' ability to function as sources of positive influence over his conduct.

The training focused on teaching Dirk respectful, assertive methods for expressing his wishes and feelings. Dirk's father was encouraged to respond more positively to his son's appropriate behavior and to listen attentively to Dirk's expressed concerns. Both parents were encouraged to state contingencies clearly, to enforce them consistently, and to work as a team. The family practiced problem solving during sessions, with the therapist focusing on helping Dirk participate constructively and on helping the parents consider Dirk's contributions without relinquishing final decision-making power.

Treatment Course and Problems in Carrying Out Interventions

Several features of this case contributed to a successful outcome. The fact that the family was capable of functioning at a high level was important. Though the parents' behavior was not effective when they entered therapy, they were highly motivated and responded well to intervention.

A crucial challenge that the therapist faced was making use of the parents' motivation to bring about some relatively rapid symptom relief. This involved balancing the need to effectively restrain Dirk's continued drug abuse and to set the machinery in motion for Dirk to learn and be rewarded for exercising more independent self-management.

An element of the treatment that seemed especially useful was the rewards that were selected to reinforce Dirk's behavior. Here, the benefit of involving the whole family in fleshing out the treatment plan paid off. These discussions led to the selection of rewards that seemed therapeutic in and of themselves. Specifically, the use of activities that were mutually valued by Dirk and his father seemed to strengthen their relationship. Further, these activities provided Dirk with opportunities to practice a more adult role and to experience feeling independent and being taken seriously (as opposed to being treated like a child), which were important alternatives to the defiant drug-using behaviors he had previously used.

However, the foundation of treatment, without which it probably could not have proceeded, was the contingency contract with the family. The importance of the contract to the success of treatment was matched by the difficulty of instituting it and keeping it functioning. During the first few weeks of therapy it was necessary to renegotiate the contract on several occasions. In one case, an emergency session had to be convened. The fact that the therapist was able to model persistence and confidence that the conflicts within the family could be resolved may have been an important factor in the family's persistence.

Outcome and Termination

After three months of treatment, the therapist met with the entire family to review progress and to decide whether termination was appropriate. Dirk showed marked improvements in decision making and in taking responsibility for himself. He reported not having used substances since the onset of treatment. Although no specific methods were used to verify Dirk's reports regarding substance use, his parents and the therapist were fairly confident that his reports were truthful for the following reasons: First, Dirk, had not previously shown a strong inclination to deceive his parents or much skill in doing so. Second, interactions within the family had become noticeably more positive and Dirk had begun to talk about himself and his future plans in ways that suggested enhanced self-esteem and greater harmony between his own personal goals and those of his parents. As a final step in treatment, the family brainstormed ways that they could encourage his continued progress.

Followup and Maintenance

A followup session was scheduled for six weeks from the final session for the purpose of checking in and reviewing progress. At the therapist's suggestion, the family formulated a list of behaviors that they would focus on practicing in the interim. These included a commitment by the parents to continue applying predetermined contingencies to Dirk's behavior. This involved a special effort on the part of Dirk's mother to resist the temptation to "make exceptions" when things seemed to be going smoothly, and a special effort on the part of Dirk's father to make approving comments to his son. For Dirk's part, the challenge was to continue exercising the problem-solving skills and assertive behaviors he had learned in therapy. The therapist encouraged the family to come in if they experienced crises or unexpected difficulties.

At the six-week followup, the family continued to be functioning well. They had decided on their own to relax some of the formal contingencies on Dirk's behavior and had done so without notable problems. The one area of continuing concern for Dirk and for the therapist was that he continued to be somewhat socially anxious and unassertive with his peers. However, he elected not to seek further therapy.

SUMMARY

Although substance abuse among children and adolescents is a serious problem, much misinformation exists. Alarmist perspectives that falsely claim increases in youthful substance abuse and that fail to discriminate between abuse and experimentation with drugs may obscure both the problem and the solutions.

Among the variables that are implicated in the etiology of substance abuse are disturbed family relationships, the modeling of drug abuse by adult family members or the peer group, poor self-esteem, and poor relationships with peers. Substance abuse frequently occurs in conjunction with other problems such as anxiety, depression, poor school performance, and juvenile delinquency.

There is a paucity of careful empirical research on treatments for substance abuse and even less on factors involved in tailoring treatments to individuals. The most promising prevention programs focus on social skills training or on an array of skills, including social skills, personal coping, and problem solving. Given the compatibility of these programs with etiological models that point to poor peer relationships, poor self-esteem, and emotional distress as important contributory factors, it makes sense that they be used in treatment as well as preventative contexts.

Although good data on what treatments are best for particular individuals have not been collected, logic suggests a careful broad-based assessment to identify factors that seem to play a role in maintaining substance abuse and an intervention plan to target these factors. When possible, including the family as at least an adjunct to treatment is indicated.

REFERENCES

Bangert-Drowns, R. L. (1988). The effects of school-based substance abuse education—A meta-analysis. *Journal of Drug Education, 18,* 243–265.

Baumrind, D. (1990, February). *Types of adolescent substance users: Antecedent and concurrent family and personality influences.* Paper presented for the Department of Psychology, Arizona State University, Tempe.

Block, J., Block, J., & Keys, S. (1988). Longitudinally foretelling drug usage in adolescence: Early childhood personality and environmental precursors. *Child Development, 59,* 336–355.

Blum, K., Noble, E. P., Sheridan, P. J., Montgomery, A., Ritchie, T., Jagadeeswaran, P., Nogami, H., Briggs, A. H., & Cohn, J. B. (1990). Allelic association of human dopamine D2 receptor gene in alcoholism. *Journal of the American Medical Association, 263,* 2055–2059.

Botvin, G. J., Baker, E., Dusenbury, L., Tortu, S., & Botvin, E. (1990). Preventing adolescent drug abuse through a multimodal cognitive-behavioral approach: Results of a 3-year study. *Journal of Consulting and Clinical Psychology, 58,* 437–446.

Botvin, G. J., Baker, E., Renick, N. L., Filazzola, A. D., & Botvin, E. M. (1984). A cognitive-behavioral approach to substance abuse prevention. *Addictive Behaviors, 9,* 137–147.

Botvin, G. J., Renick, N. L., & Baker, E. (1983). The effects of scheduling format and booster sessions on a broad-spectrum psychosocial smoking prevention program. *Journal of Behavioral Medicine, 6,* 359–379.

Bry, H. H. (1988). Family-based approaches to reducing adolescent substance use: Theories, techniques, and findings. in E. R. Rahdert & J. Grabowski (Eds.), *Adolescent drug abuse: Analyses of treatment research.* National Institute on Drug Abuse Research Monograph #77.

Califano, J. A. (1979). The secretary's forward. In U.S. Public Health Service, *Smoking and health: A report of the surgeon general.* (Department of Health Education and Welfare, U.S. Public Health Service Publication No. 79-50066). Washington, DC: U.S. Government Printing Office.

Carlson, N. R. (1988). *Foundations of physiological psychology.* Boston: Allyn Bacon.

Cook, P. S., & Petersen, R. C. (1985). Individualizing adolescent drug abuse treatment. In A. S. Friedman & G. M. Beschner (Eds.), *Treatment services for adolescent substance abusers.* National Institute on Drug Abuse, DHHS Publication No. (ADM) 85-1342.

Davidge, A. M., & Forman, S. G. (1988). Psychological treatment of adolescent substance abusers. *Children and Youth Services Review, 10,* 43–55.

Dericco, D. A., & Garlington, W. K. (1977). The effect of modeling and disclosure of experimenter's intent on drinking rate of college students. *Addictive Behaviors, 2,* 135–139.

D'Zurilla, T. J., & Goldfried, M. R. (1971). Problem-solving behavior modification. *Journal of Abnormal Psychology, 78,* 107–126.

Frederiksen, L. W., Jenkins, J. O., & Carr, C. R. (1976). Indirect modification of adolescent drug abuse using contingency contracting. *Journal of Behavior Therapy and Experimental Psychiatry, 7,* 377–378.

Harford, T. C., & Grant, B. F. (1986). Psychosocial factors in adolescent drinking contexts. *Journal of Studies on Alcohol, 48,* 551–557.

Hawkins, J. D., Lishner, D. M., Catalano, R. F., & Howard, M. O. (1986). Childhood predictors of adolescent substance abuse: Toward an empirically grounded theory. *Journal of Children in Contemporary Society, 18,* 11–48.

Horan, J. J., & Harrison, R. P. (1981). Drug abuse by children and adolescents: Perspectives on incidence, etiology, assessment, and prevention programming. In B. B. Lahey & A. E. Kazdin (Eds.), *Advances in clinical child psychology* (Vol. 4, pp. 283–330). New York: Plenum.

Horan, J. J., & Williams, J. M. (1982). Longitudinal study of assertion training as a drug abuse prevention strategy. *American Educational Research Journal, 19,* 341–351.

Horn, J. L., Wanberg, K. W., & Foster, F. M. (1983). *Guidelines for understanding alcohol use and abuse: The Alcohol Use Inventory (AUI).* Baltimore, MD: PsychSystems.

Johnston, L., Bachman, J., & O'Malley, P. (1989). Press release, University of Michigan, Ann Arbor, February 28.

Kashini, J. H., Keller, M. B., Solomon, N., Reid, J. C., & Mazzola, D. (1985). Double depression in adolescent substance users. *Journal of Affective Disorders, 8,* 153–157.

Kolko, D. J., & Milan, M. A. (1983). Reframing and paradoxical instruction to overcome "resistance" in the treatment of delinquent youths: A multiple baseline analysis. *Journal of Consulting and Clinical Psychology, 51,* 655–660.

Lam, W., Sze, P. C., Sacks, H. S., & Chalmers, T. C.

(1987). Meta-analysis of randomized controlled trials of nicotine chewing gum. *Lancet, 2,* 27–30.

Lowman, C. (1983). Drinking and driving among youth. *Alcohol Health and Research World, 7,* 41–49.

Marlatt, G. A., & Donovan, D. M. (1981). Alcoholism and drug dependence: Cognitive social-learning factors in addictive behaviors. In W. E. Craighead, A. E. Kazdin, & M. J. Mahoney (Eds.), *Behavior modification: Principles, issues and applications* (2nd ed., pp. 264–285). Boston: Houghton Mifflin.

McDonald, M. R., & Budd, K. S. (1983). "Booster shots" following didactic parent training: Effects of follow-up using graphic feedback and instructions. *Behavior Modification, 7,* 211–223.

Miller, P. M., & Eisler, R. M. (1977). Assertive behavior of alcoholics: A descriptive analysis. *Behavior Therapy, 8,* 146–149.

Murray, R. M., Clifford, C. A., & Gurling, H. M. D. (1983). Twin and adoption studies. In M. Galanter (Ed.), *Recent developments in alcoholism* (pp. 25–48). New York: Plenum.

Newcomb, M. D., & Bentler, P. M. (1989). Substance use and abuse among children and teenagers. *American Psychologist, 44,* 242–248.

Newcomb, M. D., Chou, C. C., Bentler, P. M., & Huba, G. J. (1988). Cognitive motivations for drug use among adolescents: Longitudinal tests of gender differences and predictors of change in drug use. *Journal of Counseling Psychology, 35,* 426–438.

Patterson, G. R., Reid, J. B., Jones, R. R., & Conger, R. E. (1975). *A social learning approach to family intervention. Vol. 1: Families with aggressive children.* Eugene, OR: Castalia.

Puig-Antich, J., & Chambers, W. (1978). *The schedule for Affective Disorders and Schizophrenia for School-Aged Children.* Unpublished manuscript, New York State Psychiatric Institute.

Russell, m. A. H., Merriman, R., Stapleton, J., & Taylor, W. (1983). Effects of nicotine-chewing gum as an adjunct to general practitioner's advice against smoking. *British Medical Journal, 278,* 1782–1785.

Schuster, C. R. (1986). Implications for treatment of drug dependence. In S. R. Goldberg & I. P. Stoler-man (Eds.), *Behavioral analysis of drug dependence* (pp. 357–385). New York: Academic Press.

Selzer, M. L. (1971). The Michigan Alcoholism Screening Test: The quest for a new diagnostic instrument. *American Journal of Psychiatry, 127,* 89–94.

Shedler, J., & Block, J. (1990). Adolescent drug use and psychological health: A longitudinal inquiry. *American Psychologist, 45,* 612–630.

Simpson, D. D., & Selles, S. B. (1982). *Evaluation of drug abuse treatment effectiveness: Summary of the DARP follow-up research* (pp. 1–17). National Institute on Drug Abuse Treatment Research Report, DHHS Pub. No. (ADM) 85-1209. Washington, DC: U.S. Government Printing Office.

Smith, T. E. (1983). Reducing adolescent's marijuana abuse. *Social Work in Health Care, 9,* 33–44.

Spieger, D. L., & Harford, T. C. (1987). Addictive behaviors among youth. In T. D. Nirenberg & S. A. Maisto (Eds.), *Developments in the assessment and treatment of addictive behaviors* (pp. 305–318). Norwood, NJ: Ablex.

Stanton, M. D., Todd, T. C., & Associates. (1982). *The family therapy of drug abuse and addiction.* New York: Guilford.

Stone, C. I., & Shute, R. (1977). Persuader sex differences and peer pressure effects on attitudes toward drug abuse. *American Journal of Drug and Alcohol Abuse, 4,* 55–64.

Szapocznik, J., Perez-Vidal, A., Brickman, A. L., Foote, F. H., Santisteban, D., Hervis, O., & Kurtines, W. M. (1988). Engaging adolescent drug abusers and their families in treatment: A strategic structural systems approach. *Journal of Consulting and Clinical Psychology, 56,* 552–557.

Tarter, R. E. (1990). Evaluation and treatment of adolescent substance abuse: A decision tree method. *American Journal of Drug and Alcohol Abuse, 16,* 1–46.

Vaglum, P., & Fossheim, I. (1980). Differential treatment of young abusers: A quasi-experimental study of a "therapeutic community" in a psychiatric hospital. *Journal of Drug Issues, 10,* 505–515.

CHAPTER 16

SOMATOFORM DISORDERS

Cindy L. Wigg   University of Texas at Galveston
Paul M. Cinciripini   University of Texas at Galveston

DESCRIPTION OF DISORDER

Clinical Features

The somatoform disorders are one of the most difficult groups of illnesses to evaluate and treat, both for the mental health professional and the primary care physician, who is often in the position of attempting to diagnose, treat, and/or refer these patients. Incidence of these disorders in the general population of children and adolescents has not been adequately studied, but it is clear that children often present with one or more physical symptoms that are found not to have a clearly organic basis. One only needs to review the extensive literature of "functional" abdominal pain to see the impact of this on practice of pediatricians and family practitioners.

Somatoform disorders are those in which the primary complaint is one or more physical symptoms for which no clear organic findings are present to confirm the presence of a physical illness. In addition, there is usually evidence that the symptoms are linked to psychological factors and that they are not under the patient's direct control. Historically, these disorders have been simply called "hysteria" and occupied a great deal of the literature during the time of Freud and his colleagues.

The somatoform disorders include somatization disorder, body dysmorphic disorder, conversion disorder, hypochondriasis, pain disorder, undifferentiated somatoform disorder, and somatoform disorder not otherwise specified. Of these disorders, the only ones that have been studied to any extent in childhood or adolescence are somatization disorder and conversion disorder. Therefore, this chapter will focus primarily on these two disorders. Somatization disorders have a gradual and insidious onset (Livingston & Martin-Cannici, 1985), while conversion disorders may develop precipitously. Conversion disorders often are suggestive of a neurologic disorder but can mimic most of the known diseases and may involve motor, sensory, and autonomic functions (Williams, 1985).

Associated Features

A recent area of assessment of the somatoform disorders has involved identifying clinical features associated with the illness, which can be observed by the primary care physician before a lengthy physical evaluation takes place. Many common clinical features have been associated with somatoform disorders in patients and their families. However, some of these characteristics may also be present in patients with nonpsychiatric physical disorders. For example, patients suffering from both chronic physical illness and somatoform disorders may have significant emotional and behavioral components to their illness (i.e., dysthymia, lethargy, depression, increased agitation) (Walker & Greene, 1989). Unlike the families of patients with chronic illness, the families of patients with somatoform disorders may show a higher than expected frequency of alcoholism, attention-deficit hyperactivity disorder, antisocial personality disorder, and secondary affective disorders (Routh & Ernst, 1984).

Although no single personality dimension has been found to be correlated with somatoform disorders, several authors have noted that such children and adolescents are often described as antisocial, histrionic, dramatic, seductive (Livingston & Martin-Cannici, 1985), egocentric, attention seeking, dependent, and overprotected (Prazar, 1987). Also, children with somatic complaints are often found to have experienced recent stressful life events. A careful assessment of both the patient's characteristic response to life stressors, manner of coping, and associated adoptive behaviors may be helpful not only in making the diagnosis of the disorder but also in the development of the treatment plan (Greene, Walker, Hickson, & Thompson, 1985).

Epidemiology

Prevalence of somatoform disorders in the general population of children and adolescence has been poorly studied. Shapiro and Rosenfeld (1987) reported an incidence rate of somatoform disorder in 0.08 to 0.50 percent of children and adolescents. They noted, however, that if single somatic complaints were included as criteria for the diagnosis, as many as 25 percent of the child and adolescent population may at one time present with somatoform symptoms.

Percentage of referrals to a child psychiatry clinic that are found to have a somatoform disorder have ranged from 1 to 2 percent (Goodyer & Mitchell, 1989) up to 14.5 percent in some reported studies. These differences depended on the type of psychiatric setting and how the diagnosis was made.

Older females are generally found to have two to three times the risk of males for development of a somatoform disorder, but at the younger age range the sex ratio is close to equal. Also, on inpatient units, presence of other more disruptive behaviors in males may overshadow the somatoform symptoms (Shapiro & Rosenfeld, 1987). Some authors have discussed risk factors that may be involved in the etiology of the somatoform disorders, including unresolved grief reactions (Maloney, 1980), other stressful life events (Greene et al., 1985), and modeling of somatic symptoms displayed by other family members (Prazar, 1987). The involvement of the family system in the production and maintenance of somatic complaints has also been proposed (Munuchin et al., 1975). Munuchin postulated that not only do certain types of family organizations influence development and maintenance of psychosomatic symptoms in children but that the children's symptoms play a major role in maintaining family homeostasis.

Etiology

Etiology of somatoform disorders has not been firmly substantiated or agreed upon. The early work with hysteria focused on a psychodynamic explanation for somatic symptoms. The premise was that the symptom represented a repressed conflict, and that in order to treat the symptom the underlying conflict must be identified and resolved.

There also have been attempts to identify a neurobiologic basis for the somatoform disorders. The presence of a neurophysiologic processing disorder has been suggested because of the frequent finding of neurologic symptoms in conversion disorder (Shapiro, 1987). Presence of attention-deficit hyperactivity disorder in patients and families of patients with somatoform disorders has led some to pursue the presence of an attentional dysfunction in these patients. However, no definitive results have been obtained in any of this work.

From a behavioral perspective, the symptoms of somatoform disorder can be reinforced by their role in bringing about a reduction in the patient's level of fear or anxiety or by the direct effect it has on the behavior of others. For example, unpleasant circumstances and tasks may be avoided in the presence of somatic symptoms, whereas care-taking behavior on the part of others may increase. In the absence of healthy ways to manage unpleasant tasks or effectively obtain reinforcement from one's environment, somatic complaints may serve as a powerful tool for manipulating one's environment in an effort to reduce conflict and solicit the care of others.

DIFFERENTIAL DIAGNOSIS AND ASSESSMENT

DSM-III-R Categorization

300.70   Body Dysmorphic Disorder
   a. Preoccupation with imagined defect in appearance in a normal-appearing person. If a slight physical anomaly is present, the person's concern is greatly excessive.
   b. The belief in the defect is not delusional intensity, as in delusional disorder, somatic type (i.e., the person can acknowledge the possibility that he or she may be exaggerating the extent of the defect or that there may be no defect at all).
   c. Occurrence not exclusively during the course of anorexia nervosa

300.11   Conversion Disorder
   a. A loss of, or alteration in, physical functioning suggesting a physical disorder.
   b. Psychological factors are judged to be etiologically related to the symptom because of a temporal relationship between a psychosocial stressor that is apparently related to a psychological conflict or need and initiation or exacerbation of the symptom.
   c. The person is not conscious of intentionally producing the symptom.

300.70   Hypochondriasis
   a. Preoccupation with the fear of having, or the belief that one has, a serious disease, based on the person's interpretation of physical signs or sensations as evidence of physical illness.
   b. Appropriate physical evaluation does not support the diagnosis of any physical disorder that can account for the physical signs or sensations as evidence of physical illness.

300.81   Somatization Disorder
   a. A history of many physical complaints or a belief that one is sickly, beginning before the age of 30 and persisting for several years.
   b. At least 13 symptoms from the list below must be present. To count a symptom as significant, the following criteria must be met:
      (1) no organic pathology or pathophysiologic mechanism (e.g., a physical disorder or the effects of injury, medication, drugs, or alcohol)
      (2) has not occurred only during a panic attack
      (3) has caused the person to take medicine (other than over-the-counter pain medication), see a doctor, or alter lifestyle

Symptom List

Gastrointestinal Symptoms:
   (1) vomiting (other than during pregnancy)
   (2) abdominal pain (other than when menstruating
   (3) nausea (other than motion sickness)
   (4) bloating (gassy)
   (5) diarrhea
   (6) intolerance of (gets sick from) several different foods

Pain Symptoms:
   (7) pain in extremities
   (8) back pain
   (9) joint pain
   (10) pain during urination
   (11) other pain (excluding headaches)

Cardiopulmonary Symptoms:
   (12) shortness of breath when not exerting oneself
   (13) palpitations

(14) chest pain

(15) dizziness

Conversion or Pseudoneurologic Symptoms:

(16) amnesia

(17) difficulty swallowing

(18) loss of voice

(19) deafness

(20) double vision

(21) blurred vision

(22) blindness

(23) fainting or loss of consciousness

(24) seizure or convulsion

(25) trouble walking

(26) paralysis or muscle weakness

(27) urinary retention or difficulty urinating

Sexual Symptoms for the Major Part of the Person's Life after Opportunities for Sexual Activity:

(28) burning sensation in sexual organs or rectum (other than during intercourse)

(29) sexual indifference

(30) pain during intercourse

(31) impotence

Female Reproductive Symptoms Judged by the Person to Occur More Frequently or Severely than in Most Women:

(32) painful menstruation

(33) irregular menstrual bleeding

(34) excessive menstrual bleeding

(35) vomiting throughout pregnancy

Note: The seven items in boldface may be used to screen for the disorder. The presence of two or more of these items suggests a high likelihood of the disorder.

307.80   Somatoform Pain Disorder

a. Preoccupation with pain for at least six months

b. Either (1) or (2):

   (1) appropriate evaluation uncovers no organic pathology or pathophysiologic mechanism (e.g., a physical disorder or the effects of injury) to account for the pain

(2) when there is related organic pathology, the complaint of pain or resulting social or occupational impairment is grossly in excess of what would be expected from the physical findings

300.70   Undifferentiated Somatoform Disorder

a. One or physical complaints (e.g., fatigue, loss of appetite, gastrointestinal or urinary complaints).

b. Either (1) or (2):

   (1) appropriate evaluation uncovers no organic pathology or pathophysiologic mechanism (e.g., a physical disorder or the effects of injury, medication, drugs, or alcohol) to account for the physical complaints

   (2) when there is related organic pathology, the physical complaints or resulting social or occupational impairment is grossly in excess of what would be expected from the physical findings

c. Duration of the disturbance is at least six months.

d. Occurrence not exclusively during the course of another Somatoform Disorder, a Sexual Dysfunction, a Mood Disorder, an Anxiety Disorder, a Sleep Disorder, or a psychotic disorder.

Differential Diagnosis

The most important differential diagnosis for the somatoform disorders is a nonpsychiatric illness. It is also important to evaluate the symptoms in terms of how they affect the patient's lifestyle, social interaction, responsibilities, and affective function. Absence of a physical diagnosis in itself is not sufficient to diagnose a somatoform disorder. There are specific psychological factors that should be identified, including the need for reduction of anxiety or fear, or the need for increased care taking from the environment, as previously described.

In addition, presence of a physical illness does not exclude presence of a somatoform disorder. The most prevalent example of this is pseudo-seizures in a patient with documented seizures.

A complex web of symptoms that occur both with and without underlying pathophysiology may be established quite readily in patients with bonafide illnesses who possess few coping or social skills. This may be especially relevant in children who lack the experience or vocabulary to readily articulate their emotional needs. Both patient and caregivers may have some difficulty in discriminating between the two types of events, especially when the symptoms are associated with conflicts or presence of negative affect, which can often serve as a cue for onset of the behavior.

In contrast, physical symptoms in factitious disorder are produced voluntarily by the patient for the purpose of fooling the physicians. In malingering, the symptoms are also conscious and serve to allow the patient a specific gain (i.e., work disability, etc.). Both of these conditions are very rare in children and adolescents. Children and adolescents who have major depression may also use physical symptoms to describe their feelings. A thorough history and mental status would be important to detect the presence of a primary affective disorder, as evidenced by additional symptoms of depressed mood, sleep and appetite disturbances, poor concentration, guilt, and thoughts of death or suicide.

Hypochondriasis is differentiated from the other somatization disorders by the person's fear of having a disease and then misperception of physical symptoms and signs. There is a significant component of anxiety to this disorder.

Patients with panic disorder may have associated physical symptoms; in order to make the diagnosis of a somatoform disorder, the physical symptoms must be present in the absence of a panic attack. Somatic delusions that are associated with affective disorders with psychotic features and other psychotic disorders are often intense and bizarre and will occur in the presence of other symptoms, characteristic of a thought disorder.

In psychological factors affecting physical condition, there is a documented physical illness where psychologic factors play a secondary role (e.g., stress induced angina).

Assessment Strategies

It is important to identify somatoform disorders early if we are to alter their course significantly. The more chronic the course, the poorer the prognosis (Livingston & Martin-Cannici, 1985). It is also important to minimize as much as possible the need for physical evaluations that may prove to be time consuming, expensive, dangerous, and quite possibly reinforce the symptoms. Evaluation of the disorder should include:

1. A thorough history and time line that attempts to correlate significant life events with fluctuation in symptoms.
2. Documentation of the role of family and peers in the symptom presentation—using a family interview to ascertain how parents, peers, and siblings respond to the patient's physical symptoms or presentation of distress—is especially useful.
3. Self-monitoring of the symptoms or monitoring by parents or teachers in the case of children. An emphasis should be placed on the association between changes in the patient's affect, situation, and symptoms (i.e., how do the symptoms vary at school, home, and at times of recreation, work, etc.; that is, what does the patient do in response to the symptoms and what changes take place in the environment?).

TREATMENT

Evidence for Prescriptive Treatments

Controlled studies comparing treatment effectiveness in this group of disorders are very difficult to carry out and are not available to any extent (Williams, 1985). This group of disorders presents some specific problems in attempting to compare treatment modalities.

The current grouping of somatoform disorders is diverse and has changed significantly through the various revisions of the DSM manual. Although diagnoses in this group have somatic symptoms as a primary feature, the etiology and probably the treatment strategies may not be that related.

As previously discussed, children and adolescents often will not qualify for the diagnosis criteria in DSM-III-R for many of the disorders. A clear example of this is somatization disorder, where there needs to be a lengthy pattern (several years) of multiple somatic complaints. Although adults with this diagnosis may have presented with symptoms during childhood or adolescence, it would be unlikely for them to have met the full criteria at that time.

Although the pediatric literature is full of discussion of the treatment of recurrent abdominal pain (RAP) in children, it is unclear whether these patients would fulfill the specific criteria for any of the somatoform disorders.

Another complicating factor in evaluating the treatment of these disorders is the way the patients initially present. Often they are first seen by primary care physicians who may have initiated a lengthy process to rule out specific organic causes and may well have intervened in some manner.

Given the proposed etiology of these disorders (i.e., underlying conflict expressed by somatic means and that are then environmentally reinforced), there have been unlimited discussions about the need to address the underlying conflict versus eliminating the specific behaviors; this has pitted the psychodynamicists against the behaviorists. Controlled studies in this area, especially for psychodynamic treatment, are unavailable. In addition, it is hard to find the two strategies applied to consistent diagnostic groups. Given that a great deal of the literature in this area describes the somewhat generic diagnosis as hysterical neurosis, it makes comparisons very difficult (Blanchard & Hersen, 1976).

Behavior Therapy

Behavioral treatment for somatoform disorders has proven to be very successful based on the assumptions that somatic complaints produce contingent consequences (e.g., attention, sympathy, avoidance of nonpreferred activities) that serve to reinforce the behavior.

The general procedures involved include (1) extinction to decrease or eliminate the patient's symptoms, (2) programming the patient's environment to reinforce positive behaviors while ignoring symptomatic ones, and (3) teaching the patient more effective ways of obtaining gratification from their environment (Hersen, 1983).

Relaxation may prove useful at times to provide the patient with a means for coping with a stressor and reducing any associated autonomic activations. Biofeedback has been effective in some cases, either as an aid to generalize relaxation (i.e., skin temperature feedback) or when the target symptoms have some relationship to the physiological system being monitored (e.g., frontalis EMG for tension headaches). It can also be useful in helping the patient monitor his or her physical progress (Klonoff & Moore, 1986).

Pharmacotherapy

Pharmacologic treatment for these groups of disorders has not generally been found to be effective and may actually complicate or further reinforce symptoms in some circumstances. The use of placebo is not usually effective and raises ethical questions (Prazar, 1987).

Treatment for diagnoses that may present in conjunction with these disorders (i.e., affective disorders) may include pharmacotherapy for that specific disorder. Sodium Amytal, as well as benzodiazenes, have been used in interviews of patients with suspected conversion disorder to help clarify the diagnosis.

Alternative Treatments

Family therapy, at some level, becomes an important modality in the treatment of somatoform disorders. Regardless of its proposed role in etiology, certainly with children and adolescents, the family becomes very important in the maintenance of symptoms. Therefore, attempts to eliminate reinforcers must certainly involve evaluation of and participation by family members (Munford & Chan, 1980). In addition, other people involved in the child or adolescent's environment may become very important in treatment as well. This would include extended family, teachers, counselors, coaches, and others.

Insight-oriented individual therapy may become a very important modality depending on the proposed etiology of the disorder. Certainly in patients who do not respond well to behavioral treatment alone, there needs to be a further look at the underlying issues that may be involved in the patient's illness. Simple reassurance and the use of suggestions may be helpful and efficacious in only the simplest cases but may have little effectiveness in complicated aspects, where the patterns are longstanding and environmental stressors are present.

Selecting Optimal Treatment Strategies

Since the patient often presents first to a primary care physician, use of a therapeutic prolonged evaluation in that setting may prove very helpful (Menahem, 1988). Introducing psychological factors as being important early in the evaluation not only makes it easier to get a better picture of patients and their interactions with the environment but it also makes further referral to mental health practitioners easier (Prazar, 1987).

There are several factors that are important to look at while selecting a treatment strategy. Some of these will be noted below. Many patients with somatoform disorders may also have physical disorders as well (i.e., seizures and pseudoseizures). This complicates treatment for the practitioner. In addition, some patients may have other psychiatric illnesses that need to be addressed and treated in addition to the somatoform disorder (i.e., depression, anxiety disorders, etc.). The treatment of the second disorder may in fact complicate that of the somatoform disorder. For example, side effects of antidepressant medication in a depressed patient with somatization disorder may further complicate the somatic complaints (e.g., dry mouth, dizziness, constipation, headaches).

It has been stressed that it is very important to look at the environment of the patient. In children and adolescents, this means the family, extended family, school, and friends. Interviews with teachers as well as classroom and home evaluations, are critical for a complete assessment.

The personal history of the patient may well illustrate the origin of symptoms and provide therapists with necessary leads for cognitive work that extends beyond symptom-specific intervention. For example, the finding of sexual abuse in a patient with somatoform disorder may have important implications for assessing the role of anxiety, fear, and avoidance. The age of the child and the cognitive capacity of the patient should also be considered when selecting treatment modalities. Specific limitations of the patient and the environment should be addressed.

Problems in Carrying Out Interventions

Patients with somatoform disorders can be difficult, especially for the primary care physician. Patients who come to mental health care from primary care physicians may feel rejected. Any changes in the symptom picture may lead the treating clinic to once again pursue an organic basis of the symptoms, which may further confuse patients and their families.

Relapse Prevention

Essential to the prevention of relapse in patients with somatoform disorders is to ensure that a comprehensive evaluation is carried out and that all aspects of the patient's illness are addressed and treated. Simple removal of symptoms without attention to the underlying relationship between the symptom and its role in the patient's environment may well produce relapse (Blanchard & Hersen, 1976). For many patients this involves not only behavioral treatment to reduce the symptoms but individual therapy to determine the nature of such functional reltionships. In addition, motivation and participation of family members often are essential to help the patient regain their health and achieve optimum functioning.

As patients reintegrate into their various life schemata (i.e., school, etc.) they will require assistance and training in developing new ways to identify their emotional needs and seek an appropriate response from their environments. This may therefore require social skills training and group therapy modalities. If relapses do recur, the clinician must reassess his or her initial evaluation in an attempt to look for etiological factors that may not have been addressed. Certainly, consideration of organic causes need always to be kept in mind and pursued appropriately.

CASE ILLUSTRATION

Case Description

Caroline was a 17-year-old female referred to the Child and Adolescent Psychiatry Consultation and Liaison service after several months' hospitalization on both pediatric and surgery services. At the time of psychiatric consultation, her diagnosis was idiopathic pseudo-obstructive syndrome and duodenal dysfunction. There was evidence of decreased gastric motility as well as other suggestive studies that led the medical team to make this diagnosis. The psychiatric consultation was requested to assist the medical team to identify possible stressors that may have affected the patient's physical illness and course of treatment. The planned treatment at that time was surgery, which would require that the patient be dependent on intravenous feeding for the duration of her life.

The primary symptoms at that time were constant nausea and intractable vomiting. A gastrostomy tube was in place at the time of her consultation. On consultation, Caroline reported that although she had episodes of vomiting occasionally for the last few years, the vomiting episodes became worse since the previous summer, eventually necessitating her admission to the hospital for evaluation. When asked if anything had happened to her during the summer, Caroline reported an incident where her mother discovered her with an older man in her bedroom. She reported that her mother insisted that she charge the man with statutory rape. Caroline's reluctance to do so led to a heated argument between her and her mother. Shortly, thereafter, Caroline's mother was admitted to the hospital, ostensibly for a "heart attack." Caroline's vomiting began shortly after that admission.

Differential Diagnosis and Assessment

The differential at the time of consultation included (1) psychological factor affecting physical illness and (2) possible conversion disorder. The symptoms were too limited to entertain a diagnosis of somatization disorder at that time.

Given the positive physical findings, including the evidence of decreased gastric motility by manometry, it was felt that there was a physical illness present. The treatment team, however, felt that there were some overwhelming psychological factors that contributed to the severity of the illness, leading to psychological factors affecting physical illness as the most likely diagnosis.

Treatment Selection

The recommendation was made by the consultant that Caroline be admitted to the Adolescent Psychiatry Inpatient service for further treatment. Inpatient treatment was recommended because of the severity of her symptoms and the continued need for medical management. The patient agreed. Her mother, however, was very resistant to having her daughter in a psychiatric facility. She believed that Caroline's symptoms were totally physical in nature. With the assistance of the pediatric team, it was explained to the mother how emotional factors play a significant role in the development of many physical disorders, and that further evaluation of Caroline's emotional status would assist the pediatricians in planning a more comprehensive treatment. The mother reluctantly agreed, but told Caroline that she herself might have to be rehospitalized because of how Caroline's hospitalization might affect her. Caroline then was transferred to the Adolescent Psychiatry Service.

Treatment Course and Problems in Carrying Out Interventions

On admission, Caroline, appeared to be her stated age and was well kempt. However, she wore no makeup or jewelry, and her hair was pulled back in a simple and somewhat unattractive manner. She had a heparin lock (intravenous catheter) in one forearm, and otherwise seemed fairly healthy. She appeared to be average in height and weight for her age, although her weight had decreased over the last six months. Her mood appeared euthymic and her affect was generally appropriate, except that she spoke of her upcoming surgery and the consequences of it somewhat matter-of-factly (i.e., the absence of significant concern). She denied hallucinations or delusions and her thought processes were coherent. She was well oriented and appeared to be of average intelligence.

At the time of Caroline's transfer, the initial treatment plan involved having staff specifically refrain from focusing on her physical symptoms. She was told that the pediatrician would be seeing her on a regular basis throughout her hospitalization. However, the treatment team agreed that the pediatrician's visits would not simply be based on Caroline's physical status in order to avoid reinforcing somatic complaints. Caroline was assigned an individual therapist as well as a family therapist. In addition, she was involved in the usual unit activities, including group therapy, occupational therapy, recreational therapy, and school.

Further history was obtained during the hospitalization. Caroline was the fourth of four daughters born to a mother who had never married. Caroline's three sisters shared the same father. She was the product of her mother's relationship with a married man who had other children by his marriage. Although she knew who her father was and had contact with him, he had never publicly acknowledged her as his daughter. When he visited Caroline on the pediatric ward, the nurses were told that he was her uncle.

Caroline's mother was very dependent on her daughters, both emotionally and financially. At the time of Caroline's initial hospitalization in pediatrics, she was the only daughter left in the home. However, an older sister moved back shortly thereafter to be with mother.

Caroline's mother reported that she had spent most of her late adolescence and early adulthood caring for her own parents through their prolonged illnesses and deaths. She herself admitted to having heart disease of uncertain etiology and diabetes. Caroline's family, therefore, was not one

where self-reliance, independence, and healthy conflict resolutions were reinforced.

Caroline was able to talk about her own thoughts and feelings at the time her mother was hospitalized for her so-called heart attack. She stated that she had continued to be angry at her mother about the incident with the man, but was unable to tell her mother how she felt. She reported feeling guilty about being angry at her "sick mother," and also related that she felt that she had caused her mother's heart attack. She specifically related the beginning of her vomiting episodes to this time. She was also able to recall instances during her adolescence when she would be in conflict with her family and her stomach would feel "tied up in knots," and she would occasionally vomit.

Shortly after Caroline's admission, the nausea resolved, with one brief relapse after a phone conversation with her mother. She had no vomiting episodes during the course of her hospitalization, despite daily episodes before transfer. Caroline also began to change her physical appearance. She began to wear makeup and arrange her hair attractively. She was socially reinforced on the unit for her numerous positive qualities, including her sense of humor and leadership abilities. She actively sought out treatment resources and expressed looking forward to a healthy life and planning for the upcoming summer.

Because of the unit structure, Caroline's mother was allowed only biweekly visits. The rather rapid diminution of Caroline's symptoms was correlated with the forced separation from her mother. Her primary gain was directly related to her becoming more independent of her mother and learning to relate appropriately to healthy female role models on the unit. Without the cognitive and emotional skills necessary to support her own healthy efforts at independence, the mother's presence signaled defeat in the face of adversity. Efforts at independence were punished by the mother; instead, the mother directly reinforced her daughter's helplessness and sick role behavior, in order to prevent eventual separation.

As would be expected, Caroline's mother had great difficulty with the separation from her daughter and made threats to remove Caroline from the hospital. However, after initial resolution of the symptoms, the focus shifted to individual and family therapy. In individual therapy, Caroline learned about direct ways to communicate affect to her mother, using modeling, behavior rehearsal, and roleplaying. Family therapy, as expected, was difficult. Caroline's rapid resolution of symptoms made it difficult for her mother to adhere to a purely physical explanation of the illness.

As Caroline became more confident in herself and more willing to confront her mother, she was able to directly discuss her mother's efforts to block her treatment. Caroline's mother, through family therapy, was able to tolerate the separation from Caroline, but continued to show very little awareness of her role in maintaining Caroline's illness. Although the issues that were dealt with in family therapy were too numerous to discuss, they involved identifying the mother's own needs (given her difficult life), Caroline's needs to be able to separate from her mother and expand her relationship with her father, and the tendency for all of the family members to express emotions through physical means instead of direct verbal communication.

Outcome and Termination

Caroline was discharged to her mother after multiple therapeutic passes home, during which there were no recurrence of symptoms. At the time of discharge, all of her physical tests were normal, including gastric motility and duodenal size.

Followup and Maintenance

Caroline was followed in individual and family therapy over two months and then transferred to a local community mental health clinic where she was followed for another few months. At one year, she was no longer in treatment and had no recurrence of symptoms. She was socially very active and functioning as a normal adolescent.

Her mother had received brief individual therapy at the local mental health clinic and was functioning well by her account at the time of transfer.

Case Summary

This case illustrates a conversion disorder. Presence of one symptom—vomiting—distinguishes it from a somatization disorder, where there are multiple symptoms involved over a lengthy period of time. There was some question about the possibility that in addition to the psychiatric illness, Caroline may have also had a physical disorder. However, at discharge, all repeat gastrointestinal studies were normal. Another diagnosis that might have been considered for Caroline was the one labeled psychological factors affecting physical illness. This diagnosis assumes presence of an underlying non-psychiatric physical illness. The course of Caroline's illness and response to treatment, (i.e., rapid resolution with a change in situation), however, is much more consistent with the diagnosis of conversion disorder. Specifically, the criterion that psychological factors are associated with the initiation (or exacerbation) of symptoms was met when presence or absence of the mother's influence correlated with symptom change.

There was no question of factitious disorder or malingering in this patient. The symptoms were viewed as not being under voluntary control of the patient.

The decision to treat Caroline in an inpatient psychiatric service was based on the assumption that separation from her mother would prove beneficial and that it would be easier to minimize secondary gain on a service where continuous monitoring of physical status was not the norm. Inpatient treatment, as well as providing separation, was deemed necessary because of the apparent extent of physical handicap.

The importance of inquiring about life situations when a patient presents with a physical illness is well illustrated. Despite the fact that Caroline had seen many physicians and other health care workers, the significant aspects of her personal history were never obtained. It is unclear if the "right" questions were ever asked or whether she had felt uncomfortable presenting the significant social history. Indeed, people who had contact with Caroline over her initial hospitalization recalled that they had never spoken to her without her mother present.

Our case, which ended with a very positive outcome, may have been drastically different had the psychiatric consultation not occurred. In fact, Caroline probably would have continued to surgery and would have become somewhat of an invalid for life.

Although considering the risk of missing a physical disorder when focusing on psychological issues is important, the risk of missing a psychiatric illness while focusing only on physical illness is equally important, as exemplified in this case. It is important to look at the person as a whole, whose physical well-being affects her emotional status and vice versa.

SUMMARY

Because children and adolescents with somatoform disorders present with physical complaints, they are almost always seen first by a primary care physician, whose goal often is to rule out any nonpsychiatric physical illness. Since many physical illnesses can present with a very complex symptom picture (i.e., mononucleosis, multiple sclerosis etc.), the physician may be reluctant to consider a psychological basis for the illnesses until he or she has pursued a lengthy physical evaluation. Practitioners are often worried that in pursuing a psychologic basis for an illness tht they might miss a serious underlying nonpsychiatric medical disorder. There is a similar danger, however, in not recognizing the possible psychologic basis for the physical complaints and putting the child or adolescent through unnecessary and perhaps dangerous procedures.

Many illnesses that have been found historically in adults had not been considered to be present in childhood (Weller, Weller, & Herjanic, 1983). We now recognize that this is not the case, as in the case of childhood depression. The lengthy criteria for somatization disorder in the DSM-III-R is an example of how one might have difficulty diagnosing a child or adolescent with this disorder, and yet we recognize that somatization disorder develops over a period of time and may well present in some form during childhood or adolescence. As has been the case with other psychiatric illnesses, the more cognizant we are of the possibility of a diagnosis being present, the more likely we are to adequately assess and diagnose patients with that disorder. Hopefully, early recognition and treatment of these disorders will result in improved prognoses.

REFERENCES

Blanchard, E. B., & Hersen, M. (1976). Behavioral treatment of hysterical neurosis: Symptom substitution and symptom return reconsidered. *Psychiatry Journal, 39,* 118–129.

Goodyer, I. M., & Mitchell, C. (1989). Somatic emotional disorders in childhood and adolescence. *Journal of Psychosomatic Research, 44,* 681–688.

Greene, J. W., Walker, L. S., Hickson, G., & Thompson, J. (1985). Stressful life events and somatic complaints in adolescents, *Pediatrics, 75,* 19–22.

Hersen, M. (1983). Perspectives on the practice of outpatient behavior therapy. *Outpatient Behavior Therapy: A Clinical Guide, 1,* 14–15.

Klonoff, E. A., & Moore, D. J. (1986). "Conversion reactions" in adolescents: A biofeedback-based operant approach. *Journal Behavior Therapy Experimental Psychiatry, 17,* 179–184.

Livingston, R., & Martin-Canicci, C. (1985). Multiple somatic complaints and possible somatization disorder in prepubertal children. *Journal of the American Academy of Child Psychiatry, 24,* 603–607.

Maloney, M. J. (1980). Diagnosing hysterical conversion reactions in children. *The Journal of Pediatrics, 97,* 1016–1020.

Menahem, S. (1988). The child with psychosomatic symptoms: The use of a therapeutic prolonged evaluation. *Developmental and Behavioral Pediatrics, 9,* 310–311.

Minuchin, S., Baker, L., Rosman, B., Liebman, R., Milman, L., & Todd, T. (1975). A conceptual model of psychosomatic illness in children, family organization and family therapy. *Archives of General Psychiatry, 32,* 1031–1038.

Munford, P. R., & Chan, S. Q. (1980). Family therapy for the treatment of a conversion reaction: A case study. *Psychotherapy: Theory, Research and Practice, 17,* 214–219.

Prazar, G. (1987). Conversion reactions in adolescents. *Pediatrics in Review, 8,* 279–286.

Routh, D. K., & Ernst, A. R. (1984). Somatization disorder in relatives of children and adolescents with functional abdominal pain. *Journal of Pediatric Psychology, 9,* 427–437.

Shapiro, E. G., & Rosenfeld, A. A. (1987). *The somatizing child: diagnosis and treatment of conversion and somatization disorders.* New York: Springer-Verlag.

Walker, L. S., & Greene, J. W. (1989). Children with recurrent abdominal pain and their parents: More somatic complaints, anxiety, and depression than other patient families? *Journal of Pediatric Psychology, 14,* 231–243.

Weller, R. A., Weller, E. B., & Herjanic, B. (1983). Adult psychiatric disorders in psychiatrically ill young adolescents. *American Journal Psychiatry, 140,* 1585–1588.

Williams, D. T. (1985). Somatoform disorders. *The Clinical Guide to Child Psychiatry, 10,* 192–207.

CHAPTER 17

PARASOMNIAS

Ronald Dahl   University of Pittsburgh

DESCRIPTION OF DISORDER

Parasomnia is a general term used to describe a wide range of behaviors emerging from sleep or associated with sleep. This chapter addresses a group of parasomnias that are closely related and occur commonly in children as sudden, partial awakenings from nondream sleep. These events include sleepwalking, night terrors, and confused partial arousals. (Some enuretic events can also occur as partial arousals; however, enuresis is addressed in a separate chapter.) Although the specific types of arousal (sleepwalking versus night terrors) can be considered as separate entities, these behaviors represent a spectrum of related phenomena with respect to sleep physiology. From a clinical perspective, only those behaviors associated with high arousal (e.g., full-blown night terrors or agitated sleepwalking) tend to present as problems. These *intense* events, however, merely represent the extreme end of a spectrum of partial arousal behaviors that occur in mild forms in many children. Some sections of this chapter will deal with specific types of sudden partial awakenings, whereas, in general, they will be discussed as variations on a theme.

Clinical Features

These events represent sudden, partial arousals from deep non-REM (non-rapid eye movement) sleep. The behaviors can be very mild (such as calm mumbling or a few awkward movements) or quite intense (with screaming, agitated flailing, and running). The events can last from a few seconds to 20 minutes, with an average duration of about 3 minutes. The termination of these events is usually as sudden as the initiation, with a rapid return to deep sleep. During the events, children may seem confused, often not recognizing their parents, being inconsolable, and appearing incoherent. The intense events can be accompanied by physiological hyperarousal with very rapid heart rate, dilated pupils, and rapid physical movements. Even when apparently hyperaroused, however, the child continues to be partially asleep during the event.

These partial arousals can also be accompanied by a wide range of emotional affect. Children may appear sad and crying; calm, glassy-eyed, and emotionless; laughing and happy; or extremely terrified. There are also various patterns of movements, ranging from a few slow, awkward movements, to extremely rapid and complex movements, such as running and screaming. The most intense versions of these events (such as a full-blown night terrors) are the most likely to present as clinical problems. It is important to realize that most children have very mild versions of these events, normally at the termination of their first deep sleep period. These mild events (such as talking or calmly sitting up in bed) often go unobserved by parents. Mild-to-moderate intensity arousals (such as calm sleepwalking) may be apparent to families, but usually are not regarded as problems to bring to the attention of clinicians.

The most common time for these events is in the first third of the night, at the end of the first or second deep sleep period. Since sleep cycles usually last 60 to 90 minutes, families often report that the event occurs like clockwork, at the same time every night (usually one to three hours after the child goes to sleep). Events can occur more than once a night, usually separated by intervals of 60 to 90 minutes. Later events tend to be less intense than the first event of the night. In the morning, the child usually has no memory of the events.

The peak age of occurrence for these partial arousals is 4 to 8 years of age (Klackenberg, 1987). However, they can occur as early as the first year of life, or can continue through adolescence and adulthood (but are more likely to be associated with some type of pathology in older subjects). These events are most frequent at about the time that children give up taking daytime naps, during the adjustment to longer periods of wakefulness during the day. These partial arousals are also more likely to occur during "recovery" sleep following any period of sleep disturbances or changes in schedule.

Partial arousal events also tend to occur more frequently in individuals with a positive family history for sleepwalking or night terrors (Kales et al., 1980). They are also more frequent following stressful events (Terr, 1983) and at a higher rate in children with psychological and emotional problems (Simond & Parraga, 1984). Partial arousal events are more frequent in children with Tourette's syndrome and family members of Tourette's patients (Barabas, Matthews, & Ferrari,

1984; Nee, Caine Polinsky, Eldridge, & Ebert, 1980). One study found a higher rate of parasomnias in association with school failure (Kahn et al., 1989).

Associated Features

As evident in the clinical description, there are two major themes underlying the pattern of observations concerning partial arousals in children: (1) overtiredness and (2) psychological/emotional factors. Each of these themes will be discussed briefly.

Overtiredness or any source of sleep deprivation can increase or precipitate partial arousals. Any time a child is adjusting to getting less sleep, or has disturbed nighttime sleep, the physiological compensation is to get deeper sleep (especially in the first one to two hours after sleep onset). As will be discussed in the section on etiology, such deep "recovery" sleep appears to be very fertile ground for partial arousal events. Thus, features associated with these parasomnias include a wide array of behaviors and problems that can interfere with sleep.

Difficulty falling asleep, behaviors that delay going to bed, nocturnal events that interrupt sleep, early morning awakening (or the need to get up early for structured activities), and physiological disturbances of sleep (such as obstructive sleep apnea syndrome) can all contribute to partial arousals. Other examples include erratic schedules, such as being up very late on the weekends followed by recovery sleep during the week, and the transition of giving up a daytime nap. Medications and medical illnesses that interfere with sleep are also associated with these events through similar mechanisms of leading to deep recovery sleep.

A second theme of associated features is in the realm of psychological/emotional factors. Particularly with respect to night terrors, much has been written about an association with particular psychological states, such as anxiety and repressed aggression (Klackenberg, 1982; Ferber, 1989). Stressful events and trauma are also associated with night terrors (Terr, 1983), as are general behavioral and emotional problems (Simonds & Parraga, 1984). In some cases, the psychological factors may be contributing to sleep loss. That is, emotional and behavioral problems are also associated with difficulty falling asleep, as occurs with depression and anxiety in children (Ryan et al., 1987; Dahl et al., 1990). Likewise, externalizing disorders, such as attention-deficit hyperactivity disorder and conduct disorder, can be accompanied by oppositional behaviors around bedtime, which may delay sleep onset as well as occasional difficulties falling asleep (Dahl & Puig-Antich, 1990).

Epidemiology

Prevalence estimates for these events are inconsistent. One problem is that relatively mild versions of partial arousals occur very frequently but are seldom regarded as a problem (and many events probably go unobserved by parents). Therefore, many studies measure only those events that disturb the family. Frequently, sleepwalking is considered separate from night terrors, and sudden arousals with crying may or may not be included. Such relative lack of precision and consistency in defining these events probably contributes to the wide variance in estimates. Depending on methods and definitions, estimates range from 1 to 35 percent of children having had episodes of sleepwalking. In general, interviews yield higher rates for sleepwalking than questionnaire data. One of the more in-depth studies included a longitudinal study of 212 children in Sweden, followed for 10 years with interviews and structured assessments (Klackenberg, 1982). In that study, 75 of the 212 (35 percent) reported some sleepwalking events, with 35 of the children (17 percent) with persistent sleepwalking. In 23 children (11 percent), sleepwalking persisted for at least five years, and 6 children (3 percent) had sleepwalking episodes throughout the 10 years of the study.

Genetic factors also influence prevalence estimates, as another study found that 22 percent of children had sleepwalking if neither parent was affected, 45 percent if one parent had parasomnias, and 60 percent if both parents reported a history of sleepwalking or night terrors (Kales et al., 1980). Similarly, concordance for sleepwalking in monozygotic twins has been shown to be six times higher than in dizygotic twins (Bakwin, 1970).

Since night terrors represent a less common but more severe version of sudden partial arousals, epidemiologic estimates of these events are somewhat lower than for sleepwalking. A sample of 991 cildren in a general pediatric clinic found that there were night terrors in 2.9 percent of children aged 1 to 14 years (Kurth, Gohler, & Knaape, 1965). Other studies have provided comparable estimates of 1 to 3 percent of children having night terrors (Jacobson, Kales, & Kales, 1969; Shirley & Kahn, 1958).

Both sleepwalking and night terrors are more frequent in children with Tourette's syndrome (Barabas et al., 1984) and appear to be more common in family members of Tourette's subjects (Nee et al., 1980). Increased rates of partial arousals have also been observed in children with obstructive sleep apnea syndrome (OSAS) (Guilleminault, 1987). In each of these disorders sleep disruption (related to nocturnal tics or obstructive apneas respectively) is likely to be related to the partial arousals.

Age is also an important covariate with respect to prevalence estimates. Peak age of occurrence for night terrors is approximately 4 to 6 years, with a rapid decrease by ages 8 to 9. Sleepwalking peaks slightly later and more often continues through early to midadolescence. These changes parallel roughly the decrease in deep Stage 4 sleep (which peaks at ages 3 to 5 with a fairly rapid decline until midadolescence).

Etiology

Parasomnias are sudden partial awakenings from deep sleep that appear to fragment into a mixed state of arousal. This mixed state has some aspects of being awake and some aspects of being in a deep sleep. The character of the events (whether calm or agitated and the emotional tone) may be influenced by which areas of the brain are relatively awake or relatively asleep. There appear to be at least two routes to this mixed state: (1) difficulty leaving deep sleep (stage 4) at the end of the first sleep cycle, or (2) a sudden disturbance or disruption during the middle of deep sleep. In order to better understand these factors with respect to both etiology and treatment, a brief overview of sleep physiology will help to provide some perspective.

There are three broad categories of state, including awake, rapid eye movement (REM), and non-REM sleep. Non-REM sleep is further divided into four stages: Stage 1 is a light sleep or drowsiness, State 2 is of medium depth with features of spindles and K-complexes, and Stages 3 and 4 (also called slow-wave or delta sleep) are *very* deep sleep stages. During the deepest non-REM sleep state (Stage 4), the EEG is dominated by very low-frequency, high-amplitude waves in the delta band, and children are very resistant to being awakened. If awakened from Stage 4, individuals are usually in a "fog" and require a few minutes of transition time before becoming completely alert. Most of this deep delta sleep occurs during the first one to three hours after going to sleep (prior to the first REM period). The amount and intensity of delta sleep is closely related to the length of prior wakefulness. The physiologic response to getting less sleep is to increase the very deep Stage 4 sleep. Age also influences the amount and depth of Stage 4 sleep, which reaches a peak at ages 3 to 5 years, decreases rapidly by mid-adolescence, then gradually diminishes throughout adulthood.

Sleep stages can be further understood by examining a typical *pattern* of sleep over the night. Figure 17–1 shows an example of a sleep histogram from a 10-year-old child. The vertical axis is labeled with Stages awake, 1, 2, 3, and 4 at progressively lower levels (with REM shown at an intermediate level with striped boxes). The child in the figure fell briefly into Stage 1, descended to Stage 2, and then, within a few minutes, was in deep Stages 3 and 4 (delta) sleep. This period lasted approximately 60 minutes, followed by a return to Stage 2 and a brief arousal, then a return to a second delta period for another hour. As the night progressed, this child returned to lighter Stage 2 followed by the first REM period. REM periods were then interspersed approximately every 60 to 90 minutes for the rest of the night, with longer REM periods toward the early morning. This figure demonstrates two important con-

cepts relevant to understanding sleep physiology: (1) non-REM sleep is deepest after sleep onset and gradually gets lighter as the night progresses, and (2) REM sleep is interspersed at 90-minute cycles, but tends to increase over the second half of the night.

The transition out of Stage 4 at the end of the first sleep cycle is frequently difficult (particularly in children). If the child is overly tired, or relatively sleep deprived, the transition from deep sleep to light sleep appears to be even more difficult. (This may be analogous to the difficulty we frequently experience transitioning from light sleep to full wakefulness when our alarm clocks go off when we are relatively sleep deprived.) Observations with infrared video camera show that most children have some unusual behaviors during this termination of early Stage 4. Frequently, children will mumble, have a few awkward movements or facial expressions, or even occasionally sit up, stare blankly at the wall for a few seconds, and lay back down to sleep, with no memory of these events in the morning. In a typical home, these events go completely unnoticed.

As eluded to earlier, there is a wide range of more intense behaviors that can occur during this period, including walking and/or talking, or very agitated behaviors (such as crying, screaming, running, flailing, etc.). The exact factors associated with more intense arousals during these events are not clear. Being overly tired or having an increase in Stage 4 is associated with a higher frequency of intense events. In addition, a number of sleep researchers have commented on the association of anxiety and "repressed aggression" (Ferber, 1989; Klackenberg, 1987). Clearly, there is some association with behavioral/emotional difficulties and these events as stated in the earlier sections. There are at least two possibilities for these associations. The emotional arousal itself may contribute to the identity of the event (there is some evidence that the emotional state as one falls asleep may influence one's emotional state emerging from deep sleep). It is also possible that anxiety and emotional problems may delay sleep onset, resulting in relative sleep deprivation followed by a compensatory increase in sleep depth.

In addition to the difficult transition leaving

Figure 17–1. Sleep Pattern in an Early School-Age Child

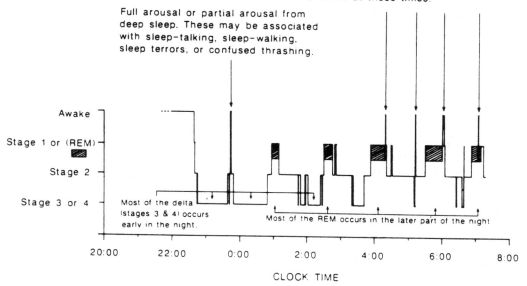

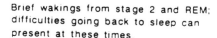

Brief wakings from stage 2 and REM; difficulties going back to sleep can present at these times.

Full arousal or partial arousal from deep sleep. These may be associated with sleep-talking, sleep-walking, sleep terrors, or confused thrashing.

Source: Ronald E. Dahl (1992). Child and adolescent sleep disorders. In D. M. Kaufman, G. E. Solomon, & C. R. Pfeffer (Eds.), *Child and adolescent neurology for psychiatrists.* Baltimore: Williams & Wilkins. © 1992, the Williams & Wilkins Co., Baltimore. Reprinted by permission.

the first deep sleep cycle, these partial arousal events can also be precipitated by external disruptions in the middle of Stage 4 sleep. In general, children are very resistant to being awakened during Stage 4 sleep. However, a sudden stimulus, such as a loud noise, can clearly precipitate partial arousals from deep sleep. Similarly, sleep-walking can be reliably induced in a sleep laboratory setting by physically lifting a child from bed during Stage 4 sleep and placing the child on his or feet. Thus, external events, such as noises, or physical disturbances occurring in the midst of a deep Stage 4 sleep can result in a partial arousal state. It is also possible that internal or physiological arousals that coincide with Stage 4 can also precipitate partial arousals. For example, children with Tourette's who have motor tics throughout the night have been observed in our labortory to have partial arousals when tics occurred during Stage 4 sleep.

There is a great deal that we do not understand with respect to the etiology of these events. It appears that these are basically two opposing forces: one trying to keep the system in a deep restorative sleep and the other producing an arousal, with a resultant mixed state of partial deep sleep and partial wakefulness. There may be many complex factors (both endogenously and exogenously) that interact in producing these states.

DIFFERENTIAL DIAGNOSIS AND ASSESSMENT

DSM-III-R Categorization

DSM-III-R separates the parasomnias into four categories: dream anxiety disorder or nightmare, 307.47; sleep terror disorder, 307.46; sleep walking disorder, 307.45; and parasomnia, not otherwise specified, 307.40.

Sleep terror disorder is designated with four main points: (1) The predominant disturbance of recurrent episodes of abrupt awakening (lasting 1 to 10 minutes) from sleep, usually occurring during the first third of the major sleep period and beginning with a panicky scream. (2) Intense anxiety and signs of autonomic arousal during each episode such as tachycardia, rapid breathing, and sweating, but no detailed dream is recalled. (3) Relative unresponsiveness to efforts of others to comfort the person during the episode and, almost invariably, at least several minutes of confusion, disorientation, and preseverative motor movements. (4) It cannot be established that an organic factor initiated or maintained the disturbance.

Sleepwalking disorder has five points highlighted in DSM-III-R. (1) Episodes of arising from bed during sleep and walking about, usually occurring during the first third of the major sleep period. (2) While sleepwalking, the person has a blank stare, is relatively unresponsive, and can be awakened only with great difficulty. (3) On awakening, the person has amnesia of the event. (4) Within several minutes after awakening, there is no impairment of mental activity or behavior. (5) It cannot be established that there is an organic factor that initiated or maintained the disturbance (e.g., epilepsy) (American Psychiatric Association, 1987).

Recently, a consensus of sleep clinicians and researchers has published the International Classification of Sleep Disorders Diagnostic and Coding Manual (American Sleep Disorders Association, 1990). In that classification system, there is a general category of confusional arousals, (307.46-2), in addition to sleepwalking (307.46.0), and sleep terrors (307.46-1). Confusional arousals encompass disorders described in older terms as sleep drunkenness or excessive sleep inertia. These events typically consist of confusion during and following arousals from sleep, most typically from deep sleep in the first part of the night. As discussed in earlier sections, all of these events (sleepwalking, confused arousals, night terrors) are closely related behaviors with similar physiological underpinnings.

Differential Diagnosis

There are at least four primary considerations in the differential diagnosis of sudden partial arousals: nightmares, nocturnal seizures, REM behavior disorder, and awake behaviors.

Nightmares versus Night Terrors

Children with nightmares usually remember dream content in vivid detail. Nightmares occur during REM sleep and thus are much more likely to occur in the last third of the night (as opposed to night terrors, which usually occur in the first third of the night). Usually, nightmares do not have major motor activity and there is less anxiety, vocalization, and autonomic discharge during a nightmare. Literally, the nightmare sufferer wakes up *after* the nightmare is over, may be troubled by the memory of vivid images, often wants parental reassurance, and typically has some trouble going back to sleep. Children with nightmares usually have normal intellectual functioning, are completely awake, and quite able to describe what they "saw."

In contrast, night terrors occur *while* the subject remains partially asleep. The child usually does not recognize the parents, cannot be reassured or easily awakened, and the event usually terminates with a sudden return to very deep sleep with no memory of the event in the morning. Occasionally, children with night terrors can describe some vague image or memory related to the event, but this contrasts with the typical nightmare description. Although the distinction between nightmares and night terrors is often straightforward in older children, it can be very difficult in a young toddler or infant.

Nocturnal Seizures

One important consideration in these sudden paroxysmal events during the night with children is a nocturnal seizure. Seizures occur *predominantly* during sleep or on a arousal from sleep in up to 50 percent of children with epilepsy (Shouse, 1989). The relationship between sleep and seizures is complex and not well understood. Sleep deprivation appears to increase seizure tendency, sleep onset can precipitate seizures, and the synchronized EEG in Stage 2 sleep appears to facilitate propagation of a seizure focus. Seizures appear to be less likely during Stages 3 and 4 sleep and much less likely during REM sleep.

It is important to note that there are rare cases when seizures occur *only* during sleep when a seizure disorder has not otherwise been considered. In children with a documented seizure disorder (or a sleep deprived 10/20 EEG suggesting epileptiform discharges), nocturnal seizures must be considered on the differential of paroxysmal events. The timing of the event is important. Seizures are most likely to occur in association with Stage 2 sleep, or at the transition at the very beginning of sleep onset, or upon awakening in the morning. Thus, a history that events always occur one to two hours after sleep onset is much more consistent with a partial arousal than a seizure. The character, pattern, and frequency of events must also be considered. Additional aspects of differentiating between nocturnal seizures and confusional partial arousals will be discussed in the section on assessment.

REM Behavior Disorder

Normally, during REM sleep there is a complete suppression of muscle tone, preventing any body movements corresponding to dream activity. A number of cases have been described in adults where this suppression seems to be abolished, resulting in "acting out" of dream activity, including punching, kicking, leaping, and so on, correlating with reported dream imagery after awakening. These cases have been given the term *REM behavior disorder* (Shouse, 1989). A similar state has been created in animal experiments by small lesions near the locus ceruleus (believed to be close to the source of the motor inhibition during REM sleep) (Jouvet & Delorme, 1965).

The well-described clinical cases of REM behavior disorder in adult humans have been associated with neurologic lesions in this area or suspected subclinical lesions in this area. There are no reported cases of REM behavior disorder in children; however, this differential should be considered in children with a suggestive history, particularly if other CNS pathology is suspected. The timing of the events (later in the night) and

memory of specific dream imagery corresponding to the actions would suggest a REM-associated behavior.

Awake Behaviors

Occasionally children may simulate sleepwalking or night terror events while actually being completely awake. The cases we have observed have been in children with previous (real) sleepwalking or night terrors. Typically, the child received considerable parental attention following a genuine partial arousal and subsequently learned to simulate the event before falling asleep at night. In some ways, these cases are analogous to children with pseudoseizures occurring in children with real seizures. That is, these are learned behaviors that persist in a simulated state because of some inadvertent reward the child receives for the behavior. These can usually be differentiated by careful observation and history (unusual timing of the event, unusual character of the event, unusual pattern of response to demands, etc.). In one case in our center, sleep studies were required to convince parents that there was no longer a physiological basis for the events and that the child was actually awake and responsive.

Assessment Strategies

A central component to the clinical evaluation is a careful history of all sleep-related habits, as well as the characteristics, pattern, and frequency of the events. This information should include average time of going to bed, estimated time to fall asleep, nighttime awakenings or disturbances, average time of awakening in the morning, and details of daytime naps. This information should encompass both weekday and weekend schedules and should assess the regularity of the schedule as well as the average schedule.

Evidence of inadequate sleep, erratic sleep schedule, or a recent change in sleep schedule is critical. Inadequate nighttime sleep is more likely to present with symptoms of irritability, impulsivity, and emotional lability, rather than frank sleepiness in prepubertal children (hypersomnolence in response to inadequate sleep usually does not become significant until adolescence

[Carskadon & Dement, 1987]). In addition, clinical assessment should address the possibility of specific sleep disturbances, such as obstructive sleep apnea syndrome (history of loud snoring, restless sleep, and labored breathing, often related to enlarged tonsils and/or adenoids) or medications that may interfere with sleep.

The pattern of events should also be assessed. Occurrence in the first third of the night and an increased frequency corresponding to periods of being overly tired are strongly suggestive of typical partial arousal events. The character of the event should also be evaluated. The following characteristics are consistent with a history for partial arousals from deep sleep: awkward movements, sudden initiation and termination of the event, duration of 2 to 10 minutes, return to deep sleep quickly after the event, amnesia for the event in the morning, difficult to console during the event, and appearing in a daze or partially asleep during the event. Often, having the family keep a *prospective* diary of the basic sleep information, as well as the timing, frequency, and characteristics of these events, will help to sort out patterns that are difficult to ascertain by retrospective history alone.

Clinical evaluation should also assess the psychological realm, including sources of anxiety or emotional disturbances. These symptoms are particularly relevant if they may be contributing to children's difficulty in falling asleep. Children often put aside their worries until bedtime, then lay awake in a tense emotional state thinking about sources of fear, sadness, or worries before going to sleep. This can prolong sleep latency as well as perhaps directly influence the likelihood of these events through emotional arousal. Sometimes, parents can be unaware of these difficulties in children who are quiet and "well behaved."

Medications and medical illnesses should also be investigated. Stimulants (such as methylphenidate or theophylline) can prolong sleep latency. Withdrawal from sedative medications can also result in sleep disturbances. Excessive caffeine intake, such as from carbonated sodas, should also be considered. Evaluation for other psychiatric illnesses, particularly Tourette's syndrome and attention-deficit hyperactivity disorder (ADHD), should be considered because of the

associations described earlier. A family history of parasomnias or other sleep disorders should also be evaluated.

The next line of assessment can include the response to simple interventions, such as increased sleep or a more regular sleep/wake schedule. If the frequency of events subsequently diminishes following an improvement in sleep/wake schedule, the events are more likely to have been simple partial arousals from deep sleep.

Formal polysomnographic (EEG) laboratory studies are rarely required. EEG sleep studies should be reserved for cases where a specific question is being addressed, such as the following situations: (1) There is significant suspicion that the event could be a nocturnal seizure. In these cases, a special type of polysomnogram with a full 10–20 EEG (in addition to the usual sleep channels) is usually necessary. (2) The partial arousals are intense, frequent, and persist despite treatment. (3) Another type of sleep disturbance (such as sleep apnea) is suspected as the cause of the partial arousals (through the mechanism of compensatory deep recovery sleep contributing to the events).

TREATMENT

Evidence for Prescriptive Treatment

Given the wide range of intensity and clinical significance to these nocturnal partial arousals, the key to therapy is matching the appropriate intervention to the degree of problem. That is, mild sleepwalking or an occasional night terror in a young child requires only some parental reassurance with general suggestions regarding improved sleep habits and the likelihood that the events will decrease over time. In contrast, frequent, repetitive, intense, and agitated arousals in an older child may require very aggressive treatments, because of the risk of self-injury during the events and the possibility of associated pathology.

Behavior Therapy

Before proceeding to specific behavioral interventions, there are general suggestions that usually are good advice for the majority of families with children having parasomnias: (1) educate the family about the events (and what to do during the actual partial arousal event); (2) encourage a regular sleep/wake schedule in the child with good sleep habits; (3) try to improve the overall quantity and/or quality of sleep of the child when applicable; (4) help the child feel safe, secure, and relaxed at bedtime; and (5) help the child identify and express sources of anxiety and fear in a supportive environment. These general recommendations will now be discussed in more detail.

One of the primary roles of the clinician is to explain what these events are and are not, as they can be extremely frightening to parents. Explaining that their child's strange behavior and nonresponsiveness is related to being partially asleep (despite looking very aroused) is often one of the most important contributions of the clinician. Parents should also be advised about what to do during the events. To some extent, parental actions should be gauged by the frequency and intensity of the events. For mild to moderate events, the parents should try to direct the child to go back to bed and back to sleep. Occasionally, a calm verbal directive to go back to bed will be obeyed by the child with calm sleepwalking. Physically taking the child by the hand and leading him or her back to bed during a mild event can also be effective. Usually, however, the event needs to take its course and will end spontaneously. During more agitated arousals, interventions trying to direct the child back to bed can result in increased arousal and can inadvertently prolong the event. In general, if mild directing of the child does not work, the parents should let the episode run its course.

One very important caveat to this advice is with respect to the need to prevent self-injury. Although self-injury is rare, it certainly can happen, and with tragic consequences. It is important to remember that the child may be partially awake (and able to open doors, walk down steps, etc.), but continues to be partially asleep and capable of accidental self-injurious behaviors. This is particularly true in agitated sleepwalking, sleep running, and some night terrors that involve running and screaming. The primary intervention is usually to take a common-sense approach with the parents

addressing specific issues in their house. Eliminating factors such as sleeping on the top bunk bed, having a bedroom near the top of the stairs, or having windows or dangerous objects in the room are major considerations. In severe cases, where partial arousals are frequent and not responding to treatment, it may be necessary to install window guards or plexiglass.

One additional caveat is that occasionally a child will wake up briefly before going back to sleep. If this happens, the parents should treat it matter of factly (unless the child is specifically upset). Often, children are embarrassed and confused by seeing their parents' concerns or having their parents describe their bizarre behavior and this can lead to greater embarrassment and anxiety. Therefore, a very nonchalant, matter-of-fact handling of the event, helping the child go back to sleep, is usually best.

The next realm of general advice for parents of children with partial arousals has to do with optimizing sleep. This includes ensuring that the child is getting sufficient sleep and is free from identifiable sleep disturbances. Following a regular schedule of bedtime and wake-up time, including weekends, is often a key aspect to this problem. The parents should consider an earlier bedtime if there is any evidence that the child is getting inadequate sleep. Specific causes of delayed bedtime or difficulty falling asleep should also be directly addressed. In some young children, the concept of reintroducing a nap should also be considered. The focus of these suggestions and specific advice should be targeted at problems elicited during the evaluation of the sleep/wake habits and schedule.

The next category of general suggestions is within the realm of psychological factors. As presented, there is some evidence that anxiety and unexpressed anger may contribute to the frequency of these partial arousal events. The family should be encouraged to facilitate their child expressing sources of anxieties, fears, anger, and conflicts in healthy ways while awake. Age-appropriate suggestions of positive family interactions within this realm can be very helpful. In some cases, specific sources of fears and anxieties may be identified by the clinician and require treatment. Examples in our clinic have included previously unidentified sexual abuse, specific phobias, and separation anxiety. In these cases, treating the primary source of anxiety seemed to allow the arousal system of the child to wind down to a lower level and was accompanied by resolution of the partial arousal.

Also, as presented earlier, the specific emotional state as the child is falling asleep seems to be relevant. Thus, behavioral interventions focused on this time interval can be crucial to positive interventions. Specifically, helping children focus on positive images, positive relaxation exercises, and family interventions to help the child feel safe and secure at bedtime can lead to decreases in sleep latency as well as a positive emotional state as the child is falling asleep (which may help partial arousal events during the night).

The role of specific behavioral interventions is best considered in the context of problem solving in the individual case consistent with the principles described so far. That is, specific treatments should target the elimination of the identified behaviors interfering with sleep. Similarly, rewarding key behaviors consistent with good sleep habits is also crucial to successful treatment.

Pharmacotherapy

Tricyclic antidepressants and benzodiazapines have been shown to have positive effects on partial arousal events. Both medications decrease arousals from sleep and lighten the deepest Stage 4 sleep. This combination of effects seems to decrease the partial arousal events from deep sleep. The difficulties with pharmacologic interventions include tolerance effects, withdrawal effects, and questions concerning possible long-term detrimental effects on sleep. That is, initially there is a strong suppression of Stage 4 sleep with these medications; however, over time, Stage 4 pressure seems to build up with tolerance effects and rebound of Stage 4.

Missed doses of medication (or discontinuation) can result in withdrawal rebound of Stage 4 and very intense partial arousals. In some ways, pharmacotherapy is really covering up events more than eliminating them. Specifically, if the primary problem is inadequate sleep, repeated disturbances of sleep, or difficulty falling asleep, covering the

partial arousal events with medication will temporarily suppress symptoms; however, they will often recur later because of the need for deep Stage 4 sleep.

The largest amount of experience with medications has been with imipramine and diazepam (Nino-Nurcia & Dement, 1987). Doses of 2 to 10 mg of diazepam at bedtime have been used successfully (Guilleminault, 1987). Imipramine is typically given at 25 to 75 mg doses at bedtime.

Although many clinicians report at least temporary success using these pharmacologic interventions, at our center we reserve pharmacotherapy for a couple specific cases: The first is to temporarily break the cycle when there is a large amount of tension/crisis in the family around the events. In some cases, the family gets so wound up around fears and concerns over these events that bedtime becomes tense for the entire family, leading to further sleep deprivation and increased events. In these cases, temporarily using imipramine to suppress the events and alleviate the tension by giving the family a couple weeks of returning to a lower arousal state can be instrumental in implementing behavioral and other treatments.

The second case for medication is when there are very frequent and severe repeated partial arousals that do not respond to behavioral treatment and optimizing sleep. We have seen individuals with multiple partial arousals, despite all interventions described above. In some of these cases (particularly when they overlap with Tourette's or obsessive compulsive disorder), we have used clonazepam at bedtime with good results. We have usually begun at a dose of 2.5 mg at bedtime.

Alternative Treatments

Hypnosis has also been used in a number of cases with positive results in treating night terrors (Kramer, 1989; Toboda, 1975). Psychotherapy has also been described as indicated in many severe cases of night terrors, especially in older adolescents and adults (Kales, Cadieux, Soldatos, & Kales, 1982).

One alternative treatment recently described involves scheduled awakenings by the parents approximately 30 minutes prior to the usual time of partial arousal events (Lask, 1988). Although the authors report good results in their experience, this approach can contribute to sleep disruption and worsen events in some cases.

Selecting Optimal Treatment Strategies

In addition to the general advice and concepts that are evident from the previous discussion, the key to optimal treatment is to target specific behaviors, problems, or sources of sleep disturbances relevant to the individual case. For example, one very common problem is oppositional behaviors around bedtime. In its mildest form, this involves multiple parental callbacks, repeated requests for additional stories or drinks of water, fears of the dark, and so on, which prolong sleep onset and decrease total sleep. In more severe forms, these involve major battles between children and parents, and escalate into high degrees of tension and conflict on a nightly basis. These behaviors may lead not only to later time of sleep onset but also to negative emotional states prior to going to sleep (which can contribute to arousal events).

Identifying the most salient features interfering with sleep onset is often the key to successful intervention. Eliminating the culprit (which may be as simple as a television in the bedroom) or changing a particular pattern of behavior at bedtime may go a long way toward addressing the problem. Conversely, the pattern of parent/child interactions may be so complex as to require a full redesigning of pre-bedtime rituals, with a specific behavioral contract of acceptable and unacceptable behaviors (with specific rewards and consequences).

One important concept in designing behavioral interventions around sleep onset is weighting the design heavily toward a reward strategy. That is, rewarding behaviors that are consistent with good sleep habits (complying with pre-bedtime rituals, going to bed and turning the lights out on time, and staying in bed for the remainder of the night) are much more likely to be effective than trying to implement punishment at bedtime (which can raise arousal levels and result in battles, which further delay sleep onset). Consequences for not complying with the program should be enforced the next day. That is, the child can be informed that he or she has lost privileges (however, if possible, the actual consequences should be enforced the next day). In younger children, this often is not possible and a time-out procedure may be necessary at the specific time. Handling the situation with emotional neutrality, rather than getting into a battle, will be less likely to interfere with sleep following the intervention.

One variant of this problem occurs in children who show little in the way of external behaviors interfering with sleep; however, their internal fears and anxieties prevent them from being able to fall asleep. Relaxation training and/or positive imagery exercises at bedtime can be essential in helping these children. The only effective way to prevent a child from focusing on negative thoughts and images that cause anxiety, fears, and the like is to help him or her actively focus on positive thoughts and images that are relaxing and associated with positive affect. Helping the family to provide structure to practice these exercises while awake will facilitate the child implementing these techniques at bedtime. Although a cassette tape of a relaxation exercise can be helpful in individual cases, in general, activities such as music and television at night are more likely to lead to difficulties going to sleep in the long run. Habits and conditioned responses are critical to both positive and negative routines. Thus, the key is to develop *strong positive routines at bedtime.*

Problems in Carrying Out Interventions

A few general categories of problems in carrying out interventions will be discussed. One general category is the overall level of chaos and disorganization in sleep and schedules across the entire family and home situation. That is, one often encounters a general family environment where the work and sleep schedules of multiple family members result in chaos and contribute to a lack of a structured schedule for the child. There physically may be a limited amount of private and quiet space for the child and the erratic hours of other family members may make it virtually impossible for the child to follow regular undisturbed bedtime hours. In addition, if parents are having difficulties following regular schedules themselves, it can be hard for them to have the organization to implement these recommendations for their children. Often, taking a more systemic approach with the entire family is essential in addressing the specific problems with the child. Again, the magnitude of intervention must be gauged to the severity of the problem in the child. On the other hand, the advantages of improved scheduling and better sleep/wake habits can also be presented to the entire family.

A second general category of difficulties involves a general lack of parenting skills concerning consistent limit setting. The parents may have trouble dealing with oppositional behaviors or temper tantrums during the day as well as at night. Having these parents try to set firm limits at night (in the absence of being able to handle temper tantrums or oppositional behaviors during the day) is not realistic. General information and advice about time-out procedures and setting consistent limits can be a prerequisite to addressing any specific bedtime or sleep-related behaviors.

Another consideration pertains to specific behavioral and emotional problems interfering with treatment. That is, specific anxiety disorders, obsessive compulsive disorders, depression, separation anxiety, or Tourette's syndrome may be the key to the sleep-related problems or behaviors. Unless the underlying disorder is identified and treated, general recommendations for good sleep/wake hygiene and improving sleep are unlikely to be successful. Therefore, as discussed earlier, *adequate clinical assessment* is often the key to successful treatment.

In an analogous manner, medical problems, as well as psychological or psychiatric problems, can complicate treatment. Obstructive sleep apnea syndrome is one example that has already been discussed; however, any medical problem that results in pain or discomfort can interfere with sleep and feed into the cycle of relative sleep deprivation, deep recovery sleep, and increased partial arousals. Thus, sickle cell anemia with painful crises, injuries, or orthopedic problems with pain, or symptoms such as nocturnal itching in children atopic dermatitis, can all be related to mild-to-moderate sleep deprivation and result in increased parasomnias. In addition to the actual medical problem, medications can interfere with sleep. Stimulant medications such as Ritalin or Theophylline can also feed into this cycle.

Relapse Prevention

The most common source of relapse is the return to sleep/wake schedules or habits that result in conditions of inadequate night time sleep. The key to relapse prevention is to help the family *anticipate* what may lead to recurrence of old habits and old schedules. It is importantfor the family to *value* adequate sleep. Having children get sufficient sleep is important not only to prevent night terrors but also for optimal daytime functioning. Inadequate sleep can lead to irritability, difficulty with concentration, and emotional lability. Thus, helping the family prioritize sleep and structured schedules can help prevent relapse of the problems. Another relapse scenario is when an acute event, such as an ear infection or an illness, will cause the family to revert back to old habits. Preventing relapse often overlaps with helping the family anticipate these types of situations and outlining with them what they will do when these arise. Another additional point about relapse is that no matter what the cause of these events or their intensity, they tend to decrease with increasing age. Thus, as children get older, there is less likelihood of a recurrence of sleep-related problems, and the frequency and intensity of these events tends to be less

CASE ILLUSTRATION: A SIMPLE CASE

Rather than focus on one case, the range of problems and treatment approaches can be best illustrated by choosing a few cases of parasomnias covering the spectrum of the disorder. Each case presented below represents a real subject seen and treated in our center.

Case Description

Brian was an 8-year-old boy brought to the clinic by his parents due to their concerns about his unusual events during the night. They described that approximately two to five times each month, they would discover Brian wandering around the house at night or find him in the morning in a different part of the house from where he went to bed. If they discovered him asleep while he was wandering around, his movements seemed to be semipurposeful, but he was in a "bizarre and possessed-like" state with a far-away look in his eyes. He appeared to be awake to his parents, but he did not recognize them and would not answer questions. Occasionally, he would seem to hear them and could be directed, but he then would suddenly become confused and think they were someone else.

At times, Brian's parents would find him in very unusual places, such as in the cellar or in his closet in the morning when they awoke, and no one would have any idea of how he got there. One morning (which had contributed to them coming into the clinic), the entire family panicked in the morning when they were unable to find him. After a lengthy search, Brian was found in a small laundry area, covered by clothes.

The sleep history revealed that Brian's "usual" bedtime was 10:00 P.M. on most nights. This bedtime was procrastinated by a variety of means, however, and often he actually went to bed at 11:00 P.M. or later. Brian was very active at night and had great difficulty winding down, but once he was in bed with the lights out, he seemed to fall asleep very quickly. The family's best estimate of when the partial arousal events occurred was around midnight to 1:00 A.M. Except for these events, the rest of the sleep history was negative for disruptions, snoring, or awakenings.

On school days, Brian got up at 6:30 A.M. to catch a 7:00 A.M. bus. It was often very difficult to wake him up in the morning, but once awake, he did not seem to be sleepy during the day. He was a very active boy, who did well in school, and, except for being a little bit "overactive," there were no other problems described by the family. Brian did not take any structured naps, although the family did note that he occasionally fell asleep during car rides.

On weekends, Brian tended to stay up even later—often until midnight—and usually slept in later, until approximately 9:00 A.M. When asked about any pattern to these events, the parents described an impression that the events were more likely to occur when he came home from spending the weekend with his grandparents where they knew he tended to be very active and get even less sleep at night.

Differential Diagnosis and Assessment

All aspects of the description are consistent with sleepwalking events, including the timing, pattern, and character of the events. In addition, there seems to be at least strong circumstantial evidence that Brian is getting barely adequate sleep and that the events are more likely to occur following sleep deprivation. Although he did not appear sleepy to his parents, he was irritable and very sensitive to sleep loss, and whenever he stopped being active (such as during car rides) he fell asleep.

Treatment Selection

The primary component to treatment was explaining what these events were to these very concerned parents. The relationship to getting less sleep was also discussed. The need for a physically safe environment was also discussed in detail. A major part of the treatment recommendations focused on trying to increase the total amounts of sleep that Brian got and particularly to regularize his somewhat erratic schedule. The parents were instructed to move his bedtime up by 15 minutes a night and have a very firm set of rules around bedtime with a point system (with rewards for compliance with this routine and limits). They were further instructed to keep a prospective diary of his sleep times, including bedtime, estimated time to fall asleep, wake-up time, and any pattern of daytime tiredness and the occurrence of the events. The goal was to increase and regularize his sleep.

Treatment Course and Problems in Carrying Out Intervention

Brian responded very well to a more structured bedtime routine and adjusted easily to early bedtimes in the short run. He increased his total amount of night sleep by approximately 45 minutes a night on school nights. He was easier to wake for school in the morning. The frequency of the events decreased dramatically to one event every other month. The parents also noted that he was less irritable and more relaxed.

Outcome and Termination

Brian continued to have the tendency to slip back to late-night schedules as soon as structure and rewards were discontinued. He also continued to have sleepwalking events following weekends or camp experiences where he was very excited and active and got less sleep. The family motivation to enforce the bedtime decreased as the events were infrequent and less concerning to them.

Followup and Maintenance

Brian continued to do well and the events disappeared completely over the next couple of years.

CASE ILLUSTRATION: A PUZZLE RESOLVED

Case Description

Beth was a 6-year-old girl brought to the clinic by her parents for sudden onset of screaming in the middle of the night, occurring almost every night for the previous month, usually occurring between 11:00 P.M. and midnight. Typically, the parents heard sudden screaming and ran into Beth's room to find her in an agitated state, with her eyes wide open, making flailing movements with her arms. She would not respond to her parents' attempted reassurances. She appeared somewhat glassy-eyed, confused, and not seeming to recognize her parents during these events. At times her heart seemed to be racing and she appeared terrified. After approximately 3 to 5 minutes (which occasionally seemed like 10 or 20), she would suddenly close her eyes, make a few mumbling sounds and awkward movements, return to a deep sleep, and remain asleep for the best of the night. In the morning, Beth would have no memory of the event, nor was she able to describe a specific nightmare that she had experienced the previous evening. She was somewhat confused and scared by her parents' descriptions of what she had done at night.

The history revealed that Beth went to bed at 9:00 P.M., following a very stable bedtime ritual including stories and similar routines. The parents reported that she went to bed easily and that they did not hear from her again until the events at about 11:00 P.M. She got up in the morning at 7:30 A.M. on weekdays for school and on weekends woke up spontaneously by 8:00 or 8:30 A.M. She was only a little difficult to wake in the morning and did not appear tired during the day; however, the parents had noticed that she seemed somewhat more irritable than usual (although they still described her as an extremely well-behaved child). She had given up her daytime nap at age 4 and had not taken any naps since that time.

The events had begun approximately two months after she had begun first grade, shortly after she had received her first report card. The parents downplayed the significance of the report card as they described her as having all A's and being very happy with school. The parents were unaware of any changes in her schedule except at the beginning of school when she did need to get up earlier. The parents did not describe any difficulties falling asleep that they had noticed, nor any other changes in Beth's psychological state.

The parents' primary concern was that the events themselves were extremely frightening to the family. Beth was normally so quiet and well behaved that these events seemed bizarre and frightening. They were concerned that these were an indication that something was very seriously wrong. They were particularly frightened by their inability to console or comfort her during the events. Additionally, the sudden onset and frequency of the events (no prior history of any partial arousals then suddenly having three to five a week) was concerning to them.

Medical and developmental history were completely unremarkable. There had been no medications or illnesses and growth and development were normal. The family history was positive for sleepwalking in an uncle until adolescence.

In the interview, Beth was extremely well behaved, was bright for her age, and sat quietly, answering questions appropriately. She did not describe any specific fears or worries and described being unaware of these events.

Differential Diagnosis and Assessment

Almost every detail of the parents' descriptions was consistent with night terrors (partial arousals of deep sleep). The timing of the event, character and length of the event, pattern, and descriptions were all consistent with this diagnosis. The puzzling questions were identifying factors with respect to sleep schedule and psychological factors and why there had been a sudden onset and high frequency of severe events.

The nature of the events and the likelihood that they were partial arousals from deep sleep were explained in detail to the parents. The description made a great deal of sense and the parents found this reassuring. They were asked to keep a prospective diary of Beth's sleep habits and events (including checking on her after they put her to bed to estimate the time she fell asleep). They were asked to chart the number of events, how long they lasted, the description of the events, the time she woke up, and any pattern of changes in daytime irritability, tiredness, and so on. In addition, the possibility of the psychological factors, such as anxieties and worries, that could be contributing were also discussed with the parents. They were encouraged to talk to Beth, have her draw pictures and discuss the pictures, and play situations to help her describe any issues of worry and conflict.

The parents returned two weeks later having complied very well with the assessment and/pretreatment attempt. Their prospective sleep diary information was very revealing in that they discovered that Beth was taking approximately 45 minutes to fall asleep after she was in bed, even though she was laying quietly with only a night light. Even more revealing was the information that the mother had discovered with respect to *a specific worry* of Beth's since getting her report card. Although Beth had received all A's, she thought that she had failed to achieve her goal of getting "straight A's" (a cousin of hers had received considerable attention from the entire family because of her reliable procurement of straight A's). Although Beth had said nothing to anyone prior to this, she thought that the A's on her report card were inferior because they were made with slanted lines (she had the idea that *straight* A's were made with block letters and vertical lines). It was also clear that this little girl was very aware of how much her family valued "straight A's" because of the amount of attention her cousin had received. She was very concerned that she had disappointed her parents, despite the praise they had given her for her report card. Clearly, this worry that she had disappointed her parents was something she had thought about at bedtime and also seemed to be contributing to her difficulty in falling asleep.

Treatment Selection

Treatment focused on the obvious factors of difficulty falling asleep and specific source of worry related to Beth's report card. The parents explained to Beth that she had achieved "straight A's" and spent some time trying to put these issues into better perspective (that is, trying to reassure her that her performance in first grade was not critical to their feelings about her). Additionally, the family was encouraged to help her feel very reassured and supported at bedtime and to help her focus on positive thoughts and feelings at bedtime. They were instructed to continue the sleep diary and estimated sleep times and number of events.

Treatment Course and Problems in Carrying Out Intervention

Beth's time to fall asleep quickly went from 45 minutes to less than 10 minutes. All partial arousal events ceased. Telephone followup over the subsequent few months indicated that she continued to be free of any partial arousals or night terrors.

Followup and Maintenance

The family was instructed to recontact the clinic if there was any recurrence of events. The general concept that their daughter's anxiety and need for reassurance may be significant (beyond the night terrors) was also presented to the family. Although it is possible that related problems may recur, or other signs of anxiety and need for reassurance may surface as she gets older, Beth is currently doing well two years later.

CASE ILLUSTRATION: SEVERE AND COMPLEX PARTIAL AROUSALS

Case Description

William was an 8½-year-old boy with a long history of night terrors and partial arousals as well as severe behavioral and emotional problems. Little was known about William's early history except that his mother reportedly had significant drug and alcohol use during her pregnancy, and his infancy and toddler years were reportedly in a very chaotic environment prior to custody being granted to his grandparents at age 3. His grandmother reports that since the age of 3, he has had severe problems with night terrors.

The events occur anywhere from 30 minutes after going to sleep up until four hours after going to sleep. They occurred from once a week to as frequently as four to five times each night. The grandparents had noted a number of changes in the frequency and intensity of events as he was put on medications for his behavioral/emotional problems (these included imipramine at bedtime, which improved the events temporarily; he had also received trials of Ritalin, Lithium, and Haldol). Although the nighttime events were severe (with extreme screaming, shouting, and running), they had received less direct attention because clinicians had focused primarily on his

severe daytime emotional and behavioral problems. The grandparents, however, had very significant concerns about the nighttime events and described how they made it that much harder to take care of William (not only was he a problem all day but they were fearful of these events at night which interfered with *their* own rest).

At times, William had fallen and hurt himself while running during these events. The grandparents had removed dangerous objects from his room and locked his bedroom door so that he could not run down the steps. One evening, they heard him banging around the room at the usual time for these events and suddenly heard the crash of a window and discovered that he had gone through the second floor window and fallen to the ground. He sustained a compression fracture of his lumbar spine as well as multiple contusions from that fall. During admission to the hospital for that event, our sleep center was consulted because of the extreme frequency and intensity of his partial arousals.

Further history revealed that he had a regular schedule for going to bed between 8:30 and 9:00 P.M., having no difficulty falling asleep, no other sleep continuity disturbances (except the partial arousals), and was only moderately difficult to wake in the morning at 8:00 A.M. He had no signs of overt daytime sleepiness, but did have very high baseline levels of irritability. His grandmother described that he was very sensitive to sleep loss and his behavior problems became very severe when he did not stay tightly to his permanently full sleep needs.

Differential Diagnosis and Assessment

Although many aspects of the history indicated that these events were likely to be partial arousals, the intensity and severity of the events were unusual. Particularly because of the history of self-injury and multiple events, despite seeming to get adequate sleep, a more comprehensive assessment was indicated. He was weaned off of all medications, and polysomnography was performed after being medication free for one week.

In the sleep lab, William was put to bed easily on his usual schedule at 8:00 P.M. and fell asleep within 8 minutes. He quickly went into Stage 4 delta sleep and within 20 minutes of going to sleep, had a sudden arousal to almost full awake for 90 seconds in which he was confused and agitated. The event ended abruptly and he quickly returned to Stage 2 sleep, followed by Stage 4. A second similar event occurred 90 minutes after sleep onset, a third event 120 minutes after sleep onset, a fourth event at 180 minutes after sleep onset, and a fifth event 280 minutes after sleep onset. The events became milder over the night, and by the fifth event, he merely sat up, talked calmly (still partially asleep and confused), but then quickly went back to deep sleep. At 6:07 A.M., he awakened spontaneously, was alert, reported feeling rested, and ready to get up for the day. He had no memory of any of the nighttime events. The first four events all occurred out of Stage 4 sleep; the fifth event came out of Stage 2. His overall sleep measures were normal except for a high percentage of delta sleep (40 percent).

Since all of the events came out of non-REM sleep, primarily Stage 4, and showed a pattern of decreasing in intensity over the night, they appeared physiologically consistent with partial arousals from deep non-REM sleep. There was no indication of any seizure-like activities (although to be ruled out completely, a full 10/20 EEG with a faster paper speed would have been required). The events were clearly not REM-related phenomena. There was one other unusual feature evident from this polysomnographic recording. In addition to the 5 arousals described above, there were another 11 paroxysmal arousals scattered across other sleep stages, including REM and light Stage 2. These arousals also occurred suddenly and lasted about 90 to 120 seconds, but were not accompanied by behavioral manifestations of partial arousals. Literally, there appeared to be a sudden arousal, approximately every 20 minutes throughout the night, of unclear etiology. When these arousals corresponded with deep non-REM sleep, they resulted in partial arousals. When they coincided with REM or light Stage 2, they resulted in full arousal and then a quick return to sleep.

A second night of sleep was recorded with a trial of Imipramine, 75 mg, at bedtime. On Imipramine, the sleep study showed six arousals with only two partial arousals—one at 45 minutes after sleep onset, the second 110 minutes after sleep onset. In each of the partial arousal events, William had only a moderate increase in heart rate and no other signs of autonomic hyperarousal and was easily redirected back to bed and returned to sleep easily.

Treatment Selection

Treatment included counseling and education of the grandmother about continuing to ensure optimal nighttime sleep, continuing to prioritize the regular sleep/wake schedule and a variety of factors in the house for physical safety of the environment. Pharmacologic treatment decisions included considerable discussion of the past history, which clearly had shown that imipramine had not been effective at controlling these episodes, nor had it eliminated them in the laboratory (it only decreased them from five events to two events). Clonazepam (a benzodiazapin) was felt to be a more powerful suppressant of these events and a trial of clonazepam was recommended.

Treatment Course and Problems in Carrying Out Interventions

Although clonazepam initially and dramatically decreased these events, there were considerable problems with tolerance and withdrawal. That is, tolerance developed quickly, and there was a need to increase the dosage of the medication; furthermore, when a dose of medication at bedtime was missed for any reason, William often showed severe rebound partial arousals. Because of these difficulties, a trial of Tegretol was attempted. The nighttime dose of Tegretol also seemed to be effective at decreasing the frequency and intensity of events (but did not eliminate them entirely).

Outcome and Termination

William continues to have intermittent severe partial arousals, but these have been less intense and less frequent while he has been on the Tegretol. With the added physical safety features, he has had no further self-injury. Although he continues to have significant behavioral and emotional problems, the problems with the partial arousals at least seem to be contained.

SUMMARY

Sudden partial arousals from deep sleep are common occurrences in children. These sudden arousals result in a mixed state of being partially asleep and partially awake. The events can range physically from a few awkward movements to very complex and agitated behaviors with a wide spectrum of emotional affect. They occur most frequently in children between the ages of 4 and 8, and in association with relative sleep deprivation or being overtired. Family history of partial arousals increases the likelihood of events, and there is a clear association with emotional and behavioral problems in children and adolescents. The etiology of partial arousals appears to be related to difficulty leaving the first deep sleep cycle or a sudden disruption in a deep sleep cycle.

The differential diagnosis includes nightmares, nocturnal seizures, REM behavior disorder, and awake behaviors. A major component of assessment is a careful and thorough history covering sleep habits and the details and patterns of the partial arousal events. Behavioral therapy is the mainstay of treatment. Pharmacologic treatment can be an adjunct to treatment and is also indicated in some severe recurrent cases. Optimal treatment requires correctly identifying contributing components to the problem and targeting these components, including increasing the amount of sleep, improving the quality of sleep, and regularizing these components. Increasing the amount of sleep, improving the quality of sleep, and regularizing the sleep/wake schedule can result in dramatic resolution of partial arousals. Behavioral interventions to regularize bedtime hours, encourage relaxation at bedtime, and the elimination of anxiety-provoking thoughts at bedtime have also been shown to be helpful.

Our understanding of the psychophysiology of partial arousals is limited. There is a need for more research to provide a better understanding of these complex behaviors and their relationship to psychopathology in children and adolescents.

REFERENCES

Abe, K., & Shimakawa, M. (1966). Predisposition to sleep walking. *Psychiatric Neurology, 152,* 306–312.

American Psychiatric Association. (1987). *Diagnostic and statistical manual of mental disorders* (3rd ed., rev.). Washington, DC: Author.

American Sleep Disorders Association in Association with the European Sleep Research Society, the Japanese Society of Sleep Research and the Latin American Sleep Society. (1990). *The international classification of sleep disorders diagnostic and coding manual.* Lawrence, KS: Allen Press.

Bakwin, H. (1970). Sleep walking in twins. *Lancet, 2,* 446–447.

Barabas, G., Matthews, W. S., & Ferrari, M. (1984). Disorders of arousal in Gilles de la Tourette's syndrome. *Neurology, 34,* 815–817.

Carskadon, M. A., & Dement, W. C. (1987). Sleepiness in the normal adolescent. in C. Guilleminault (Ed.), *Sleep and its disorders in children* (pp. 53–66). New York: Raven Press.

Cirignotta, F., Zucconi, M., Mondini, S., Lenzi, P. L., & Lugaresi, E. (1983). Enuresis, sleep walking and nightmares: An epidemiological survey in the Republic of San Marino. In C. Guilleminault & E. Lugaresi (Eds.), *Sleep/wake disorders: Natural history, epidemiology and long-term evolution* (pp. 237–241). New York: Raven Press.

Dahl, R. E., & Puig-Antich, J. (1990). Sleep disturbances in child and adolescent psychiatric disorders. *Pediatrician, 17,* 32–37.

Dahl, R. E., Puig-Antich, J., Ryan, N. D., Nelson, B., Dachille, S., Cunningham, S. L., Trubnick, L., & Klepper, T. P. (1990). EEG sleep in adolescents with major depression: The role of suicidality and inpatient status. *Journal of Affective Disorders, 19,* 63–75.

Ferber, R. (1989). Sleepwalking, confusional arousals, and sleep terrors in the child. In M. H. Kryger, T. Roth, & W. C. Dement (Eds.), *Principles and practice of sleep medicine* (pp. 640–642). Philadelphia: Saunders.

Guilleminault, C. (1987). Disorders of arousal in children: Somnambulism and night terrors. In C. Guilleminault (Ed.), *Sleep and its disorders in children* (pp. 243–252). New York: Raven Press.

Halstrom, R. (1972). Night terror in adults through three generations. *Acta Psychiatrica Scandinavica, 48,* 350-352.

Jacobson, A., Kales, J. D., & Kales, A. (1969). Clinical and electrophysiological correlates of sleep disorders in children. In A. Kales (Ed.), *Physiology and pathology: A symposium* (pp. 109-118). Philadelphia: Lippincott.

Jouvet, M., & Delorme, F. (1965). Locus coeruleus et sommeil paradoxal. *Social Biology, 159,* 895-899.

Kahn, A., Van de Merckt, C., Rebuffat, E., Mozin, J. J., Sottiaux, M., Blum, D., & Hennart, P. (1989). Sleep problems in healthy preadolescents. *Pediatrics, 84,* 542-546.

Kales, J. D., Cadieux, R. J., Soldatos, C. R., & Kales, A. (1982). Psychotherapy with night terror patients. *American Journal of Psychotherapy, 36,* 399-407.

Kales, A., Soldatos, C. R., Bixler, E. O., Ladda, R. L., Charney, D. S., Weber, G., & Schweitzer, P. K. (1980). Hereditary factors in sleep walking and night terrors. *British Journal of Psychiatry, 137,* 111-118.

Klackenberg, G. (1982). Somnambulism in childhood: Prevalence, course and behavioral correlation. *Acta Paediatrica Scandinavica, 71,* 495-499.

Klackenberg, G. (1987). Incidence of parasomnias in children in a general population. In C. Guilleminault (Ed.), *Sleep and its disorders in children* (pp. 99-113). New York: Raven Press.

Kramer, R. L. (1989). The treatment of childhood night terrors through the use of hypnosis — A case study. *The International Journal of Clinical and Experimental Hypnosis, 37,* 283-284.

Kurth, V. E., Gohler, I., & Knaape, H. H. (1965). Untersuchungen uber der parvor nocturnus bei kindern. *Psychiatric Neurologie Und Medizinische Psychologie, 17,* 1-7.

Lask, B. (1988). Novel and non-toxic treatment for night terrors. *British Medical Journal, 297,* 592.

Nee, L. E., Caine, E. D., Polinsky, R. J., Eldridge, R., & Ebert, M. H. (1980). Gilles de la Tourette Syndrome: Clinical and family study of 50 cases. *Annals of Neurology, 7,* 41-49.

Nino-Nurcia, G., & Dement, W. C. (1987). Psychophysiological and pharmacological aspects of somnambulism and night terrors in children. In H. Y. Meltzer (Ed.), *Psychopharmacology: The third generation of progress* (pp. 873-879). New York: Raven Press.

Ryan, N., Puig-Antich, J., Rabinovich, H., Ambrosini, P., Robinson, D., Nelson, B., Iyengar, S., & Twomey, J. (1987). The clinical picture of major depression in children and adolescents. *Archives of General Psychiatry, 44,* 854-861.

Shirley, A. F., & Kahn, J. P. (1958). Sleep disturbances in children. *Pediatric Clinics of North America, 5,* 629-643.

Shouse, M. N. (1989). Epilepsy and seizures during sleep. In M. H. Kryger, T. Roth, & W. C. Dement (Eds.), *Principles and practice of sleep medicine* (pp. 364-376). Philadelphia: Saunders.

Simonds, J. F., & Parraga, H. (1984). Sleep behaviors and disorders in children and adolescents evaluated at psychiatric clinics. *Developmental and Behavioral Pediatrics, 5,* 6-10.

Terr, L. (1983). Chowchilla revisited: The effects of psychic trauma four years after a school-bus kidnapping. *American Journal of Psychiatry, 140,* 1543-1550.

Toboda, E. L. (1975). Night terrors in a child treated with hypnosis. *American Journal of Clinical Hypnosis, 17,* 270-271.

CHAPTER 18

TIC DISORDERS

Lori A. Head   Medical University of South Carolina

Floyd R. Sallee   Medical University of South Carolina

Mitsuko P. Shannon   Medical University of South Carolina

DESCRIPTION OF DISORDER

Clinical Features

Tics are rapid, sudden, purposeless movements that are involuntary, repetitive, and stereotyped in nature. Tics are highly distinct from other movement disorders of childhood. These disorders are classified by age of onset, duration of symptoms, and presence or absence of vocal or phonic tics along with the usual motor tics. Key clinical features are their occurrence at random intervals and apparent voluntary suppression for varying periods of time. Some patients frequently describe a premonitory sensory urge for which tics are voluntarily performed to relieve the urge. The norm is for the tic to occur without apparent cause. Tics are sometimes triggered by environmental stimuli and are exacerbated by stress, fatigue, or underlying medical illness. A waxing and waning course in severity as well as a change in anatomical location from time to time are also common features.

Motor tics are further subdivided into simple or complex types. Simple motor tics are fast, darting, meaningless muscular movements that occur in isolated muscle groups or in one anatomical location. They can be embarrassing and sometimes physically painful, such as jaw snapping or blepharospasm. Complex motor tics are often slower and more purposeful in appearance. These include hopping, clapping, tensing of multiple muscle groups, touching objects or people, making obscene gestures, or engaging in socially inappropriate acts. Frequently, complex motor tics are difficult to separate from compulsions when the activity is organized and ritualistic in character. Self-destructive behaviors, such as head banging, eye poking, or biting are complex tics that require immediate intervention.

Simple vocal tics are sounds and noises, such as hissing, coughing, barking, or spitting. The tics of the sniffing and throat clearing variety precipitate investigations for allergy, upper respiratory infections or sinusitis, and other ENT abnormalities. Complex vocal tics involve meaningful words or phrases (e.g., "Oh boy," "That's right"). Dysfluencies of speech that resemble stammering or undue word emphasis and/or alterations in speech volume and phrasing can also be complex vocal tics. Frequently, speech blocking during speech initiation or at transition phrases is quite common. The most dramatic and distressing complex vocal symptom is coprolalia. This is an explosive occurrence of foul or "dirty" words that are usually of a sexual or aggressive nature. Coprolalia is present in only a minority of Tourette's patients (from 5 to 20 percent), but is by far the most dramatic. It is not necessary to have coprolalia for a diagnosis of Tourette's, and linguistic context frequently determines the presence or absence of coprolalia. Other bizarre and unusual symptoms present in Tourette's patients include a tendency to imitate what they have seen (echopraxia), heard (echolalia), or said (palilalia). These more unusual symptoms are present in a series of patients with very low frequency.

Associated Features

Associated clinical features of tic disorders include psychiatric and cognitive dysfunctions. These are frequently encountered in patients with more severe tic disorders, such as in Tourette's disorder (TD). Attention-deficit hyperactivity disorder (ADHD) and obsessive-compulsive disorder (OCD) are two of the more frequently comorbid psychiatric dysfunctions. Comings and Comings (1984, 1985) report that in 250 cases of Tourette's disorder, ADHD was present in 54 percent. In the more severely disordered Tourette's patients, incidence of concurrent ADHD increases to 70 to 80 percent. Even in mild cases of Tourette's patients, incidence of ADHD is 78 times that of the general population. Learning disabilities are present in a large portion of patients, but it is presently unknown to what extent these learning problems exist in the absence of ADHD. Hagin and Kugler (1988) reported a series of Tourette's disorder patients that have lower than expected school achievement in mathematics and reading comprehension.

Though OCD is genetically linked to tic disorders, there is considerable controversy as to its incidence or comorbidity in patients with TD. Frankel and associates (1986) found an incidence of OCD in adult TD patients of 51 percent using the Leyton Obsessional Inventory (LOI) (Cooper, 1970). An epidemiologic study of 431 patients diagnosed with Tourette's disorder commissioned by the Ohio Tourette's Syndrome Association found a point prevalence of 74 percent for OCD at some time during their illness (Stefl, 1983). In children, Grad, Pelcovitz, Olsen, Matthews, and Grad (1987) found that 7 of 25 patients with an average age of 11 years met criteria for OCD based on the child version of the LOI (Berg, Rapoport, & Flament, 1986). Other personality traits, such as aggression, hostility, and depression, have been found in samples of TD patients in addition to obsessive-compulsive behavior (Stafl, 1983).

Epidemiology

Tics are the most common movement disorder of childhood, and the prevalence of tics is estimated at 5 to 18 percent of school-aged children between the ages of 6 and 16 (Achenbach & Edelbrock, 1981). Stress is counted as the major factor in tic onset for transient tic disorders of childhood. TD, thought once to be uncommon, occurs in 1 person in every 2,500 in its complete form and approximately 3 times that number in partial expressions that include chronic motor tics (Brunn, 1984, 1988). From a large epidemiologic study by Caine, McBride, and Chiverton (1988), point prevalence of TD in children under the age of 17 is approximately 3 per 10,000. Because the incidence of transient tics is quite common in the population, the task of the clinician is to determine when tics are likely to be a more progressive and debilitating syndrome leading to TD.

No pathophysiologic factors have yet been identified in the etiology of tics, although genetic factors play a significant role in a subset of patients (Pauls & Leckman, 1986). At present there is no definitive diagnostic test other than careful clinical evaluation. Diagnosis is based solely on observable signs and symptoms. Secondary tics, however, can be the result of postencephalitic or traumatic injury and can sometimes be drug induced (e.g., stimulants, levodopa neuroleptics, carbamazepine, phenytoin, and phenobarbital). (Carbon monoxide poisoning or chorea resulting from traumatic insult can also lead to tic-like clinical features.) The bulk of tic disorders are idiopathic, and a genetic basis can be found only in approximately 50 percent of cases.

Etiology

The pathophysiologic basis of Tourette's syndrome has yet to be described, but the most compelling hypothesis concerning the origin of tics involves an overactivity of central dopaminergic systems. Dopamine is the primary negative feedback control of an inhibitory loop of the caudate putamen to globus pallidus involving the basal ganglia gabaminergic system. An overactivity of dopamine in this negative feedback loop allows the escape of these areas, resulting in uncoordinated rapid motoric outbursts recognized as tics. The evidence for central dopamine overactivity comes from three sources: biochemical, pharmacologic, and clinical observation.

Biochemical evidence comes by examination of the cerebrospinal fluid breakdown products of dopamine, homovanillic acid (HVA). HVA is consistently decreased in Tourette's Syndrome patients (Singer, Tune, Butler, Zuczek, & Coyle, 1982), indicating decreased central turnover of dopamine perhaps mediated by supersensitive dopamine receptors. *Pharmacologic evidence* comes from administration of dopamine agonists such as L-Dopa, which can exacerbate tics or precipitate a toxic Tourette's Syndrome. Inhibitors of dopamine synthesis (a-methyl-p-tyrosine) decrease tics as well. *Clinical evidence* of a role for dopamine in tic pathophysiology consists of the tremendous clinical efficacy of dopamine-blocking drugs such as the neuroleptics.

Only recently have attempts been made to understand the involvement of noradrenergic or cholinergic neurochemical systems and to apply this knowledge to the treatment of Tourette's Syndrome and related tic disorders (Leckman et al., 1991). Specifically, much attention has been directed to researching the efficacy of clonidine, an alpha-2-adrenergic agonist. Cohen, Young, and Nathanson (1979) were the first to report beneficial effects of clonidine in the treatment of TS. Since then, clonidine has been widely used in clinical practice and is recommended as an alter-native to neuroleptics. The mechanism of action of the effects of clonidine has not been firmly established yet. However, previous reports have speculated that the effectiveness of clonidine in treating TS may be due to the ability of the alpha-2-adrenergic receptor agonist to reduce the firing rate and the release of catecholamines from central noradrenergic and dopaminergic neurons (Cohen et al., 1979). There is also increasing evidence to support heterogeneity among the alpha-2 class of adrenergic receptors and their distinctive distribution within relevant brain regions, which may account for differences in patient response of the particular symptoms of tic disorders to clonidine treatment (Bylund, 1985).

DIFFERENTIAL DIAGNOSIS AND ASSESSMENT

DSM-III-R Categorization

The DSM-IV categorization is unchanged from that of DSM-III-R (APA, 1987) with durational criteria separating transient tic disorders from both chronic motor tic and TD. To meet criteria for transient tic disorder, tic symptoms should persist no longer than 12 consecutive months. This distinction, however, in some children, is complicated by the fact that transient tics may recur over several years but the tics themselves tend to be mild and not persist for longer than a few weeks or months. Chronic motor vocal tic disorders are characterized by stability of their symptomatology, which persists in the same anatomic location with the same phenomenology over a long period of time from childhood into adult life. Chronic motor tics are far more common than chronic vocal tics. Chronic motor tics of a mild degree are seen in the community as "habits" that do not often precipitate medical intervention. A family genetic study suggests that chronic motor or chronic vocal tic disorder is two to three times more prevalent than TD (Comings, Comings, Devor, & Cloniger, 1984) and that an etiologic relationship between chronic motor tic disorder and TD is supported (Pauls & Leckman, 1986).

Differential Diagnosis

A diagnosis of Tourette's disorder is clearly delineated in DSM-IV diagnostic criteria, but assessment of durational criteria is sometimes difficult. Both multiple motor and one or more vocal tics must be present for some time during the illness, although not necessarily concurrently. Tics must occur many times a day and nearly every day or intermittently throughout a period of more than one year. The anatomical number, frequency, and complexity of tics are noted to change over time and the onset must be before age 21. Furthermore, occurrence of tics should not be exclusively during psychoactive substance intoxication or as a result of known central nervous systems disease, such as Huntington's chorea or postviral encephalitis. Differential diagnoses include postencephalitic tics, head injury, carbon monoxide poisoning, neuroacanthocytosis, and drug-induced (e.g., stimulant, Levodopa, neuroleptic) toxicity.

Assessment Strategies

Assessment strategies should include a clinical interview, a neurologic examination, and assessment instruments such as parental self-report inventories (e.g., Tourette's Syndrome Questionnaire [TQ], Tourette's Syndrome Symptom List, Latent Obsessional Inventory, Child Version, or Child Behavior Checklist and Profile). Tics are difficult to objectively quantify reliably due to their heterogeneous presentation. Tics, such as simple eye blinks and grins, must be measured along with copropraxia and coprolalia, although the latter are far more distressing in a social context. Complicating assessment is the tendency for symptoms to wax and wane irrespective of treatments or interventions. Self-reports concerning the global assessment of tics are fairly reliable, but comparing last week's eye blink to this week's shoulder shrug may be problematic in a clinical setting.

Patients during clinical interviews are known to suppress or to cover up tics. Goetz, Tanner, Wilson, and Shannon (1987a) found that in 30 patients the motor tics recorded with an examiner present was only 27 percent of that recorded in the absence of an examiner. For 7 of 30 patients with flagrant tics, no observable tics were noted with the examiner present. Therefore, part of the assessment should include videotaping with the patient alone in the examination room and without the bias of an interview situation.

The clinical assessment should document the location, number, frequency, intensity, complexity, and degree of disruption associated with motor and phonic tics. The assessment should substantiate clinical waxing and waning of the disorder and its duration of severe tic symptoms along with factors associated with their exacerbation or improvement. An assessment should also be made of the risk to self-injury due to the presence of tics (e.g., eye poking or biting tics). A past medical/developmental history relevant to onset of tics for documentation of prenatal birth injury, developmental delay, medication exposures, or head injuries is also important in the assessment of a patient presenting with tics. A documentation of life events associated with onset and exacerbation of tic symptoms, stability of family life, coping skills, and social support available to the patient are necessary. A genetic family history of other relatives or family members with unusual movement problems or obsessive compulsive behaviors should be taken.

Neurologic Examination

Tics are rarely confused with other forms of hyperkinetic movement disorders. Both clonic and tonic tics occur but most often tics are brief and are of the clonic variety. Clonic tics can sometimes be confused with myoclonus and chorea. Tonic tics can be confused with dystonic movements. Buccolingual tics can be problematic in patients treated with neuroleptics, as it is difficult to distinguish readily these movements from neuroleptic-induced dyskinesias. Tics often involve ocular movements, rarely seen in other movement disorders of childhood. Characteristics of abruptness, suppressability, and the influence of stress or relaxation on movement should help the clinician determine that a tic is present.

A careful neurologic workup should be done so as not to miss metabolic conditions (e.g., Wilson's disease), which may produce tremors sometimes confused with tics. The neurologic examination of Tourette's patients frequently reveal minor motor asymmetries or unilateral impairment of rapid alternating movements in approximately half of the patients examined (Sweet, Solomon, Wayne, Shapiro, & Shapiro, 1973). From 12 to 38 percent of patients frequently have EEG abnormalities such as nonspecific slowing (Bergen, Tanner, & Wilson, 1982). Neuroimaging of patients presenting with tics has been nonspecific with reports of asymmetrical lateral ventricles or prominent cortical sulci, particularly in TD patients (Caparulo et al., 1981; Lees, Robertson, Trimble, & Murray, 1984). At present, in the absence of localized findings on neurologic examination, an extensive neurophysiologic or neuroanatomic workup is not routinely performed in the evaluation of tic disorders.

Rating Scales

A systematic collection of self-report data from parents and patients is advantageous to the clinicians because of sampling across multiple settings and to obviate observer bias. Structured parental and/or self-reports have been used in epidemiologic, genetic, and research studies. The best of these questionnaires include the Tourette's Syndrome Questionnaire (TSQ) and the Tourette's Syndrome Symptom List (TSSL) (Cohen, Leckman, & Shaywitz, 1984). Adjunctive symptoms of inattention, impulsivity, and motoric hyperactivity are best delineated by the relevant scales or by using the Child Behavior Checklist and Profile (Achenbach & Edelbrock, 1983). Some type of clinician-utilized rating scale is frequently helpful in assessing visit to visit variability and tic symptoms and for also assessing treatment progress. The most useful of these scales are the Tourette's Symptoms Severity Scale (TSSS) developed by Shapiro and Shapiro (1984) and the Tourette's Syndrome Global Scale (TSGS) (Harcherick, Leckman, Detlor, & Cohen, 1984).

A newly developed unified ratings scale sponsored by the Tourette's Syndrome Association, called the Unified Tic Rating Scale (UTRS), integrates a number of strategies and rating scales. The UTRS consists of six parts, including a symptoms checklist, historical ratings, examiner ratings, tic counts, and overall impairment ratings, and

global disability ratings (Peter Como, personal communication). The videotaped assessment can either be formalized by using a rating scale developed by Goetz and colleagues (1987a) or can simply be a method for following patients in clinical treatment (Goetz, Tanner, Wilson, Carroll, Como, & Shannon, 1987b). The drawbacks of videotaping include the need for expensive and cumbersome equipment; however, the benefit cannot be underestimated for reviewing treatment-emergent side effect symptoms after the employment of neuroleptics. Videotapes can be examined to determine if a movement problem is due to underlying tic disorder or neuroleptic usage.

TREATMENT

Evidence for Prescriptive Treatments

Treatment of Tourette's disorder and other tic disorders has been problematic and, in many cases, disappointing. The treatment strategies must be decided on a case-by-case basis, reflecting the heterogeneity of tic symptoms and/or their behavioral sequelae. Behavior therapy, pharmacotherapy principally with neuroleptics and/or clonidine, and some adjunctive treatments involving medications, family work, school or work consultation, and psychotherapy should all be considered. Treatment success depends on a multimodal approach that considers quality-of-life issues, not simply tic suppression alone.

Behavior Therapy

Since 1958, a variety of behavioral techniques have been employed in the treatment of tic disorders (Ollendick, 1981). To date, the most effective techniques include self-monitoring and habit-reversal procedures. In several case studies (Maletzky, 1974; Thomas, Abrams, & Johnson, 1971; Ollendick, 1981), self-monitoring was reported to decrease tics and was associated with long-lasting remission of symptoms. In addition to self-monitoring, habit reversal is usually employed. This is done by employing a competing response on awareness of the onset of the tic. For example, the client may tense a muscle group antagonistic of the tic (Ollendick, 1981). At this time, no controlled studies of these practices have been performed; therefore, it is difficult to assess the reliability of behavior therapy in children. It is felt that behavior therapy alone may be an effective treatment in only mild cases of tic disorders. In the more severe cases, behavior therapy in combination with medications is thought to have the best chance for success. The evaluation of treatment progress in behavior therapy also should consider the waxing and waning course of the illness.

Pharmacotherapy

Pharmacotherapy is the mainstay of treatment for most tic disorders. It is now possible to decrease tic symptomatology by up to 95 percent in most cases by use of neuroleptic drugs with dopamine receptor-blocking activities. By blocking the dopamine receptors, the dopaminergic overactivity is temporarily corrected. Neuroleptics seem to differ in their receptor affinities. Most classical neuroleptics, such as haloperidol and pimozide, have a high affinity to dopamine D2 receptors, but the thioxanthines and phenothiazines have relatively more affinity to D1 receptors. This finding has been correlated to the ability of these drugs to induce neurologic side effects and effect hyperkinetic symptoms. It has been claimed that a drug with a high D2 affinity would most likely be able to improve symptoms of Tourette's Syndrome (Stahl & Berger, 1982), but not without a significant side effect profile. Recent confirmation of this theory has been the success of sulpiride, an exclusive D2 blocking agent (Robertson, Schnieden, & Lees, 1990). Unfortunately, no sulpiride-like drug is currently available for use in the United States.

Haloperidol, a selective D2 blocker, is the drug of first choice to treat patients with Tourette's disorder and related tic disorder since its successful use in 1961 (Shapiro et al., 1989). Haloperidol is effective in 90 percent of cases with tic symptom reduction in the range of 60 to 80 percent (Bruun, 1984; Shapiro, Shapiro, & Eisenkraft, 1983; Shapiro, Shapiro, & Wayne, 1973). Unfortunately, haloperidol is difficult to use because of a narrow therapeutic window. The dosage must be titrated against an endpoint of incapacitating side effects in motor (extrapyramidal), cognitive (attention, memory, learning), and affective (lethargy, phobia, depression) domains in a high percentage of patients.

In 60 percent of patients treated with haloperidol, significant side effects either interfere with therapeutic effects of nullify them to the degree that they must be removed from the medication (Shapiro et al., 1973). Haloperidol may impair motivation, decrease attention, and impair learning; however, quality studies are few (Comings & Comings, 1987; Mikkelsen, Detlor, & Cohen, 1981; Shapiro et al., 1989). In a more recent study by Shapiro and colleagues (1989), 20 percent of the patients treated with a mean daily dose of haloperidol of 4.5 ± 2.7 mg reported moderate or marked loss of motivation, depression, and/or cognitive dulling. However, Bornstein and Yang (1991) compared Tourette's disorder patients who were taking neuroleptics to Tourette's disorder patients who were not taking medication and found that they did not perform differently in terms of educational, intellectual, and neuropsychological tests. Although these results are encouraging, haloperidol has definite side effect limitations. Despite these limitations, haloperidol is still considered the single most successful treatment for TD.

At this time, no precise dosage range for the use of haloperidol for the treatment of tic disorders has been established. The dosage required for the treatment of patients with tics is considerably less than that used to treat psychoses. Studies on blood levels done by Erenberg (1988) corroborate that the levels necessary are only one seventh of that needed to treat other psychiatric disorders. There is, however, no definitive relationship between blood level and tic symptom reduction or side effects. Plasma half-lives have no clinical correlation to biologic half-lives for neuroleptic drugs. The plasma half-life for haloperidol has been reported as 13 to 35 hours. Of more clinical importance than half-life is the attainment of steady-state CNS levels (which takes approximately four days) that allow for once daily dosing. Based on this, the medication should be increased weekly in order to more completely evaluate the impact of the most recent change. Also, the medication should first be given on a twice daily schedule. This can be later moved to a more convenient once a day regimen.

The initiation of a neuroleptic medication can be associated with acute extrapyramidal side effects. This can be avoided by starting the medication at a very low dose and increasing by slow, steady increments. If an acute reaction is suspected, treatment with an antihistamine or anticholinergic medications can rapidly and safely reverse the reaction. Although many exceptions exist, most frequently the pediatric patient receives 0.05 mg/kg per day (Erenberg, 1988). In light of the fact that haloperidol is effective but carries with it many deleterious side effects, a principal goal of clinical research in TD is to find a therapeutic agent with the same or greater efficacy as haloperidol, but with fewer side effects and greater acceptability among patients.

The drug of second choice is pimozide, a diphenylbutylpiperidine (Shapiro et al., 1983; Shapiro, Shapiro, & Fulop, 1987). Like haloperidol, pimozide preferentially binds the D2 receptor, but in several trials on different hyperkinetic diseases, it was found to have fewer akinetic and sedative side effects (Regeur, Pakkenberg, Fog, & Pakkenberg, 1986). In a study carried out by Shapiro and associates (1989), haloperidol, pimozide, and placebo were compared for efficacy and side effects in a double-blind, cross-over design. The results of this controlled study of the treatment of 57 patients with Tourette's disorder suggested that both haloperidol and pimozide were more effective than placebo, but that haloperidol was slightly more effective than pimozide. Contrary to previous beliefs, the authors found no statistical differences in the side effects of haloperidol versus pimozide, including akinesia and sedation.

Furthermore, electrocardiogram (ECG) results were compared and revealed statistically significant prolongation of the QTc for pimozide versus haloperidol. The clinical significance of this QTc abnormality is thought to be minimal. Thus, the results of this study, which is the only double-blind, placebo-controlled study of haloperidol versus pimozide to date, suggest that, since haloperi-

dol is slightly more effective than pimozide, with a similar pattern of adverse effects, and because pimozide has the potential for prolonged QTc intervals requiring routine ECG monitoring, haloperidol is still the treatment of first choice for TD. However, in patients who do not respond adequately to haloperidol, a therapeutic trial of pimozide may be indicated.

In terms of dosage and administration, pimozide is similar to that of haloperidol. When adverse reactions occur, they are exactly the same as other neuroleptics, requiring the same management. The relative potency is 2.0 to 2.5 mg of pimozide is equivalent in action to 1 mg of haloperidol (Erenberg, 1988). The current recommendation is that a dosage regimen of pimozide start with a low initial dose (0.5 to 1.0 mg/d) to be increased every four to seven days by 0.5 to 2.0 mg/d until clinical efficacy is achieved to a usual maximum of 10 mg/d or 0.2 mg/kg/d of pimozide. Adolescents and adults may receive a maximum of 20 mg/day. Salee and associates (1987) conducted a study to characterize the pharmacokinetics of pimozide in adults and children with Tourette's disorder. The results indicate extreme intersubject variability and a trend for the biologic half-life of pimozide in children to be shorter than that of adults. However, more study is warranted.

Clonidine is the drug of first choice when dealing with mild and transient tic disorders. It is also indicated alone or in conjunction with a neuroleptic when attentional problems or an ADHD-like syndrome is part of the clinical presentation. The opinion that clonidine has a place in the treatment of tic disorders is widespread, but it is not yet conclusive. Some studies have concluded that up to 62 percent of the patients have responded favorably (Leckman et al., 1985), whereas one author found clonidine to be no better than placebo (Goetz et al., 1987b). Clonidine has also been reported to have a beneficial effect on behavior and impulsivity in subjects with TD. This effect seems to be independent of its effect on motor tic behaviors (Leckman et al., 1991). The potential for improving comorbid behavioral problems and decrease tic activity is appealing. In general, the neuroleptic agents do not improve behavior. The side effects of clonidine include dizziness, nausea, and orthostatic hypotension. Clonidine does not cause extrapyramidal side effects.

In general, treatment with clonidine is started at 0.05 mg twice daily. The response to clonidine is delayed, even up to several weeks. If the initial dose is tolerated, it can be increased by 0.1 mg twice daily. After four weeks, the dosage can again be increased. The increase can be continued until sedation or dizziness is reported. The usual daily dose is 5.5 ug/kg per day (Erenberg, 1988). If compliance is an issue, a clonidine transdermal patch is available. If the clonidine is to be discontinued for any reason, it must be tapered off slowly, over a minimum of one week.

Alternative Treatments

The search for alternative treatments for tic disorders continues. Many other dopamine receptor blocking agents have been tried (fluphenazine, sulpiride, piquindone, a selective D1 receptor agonist). To date, fluphenazine and sulpiride look the most promising. Fluphenazine, a piperazine phenothiazine, is thought to be an alternative treatment for patients with multiple tics who cannot tolerate haloperidol. Side effects often diminish without loss of tic control (Goetz, Tanner, & Klawans, 1984). Sulpiride, a substituted benzamide, with selective D2 receptor blocking effects, has been reported to have a lower incidence of extrapyramidal side effects than traditional neuroleptics. In a retrospective study done by Robertson and associates (1990), sulpiride proved useful in the control of motor and vocal tics. Sulpiride, which is currently used widely in Europe, is said to have less deleterious effects on memory and learning than haloperidol (Robertson et al., 1990). Double-blind, placebo-controlled, long-term, prospective studies need to be done to more clearly establish the role of fluphenazine and sulpiride in the treatment of this patient population.

Unfortunately, in the treatment of Tourette's disorder and related tic disorders, there is no "magic bullet." The neuroleptic agents now available are the most effective for tic symptom reduction; however, the possibility of significant side effects is quite high. No alternative methods to date have proved to be as efficacious in ameliorating severe tic symptomatology. Successful treatment of this disorder not only takes skilled clinicians to manage the pharmacotherapy but also hard work and understanding on the part of the patient and the patient's family or support system.

Recently, the association between multiple tics and obsession and compulsions has attracted much interest. Although the proposed etiologies of tic disorders and OCD are quite similar, their pharmacotherapies are quite different. To date, there are only case reports in the literature supporting the use of anti-OCD drugs such as fluoxetine and clomipramine in combination with neuroleptics in the treatment of tic disorders (Ratzoni, Hermesh, Brandt, Lauffer, & Munitz, 1990).

In the case report involving the use of clomipramine, the OCD and tic symptomatology abated. In the three case reports of fluoxetine, the obsessive-compulsive symptoms were markedly improved in all patients; tics improved in one patient, worsened in one, and were unchanged in the other (Riddle, Hardin, King, Scahill, & Woolston, 1990).

Attention-deficit hyperactivity disorder is also more prevalent in patients with tic disorders than the general population. If the ADHD is severe enough to raise the issue of pharmacologic treatment, a trial of clonidine alone or in combination with a neuroleptic is appropriate. The administration of psychostimulant drugs to a child with a tic disorder is indicated in only very rare cases (Golden, 1990).

Psychotherapy and stress management are also very valuable adjunctive tools to medication management, and in many cases imperative to a positive outcome. In moderate to severe cases of the tic syndromes, psychotherapy alone or medication alone is responded to less favorably than the combination of these therapies. It is also known that during periods of stress, tic symptomatology is exacerbated. In fact, even when the tic disorder has been in remission for years, stressful times can cause recurrence of the hyperkinesis. Stressful situations cannot always be avoided; therefore, in order to prevent unnecessary relapse, it is important that the patient learn stress management techniques.

Selecting Optimal Treatment Strategies

Selecting optimal treatment strategies must be done on a case-by-case basis. It is important to point out that none of the available medications is curative and that all are designed for palliative measures. Also, there is no evidence to indicate that early treatment with medication will alter the course of the disorder in any way. Therefore, use of medication should be reserved for moderate to severe cases.

In the milder cases (about 50 to 65 percent) of Tourette's disorder and related tic disorders, the best treatment is nonpharmacologic. Because of the potential for side effects, medication should be avoided. However, there is no evidence that early intervention is unnecessary. The patient should begin immediately to understand the nature of the disorder. In addition, because the tics are frequently more bothersome to the parents and family members than the involved children, it is imperative that the family be educated as well. If the patient has comorbid behavior and/or attention deficits, these must also be confronted.

When the tics become disruptive to the point of causing psychosocial impairment, pharmacologic intervention should begin. Since the tolerance of tic behavior varies from family to family, it is important that families become a part of the decision-making process and that each case be assessed individually. It is also important to stress that the medication will only provide partial symptomatic relief. Because therapeutic and toxic dosages are so close, it is generally considered best to keep the total dosage at an amount that will decrease symptoms by approximately 75 percent (Erenberg, 1988). Those concerned must also be educated on the characteristic waxing and waning of the disorders and that it may not be due to the medication.

In making specific medication decisions, many issues must be considered and there are many different schools of thought. The most widely used approach is to initiate treatment with clonidine in those patients who have tics of mild to moderate severity. Although the success rate with clonidine is below that of the neuroleptics, the side effect profile is generally insignificant, especially with transdermal delivery. A trial of clonidine often leads to long-term benefits and reduces the need for neuroleptics. There is also the potential for behavioral improvements, if this is an issue.

The threshold for the use of neuroleptics should be quite high, given their potential for side effects and long-term sequelae. However, if the tics are severe or causing significant impairment, they should not be withheld. When a neuroleptic drug is indicated, haloperidol or pimozide are currently the drugs of choice with similar efficacy and side effect profile. Some investigators feel pimozide is associated with less sedation and akinesia. In some refractory cases, combinations of clonidine, pimozide, or haloperidol can be used.

Problems in Carrying Out Interventions

Not only are the available treatments not optimal but there are many problems in carrying out both pharmacological and nonpharmacological interventions. The biggest obstacle to face is that of compliance. Compliance usually is more of an issue with the parents than with the involved child. The most common form of noncompliance is the refusal to medicate, even when indicated. This is due to the stigma that has been placed on the use of "psychiatric" medications. Also, parents often see many untoward side effects at the initiation of therapy and promptly discontinue the drug without consulting the physician. Many parents feel that medications leave their child appearing "drugged up." Furthermore, as we know, the nature of tic disorder is that of a waxing and waning with periods of remission. When a child's tics are less severe, the parents many times will want to stop the medicine, the feeling being that it is no longer needed. Abrupt withdrawal of many of these medications can lead to relapse and significant discomfort.

On the other spectrum, noncompliance can also

take the form of overuse of medications. As stated earlier, many times the tics are more bothersome to the parents and family members than to the affected child; therefore, the parents have a tendency to overmedicate. Compliance with psychotherapy is also a problem. It is almost inevitable that some time throughout the course of the child's life, psychotherapy in some form will be necessary. There is also a stigma around therapy per se and many families will refuse to attend.

Another major problem in carrying out interventions occurs in less fortunate situations when the family is not invested in the well-being of the affected child. A child with a tic disorder needs a great deal of support for normal psychosocial development. The child already faces many hurdles in peer groups and very badly needs a stable home environment. However, it is important to not overprotect the child as to disrupt the normal maturation process as well as the rest of the household.

Relapse Prevention

Even in the worst case scenario, there are several things that can be done to prevent unnecessary relapse and complications. The most important preventive measure is education. The child must be educated about the disorder. The child must also be kept informed and involved in decisions as to all aspects of the illness. The child must learn how to monitor his or her symptoms and side effects of the medications if capable. The child must also learn behavioral strategies that will hopefully decrease hyperkinesis. Parents and other family members must also be involved in medication and therapy decisions. In most cases, the parents are the primary caregivers of the child and must be able to titrate the medication if necessary. The parents must also know what to do in the event of acute side effects. The parents and family members must also learn coping skills in dealing with this syndrome. It is never easy to see a loved one in distress. The child's teachers, clergy, coaches, friends, and so on all must be educated about the disorder and given some practical advice for dealing with some of the bizarre behaviors that they will witness.

Support is the second key to preventing comorbid behavioral problems and relapse, and can come from many different sources. In most cases the major support system usually comes from the family. However, not all children with tic disorders have this resource. A second avenue for support is from the child's physician. Most clinicians who are treating tic disorders are quite invested in the care of their patients and are willing to lend support whenever necessary. In addition, there are many support groups around the country that provide counseling. This also gives children and parents a chance to learn that they are not alone, and therefore they can share experiences.

CASE ILLUSTRATION

Case Description

Jeff, a 13-year-old white male, with a five-year history of severe motor and vocal tics, was referred for inpatient psychiatric evaluation exhibiting aggressive and hypersexual behavior. This behavior included hitting a camp counselor without provocation, running away from camp, explosive outbursts of singing "The Star Spangled Banner," and exposing himself to peers after making sexually provocative statements. The patient has a long psychiatric history that started at the age of 3, with inattention and increased motor activity.

Dextroamphetamine was initially started and changed to methylphenidate by Jeff's pediatrician over the course of two years. Good results were achieved, and the patient did well until motor tics, which included eye blinking, were noticed. It was felt that results achieved on the methylphenidate outweighed the motor tic problem and the medication was continued. Approximately one year later, a mathematics learning disability was diagnosed. Jeff continued to do well until the fourth grade, at which time the motor tics developed into vocal throat noises and a "flap" of the arms that caused him to be teased by other children. The methylphenidate was discontinued. The patient's motoric behavior returned as well as the inattentiveness, and his grades dropped.

Due to the continued motor tics, a neurologic evaluation was sought by the family. Clonidine was started by the neurologist with only slight tic resolution. Methylphenidate was again instituted with only minimal exacerbation of tics. Two years later, behaviors surfaced that included an extreme need for order in the patient's room, to shower at certain times of the day, and an extreme desire to call and be around a fellow classmate to the point of obsession. At this juncture, a psychiatric evaluation was requested and obsessive-compulsive disorder was diagnosed. Jeff was then placed on clomipramine. One year later, at age 13, the motor tics became markedly elevated and the patient began exhibiting hypersexualized behaviors. He would feel compelled to expose his genitalia in public and have an overwhelming compulsion to touch the genitalia of his peers.

The patient's prenatal course was complicated by the fact that his mother was a type I diabetic, resulting in polyhydramnios. Delivery was complicated by a shoulder presentation, which necessitated a fractured clavicle. Developmentally, the patient's milestones were all delayed. Current school functioning is compromised by behavior problems with a continued need for remedial math secondary to his learning disability. Family psychiatric history included one older brother who was also diagnosed with OCD; the patient's father was described as hyperactive as a child.

Neurological examination revealed an ambidextrous 13-year-old white male with a continuous facial tic of eye squinting. The eye-squinting tic was present both when videotaped alone and with the examiner present. Jeff also exhibited a complex tic of holding his right hand up in the air as if to brush his hair, then coming out towards the examiner. No vocal tics were heard. The remainder of the exam revealed a poor tandem gait with intention tremor and posturing on stressed gait. A Tourette's Symptom Global Scale (TSGS) was administered with a score of 44, reflecting both the motor component and Jeff's severe behavior and learning difficulties.

Mental status revealed an inattentive male with labile affect. Jeff was obsessed with his need to pull his pants down. At the same time he felt remorse about his socially inappropriate behavior,

he was fascinated with the subject. He had no disorganization of speech or thought. His judgment was intact as he knew his exposing behavior to be socially inappropriate.

A full assessment was performed, which included routine laboratory studies, MRI, EEG, EKG, and psychometrics. The abnormal studies were as follows: The EEG revealed background slowing with generalized cerebral dysfunction. The MRI showed a cystic midline structure in the cerebellum consistent with a congenital Dandy-Walker posterior fossa cyst. A WISC-R revealed a Verbal IQ of 104 and a Performance IQ of 84.

Differential Diagnosis and Assessment

This complex case presents with typical movement problems of tics but includes more unusual behavior in the compulsive spectrum. These compulsions of exposure include a willful knowledge of the act but no seeming control over completion of the exposure. This is akin to the induction of self-injurious behavior in patients with TD who feel compelled to put their hand in a fan or on a hot stove despite the known result. There is a limbic release quality to these accounts, in that despite known cues from the environment, the patient is unable to modify his behavior. Jeff also presents with the frequent prodromal and often comorbid ADHD syndrome for which methylphenidate is often given, leading to tic exacerbation.

In this case, methylphenidate was not causative, and its use later in the clinical course did not seem to exacerbate tics and in fact was palliative with regard to the patient's ADHD. The patient's learning disability was a specific one in the math area and was not solely due to ADHD. The patient's OCD symptoms appeared late in the course of tic disorder. Despite treatment with clomipramine, his obsession with self-exposure and his compulsion to engage in this were not ameliorated. Jeff's case was further complicated by the finding of a cerebellar cyst. It is unknown to what extent this static structural anomaly contributed to the onset of tic symptoms. Essentially, the finding of a structural anomaly does not alter the course of pharmacotherapy. This case illustrates the advantage, however, of both a neurologic and psychiatric workup.

Treatment Selection

Treatment focused on the most salient and problematic symptom of self-exposure. Treatment consisted of behavioral consequences for each act and an increase in Jeff's dose of clomipramine to 250 mg/day, or approximately 5 mg/kg/day. Pimozide at 2 mg/day was also utilized to decrease motor tics. At such a low dose of neuroleptic, it was felt that clonidine 0.1 mg twice per day would be needed to work synergistically with pimozide as well as to afford some measure of treatment for Jeff's ADHD symptoms.

Treatment Course and Problems in Carrying Out Interventions

A reasonable length of time would be needed in order for the clonidine to reach maximum benefit. This could be as long as one to two months, leading to two problems: (1) parents as well as children lack the patience necessary in waiting for the benefits to occur and (2) because of the delayed onset of action, compliance is a problem, particularly in the adolescent age group. Pimozide and clomipramine together are quite sedating, so that medication would need to be adjusted as not to interfere with Jeff's known learning disability.

Outcome, Termination, Followup, and Maintenance

Jeff did marginally well on a combination of pimozide, clomipramine, and clonidine, with a reduction in compulsive behavior, inattentiveness, and tics. Followup after the initiation of treatment included regular medication checks every two weeks, until the clonidine reached maximum efficacy, in about eight weeks. Side effects should be closely noted, as well as any physiologic changes that would include pulse and blood pres-

sure changes. After maximum benefit is achieved, as well as maximum dosage, monthly followup is usually sufficient. Treatment of ADHD and tic disorders is usually continued for a period of time, which will enable the patient to reestablish a level of functioning both socially and academically. It would then be prudent after a sufficient period of time, typically 6 to 12 months, for the clinician to begin tapering medication in anticipation of a medication-free period, if possible.

SUMMARY

The tic disorders, which are the most common movement disorders of childhood, remain quite problematic to the patient, the patient's family, the community, and the clinician. Although progress has been made over the last several years in the assessment, diagnosis, and treatment of tic disorders, much more research is necessary to effectively manage this difficult patient population.

The advances that have been made in the diagnosis and assessment of tic disorders are primarily due to the development of reliable and repeatable rating scales, such as the TSSS, TSGS, and the UTRS. The advantage of such measures is that they can be easily adapted for treatment management and for patient followup. The disadvantage of these global measures is that they force the examiner to integrate disparate features of the syndrome that may fluctuate widely over the assessment period of interest. Strategies to combine successful rating scales and assessment tools into a unified approach holds promise for accurate determination of the symptomatology in tic disorders. Assessment and diagnosis of associated psychiatric symptoms, such as OCD and ADHD, is also vital for appropriate patient care.

Advances in the treatment of tic disorders have also been made. Unfortunately, however, to date, no ideal treatment regimen is available. Only a few medications (e.g., haloperidol, pimozide, clonidine) have been found useful in tic symptom reduction. Although effective, these medications have several drawbacks: (1) haloperidol and pimozide can have deleterious side effects, (2) none is successful in all cases, and (3) none is curative and can provide only symptomatic relief.

More recent advances have been made in treating associated psychiatric symptoms, such as ADHD and OCD. These treatments include the use of fluoxetine and clomipramine for OCD, and clonidine for ADHD. Depending on the clinical presentation, many times the combination of haloperidol or pimozide with clomipramine and/or clonidine is an effective regimen for improving associated behavioral difficulties and suppression of tic activity. Furthermore, due to the psychological sequelae of the tic disorders, adjunctive therapies such as psychotherapy, family therapy, school counseling, and stress management are quite relevant to a positive course.

Even with the best clinical management, approximately one third of patients with significant tic disorders will not benefit from the currently available treatment approaches (Erenberg, 1988). This has motivated researchers all over the world. Hopefully, in the near future, a larger number of safe and effective treatments will be available.

REFERENCES

Achenbach, T. M., & Edelbrock, C. S. (1981). Behavioral problems and competencies reported by parents of normal and disturbed children aged four through sixteen. *Monographs of the Society for Research in Child Development, 46.*

Achenbach, T. M., & Edelbrock, C. S. (1983). *Manual for the Revised Child Behavior Checklist and Profile.* Burlington, VT: University Associates in Psychiatry.

American Psychiatric Association. (1987). *Diagnostic and statistical manual of mental disorders* (3rd ed., rev.). Washington, DC: Author.

Berg, C. J., Rapoport, J. L., & Flament, M. F. (1986). The Leyton Obsessional Inventory-Child Version. *Journal of the American Academy of Child Psychiatry, 25,* 84–92.

Bergen, D., Tanner, C. M., & Wilson, R. (1982). The electroencephalogram in Tourette syndrome. *Annals of Neurology, 11,* 638–641.

Bornstein, R. A., & Yang, V. (1991). Neuropsychological performance in medicated and unmedicated patients with Tourette's disorder. *American Journal of Psychiatry, 148,* 468–471.

bruun, R. D. (1984). Gilles de al Tourette's syndrome: An overview of clinical experience. *Journal of the American Academy of Child Psychiatry, 23,* 126–133.

Bruun, R. D. (1988). The natural history of Tourette's syndrome. In D. J. Cohen, R. D. Bruun, & J. F. Leckman (Eds.), *Tourette's Syndrome and tic disorders: Clinical understanding and treatment* (pp. 22–39). New York: Wiley & Sons.

Bylund, D. B. (1985). Heterogeneity of alpha-2 adrenergic receptors. *Pharmacology and Biochemical Behaviors, 22,* 835–843.

Caine, E. D., McBride, M. C., & Chiverton, P. (1988). Tourette's syndrome in Monroe County school children. *Neurology, 38,* 472.

Caparulo, B. K., Cohen, D. J., Rothman, S. L., Young, D. G., Katz, J. D., Shaywitz, S. E., & Shaywitz, B. A. (1981). Computed tomographic brain scanning in children with developmental neuropsychiatric disorders. *Journal of the American Academy of Child Psychiatry, 20,* 388–397.

Cohen, D. J., Leckman, J. F., & Shaywitz, B. A. (1984). The Tourette syndrome and other tics. In D. Shaffer, A. A. Ehrhardt, & L. Greenhill (Eds.), *The clinical guide to child psychiatry.* New York: Free Press.

Cohen, D. J., Young, J. G., & Nathanson, J. A. (1979). Clonidine in Tourette's syndrome. *Lancet, 2,* 551–553.

Comings, D. E., & Comings, B. G. (1984). Tourette's syndrome and attention deficit disorder with hyperactivity: Are they genetically related? *Journal of the American Academy of Child Psychiatry, 23,* 138–146.

Comings, D. E., & Comings, B. G. (1985). Tourette syndrome: Clinical and psychological aspects of 250 cases. *American Journal of Human Genetics, 37,* 435–450.

Comings, D. E., & Comings, B. G. (1987). A controlled study of Tourette syndrome. I. Attention-deficit disorder, learning disorders, and school problems. *American Journal of Human Genetics, 41,* 701–741.

Comings, D. E., Comings, B. G., Devor, E. J., & Cloninger, C. R. (1984). Detection of major gene for Gilles de la Tourette syndrome. *American Journal of Human Genetics, 36,* 586–600.

Cooper, J. (1970). The Leyton obsessional inventory. *Psychological Medicine, 1,* 48–64.

Erenberg, G. (1988). Pharmacologic therapy of tics in childhood. *Pediatric Annals, 17,* 395–404.

Frankel, M., Cummings, J. L., Robertson, M. M., Trimble, M. R., Hill, M. A., & Benson, D. F. (1986). Obsessions and compulsions in Gilles de la Tourette's Syndrome. *Neurology, 36,* 378–382.

Goetz, C. G., Tanner, C. M., & Klawans, H. L. (1984).

Fluphenazine and multifocal tic disorders. *Archives of Neurology, 41,* 271–272.

Goetz, C. G., Tanner, C. M., Wilson, R. S., & Shannon, K. M. (1987a). A rating scale for Gilles de la Tourette's syndrome: Description, reliability, and validity data. *Neurology, 37,* 1542–1544.

Goetz, C. G., Tanner, C. M., Wilson, R. S., Carroll, V. S., Como, P. G., & Shannon, K. M. (1987b). Clonidine and Gilles de la Tourette's syndrome: Double-blind study using objective rating methods. *Annals of Neurology, 21,* 307–310.

Golden, G. S. (1990). Tourette syndrome: Recent advances. *Neurology Clinics, 8,* 705–714.

Grad, L. R., Pelcovitz, D., Olson, M., Matthews, M., & Grad, G. (1987). Obsessive-compulsive symptomatology in children with Tourette's syndrome. *Journal of the American Academy of Child Psychiatry, 26,* 69–74.

Hagin, R. A., & Kugler, J. (1988). School problems associated with Tourette's syndrome. In D. J. Cohen, R. D. Bruun, & J. F. Leckman (Eds.), *Tourette's syndrome and tic disorders: Clinical understanding and treatment* (pp. 224–236). New York: Wiley & Sons.

Harcherick, D. F., Leckman, J. F., Detlor, J., & Cohen, D. J. (1984). A new instrument for clinical studies of Tourette's syndrome. *Journal of the American Academy of Child Psychiatry, 23,* 153–160.

Leckman, J. F., Detlor, J., Harcherik, D. F., Ort, S., Shaywitz, B. A., & Cohen, D. J. (1985). Short- and long-term treatment of Tourette's syndrome with clonidine: A clinical perspective. *Neurology, 35,* 343–351.

Leckman, J. F., Hardin, M. T., Riddle, M. A., Stevenson, J., Ort, S., & Cohen, D. J. (1991). Clonidine treatment of Gilles de la Tourette's syndrome. *Archives of General Psychiatry, 48,* 324–328.

Lees, A. J., Robertson, M., Trimble, M. R., & Murray, N. M. F. (1984). A clinical study of Gilles de la Tourette's syndrome in the United Kingdom. *Journal of Neurology, Neurosurgery, and Psychiatry, 47,* 1–8.

Maletzky, B. M. (1974). Behavior recording as treatment: A brief note. *Behavior Therapy, 5,* 107–111.

Mikkelsen, E. J., Detlor, J., & Cohen, D. J. (1981). School avoidance and social phobia triggered by haloperidol in patients with Tourette's disorder. *American Journal of Psychiatry, 138,* 1572–1576.

Ollendick, T. H. (1981). Self-monitoring and self-administered overcorrection: The modification of nervous tics in children. *Behavior Modification, 5,* 75–84.

Pauls, D. L., & Leckman, J. F. (1986). The inheritance of Gilles de la Tourette syndrome and associated behaviors: Evidence for an autosomal dominant transmission. *New England Journal of Medicine, 315,* 993–997.

Ratzoni, G., Hermesh, H., Brandt, N., Lauffer, M., & Munitz, H. (1990). Clomipramine efficacy for tics, obsessions, and compulsions in Tourette's syndrome and obsessive-compulsive disorder: A case study. *Biological Psychiatry, 27,* 95–98.

Regeur, L., Pakkenberg, B., Fog, R., & Pakkenberg, H. (1986). Clinical features and long-term treatment with pimozide in 65 patients with Gilles de la Tourette's syndrome. *Journal of Neurology, Neurosurgery and Psychiatry, 49,* 791–795.

Riddle, M. A., Hardin, M. T., King, R., Scahill, L., & Woolston, J. L. (1990). Fluoxetine tretment of children and adolescents with Tourette's and obsessive compulsive disorder: preliminary clinical experience. *Journal of the American Academy of Child and Adolescent Psychiatry, 29,* 45–48.

Robertson, M. M., Schnieden, V., & Lees, A. J. (1990). Management of Gilles de la Tourette syndrome using sulpiride. *Clinical Neuropharmacology, 13,* 229–235.

Sallee, F. R., Pollock, B. G., Stiller, R. L., Stull, S., Everett, G., & Perel, J. M. (1987). Pharmacokinetics of pimozide in adults and children with Tourette's syndrome. *Journal of Clinical Pharmacology, 27,* 776–781.

Shapiro, A. K., & Shapiro, E. (1984). Controlled study of pimozide vs. placebo in Tourette's syndrome. *Journal of the American Academy of Child Psychiatry, 23,* 161–173.

Shapiro, A. K., Shapiro, E., & Eisenkraft, M. A. (1983). Treatment of Gilles de la Tourette syndrome with pimozide. *American Journal of Psychiatry, 140,* 1183–1186.

Shapiro, A. K., Shapiro, E., & Fulop, G. (1987). Pimozide treatment of tic and tourette disorders. *Pediatrics, 79,* 1032–1039.

Shapiro, A. K., Shapiro, E., & Wayne, H. (1973). Treatment of Tourette syndrome, with haloperidol, review of 34 cases. *Archives of General Psychiatry, 28,* 92–97.

Shapiro, E., Shapiro, A. K., Fulop, G., Hubbard, M., Mandeli, J., Nordlie, J., & Phillips, R. A. (1989). Controlled study of haloperidol, pimozide, and placebo for the treatment of Gilles de la Tourette's syndrome. *Archives of General Psychiatry, 46,* 722–730.

Singer, H. S., Tune, L. E., Butler, I. J., Zuczck, & Coyle, J. T. (1982). Dopaminergic dysfunction in

Tourette syndrome. *Annals of Neurology, 12,* 361–366.

Stahl, S. M., & Berger, P. A. (1982). Cholinergic and dopaminergic mechanisms in Tourette syndrome. In A. J. Friedhoff & T. N. Chase (Eds.), *Gilles de la Tourette syndrome* (pp. 141–149). New York: Raven Press.

Stefl, M. E. (1983). *The Ohio Tourette study.* School of Planning, University of Cincinnati.

Sweet, R. D., Solomon, G. E., Wayne, H. L., Shapiro, E., & Shapiro, A. K. (1973). Neurological features of Gilles de la Tourette's syndrome. *Journal of Neurology, Neurosurgery, and Psychiatry, 36,* 1–9.

Thomas, E. J., Abrams, K. S., & Johnson, J. B. (1971). Self-monitoring and reciprocal inhibition in the modification of multiple tics of Gilles de la Tourette's syndrome. *Journal of Behavior Therapy and Experimental Psychiatry, 2,* 159–171.

CHAPTER 19

TRICHOTILLOMANIA

Lee Baer   Harvard Medical School
Deborah Osgood-Hynes   Harvard Medical School
William E. Minichiello   Harvard Medical School

DESCRIPTION OF DISORDER

Clinical Features

Trichotillomania is a disorder of chronic hair pulling resulting in alopecia. The major clinical features of trichotillomania include pulling of hair from the scalp, eyebrows, and eyelashes (which may be totally or partially lost), usually symmetrically and occasionally pulling of pubic hair and other bodily hair (Muller, 1987). It is common for the self-inflicted nature of the hair loss to be denied, with the rate as high as 84 percent in one sample of 19 patients (Greenberg & Sarner, 1965).

Most of the clinical features described above have been derived from experience with small groups of patients or single patients. A recent study of the clinical characteristics of adult hair pullers, most of whom began before age 12 (Christenson, Mackenzie, & Mitchell, 1991) was the first to examine the clinical characteristics of a large sample ($n = 60$) in a scientific way. This sample reported pulling hair from a variety of sites: 38 percent pulled from one site only, 62 per-

cent pulled from two or more sites, and 33 percent from three or more sites. Hair pulling was most frequently reported from the scalp (75 percent), eyelashes (53 percent), eyebrows (42 percent), and pubic area (17 percent). Surprisingly 8 percent spontaneously reported having pulled hair from a child's scalp or eyelashes, and 3 percent had pulled hair from a spouse or significant other (Christenson et al., 1991). Consistent with our own clinical observations that patients are more likely to pull out hairs that "don't feel right," 57 percent of this sample reported tht coarse or thick hairs were more likely to be pulled. Others reported increased gratification with gray hairs or hairs with a complete root. Only 28 percent of patients in this group usually felt pain while pulling their hair.

Eating of pulled hair has been reported, with opinion varying as to whether this is a rare associated feature (Muller, 1987) or more common (Jillson, 1983); this is important because trichophagy can lead to the serious and life-threatening complication of trichobezoars developing in the stomach or intestines. In the study by Christenson and colleagues (1991), 48 percent reported at lest one oral behavior associated with hair pulling: rubbing hair around the mouth, licking the hair, eating the hair, and chewing or biting off the ends of the hair. However, no subjects reported a history of abdominal symptoms or trichobezoars.

Hair pulling occurs most frequently during sedentary activities (e.g., watching television, reading, talking on the telephone, and lying in bed), and is usually worse in the evening or just before falling asleep (Christenson et al., 1991; Greenberg & Sarner, 1965; Jillson, 1983).

Associated Features

Trichotillomania has been reported to occur in a wide variety of psychiatric disorders, including obsessive-compulsive disorder (OCD), mental retardation, schizophrenia, borderline personality disorder, and depression (Krishnan, Davidson, & Guajardo, 1985), although no data were presented. It has also been reported that trichotillomania is often observed in children in association with thumb sucking, nail biting, nose picking, masturbation, poor peer relationships, and academic problems (Krishnan et al., 1985).

Regarding comorbid conditions, Greenberg and Sarner (1965) reported that of their sample of 19 patients, 68 percent were moderately to severely depressed, and gave a history of depressive episodes (although diagnostic criteria were not specified). They also reported that 74 percent of these patients (child, adolescent, and adult) had developed moderate to severe school problems subsequent to hair pulling. These authors also noted that 63 percent of their nonobese female patients (but none of the males) showed "a striking overconcern with their weight which extended far beyond the usual American woman's concern with slimness, and which amounted to a true somatic preoccupation" (p. 484). A recent letter to the editor (George, Brewerton, & Cochrane, 1990) similarly commented on the presence of classical trichotillomania in three of five females with bulimia nervosa.

In their sample, Christenson and associates (1991) examined DSM-III-R lifetime diagnosis of Axis I disorders, and found a 55 percent lifetime prevalence for major depressive disorder, and 20 to 32 percent prevalence of panic disorder (with or without agoraphobia), generalized anxiety disorder, simple phobia, eating disorder, and substance use disorder. No control group was provided for comparison of lifetime prevalence rates.

Epidemiology

There are no epidemiologic studies of the incidence and prevalence of trichotillomania. Fabbri and Dy (1974) reported that fewer than 100 cases had been reported in the literature. Some have estimted its prevalence to be very rare; for example, Mannino and Delgado (1969) found only 7/1,368 (0.5 percent) patients at a mental health center. Anderson and Dean found 3/500 (0.6 percent) patients at a child guidance clinic (Mannino & Delgado, 1969), and Schacter (Mannino & Delgado, 1969) found only 5/10,000 cases (0.05 percent) of trichotillomania in children with psychiatric disorders. At the other extreme, Azrin and Nunn (1978) estimated that up to 8 million Americans may be affected (2 to 3 percent), which would make trichotillomania as common as obsessive-compulsive disorder (Jenike, Baer, & Minichiello, 1990). Christenson and associates noted that "trichotillomania appears to be more common than previously expected, as evidenced by the availability of a large number of subjects" (1991, p. 370). Similarly, Muller (1987) reported that he saw 15 to 20 patients with trichotillomania per year in a general dermatologic practice at Mayo Clinic.

Low estimates of prevalence may be related to the frequent denial of these patients (Greenberg & Sarner, 1965) and lack of tretment seeking for trichotillomania as a presenting psychiatric complaint. Similarly, in a recent letter to the editor, Friman and Rostain (1990) suggested that hair pulling in children rarely poses as severe a problem as it does in cases reported in the psychiatric literature, and that most cases present as a benign habit easily treated with various interventions.

There is general agreement as to the preponderance of females in the sex ratio of trichotillomania: Christenson and colleagues (1991), Mannino and Delgado (1969), Oranje, Peereboom-Wynia, and De Raeymaecker (1986), and Greenberg and Sarner (1965) found 93 percent, 78 percent, 71 percent, and 84 percent of their respective samples were female. Muller (1987), reporting on 145 patients, found 70 percent females, although 62 percent of the affected preschool-aged children were boys. A few studies (Bartsch; Butterworth & Strean [cited in Mannino & Delgado, 1969]) found no sex ratio difference.

Christenson and associates (1991) reported a mean age of onset of 13 ± 8 years (with median = 12 and range = 1–39 years). Greenberg and Sarner (1965) similarly reported the most common age of onset between the eleventh and sixteenth year.

Etiology

The etiology of trichotillomania is unknown. Christenson and colleagues (1991) found only 5 percent of their subjects began to pull their hair out in response to a skin or scalp disease.

The trichotillomania literature has largely been dominated by psychoanalytic theories of etiology, viewing the symptom as related to problems in psychosexual development, and symbolizing self-hatred, self-castration, or masturbation (Friman, Finney, & Christopherson, 1984). Behavioral theories of etiology have viewed hair pulling as an anxiety-reducing habit comparable to thumb sucking, nose picking, or fingernail biting (Azrin & Nunn, 1973). To date, no single theory of etiology appears to explain trichotillomania.

Trichotillomania can also be viewed as a disruption of the normal grooming response present in all primates (often involving oral grooming behaviors), which has been linked to a variety of homeostatic processes, including removal of parasites, tension reduction, increasing arousal, and preparation for a sleep (Colbern & Gispen, 1988).

DIFFERENTIAL DIAGNOSIS AND ASSESSMENT

DSM-III-R Categorization

The term *trichotillomania* was given by the French dermatologist Hallopeau in 1889 (Hallopeau, 1959) to describe a compulsion to pull out hair. Although trichotillomania has been described as a dermatologic disorder, and Hallopeau apparently believed that patients with this disorder were otherwise sane, trichotillomania has in recent years come to be viewed as a psychiatric disorder of psychogenic origin. Several dermatologists have suggested that the name *trichotillomania* is a nisnomer, since *mania* implies the presence of a serious psychiatric disorder or a psychosis; however, such an association may frequently be lacking, especially in young children and in mild cases such as those frequently seen by dermatologists (Jillson, 1983; Muller, 1987). The alternate term, *trichotillohabitus* has been suggested (Jillson, 1983), denoting a similarity to other habits such as nail biting and finger sucking.

Today, trichotillomania is categorized in the DSM-III-R as an Impulse Control Disorder, with the following diagnostic criteria:

1. Recurrent failure to resist impulses to pull out one's own hair, resulting in noticeable hair loss
2. Increasing sense of tension immediately before pulling out the hair
3. Gratification or a sense of relief when pulling out the hair
4. No association with a preexisting inflammation of one's skin, and not a response to a delusion or hallucination.

Christenson and associates (1991) studied these DSM-III-R criteria in their sample and found moderately good agreement: 95 percent reported an increasing sense of tension before pulling out their hair, 88 percent reported gratification or a sense of relief afterward, and 100 percent had one of these two characteristics. However, 7 percent of their subjects did not satisfy all DSM-III-R criteria for trichotillomania.

Although there has been increased discussion recently regarding the similarities between trichotillomania and OCD (classified as an Anxiety Disorder in DSM-III-R) in their response to clomipramine (Swedo et al., 1989), it appears that trichotillomania is likely to remain as a distinct disorder, remaining classified under Impulse Control Disorders in DSM-IV (Jenike, personal communication, June 24, 1991).

Differential Diagnosis

Trichotillomania must be differentiated from dermatologic disorders causing hair loss. Muller noted,

> Trichotillomania can mimic alopecia areata, common baldness (androgenetic alopecia), tinea capitis, hereditary disorders of keratinization such as monilethrix and pili torti, as well as other forms of traumatic alopecia, such as these caused by the use of excessively tight rollers and hairpins, or special pseudopelade-like alopecia. The traumatic types of alopecia caused by vigorous scratching of atopic dermatitis, seborrheic dermatitis, and other severely pruritic dermatoses should not be considered forms of trichotillomania. (1987, p. 598)

But in most cases, the diagnosis of trichotillomania is easily made from the clinical presentation and history. In all the cases that have presented to our Obsessive-Compulsive Disorders Clinic, patients have either readily admitted to hair pulling (not secondary to a scalp condition) or, in those few cases where a child has denied this, a parent or teacher has observed them pulling their hair. In cases where a patient denies hair pulling, and there has been no observation of this behavior, dermatologists may use punch biopsies of the affected scalp to confirm the diagnosis of trichotillomania (Muller, 1987).

In the psychiatric differential diagnosis, DSM-III-R requires that the hair pulling not be in response to a delusion (such as that the hair is infested with insects) or a (command) hallucination to pull the hair. Compared to OCD, patients with trichotillomania rarely have obsessive thoughts characteristic of OCD (themes involving contamination, doubting, symmetry, sex, violence, or blasphemy), nor are their compulsions performed for a particular reason (such as to prevent harm to another or for cleanliness), as is common in OCD (Jenike et al., 1990).

Assessment Strategies

The most rigorous assessment of trichotillomania has usually been in the context of behavior therapy interventions. The majority of these assessments have been self-recordings of the frequency of hair pulling (e.g., number of hairs pulled) (Friman et al., 1984). This has been accomplished both with pencil and paper, or by clicking a hand-held counter each time a hair is pulled (Ottens, 1981). However, this self-assessment method may be prone to poor compliance and low validity in a disorder with high rates of denial. As a result, several behavioral studies have added additional "natural" measures, including saving all hairs pulled in a week (which is also subject to low validity, since subjects can easily "fake good"), or measurement of hair length, or both (Friman et al., 1984). It has been suggested (Bayer, 1972) that collection of hairs by the patient, to be brought to the therapist, is more effective than simple paper-and-pencil recording. Friman and colleagues (1984) have criticized the lack of vigor of self-report measures alone, recommending instead "natural" measures, accompanied by estimates of interobserver reliability.

Bernard, Kratochwill, and Keefauver (1983) combined several of these assessment strategies in a successful single case study of a 17-year-old girl who pulled her hair while studying: She recorded on a self-monitoring chart the number of hairs pulled during each study session, then deposited the hairs pulled out during each session in individual envelopes. In addition, her mother was asked (with the patient's consent) to covertly monitor her daughter's frequency of hair pulling for brief periods while she was studying.

Dahlquist and Kalfus, noting the difficulties of reliable self-monitoring, developed a laborious but apparently reliable measure of hair pulling:

> For assessment purposes, "baldness" was operationally defined as an area of scalp 0.3 cm diameter containing 3 or less hairs. The size and parameters of her bald patches were then measured in order to construct a paper pattern the size of the bald area. Three holes 0.3 cm in diameter were randomly cut in the pattern to allow for sampling the number of hairs in the front, middle, and back areas of the bald spot. . . . Inter-observer agreement was 100 percent. (1984, p. 48)

The patient was not allowed to see the pattern, so she was unaware of which areas of her scalp would be counted each week.

Most case reports, especially of nonbehavioral treatment, have relied on the clinician's judgment of regrowth of hair as an indicator of improvement. This approach is adequate in the case of a large treatment response, but it does not permit quantification of smaller changes or assessment of rates of change.

In their double-blind trial of clomipramine and desipramine in trichotillomania, Swedo and colleagues (1989) took the first step in the psychometric assessment of this disorder. They developed three measures based on scales used to rate OCD symptoms. One scale was a five-item assessment of symptom severity on a 0 (none) to 5 (most severe scale). The five questions included the amount of time spent pulling hair, the strength of the urge, the discomfort, and interference with activities. A second scale "trichotillomania impairment scale," was a 0–10 analog scale rating severity of impairment. The third scale was a clinician-rated scale of progress, with 0 representing the absence of symptoms, 10 designating the pretreatment baseline level, and 20 showing a state of total incapacitation. Interrater reliability for two rates was acceptable, ranging from 0.78 to 0.81 for the three measures (Swedo et al., 1989). The trichoillomania impairment scale and the clinician-rated progress scale were both sensitive to differences between the two treatment groups.

The Yale-Brown Obsessive-Compulsive Scale (Goodman, Price, & Rasmussen, 1989) is a standard instrument in OCD trials, and despite the differences between OCD and trichotillomania, we have found it useful in the clinical assessment of trichotillomania when combined with other meaures. A child version (CY-YBOCS) is also available.

TREATMENT

Evidence for Prescriptive Treatments

Behavior Therapy

The earliest case reports of successful treatment of trichotillomania by behavior therapy methods were of adult hair pullers. Our review of the adult literature found six single case reports of successful treatment (e.g., usually complete control of hair pulling) with a variety of behavioral methods: thought stopping (e.g., when the patient's hands started to move, she told them, "No, stay where you are") (Taylor, 1963); self-monitoring, including saving the pulled hairs and bringing them to the therapist weekly (Bayer, 1972); increasing awareness of the habit and use of a competing response (e.g., grasping an object or fist-tightening) to the urge (Azrin & Nunn, 1973); self-monitoring by hair saving, relaxation training, and systematic desensitization to the situations that elicit hair pulling (Bornstein & Rychtarik, 1978); increasing awareness of the habit, relaxation, competing response, coping self-instructions (Ottens, 1981); increasing awareness of the habit, thought stopping via rubberband snapping and substitution of positive self-statements (Stevens, 1984); and increasing awareness of the habit and competing response (e.g., grasping objects) contingent on the urge (but not effective noncontingently) (Miltenberger & Fuqua, 1985).

In addition to these successful adult single case reports, the literature contains three multiple case comparisons of the method of habit reversal for adult hair pullers (Azrin & Nunn, 1978 — composed of most of the components found successful in the case reports above, and described in detail in the case example later in this chapter). Azrin, Nunn, and Frantz (1980) found in 34 subjects that a single two-hour session of habit-reversal training produced complete elimination of hair pulling for most subjects, and was significantly better than the method of negative practice (e.g., sitting in front of a mirror and acting out the motions of hair pulling on an hourly schedule). Rosenbaum and Ayllon (1981) also found habit reversal highly effective in a multiple baseline study of four subjects. Greenberg and Marks (1982) found habit reversal and response cost highly effective in four of six subjects in a an A-B design, with results maintained at one-month followup.

Although these findings suggest at least the short-term efficacy of behavior therapy for adult hair pullers, what are their implications for the treatment of children and adolescents with trichotillomania? Among the group studied by

Rosenbaum and Ayllon (1981) was a 10-year-old girl, who, like the adults, responded rapidly to the habit reversal method and maintained complete control of the habit at 12-month followup. Similarly, among Azrin and colleagues (1980) group were a 14-year-old adolescent male, two 14-year-old adolescent females and one 17-year-old adolescent females. Similar to the adults in this report, all four adolescents showed complete control of their hair pulling after habit-control training, and maintained these gains at four-week followup. Although these authors report that 67 percent of subjects followed at 22 months maintained no hair pulling, no details are provided about the ages of these patients. Adding to the evidence for the efficacy of behavior therapy for child and adolescent trichotillomania are a number of successful single case reports that have recently appeared in the literature. These reports have used a variety of behavioral methods, and their details are summarized in Table 19–1.

The successful case report and 18-month followup by Rosenbaum (1982) suggested an abbreviated habit reversal technique suitable for pediatric settings, consisting mainly of awareness training and use of a competing response.

Pharmacotherapy

There are case reports of effective treatment of adult trichotillomania with chlorpromazine (Childers, 1958), isocarboxazid (an MAOI; Krishnan, Davidson, & Miller, 1984), amitriptyline (Snyder, 1980), and imipramine (Sachdeva & Sidhu, 1987). In the cases of isocarboxazid and imipramine, both patients had trichotillomania associated with depression.

To date, the only controlled trial of medication in trichotillomania is a comparison of the anticompulsive serotonergic medication, clomipramine, to desipramine in a 10-week double-blind cross-over trial with 14 women meeting criteria for trichotillomania without primary affective illness (Swedo et al., 1989).

The mean maximal clomipramine dose was 180 ± 50 mg/day (range 100 to 250 mg). For desipramine, the mean dose was 173 ± 33 mg/day (range 150 to 200 mg). Clomipramine proved superior to desipramine on two of the three outcome measures (described above). On the trichotillomania assessment scale, there was a statistically significant difference between the drug groups, with the magnitude of 0.91 SD's representing a "large" effect size (Cohen, 1988). On the clinical progress scale, there was a larger statistically significant difference between the drug groups of 1.42 SD. Swedo and colleagues (1989) note that "12 of the 13 patients had significant symptomatic improvement while they were taking clomipramine; three patients had total remission of their hair-pulling symptoms" (p. 500).

Clomipramine also resulted in statistically greater reduction in both depression and anxiety than desipramine—a finding interpreted by the authors as indicating that these symptoms improved secondary to hair pulling. This study found that patients who received clomipramine first showed clinical deterioration when switched to desipramine, indicating that continued pharmacotherapy may be required for maintenance of improvement. There was no followup beyond the 12-week study period.

Recently, Swedo (1990) summarized the results of a two-year followup of 20 trichotillomania patients treated with either clomipramine or fluoxetine (another anticompulsive serotonergic medication). She found that overall there was a 40 percent decrease in symptoms, with 4 patients showing marked improvements (80 to 100 percent), and 7 unchanged from baseline. Swedo also described "a few patients who took climipramine for 4–5 months and their hair-pulling didn't come back when they stopped the medication" (p. 5).

Thus it appears tht the same serotonergic antidepressant medications useful in OCD are also useful in trichotillomania. Some patients, however, are unable to tolerate their side effects, including weight gain, dry mouth, sexual dysfunction, agitation, and trouble sleeping (Swedo, 1990).

There are as yet no controlled trials of medication and research experience in OCD has indicated that the same serotonergic medications effective in adult OCD have also proven effective in treating children and adolescents with this disorder (Jenike et al., 1990); our very preliminary clinical experience in trichotillomania suggests that this may be true for hair pulling as well as OCD.

Table 19–1. Summary of Behavior Therapy Case Studies in Child and Adolescent Trichotillomania

REFERENCE	SUBJECTS AGE AT TIME OF TREATMENT	ASSESSMENT	DESIGN AND PROCEDURES	DURATION OF PULLING PRETREATMENT	LOCATION OF PULLING (EXTENT OF PULLING AT BASELINE)	LENGTH OF TREATMENT	RESULTS AND FOLLOWUP
Child Single Case Studies							
Evans (1976)	8½-year-old female		Time out and positive reinforcement				Elimination of pulling
Anthony (1978)	9-year-old male	Self-recording and measurement of hair length (without reliability)	• Case study (B only) • Self-monitoring (wrist counter) • Plus response prevention	2 years			Decrease to zero rates. Increase in hair length. Zero rates at 8-week and 6-month followup.
Sanchez (1979)	27-month-old male	Parent monitoring of pulling incidents (wrist counter) (without reliability)	A-B • Differential reinforcement of other behaviors plus time out (A) • Response chain interruption plus treatment A(A + B)	1 year 9 months	Scalp (1.2 hairs per hour)	15 weeks	Gradual decrease to zero hairpulling. Gradual increase in percent of scalp area in recovery to 100 percent. Six- and 12-month followup showed no recurrence of pulling.
Barrett & Shapiro (1980)	7½-year-old female (severely retarded)	Direct observation of mean frequency of pulling incidents (with interrater reliability)	A-B • Reversal to baseline • Positive practice • Verbal warning plus positive practice		Scalp (30 incidents per day)	90 days	Gradual reduction to low rate. Zero rates at 6-, 9-, and 12-month followup
Rosenbaum (1982)	7-year-old male	Parent monitoring (without reliability)	A-B modified habit reversal	2 years	Eyebrow (5 incidents per day)	1 20-minute session	Decrease to zero rates. Increase in eyebrow fullness at 18 months.

Table 19–1. (Continued)

REFERENCE	SUBJECTS AGE AT TIME OF TREATMENT	ASSESSMENT	DESIGN AND PROCEDURES	DURATION OF PULLING PRETREATMENT	LOCATION OF PULLING (EXTENT OF PULLING AT BASELINE)	LENGTH OF TREATMENT	RESULTS AND FOLLOWUP
Nelson (1982)	7-year-old male	Parent monitoring (without reliability)	A-B positive practice	2 years	Scalp (average 3 incidents per day)	44 days	Rapid reduction to zero rate at day 20. Maintenance of zero rate at 3- and 10-month followup.
Dahlquist & Kalfus (1984)	9-year-old female	Parent monitoring (without reliability), size and parameters of bald patches (interrater reliability)	A-B • Disregard pulling • Positive practice • Response prevention • Contingency contracting	6 months	Scalp (bald area, 27.5 cm2)	7 sessions	Gradual increase in hair growth; by session 4, no bald areas. Results maintained at 6- and 10-month followup.
Mathew & Kumaraiah (1988)	8½-year-old female	Self-monitoring (without reliability)	A-B • Differential reinforcement of other behaviors • Mild aversive conditioning	6½ years	Scalp (18 incidents per day)	12 session	Gradual decrease to total extinction. Zero rate of pulling at 7-month followup.

Adolescent Single Case Studies

REFERENCE	SUBJECTS AGE AT TIME OF TREATMENT	ASSESSMENT	DESIGN AND PROCEDURES	DURATION OF PULLING PRETREATMENT	LOCATION OF PULLING (EXTENT OF PULLING AT BASELINE)	LENGTH OF TREATMENT	RESULTS AND FOLLOWUP
Stabler & Warren (1974)	14-year-old female	Hair count (without reliability)	A-B • Behavioral contracting • Token reinforcement and mild response cost	2 years	Scalp (25 hairs per day)		Rapid decrease to zero rates. No recurrence at 6-month followup. 26 weeks
McLaughlin & Nay (1975)	17-year-old female	Number of hairs pulled; length of hair (without reliability)	A-B • Relaxation and competing response training	14 years	Scalp (110 hairs over 2-week period)	26 weeks	Gradual decrease to zero rates by week 18.

Table 19-1. (Continued)

REFERENCE	SUBJECTS AGE AT TIME OF TREATMENT	ASSESSMENT	DESIGN AND PROCEDURES	DURATION OF PULLING PRETREATMENT	LOCATION OF PULLING (EXTENT OF PULLING AT BASELINE)	LENGTH OF TREATMENT	RESULTS AND FOLLOWUP
DeLuca & Holborn (1984)	17-year-old female	Self-monitoring; number of hairs pulled (without reliability)	A-B • Relaxation and competing response training	14 years	Scalp (107.5 hairs per day)	68 days	Gradual decrease during baseline self-monitoring. Further decrease following relaxation training. Upon relapse and gradual increase, competing response training led to zero rate of pulling. No recurrence at frequent followups up to 24 months.
Tarnowski et al. (1987)	11-year-old female	Area of baldness (interrater reliability); photographs	A-B modified habit reversal	2 years	Scalp	2 sessions	Gradual increase in hair growth and decrease in area of baldness. Three- and 12-month followup showed maintenance of results.

Finally, we know from animal studies that grooming behaviors can be increased by opiate administration and blocked by anxiolytics (such as diazepam) and clomipramine in rats (Colbern & Gispen, 1988). The implications, if any, for human trichotillomania are as yet unclear.

Alternative Treatments

There have been a handful of case reports of successful treatment of trichotillomania in children by psychoanalysis and intensive psychotherapy (with treatment lasting from "a short period" to two years) (reviewed by Mannino & Delgado, 1969). However, some authors using these methods have commented on the "malignant and chronic nature of the illness and on frequent exacerbations and remissions" (Mannino & Delgado, 1969).

There are also several case reports of the successful use of hypnosis in the treatment of adults with trichotillomania (Barabasz, 1987; Spiegel & Spiegel, 1978). The general conclusion from reviewing these reports is that a variety of hypnotic suggestions can be effective, but hypnosis is most likely to succeed with a patient of high hypnotic ability (as measured by a standardized scale, such as the Stanford Hypnotic Clinical Scale [Morgan & Hilgard, 1975]). However, since the majority of children have relatively high hypnotic ability, this may be a useful adjunctive technique in this age range.

The only report of hypnosis for childhood trichotillomania was by Gardner (1978), who used hypnosis with a 10-year-old female. At the initiation of hypnosis and awareness training, hair pulling appeared to be decreasing. During hypnosis, the subject was reminded of her wish to have pretty hair and was given suggestions for good hair grooming. It was also suggested that she would become increasingly aware of the behavior whenever it began. As her hand approached her head to twist, pull, or scratch, she could be aware of a powerful thought from the part of her that wanted pretty hair: "Stop. Please do not hurt." Self-hypnosis was taught and daily practice encouraged. Following three sessions, no further hair pulling was reported and new hair growth was seen.

Bernard and associates (1983) used cognitive therapy to treat a 17-year-old female with trichotillomania. Self-monitoring of the number of hairs pulled and saving the hairs was followed by rational-emotive therapy (RET). This consisted of disputation, which emphasized irrational cognitions associated with problematic situations found to be antecedent of pulling behaviors (primarily during studying time). This led to a modest decrease in hair pulling, from an average 1.5 hairs pulled out per minute. After three weeks/three sessions, a return to baseline showed a slight increase in pulling. RET was again instituted for two more sessions, resulting in a decrease and relative plateau of hair pulling.

At this point, self-instructional training (SIT) was introduced. Along with RET, SIT consisted of the therapist modeling a cognitive problem-solving dialogue that the subject progressively internalized. The subsequent introduction of SIT combined with RET for three sessions resulted in a decrease in the average number of hairs pulled out to 0.12 hair per minute. The reintroduction of SIT and RET (following a brief return to RET alone) led to a total cessation of all hair pulling which continued through followup at 20 and 36 weeks. It was speculated that, when working with younger, less verbally sophisticated individuals, RET disputational training aimed at changing a belief system may be insufficient to produce change.

Selecting Optimal Treatment Strategies

Based on the current literature, given its lack of side effects and its brief nature, behavior therapy should be a first-line treatment for the treatment of childhood or adolescent trichotillomania. There is not enough evidence to suggest the efficacy of nonbehavioral psychotherapies for this disorder.

Although a variety of behavior therapy techniques have reduced or eliminated hair pulling, the method that appears to be most effective—in terms of number of clients treated, favorable comparison to other treatments, and experimental evaluation — is that of habit reversal. A benefit of the habit-reversal method is that this multimodal behavioral approach includes most or all of the individual components that have been found to be effective for trichotillomania (e.g., self-monitoring, awareness training, relaxation training, and competing response training). The studies of habit reversal and its effectiveness by Azrin and colleagues (1980), Rosenbaum and Ayllon (1981), Tarnowski, Rosen, McGrath, and Drabman (1987), and Rosenbaum (1982) showed rapid decreases in hair-pulling behavior, as well as relative brevity of treatment (range one to three of treatment sessions). It has also been suggested that habit reversal is good for the treatment of both severe and mild cases of hair pulling (Tarnowski et al., 1987).

For patients who are assessed as having excellent hypnotic ability by means of a standardized scale, then hypnosis may be used, either alone or as an adjunct to a behavioral treatment such as habit reversal. For example, we often use hypnosis to reinforce the awareness training and relaxation components of habit reversal. If behavioral analysis indicates obvious cognitive distortions, then a cognitive therapy approach such as RET may help both outcome and maintenance.

Finally, if the patient is unable to comply with any behavior therapy method because of the strength of the urge to pull out hairs, then evaluation for treatment with a serotonergic antidepressant medication like clomipramine or fluoxetine is indicated. Some patients who have been unable to comply with a trial of habit reversal are later able to do so while taking one of these medications.

Problems in Carrying Out Interventions

The major reason for treatment failure in the behavioral treatment of trichotillomania, like other disorders such as OCD, is noncompliance. The issue of treatment acceptability is important because intervention methods that the client views negatively (e.g., saving hairs, aversive conditioning) are likely to be met with noncompliance.

Treatment acceptability should be routinely assessed in order to minimize such difficulties (Tarnowski et al., 1987). If hair pulling occurs only when the child is alone, and he or she is not motivated or able to exercise self-control strategies, then difficulty in treatment implementation may result. In these cases, a token reinforcement system (e.g., earning and exchanging points by compliance) is usually necessary.

When considering the application of habit reversal, modified habit reversal, or other treatment intervention, it is important to assess:

1. The child's level of verbal functioning and ability to follow directions
2. The extent to which the child and parents are motivated to control the problem behavior
3. The extent to which the child and parents are motivated to control the problem behavior
4. The parent's ability to carry out the treatment regimen (Azrin et al., 1980)

As previously noted, hypnosis and anticompulsive medications can also help patients comply better with behavioral treatment (see the clinical example later in this chapter).

Relapse Prevention

Only a few of the case studies for any treatment modality have provided very long-term (e.g., greater than one year) followup of maintenance of effect after the treatment is terminated. This is especially true of medication treatment. This is unfortunate, since clinical observation indicates that patients with this disorder may be subject to relapse. The habit-reversal method has several components built in to enhance generalizability and reduce relapse:

1. Practice of methods in everyday situations.
2. Symbolic rehearsal procedure by Azrin and Nunn (1973), in which the subject imagines common habit-dictating situations and imagines that a pulling moment has been detected, and the subject is performing the required exercise.

3. Application of habit-reversal components to a variety of high-risk situations.

We have found it helpful to schedule in advance a number of followup sessions to immediately address any relapse of hair pulling and to avoid more extensive relapse. Tarnowski and associates (1987) also recommended several spaced treatment and followup sessions.

Azrin and colleagues (1980) reported that following treatment with habit reversal, subjects indicated that their pulling habit was not just actively suppressed but eliminated, both as an overt act and a compulsive urge. Nor did the competing clenching-grasping action persist as a habit, substituting for the hair pulling. No new habit appeared as hair pulling ceased. However, for those who pulled eyelashes, several reported a desire to reinitiate pulling because of local sensitivity when the lashes began regrowing after the initial cessation of eyelash pulling. We have seen a similar phenomenon in patients who are dismayed by the short, fine hairs that regrow in bald areas; it is critical to alert patients to what the returning hair will feel and look like to prevent relapse due to these "new" experiences during recovery.

CASE ILLUSTRATION

Case Description

Jane, a 17½-year-old academically talented high school senior, was referred for behavioral treatment of trichotillomania by her psychiatrist. At the time of referral, the patient was being treated with fluoxetine 20 mg/day, reduced from 60 mg/day due to her inability to tolerate side effects. She attributed a 25 percent reduction in hair plucking to her medication response. Concurrently, she was in treatment biweekly with a clinical psychologist for supportive psychotherapy centering around adolescent problems caused by her shyness. The patient resided at home with her parents and 14-year-old sister, with whom she had a very positive, supportive relationship.

The age of onset for her trichotillomania was 9 years old. Initially her plucking was of her eyebrows and eyelashes only. She reported remission of this behavior at age 12. This was accomplished without formal treatment; the patient attributed her success to sheer willpower, aided by her parents' suggestion that she wear gloves to bed and sit on her hands whenever she had the urge to pluck. At age 16, her trichotillomania reappeared and consisted solely of plucking the hair on the crown of her head. When she presented for treatment, the crown of her head had a bald spot eight inches in diameter. At age 17, she also began plucking her pubic hair. This behavior took place an average of 15 minutes per day and occurred only when she was in the bathroom.

Differential Diagnosis and Assessment

Since Jane readily admitted to the self-inflicted nature of her hair loss, had no scalp disease, had no delusions or hallucinations causing her hair pulling, and met DSM-III-R criteria for trichotillomania, the diagnosis was straightforward. Baseline data collected by paper-and-pencil recording of frequency and duration of hair pulling indicated that Jane touched, twisted, and/or plucked the hair on the crown of her head for two hours and 45 minutes per day. Behavioral assessment also indicated that Jane would touch, twist, or pluck her hair whenever she was anxious, especially if the anxiety was triggered by social interactions with people she did not know well, whenever she met another person for the first time, or whenever a family member or friend expressed disapproval or anger toward her.

Other situations that triggered the urge to pull were whenever she felt bored or fatigued. Jane reported that her parents and younger sister, in attempting to help Jane, unwittingly reinforced her trichotillomania by nagging her about plucking her hair whenever she was observed doing it. Jane denied that any personal positive or negative reinforcement was gained from plucking her hair (e.g., no secondary gains).

Treatment Selection

After analyzing the data gathered by Jane after the initial behavioral assessment regarding the frequency, duration, antecedents, and consequences of her hair pulling, it was decided to initially orient her parents to the behavioral treatment of trichotillomania and seek their cooperation and assistance. They were instructed in reinforcement theory and asked to refrain from unwittingly reinforcing Jane's hair pulling by refraining from nagging or calling attention to her plucking. Since Jane appeared motivated to control her hair pulling, habit reversal—which is now our behavior therapy method of choice for trichotillomania—was selected.

Treatment Course and Problems in Carrying Out Interventions

Based on the data gathered by Jane about the antecedents to her hair plucking and the frequency and intensity of anxiety as the trigger to her hair pulling, she was next trained in relaxation (including diaphragmatic breathing) as a self-control procedure (Minichiello, 1987) as a more adaptive alternative to hair pulling whenever she experienced anxiety.

When Jane returned for her next session, the frequency of hair pulling was reduced, to which she partially attributed her newly acquired relaxation skill. However, she was still unable to control her hair-pulling urge once it was triggered. Treatment proceeded next to training in habit reversal. The 13 major components of habit reversal, as specified by Azrin and associates (1980) are:

1. Competing response training: The subject learns the competing and preferably inconspicuous response of grasping or clenching the hands for three minutes whenever hair pulling has occurred or is likely to occur.
2. Awareness training: The subject learns to be aware of the specific movements involved in hair pulling. This is helped by observing herself in a mirror.
3. Identifying response precursors: A common response that is a precursor to hair pulling is face touching or hair straightening.
4. Identifying habit-prone situations: The subject learns to identify which situations lead to hair pulling, such as watching TV, studying, or being alone.
5. Relaxation training.
6. Prevention training: The subject practices the competing reaction for three minutes, grasping or clenching whenever nervousness, a response precursor, or a habit-prone situation exists.
7. Habit interruption: The subject practices using the competing grasping or clenching reaction to interrupt the hair pulling immediately.
8. Positive attention/overcorrection: The subject practices positive hair care, such as combing or brushing the hair, after each episode of pulling.
9. Daily practice of competing reaction: The subject practices the competing response before a mirror at home.
10. Self-recording: The subject records each instance of hair pulling and each compulsion to hair pull to provide greater awareness and give feedback for progress in hair pulling.
11. Display of improvement: The subject seeks out those situations previously avoided.
12. Social support: A significant other is taught how to encourage and remind, in a positive manner, the person to stop pulling hair.
13. Annoyance review: The subject lists and discusses the various problems caused by hair pulling, serving to increase motivation for treatment and to identify sources of reinforcement for controlling hair pulling.

Our focus was primarily on elements 1 and 2.

With the therapist modeling the habit-reversal technique, Jane was instructed to clench her fists together tightly if she had the urge to pluck while walking or standing and talking to a person. She was instructed to grasp tightly the armrests or seat of the chair if she had the urge to pluck while seated; to grasp tightly the sides of the book she was reading if she had the urge to pull her hair while reading; and to grasp tightly her pen and the paper on which she was writing if she had the urge to pluck while writing. At the conclusion of the session, Jane had rehearsed habit reversal as a competing response to hair pulling in all situations encountered in the past that resulted in the touching, twirling, or pulling her hair. She was instructed to initiate the habit reversal at the onset of the urge to pull and to maintain it until the urge had passed.

Upon her return for the next treatment session, her record keeping indicated a significant reduction in the frequency and length of time involved in hair pulling, reduced from a mean of 165 minutes per day at baseline to 24 minutes per day. Jane was a highly motivated young lady who was very faithful in initiating habit reversal as soon as she had the urge to move her hand in the direction of her face. Such excellent compliance with habit reversal is common among the adolescents we have treated.

Often one must be very creaive in designing a method that results in crrying out the principles of habit reversal. A recent example was an adolescent patient who had a poor record of compliance with habit reversal. This female patient was a fan of the singer Madonna and her music. She found it very rewarding to "lip synch" the words while a Madonna recording was playing on her stereo. Her compliance with habit reversal was increased significantly when we suggested that, whenever she had the urge to pluck her hair or eyebrows while at home, she should go to her bedroom, grasp her portable microphone in her hands, and lip synch the words and act out the Madonna song playing on her stereo (e.g., a competing response).

After further analysis of the data collected whenever Jane was not totally successful with habit reversal, it was decided to initiate systematic desensitization (Wolpe, 1975) to the situations requiring social interactions with people she was unfamiliar with and situations in which she was criticized.

When Jane returned for the next treatment session, her records indicated almost complete control of her trichotillomania. Her compliance and success with habit reversal was almost perfect. She plucked an average of 1.3 minutes per day. She also reported that she was now taking clomipramine, 100 mg per day, and found it significantly easier to comply with habit reversal. Systematic desensitization initiated at the previous session was completed at this session. A portion of the session was also set aside to help the patient problem solve (Goldfried & Davison, 1976) a relationship problem that had arisen during the week. Situations of this nature will periodically arise when treating adolescents for trichotillomania, and it is important to set aside time to help the patient deal with these problems rather than try to adhere to a rigid format for treating trichotillomania in isolation.

At the next treatment session two weeks later, Jane's homework data indicated complete control of her trichotillomania. She was employing all her self-control procedures effectively and had not plucked her hair at all. She related an example of how effectively she employed her self-control procedures of relaxation, diaphragmatic breathing, and habit reversal when she became lost for two hours in a large city museum but did not touch, twirl, or pull her hair.

Outcome and Termination

Telephone followup was initiated for the next month at two-week intervals, which coincided with two stressful events — college acceptance notification and senior prom preparation. Jane continued to maintain her rate of zero plucking of her hair and continued to employ her self-control procedures. Her dosage of clomipramine had been increased to 125 mg/day.

Followup and Maintenance

A final treatment session was held one month later. Jane's homework data continued to reflect a zero rate of hair plucking, and telephone followup was arranged for one- and two-month intervals. She continued to take clomipramine and will attempt to taper off it during the next year.

SUMMARY

Trichotillomania is a disorder of chronic hair pulling resulting in alopecia. The clinical features of trichotillomania include pulling of hair from the scalp, eyebrows, and eyelashes (which may be totally or partially lost), usually symmetrically and occasionally include pulling pubic hair and other bodily hair. Trichotillomania has been reported to occur in a wide variety of psychiatric disorders, and patients with trichotillomania may be more likely to have a lifetime diagnosis of depressive, anxiety, eating, or substance abuse disorders, although the research in this area is uncontrolled. There are no epidemiologic studies of the prevalence of trichotillomania, and estimates have ranged from very rare (0.05 percent) to very common (2 to 3 percent). Most studies have found between 70 and 93 percent of sufferers are female, with age of onset usually between the eleventh and sixteenth year.

The etiology of trichotillomania is unknown. Psychodynamic, behavioral, and biological theories have been postulated but, to date, no single theory of etiology appears to explain trichotillomania.

Trichotillomania is currently categorized in the DSM-III-R as an Impulse Control Disorder. It must be differentiated from dermatologic disorders causing hair loss, and from psychiatric disorders such as schizophrenia and obsessive compulsive disorder.

Based on the current literature, albeit mostly case reports, behavior therapy techniques such as habit reversal should be a first-line treatment for the treatment of childhood or adolescent trichotillomania, due to their brief nature and lack of side effects. There is not enough evidence to suggest the efficacy of nonbehavioral psychotherapies for this disorder. Serotonergic medications such as clomipramine and fluoxetine appear to be effective in adult trichotillomania, and may also be effective in children and adults with this disorder. These medications are often used in combination with behavior therapy treatment. Regardless of the treatment modality used, relapse prevention after discontinuation of the treatment is an important consideration in this disorder.

REFERENCES

Anthony, W. (1978). Brief intervention in the case of childhood trichotillomania by self-monitoring. *Journal of Behavior Therapy and Experimental Psychiatry, 9,* 173–175.

Azrin, N. H., & Nunn, R. G. (1973). Habit reversal: A method of eliminating nervous habits and tics. *Behaviour Research and Therapy, 11,* 619–628.

Azrin, N. H., & Nunn, R. G. (1978). *Habit control in a day.* New York: Simon and Shuster.

Azrin, N. H., Nunn, R. G., & Frantz, S. E. (1980). Treatment of hairpulling (trichotillomania): A comparative study of habit reversal and negative practice training. *Journal of Behavior Therapy and Experimental Psychiatry, 11,* 13–20.

Barabasz, M. (1987). Trichotillomania: A new treatment. *International Journal of Clinical and Experimental Hypnosis, 35*(3), 146–154.

Barrett, R. P., & Shapiro, E. S. (1980). Treatment of stereotyped hair-pulling with overcorrection: A case study with long-term followup. *Journal of Behavioral and Experimental Psychiatry, 11,* 317–320.

Bayer, C. A. (1972). Self-monitoring and mild aversion treatment of trichotillomania. *Journal of Behavior Therapy and Experimental Psychiatry, 3,* 139–141.

Bernard, M. E., Kratochwill, T. R., & Keefauver, L. W. (1983). The effects of rational-emotive therapy and self-instructional training on chronic hair pulling. *Cognitive Therapy and Research, 7*(3), 273–280.

Bornstein, P. H., & Rychtarik, R. G. (1978). Multicomponent behavioral treatment of trichotillomania: A case study. *Behaviour Research and Therapy, 16,* 217–220.

Childers, R. T. (1958). Report of two cases of trichotillomania of longstanding duration and their response to chlorpromazine. *Journal of Clinical and Experimental Psychopathology, 19,* 141–144.

Christenson, G. A., Mackenzie, T. B., & Mitchell, J. E. (1991). Characteristics of 60 adult chronic hair pullers. *American Journal of Psychiatry, 148*(3), 365–370.

Cohen, J. (1988). *Statistical power for the behavioral sciences* (2nd ed.). Hillsdale, NJ: Erlbaum.

Colbern, D. L., & Gispen, W. H. (Eds.). (1988). Neural mechanisms and biological significance of grooming behavior. *Annals of the New York Academy of Sciences* (Vol. 525). New York: New York Academy of Sciences.

Dahlquist, L. M., & Kalfus, G. R. (1984). A novel approach to assessment in the treatment of childhood trichotillomania. *Journal of Behavior Therapy and Experimental Psychiatry, 15*(1), 47–50.

DeLuca, R. V., & Holborn, S. W. (1984). A comparison of relaxation training and competing response training to eliminate hair pulling and nail biting. *Journal of Behavior Therapy and Experimental Psychiatry, 15*(1), 67–70.

Evans, B. (1976). A case of trichotillomania in a child treated in a home token program. *Journal of Behavior Therapy and Experimental Psychiatry, 7,* 197–198.

Fabbri, R., & Dy, A. J. (1974). Hypnotic treatment of trichotillomania: Two cases. *The International Journal of Clinical and Experimental Hypnosis, 22*(3), 210–215.

Friman, P. C., Finney, J. W., & Christopherson, E. R. (1984). Behavioral treatment of trichotillomania: An evaluative review. *Behavior Therapy, 15,* 249–265.

Friman, P. C., & Rostain, A. (1990). Trichotillomania (hair pulling). Letter to the editor. *New England Journal of Medicine, 322*(7), 471.

Gardner, G. G. (1978). Hypnotherapy in the management of childhood habit disorders. *Journal of Pediatrics, 92*(5), 838–840.

George, M. S., Brewerton, T. D., & Cochrane, C. (1990). Trichotillomania (hair pulling). Letter to the editor. *New England Journal of Medicine, 322*(7), 470–471.

Goldfried, M. R., & Davison, G. C. (1976). *Clinical behavior therapy.* New York: Holt, Rinehart and Winston.

Goodman, W. K., Price, L. H., Rasmussen, S. A. et al. (1989). The Yale-Brown Obsessive-Compulsive Scale (Y-BOCS). Part I: Development, use and reliability. *Archives General Psychiatry, 46,* 1006–1011.

Greenberg, D., & Marks, I. (1982). Behavioural psychotherapy of uncommon referrals. *British Journal of Psychiatry, 141,* 148–153.

Greenberg, H. R., & Sarner, C. A. (1965). Trichotillomania. *Archives of General Psychiatry, 12,* 482–489.

Hallopeau, M. (1959). Alopecie par grattage: Trichotomanie ou trichotillomanie. *Ann Derm Syph, 10,* 440.

Jenike, M. A., Baer, L., & Minichiello, W. E. (Eds.). (1990). *Obsessive-compulsive disorders: Theory and management.* (2nd ed.). Chicago: Year Book Medical Publishers.

Jillson, O. F. (1983). Alopecia. II. Trichotillomania (trichotillohabitus). *Cutis, 31,* 383–389.

Krishnan, K. R. R., Davidson, J. R. T., & Guajardo, C. (1985). Trichotillomania — A review. *Comprehensive Psychiatry, 26,* 123–128.

Krishnan, K. R. R., Davidson, J. R. T., & Miller, R. (1984). MAO inhibitor therapy in trichotillomania associated with depression: A case report. *Journal of Clinical Psychiatry, 45,* 267–268.

Mannino, F., & Delgado, R. A. (1969). Trichotillomania in children: A review. *American Journal of Psychiatry, 126*(4), 505–511.

Mathew, A., & Kumaraiah, V. (1988). Behavioural intervention in the treatment of trichotillomania. *Indian Journal of Pediatrics, 55,* 451–453.

McLaughlin, J. G., & Nay, W. R. (1975). Treatment of trichotillomania using positive coverants and response cost: A case report. *Behavior Therapy, 6,* 87–91.

Miltenberger, R. G., & Fuqua, R. W. (1985). A comparison of contingent vs. non-contingent competing response practice in the treatment of nervous habits. *Journal of Behavior Therapy and Experimental Psychiatry, 16*(3), 195–200.

Minichiello, W. E. (1987). In A. H. Gorol, L. A. May, & A. G. Mulley (Eds.), *Primary care medicine.* Philadelphia: Lippincott.

Morgan, A., & Hilgard, J. R. (1975). Stanford Hypnotic Clinical scale (SHCS). In E. P. Hilgard & J. R. Hilgard (Eds.), *Hypnosis in the relief of pain* (pp. 209–221). Los Altos, CA: Kaufman.

Muller, S. A. (1987). Trichotillomania. *Dermatology Clinics, 5*(3), 595–601.

Nelson, W. M. (1982). Behavioral treatment of childhood trichotillomania: A case study. *Journal of Clinical Child Psychology, 11*(3), 227–230.

Oranje, A. P., Peereboom-Wynia, J. D. R., & De Raeymaecker, D. M. J. (1986). Trichotillomania in childhood. *Journal of the American Academy of Dermatology, 15*(4), 614–619.

Ottens, A. (1981). Multifaceted treatment of compulsive hair pulling. *Journal of Behavior Therapy and Experimental Psychiatry, 12*(1), 77–80.

Rosenbaum, M. S. (1982). Treating hair pulling in a 7-year old male: Modified habit reversal for use in pediatric settings. *Developmental and Behavioral Pediatrics, 3*(4), 241–243.

Rosenbaum, M. S., & Ayllon, T. (1981). The habit reversal technique in treating trichotillomania. *Behavior Therapy, 12,* 473–481.

Sachdeva, J. S., & Sidhu, B. S. (1987). Trichotillomania associated with depression. *Journal of the Indian Medical Association, 85,* 151–152.

Sanchez, V. (1979). Behavioral treatment of chronic hair

pulling in a two year old. *Behavior Therapy and Experimental Psychiatry, 10,* 241–245.

Snyder, S. (1980). Trichotillomania treated with amitriptyline. *Journal of Nervous and Mental Disease, 168,* 505–507.

Spiegel, H., & Spiegel, D. (1978). *Trance and treatment: Clinical uses of hypnosis.* New York: Basic Books.

Stabler, B., & Warren, A. (1974). Behavioral contracting in treating trichotillomania: A case note. *Psychological Reports, 34,* 401–402.

Stevens, M. J. (1984). Behavioral treatment of trichotillomania. *Psychological Reports, 55,* 987–990.

Swedo, S. E. (1990). Trichotillomania: An update from the National Institute of Mental Health. *OC Foundation Newsletter, 4*(5), 5.

Swedo, S. E., Leonard, H. L., Rapoport, J. L., Lenane, M. C., Goldberger, E. L., & Cheslow, D. L. (1989). A double-blind comparison of clomipramine and desipramine in the tretment of trichotillomania (hair-pulling). *New England Journal of Medicine, 321*(8), 497–501.

Tarnowski, K. J., Rosen, L. A., McGrath, M. L., & Drabman, R. S. (1987). A modified habit reversal procedure in a recalcitrant case of trichotillomania. *Journal of Behavior Therapy and Experimental Psychiatry, 18*(2), 157–163.

Taylor, J. (1963). A behavioral interpretation of obsessive compulsive neurosis. *Behaviour Research and Therapy, 1,* 237–244.

Wolpe, J. (1975). *The practice of behavior therapy* (2nd ed.). New York: Pergamon.

CHAPTER 20

FIRE SETTING

Robert Cole   University of Rochester

Wendy Grolnick   Clark University

Paul Schwartzman   National Fire Service Support Systems, Inc.

DESCRIPTION OF PROBLEM

Core Features

The term *childhood fire setting* has been used to describe a wide range of behaviors associated with the nonsanctioned, noninstrumental use of fire in children and adolescents. Included under this heading are such diverse behaviors as the inadvertent starting of a fire by a child playing with matches and the deliberate and repeated setting of fires in order to cause damage or injury. We prefer to reserve the term *fire setting* for intentional acts designed to create a disturbance or to inflict damage or harm, and to use the term *fire play* to describe other involvement with fire and fire materials.

Since the issues underlying such different behaviors vary considerably, specifying the context and type of firesetting is crucial in order to determine a diagnosis and choose a treatment strategy. Among the considerations that are useful in classifying children's involvement with fire are intent or motive, frequency, and age. Children frequently start fires accidentally, but they also do

so deliberately, for revenge or to call attention to significant personal, interpersonal, or family problems (Cole et al., 1986; Wooden & Berkey, 1984). Also, the frequency of children's fire setting is a key factor in understanding the meaning of children's fire involvement, especially given the findings from the delinquency literature that the number of convictions children receive is highly predictive of their level of disturbance and subsequent outcome (Rutter & Garmezy, 1983; West & Farrington, 1973). In addition, the nature of children's fire involvement may change. While a first fire may start as an accident or as a result of curiosity, subsequent fires may be started deliberately, giving them a different psychological meaning.

An additional factor is the children's developmental level. Children's understanding of fire may not be firmly established even by the age of 10 (Grolnick et al., 1990). Thus, younger children may not be aware of the possible consequences of their interaction with fire. Using these three factors, it is possible to describe the characteristics of children who engage in fire setting.

While early accounts of juveniles who set fires describe a single profile of very disturbed children with symptoms of enuresis and cruelty to animals, recent research recognizes that children who start fires are a heterogeneous group. The most common profile describes a child who acts primarily out of curiosity. The few studies that have examined representative samples of children who start fires, by assessing *all* children who come in contact with the fire department for having started a fire, converge on this point. Fineman (1980) described the majority of children who start fires as doing so in the course of experimentation and suggested that these children may not have other psychological problems. Cole and colleagues (1986) studied all children who came in contact with the fire department for having started a fire within a 3½-year period. Some 617 children were involved in 474 fire incidents. Over 60 percent of the children could be characterized as having started the fire as a result of curiosity. These children tended to be young, most typically between 5 and 9 years of age, and to be involved in only one reported fire incident.

Given that many of the children involved in reported incidents were not particularly disturbed, it becomes important to ask how prevalent fire involvement is in the general population. Kafry (1978) conducted a normative survey of young boys in which she found that interest in fire is almost universal. Further, 40 percent of the children had engaged in fire play, a number remarkably similar to that reported in the large-scale survey conducted by Grolnick and associates (1990).

While this curiosity-driven fire play is not necessarily pathological, it is nevertheless potentially very dangerous and a concern. There are familial and environmental factors that predict whether children engage in fire play and that serve as rules to preventive intervention. Grolnick and associates (1990) found that (1) access to ignition materials, (2) a perception that parents would not punish those caught playing with fire, and (3) exposure to and responsibility for activities involving fire, were all associated with fire play.

The positive association between fire play and responsibility for activities involving fire has forced us to reconsider the common use of the term *curiosity* when describing children's fireplay.

Following Kafry (1980), we characterize these children as mischievous rather than as simply curious. Children who engage in fire play tend to test limits, confident in their ability to evade, or, in some cases, perceiving that there will be no consequences for their behavior. There is evidence (Grolnick et al., 1990) that children given more responsibility for fire activities such as cooking and tending a fire are more confident in their ability to control fire than are those without such responsibility. We have hypothesized that these children might have been given these responsibilities too young, before they are developmentally capable of understanding the seriousness of their responsibility and the power and potential destructiveness of fire of even a single match.

Preadolescent children (or more precisely, children who have not yet attained the cognitive stage of formal operations) have difficulty entertaining "what'if" propositions. Their understanding of future events is limited by what they have observed and, in most cases, what they have observed is that fire is small, attractive, and fragile. The extremely rapid transformation of a single match to a burning bedroom is almost incomprehensible to most preadolescents (and in fact to many adolescents and adults). The assignment of responsibility for fire activities to these children reinforces their confidence in their ability to manage these activities. This false sense of security, coupled with a mischievous nature, typically accounts for what has been called *curiosity fire play*.

Supporting this position, Kafry (1980) found that the children who played with fire were described by their mothers as more disobedient and as having more accidents than those who did not play. Thus, supervision, limit setting, and the appropriate assignment of responsibilities for fire activities appear to be issues involved in children's fire play.

A second group of children who are involved with fire are motivated by something other than curiosity, and their fire setting is intentional. These children have been described by Fineman (1980) as pathological fire setters. Wooden and Berkey (1984) classified three types of children (aside from those playing with matches): (1) those whose fire setting represents a call for help, (2) those whose fire setting is part of a pattern of juvenile delinquency, and (3) those who are seriously disturbed. Children from all of these groups tend to be older than those starting fires out of curiosity and tend to have set more than one fire.

Most of the research on children and fire has focused on pathological or noncuriosity fire setting. In this research, children have typically been identified through mental health agencies, either in residential psychiatric facilities (most frequently) or outpatient clinics. Thus, these samples are select and represent the most disturbed children. Several of these studies have suggested that fire setting among children receiving psychiatric care is part of a larger constellation of conduct and aggressive problems (Kolko, 1985). Fire setters in inpatient and outpatient clinics are most typically diagnosed as having a conduct disorder (Heath, Hardesty, Goldfine, & Walker, 1983; Kazdin & Kolko, 1986), with a proportion receiving the diagnosis of attention deficit-hyperactivity disorder (Kuhnley, Hendren, & Quinlan, 1982), and a very small proportion pyromania (Kolko, 1990; Kuhnley et al., 1982).

Associated Features

In a study of hospitalized firesetters, Kolko, Kazdin, and Meyer (1985) found that these children evidenced greater delinquency, aggressiveness, and hyperactivity relative to a control group of hospitalized children. Further, relative to hospitalized conduct-disordered children with no history of fire setting, these authors found that the fire setters were less socially skilled and more aggressive. The fact that activities such as stealing, lying, running away, and truancy have been found to exist together in delinquent and pathological firesetters has led Kolko (1990) to suggest that firesetting may be conceptualized as a "concealed behavior." Other researchers have found a lack of assertiveness and/or lack of social skills (Kolko et al., 1985; Sakheim, Vigdor, Gordon, & Helprin, 1985) in fire setters, thereby supporting this theory, although there is little research specifically focusing on it.

There is significant evidence for parental and family problems in families of children whose involvement with fire is attributable to motives other than curiosity (Heath, Gayton, & Hardesty, 1976; Kazdin & Kolko, 1986). Their parents have been described as depressed, low in affection (Kazdin & Kolko, 1986), unavailable (Macht & Mack, 1968), and lacking in supervision and monitoring (Kazdin & Kolko, 1986; Fine & Louie, 1979). Relative to parents of other hospitalized children, Kazdin and Kolko (1986) found that parents of fire setters had more psychiatric symptoms and displayed less affection and consensus in their marital relationships.

Moving beyond the study of hospitalized children, Cole and associates (1986) found that among all fires reported to the fire department, the presence of serious family problems was the best predictor of recidivism. Two specific family problems accounted for this relationship: (1) verified current or prior child abuse or neglect and (2) prior family contact with the police. Among the full sample of families whose children had been involved in fire incidents reported to the fire department, 14 percent had had a verified incident of abuse or neglect. Among the recidivists, 45 percent of the families had a history of abuse or neglect. Similarly, 13 percent of the full sample of families had a history of police contact, while 35 percent of the families of the recidivists had prior police contact.

Investigators have also suggested that children who set fires are under stress (Wooden & Berkey, 1984). Recent separations, divorces, and deaths in family members have all been identified in fire setters (Fineman, 1980; Gruber et al., 1981). These data together strongly suggest that family dysfunction — inadequate supervision, inappropriate assignment of responsibility, depression, reduced involvement, loss, divorce, abuse, and neglect — is strongly implicated in noncuriosity fire activity.

Epidemiology

The problem of children and fire can be described at many levels. From a community perspective, the problem is clearly serious. Incendiary (deliberately set) and suspicious (probably set) fires accounted for $1.5 billion in damages to structures and $135 million in other property damage in 1987 alone. in that year, 730 lives were lost due to arson fires. Over several reporting years, it has been estimated that juveniles account for approximately 38 to 40 percent of all *arson* arrests (Hall, 1988). One of every 14 persons arrested for arson is under age 10 and one of every four is under age 15. These statistics, while striking, represent only part of the problem of children and fire since only a small proportion of children identified as having set a fire are charged with arson and even fewer are arrested. Experts estimate that between 50 percent (U.S. Department of Justice, 1989) and 60 percent (Mieszala, 1981) of incendiary and suspicious fires in large cities are caused by children under the age of 18.

Findings from large-scale surveys of normative samples of children suggest that fire play is quite common among children and is not limited to the small portion of children who account for the more serious fires reported above or for the high frequency of arson in children. In a survey of 771 elementary and junior high school students, Grolnick, Cole, Laurenitis, and Schwartzman (1990) found that over 50 percent of children reported having engaged in fire play at some point in their lives. It is not surprising, then, that fires and burns rank third among causes of death for 5- to 14-year-olds.

The problem of children and fire can also be examined from a mental health perspective. Studies have been somewhat inconsistent in describing the percentage of children involved in fire play or deliberate fire setting among children in various mental health settings. Vandersall and Weiner (1970) reported an incidence rate of 2.3 percent in a hospital clinic and private practice. Stewart, Meardon, and Cummings (1980) found a rate of 12 percent. Others have reported similar rates (e.g., 17 percent: Gruber, Heck, & Mintzer, 1981; and 14.3 percent: Stewart & Culver, 1982. Achenbach and Edelbrock (1981), in a normative sample of children, found that 3 percent of non-referred children and between 6 and 20 percent of referred children (depending on age) had a history of fire setting.

DIAGNOSIS AND ASSESSMENT

Diagnostic Issues

Fire play, and some of what is classified as fire setting, does not by itself have important psychological significance. It may simply be an act of what has traditionally been called curiosity, a reckless act with no deliberate attempt to harm. Conversely, it may be an indication of the level of distress or disturbance of a child or family. A careful assessment of the incident itself, the context in which it occurred, and the child and his or her family are essential to understand this behavior and guide the choice of a therapeutic intervention. Many children need only education, and their parents need only a reminder to (1) keep fire materials out of their children's reach, (2) assign only age-appropriate responsibilities for fire, and (3) tighten their supervision. Other children need much more intensive intervention.

Several questions need to be addressed during assessment of the child and family:

1. Was the fire deliberately set? If not, was it the result of a reckless act that suggests extremely poor judgment or impulsivity?
2. What was the child's stated intention and motivation? Do the circumstances of the fire fit with the child's stated motive?
3. Is there a pattern of repeated incidents, even after a deliberate educational intervention by the parents, the fire department, or another agency?
4. What was the child's reaction to the fire?
5. Did he attempt to extinguish it? Did she get help? Was he remorseful? Did she tell the truth about what happened?
6. Were other children involved?
7. Is there any evidence of extreme peer pressure or gang activity?
8. What was the family's reaction to the fire?
9. Were they concerned? Did they have any insight into the circumstances contributing to the incident—for example, availability of fire materials, inadequate supervision, short-term or chronic stressors, temperament, and so on? Were they cooperative? Were they truthful?

10. Is there other evidence of family dysfunction?
11. Do they appropriately safeguard fire-ignition materials? Do they provide adequate supervision? Do they demonstrate an understanding of the child's developmental level and appropriate judgment in the assignment of responsibility? Is there evidence of physical or sexual abuse or neglect? Does the family exhibit harsh or punitive attitudes toward the child? Is there evidence of other criminal behavior or alcohol or drug abuse? Do they provide an otherwise safe and adequate environment?
12. Is there evidence for a diagnosable childhood psychological disorder, most likely a conduct disorder, attention deficit-hyperactivity disorder, or adjustment disorder?
13. Is there evidence for pyromania? This is extremely rare, but a possibility. Independent of a diagnosable disorder, is there evidence of inadequate interpersonal skills or emotional management strategies? Does the child have the skills to communicate his or her distress in other, less drastic ways?

Assessment Strategies

There are three major sources of data upon which to base the assessment: review of the incident, psychiatric interview of the child, and family assessment.

Review of the Incident

The characteristics of the incident(s) and the child's and family's response to it contains valuable information about the psychological status of the child. if the referral originated from the fire department, or if the fire department has investigated a recent incident, they may be in a position to provide this information. If any of the incidents were reported to the fire department, they may have conducted an investigation. If so, they have had the opportunity to observe the family during a time of stress, if not crisis, to assess the truthfulness of the child's and parent's accounts of the incident, to interview neighbors and witnesses, and to obtain other agency records that

help to rapidly establish the typical pattern of child and family behavior.

As a result of a growing awareness of the prevalence of juvenile involvement in fire, a large number of local fire departments are training their investigators to recognize and report juvenile involvement, to interview children and their families, and to facilitate referrals to appropriate community social services and mental health agencies. Appropriately trained investigators will have information designed to address the questions outlined above.

There are several facts about the fire incident itself that are helpful to understanding the child, and in turn to treatment planning.

Where did the incident occur?   Most fire incidents occur where children typically play, in their bedrooms, in other areas of their house, or outside. This is consistent with a pattern of curious or mischievous fire play. In some cases the locations are carefully selected to place particular people or their property at risk (e.g., under a siblings' crib) or, conversely, to create a disturbance while attempting to minimize risk to others. Cole and colleagues (1986) found that 75 percent of all fires started by children are started at home, mostly in bedrooms and closets. This is especially likely to be true of young children. Children feel secure in their bedrooms and use them for experimentation. Equally important, parents feel safe when their children are in their rooms and perhaps check on them less frequently. This gives the children an opportunity to experiment.

Who was there? Was the child acting alone or was the child with friends?   Peer pressure and gang activity are sometimes a factor in fire play. Children may show off in front of their friends by displaying their control of a powerful force. Occasionally fire setting is part of gang initiation. One city has reported that prospective gang members must set fire to a vacant building prior to initiation. Gang status can also be related to the size or destructiveness of the fire.

What was the ignition source and how was it obtained?   The vast majority of fires started by children are started with matches or lighters. How easily these materials can be obtained is informative. In most incidents matches and lighters are immediately available and all too frequently in view (e.g., on the coffee table, on the kitchen counter). The availability of ignition materials, when considered in combination with the ages of the children in the house and their history of fire play, is a useful indicator of the level of judgment of the family and to its ability to maintain some level of organization. On occasion, children will use an accelerant (e.g., gasoline) when starting a fire. This often signifies something more than simple curiosity or mischief. At a minimum, it suggests very poor judgment and more likely a deliberate attempt to cause harm. If young children are involved, it may also signify poor family judgment.

What was burned? Very often nothing is burned—a child has been lighting matches or lighters just to watch them burn. Similarly, children often burn nothing more than paper or cardboard, although carpets, bedding, and curtains become involved if the fire gets out of control. Occasionally, however, toys, clothing, or other objects are burned. The nature of the burned objects also provides some information regarding motivation. Burning larger objects or others' possessions indicates poor impulse control, anger, or a deliberatge attempt at revenge or harm.

What was the child's reaction to the fire? The two most common reactions to a fire out of control are to (1) run to get help and (2) hide. Running to get help is the more constructive response and suggests greater maturity and presence of mind. Hiding might be protective, or it might suggest a fear of the disciplinary consequences when the fire is finally discovered. Hiding certainly puts a child at great risk but does not necessarily suggest dysfunction. *Staying to watch* a fire that is out of control is a sign of much greater concern and occurs much less frequently. A new appreciation of the consequences of fire play, acceptance of responsibility for what happened, and sincere remorse all suggest that the behavior was not intentional and will not be repeated. In fact, recidivism is extremely low among children involved in fire play (Cole et al., 1986).

Psychiatric Interview of Child

Because fire play and fire setting have been associated with such a wide variety of child and family problems, a structured diagnostic interview such as the Diagnostic Interview for Children and Adolescents (DICA) is strongly recommended. This ensures adequate coverage of all possibly relevant issues regardless of the initial presentation. If a diagnosis is warranted, one would expect to find one of the three disorders most commonly associated with fire setting: conduct disorder, attention deficit-hyperactivity disorder, or adjustment disorder.

Family Assessment

Given the large number of family factors associated with fire play (access, supervision, assignment of responsibility), with deliberate fire setting (separation, loss, divorce, parental involvement, depression, hostility, punitive attitudes), and recidivism (abuse, neglect, criminal activity), a comprehensive family assessment is essential. A home visit is also highly desirable. It permits the direct assessment of the safety and adequacy of the environment, the availability of ignition materials, and the opportunity to observe parents at home interacting with their children.

TREATMENT

Evidence for Prescriptive Treatments

As stated earlier, fire play and fire setting occur in a variety of settings with a variety of motivations. Systematic research in normative samples of children and adolescents indicates that experimentation with fire is relatively common and by itself does not indicate psychopathology. It is therefore crucial to conduct a careful assessment of the incident, the child, and the family, as previously delineated. If the only motive in starting a fire is curiosity or mischievousness, then a timely educational intervention by well-trained personnel along with a family discussion of appropriate fire safety will likely curtail fire play. Fire setting that is motivated by something other than curiosity or is repeated requires further intervention or treatment. Treatment is directed at intrapersonal, interpersonal, and family factors. In general, treatment is not particularly different from existing recognized approaches to psychotherapy but does require additional coordination and networking to ensure that fire use does not continue.

In this section, we will start by describing intervention strategies appropriate to *all* children who start fires, coordination with other agencies, education, and parent counseling about fire safety. We will then move on to a discussion of treatment strategies for children whose fire setting is motivated by something other than curiosity.

Coordination with Fire Department

In all cases, therapists should not work in isolation. Because of the danger to the community posed by the child setting fires, the therapist has an obligation to work cooperatively with all of the community agencies that share responsibility for the community as well as the child's welfare. This certainly includes the fire department. It may also include the police, depending on the fire and police departments' delineated responsibilities and on the circumstances of the case. It may include child protective services or community mental health or public health nursing that provide community outreach, home visits, or case management services.

If the child and family are cooperative, regularly attending therapy sessions, then the role of these other agencies may be simply advisory. These agencies may also supplement and support what the individual therapist is able to provide by conducting investigations and by providing educational, case management, and home visit services. If the family is uncooperative, or is too disorganized, overwhelmed, or dysfunctional to benefit from traditional outpatient individual or group modes of treatment, then a higher level of restrictiveness or coerciveness may need to be instituted. This may require hospitalization, or even legal action. The therapist's responsibility to the community is more immediate with fire setting than it is with most other problems. Fortunately, an increasing number of communities are developing an awareness of the problem and mechanisms for a coordinated response.

Education

Regardless of the seriousness of the incident or motive of the child in starting a fire, education regarding fire must be part of the intervention strategy. If the fire department has been involved, an educational intervention may have already been conducted and this information can be reinforced by the therapist. If the fire department has not been involved, the therapist may wish to enlist the aid of the fire department in having a trained educator talk with the child about fire safety.

Content of the educational intervention for the child is a function of developmental level. Several fire education programs, designed for specific ages, are available and can be obtained from the local fire department. Included should be information about the nature of fire, how rapidly it spreads, and its potential for destructiveness. It is often helpful to ascertain the child's own beliefs about fire and to specifically address the accuracy of these beliefs. Children should also be taught appropriate procedures to follow if a fire should occur (e.g., to call the fire department from a neighbor's house). Information should be presented seriously, although without scaring the child, which tends to undermine learning.

Parent Counseling

Fire safety must also be reviewed with parents. If the family does not have a significant dysfunction, the intervention should focus on access to matches and lighters, the importance of not giving children responsibility for fire before they are ready, and constant and appropriate supervision (Grolnick et al., 1990).

Intervention Settings for Noncuriosity Fire Setting

Treatment for fire setting generally follows the traditional mental health hierarchy giving priority to the least restrictive intervention:

1. Outpatient treatment with other agency support
2. Day treatment programs with other agency support

3. Hospitalization
4. Placement outside the family (e.g., foster care, residential treatment)

The degree of restrictiveness depends on the likelihood of continued fire play or fire setting and the family's functioning, cooperation, and resources. Outpatient counseling is generally effective where the fire setting was attention seeking and not a deliberate attempt to physically harm someone.

Some children who set fires present an imminent risk to themselves or others and may require hospitalization. The hospital provides an environment that can provide constant supervision. In addition, emotional stimulation can be regulated and intensive multidisciplinary assessments and services can be quickly provided.

Therapeutic Strategies

To date, there has been little systematic research on therapeutic techniques with childhood fire setters. The majority of research takes the form of case studies. While of benefit in generating promising treatments, the techniques explored cannot be assumed to be successful across children and, especially, across as heterogeneous population. A number of possible strategies and their rationales are presented here. It should be noted that the most successful therapies employ multiple strategies to address the many problems facing children and their families.

Techniques Designed to Identify Antecedents of Fire Setting

The rationale for these techniques is that the child and family must recognize the ways in which fire setting has become a mechanism for the child to express his or her feelings. The specific feelings that lead to fire setting and the events that stimulate these feelings are assumed to require identification and labeling.

To specifically identify events that lead to fire setting, the fire incident is discussed in detail. This helps the child experience, identify, and label the emotions present immediately prior to, during,

and following the fire. Typically, an event sets into motion "a sequence of sad, lonely feelings replaced by intense, angry feelings that are partially controlled by a destructive urge or fantasy and significantly reduced by setting a fire" (Bumpass, Fagelman, & Brix, p. 331). Exploration of the sequence of events occurs best after the therapist has established a comfortable rapport with the child. Timing is an important consideration. Prior to therapy the child will undoubtedly have been subject to a barrage of threatening, blaming, and guilt-inducing questions like, "Why did you do this? What were you thinking of?" It may take some time for the child to be able to explore these feelings in a nondefensive manner.

An effective method for exploring these feelings is to have the child describe what happened in as much detail as possible. It is considerably easier for children to describe an event than to explain their feelings. During this process, the therapist can observe feelings and help the child to label them.

Bumpass and colleagues (1983) have developed a graphing method that expands on this idea by incorporating a charting process in which the child can concretely visualize the events causing particular feelings leading up to fire setting. This is essentially a graph with the events and feelings, in chronological order, written along the X-axis, and the magnitude of the emotion indicated along the Y-axis. Once the child and parents understand and can identify this sequence, alternative responses and behaviors can be explored. In a study of 29 patients treated with this method, Bumpass and colleagues (1983) reported that only two set subsequent fires. Followup periods were from 6 months to 8 years with an average of 2½ years.

Techniques to Develop Communication and Social Skills

In families where children resort to fire setting, communication and problem-solving skills are often compromised. Children often have difficulty with assertiveness and the appropriate and controlled expression of anger. Social skills techniques help to contribute to effectiveness of peer relationships and help children cope effectively with the environment (Koles & Jensen, 1985), including teaching alternatives to angry outbursts in challenging situations (Kolko, Dorsett, & Milan, 1981). McGrath, Marshal, and Prior (1979) used social skills training, along with other methods (including covert sensitization and fire safety training) with positive results. Similarly, Koles and Jensen (1985) included social skills training along with other techniques in the successful treatment of a 10-year-old boy.

Kolko and Ammerman (1988) combined the charting method described above to identify feelings and thoughts precipitating angry outbursts with intervention designed to inhibit antisocial responses and replace them with adaptive responses. Included was discussion of and practice in problem solving to promote more positive interpersonal interactions. Significant improvement in fire setting was noted.

Depending on the age of the child and the style of the therapist, several techniques can be used to teach these skills. Didactic discussion illustrated with videotaped examples are often helpful. Roleplay and rehearsal are also useful. These techniques can be employed in a family setting as families need opportunities to practice these skills under therapist guidance.

Group sessions for both parents and children can be especially effective for developing these skills. Having the benefit of other group members' experiences tends to reduce resistance to change and to provide support from credible sources other than the therapist.

Contingency Management Strategies

One of the more frequently used techniques involves using positive reinforcement for nonfire setting and aversive responses for fire-setting behavior. Carstens (1982) applied a work penalty (one hour of labor, such as scrubbing the back porch) to control a 4-year-old's fire-setting behavior. He reported no further fire setting during a six-month followup. One promising method to enhance maintenance and generalization of change is to use the parent as therapist (Holland,

1969). Kolko (1983) applied a token reinforcement procedure with a 6-year-old child. In this procedure, the mother was taught to provide one piece of a puzzle each day a fire was not set. The puzzle could later be exchanged for a desired object.

Assisting parents more generally to develop appropriate behavior management techniques is also important. Helping parents to acknowledge positive behavior, give praise, offer suggestions, ask for behavior change, and appropriately express negative feelings will enhance their children's self-esteem, reduce anger, and support their own expressions of anger and frustration.

In our own experience with these families, we find that parents oftenlack perspective and judgment when setting limits and establishing consequences for misbehavior. Their expectations are too general, vague, unclear, or contradictory. They often are developmentally inappropriate, requiring much more self-discipline and self-monitoring than their children can attain. This is most clearly evidenced in the inappropriate assignment of responsibility to their children. Primary-school children in grades 3 and 4 are not uncommonly asked to babysit for their younger siblings and to cook for them. Even otherwise responsible teenagers are sometimes given overwhelming responsibilities. One serious incident occurred when a teenaged babysitter was unable to monitor the activities of several preschool and school-aged children, including a 2-year-old who was playing with his toys on the stove.

Very often parents in these families were victims of abuse and neglect themselves and perpetuate what they know. Helping parents explore their own values and priorities is the first step in establishing clear limits. Emphasizing issues that are of primary importance to the children and their parents removes considerable pressure by lessening what the parents need to monitor and reinforce. In addition, this discussion of priorities facilitates consistency by helping everyone to better understand the family's shared expectations.

Parents need to learn how to apply minimal, effective consequences. Recall that one of the factors associated with fire play was the children's perception that nothing would happen to them if they were caught playing with matches or lighters.

In part, this perception is based on the children's feelings that their parents trust them, as evidenced by the responsibilities they have been assigned involving fire. In part, however, this perception may arise from the knowledge that only rarely does anything happen to them. Many parents warn but offer no consistent follow-through. Only occasionally is there a consequence, which by the time it occurs is only remotely related to fire play and also is likely to be harsh and punitive, leading to feelings of revenge and resentment.

Family Problem-Solving Techniques

Families experiencing problems with childhood fire setting may have difficulty communicating and solving problems, both individually and as a family. In such cases, family problem-solving techniques, which have been used and evaluated in a variety of settings and with a variety of clinical populations, may be effective.

One program (Ritchey & Jankowski, 1989) uses a seven-step problem-solving technique. The steps are (1) define the problem, (2) brainstorm possible solutions or alternatives, (3) evaluate the solutions or alternatives, (4) select a solution, (5) plan the implementation, (6) try it, and (7) evaluate the effectiveness of the plan. Families are taught to follow each step and are urged to practice in working out problems together.

Satiation Approaches

Satiation, or overpractice, involves forcing a child to light hundreds of matches in a controlled setting. This is often suggested as a therapeutic intervention. The rationale is that this experience will make fire less reinforcing. A number of case studies (e.g., Koles & Jensen, 1985; Kolko & Ammerman, 1988; Welsh, 1971; Wolff, 1984) have utilized this technique apparently successfully, although followup periods tended to be short and the technique was most frequently used along with other interventions, so it is not possible to ascertain whether satiation played any role in reducing fire-setting behavior. Given recent data

(Grolnick et al., 1990) there is some concern about the use of this technique. Children who play with matches tend to have more experience with fire activities than those who do not play with matches. This satiation technique may actually reinforce their fire setting by enhancing their already overstated sense of control.

Other Alternatives

Another alternative, and a useful addition to the general strategies outlined above, is to teach children relaxation exercises and other self-soothing techniques to assist them in controlling their emotions. Relaxation techniques have been used successfully with hyperactivity (Mash & Dalby, 1979) and have been found to be useful with fire setters (Koles & Jensen, 1985). Understanding, support, communication, and appropriate behavior management may not be enough for children who cannot manage their emotions and find safe and socially acceptable outlets for their frustration and anger.

Covert sensitization has also been utilized with fire setters. Stawar (1976), for example, used operant techniques to structure a 7-year-old boy's fantasies. The boy was told a story about a boy finding matches and giving them to his mother. He was rewarded for accurately relaying the story. At seven-month followup, there was no repeat of the fire setting.

Hospitalization

Geffen (1991) has developed a hospital-based program to treat children with compulsive fire-setting behavior. The program's primary goal is to teach children to talk about their emotions and reject fire as a means of expressing themselves. The program generally employs the treatment strategies described below with the addition of a technique to assess the children's ability to avoid fire setting under stress.

In the Geffen (1991) technique, once a therapeutic relationship is established and there is a thorough understanding of the behavioral and emotional antecedents of the fire setting, these conditions and emotions are recreated in the therapy session. At the peak of the child's emotional arousal, the therapist is called away, leaving the child alone. The room is arranged with age-appropriate materials and matches are hidden among these materials. The child is observed through a one-way mirror. If the child chooses the matches, the therapist immediately returns. If not, the child is left for approximately 15 minutes. Afterwards, the child's response is discussed. After this process is successfully repeated in the hospital setting three times, it is repeated outside the hospital. When the child has passed all these tests and there has been significant progress in individual and family therapy, the child is discharged. Geffen stated that this normally can be accomplished within a month. Families with more serious history of abuse obviously take longer.

Hospitalization is most appropriate when there is significant child pathology and family dysfunction. Cole and colleagues (1986) described several children whose fire-setting behavior was motivated by severe parental dysfunction, which included child abuse and neglect. In these cases, the children were removed from the home and placed in foster care or other residential programs to protect them from the abusive environment. Strategies to treat children who are victims of abuse and neglect are discussed elsewhere in this volume (see Chapter 23) and clearly apply to this population of children.

CASE ILLUSTRATION

Ray, an 11-year-old white male, was seen igniting gasoline in the brick barbecue in his backyard by a neighbor. The neighbor notified his parents, and his parents, uncertain about what to do, called the local fire department and asked them to speak with Ray. The parents explained to the youth officer that Ray was often "a handful." He frequently refused to follow rules and engaged in activities that his parents felt were unsafe. Ray also had difficulty in school. He was classified as learning disabled and was taking special classes. The youth officer interviewed Ray and felt counseling would be appropriate. He told the family that he would refer them to a therapist who works with families of children who use fire and would

ask the therapist to call the family to arrange an appointment. The therapist was asked to make the initial contact to increase the likelihood of follow-through, given the risk involved in the fire-setting behavior.

In the initial session, including Ray and his parents, the therapist explained that in his experience, children use fire for different reasons. Sometimes fire use is motivated by curiosity and lack of understanding and sometimes it is a signal that there are other concerns or problems that children and families may be experiencing. He stated that it was his goal to help them better understand Ray's reasons and to offer assistance in helping them to find positive, safer ways to address concerns they might have. Background information about the family and the fire was then elicited.

Ray's parents had been married for 14 years and had two children, Ray, age 11, and Robert, age 9. Both parents were college graduates and held full-time managerial positions in a major, local corporation. The mother had arranged flex time at work so that she could be at home with the boys after school. The father worked long hours and traveled regularly. This was shared with obvious annoyance by both the mother and Ray.

The family lives in a single-family home in a middle-class suburban neighborhood. Ray and Robert attend the public school nearby. Both parents grew up in the area. Their extended families live nearby and see each other regularly. In fact, visits to grandparents and uncles were the only regular family activities they reported.

While Ray waited outside, his parents willingly shared their deep concern about Ray. They acknowledged that they needed help. They sensed that everything was very difficult for Ray and that he would often become very frustrated and angry. When this happened at home, he would throw and break things. It took quite some time for Ray to regain his composure and even then he was quite irritable. Both parents showed very little affect as they described this behavior. They felt that their marital relationship was secure but that their work demands and their difficulties with Ray were wearing on them. The father added that he felt very alienated from Ray. Ray refused to participate in activities that the father initiated, which made him upset.

Ray's parents discussed their son's school difficulties. Ray had been diagnosed as learning disabled in third grade. His school records indicated that Ray was of above average intelligence but had a significant deficit in his ability to process information. He could understand verbal information and directions but had considerable difficulty formulating his ideas on paper. Ray's failure undermined his self-esteem and made him vulnerable to ridicule by his peers. He resisted extra help in school because of the reaction he got from his peers. Both parents put pressure on Ray to work harder in school, feeling that if he studied harder, he would do better. This made Ray quite angry.

The parents mentioned that the relationship between Robert and Ray was very strained. They both felt rather powerless when dealing with the boys. A typical response to the boys' fighting was to yell at them and send them to their rooms. The parents also disagreed about how to discipline the boys. The father felt the mother was too lenient and she felt he was too harsh. The mother also resented her husband's regular absence due to his travel. When Ray was discovered to be setting fires, his parents scolded him and told him about the danger of his behavior. He did not react, and with an increasing sense of frustration, they decided to call the fire department.

When alone with the therapist, Ray did not see any reason why the family should be seeing a therapist. He minimized his parents' concerns, explaining that all brothers fight and all kids disagree with their parents.

As the session continued, Ray shared that he liked to fish and hunt and did so occasionally with an uncle. He added that his father did not enjoy hunting and fishing. Ray went on to share his distaste for school. He described school as boring and irrelevant. Ray did say that he enjoyed gym class and had a few friends with whom he liked to spend time. Ray said he used to play baseball and felt that he had some ability, but he stopped because his father insisted on trying to teach him how to play better. His father attended all of his games.

Ray echoed his parents' description of his relationship with Robert. He acknowledged that they do not get along, that they fight regularly, and that his parents could not do much about it. There was some satisfaction in his voice about having this power. Ray explained that he and Robert fight about sharing, what to watch on television, and whose turn it is to feed the dog. The fights can get quite physical but as yet no one has been hurt.

Ray described his fire involvement in a familiar fashion. He did not see it as dangerous, indicating a strong sense of power and control. He reported that he has played with matches and lighters for a long time, usually with other children in the neighborhood. Prior to the barbecue fires, he had started small paper fires in the woods behind his home and sometimes used fire while playing with army figures.

When challenged about the danger of using gasoline to start fires, he continued to minimize the risk and explain his ability to handle it. He shrugged his shoulders when asked about his parents and their reaction. Ray was not able to describe a specific incident or trigger that led to his desire to start a fire but he appeared to experience some satisfaction about being able to force his parents to react.

Ray was fascinated by fire and its power but stated that it was not anything that he thought very much about. The fires were set impulsively; they were not planned. Ray was attracted by a number of activities that involved risk and force, as illustrated by his interest in hunting, guns, motorcycle racing, and fire. They were activities that demonstrated his own power and competence, unlike school. They were also activities that his parents did not support.

At the conclusion of the session, the therapist summarized for Ray and his parents the issues that arose in their discussion and proposed an initial plan to address his concerns. It was agreed that weekly sessions would be scheduled and that participation would vary, depending on the concern being addressed. The critical issues identified were (1) Ray's alienation from school and the impact that has on his self-esteem, (2) his relationships with others, (3) his parents' inability to establish appropriate standards and guidelines and to implement effective consequences, and (4) his family's inability to clerly communicate and problem solve. The family agreed that these were central issues and that they would cooperate with this plan.

The initial course of treatment focused on engaging Ray in the therapeutic process. Individual sessions were held with Ray to continue to build rapport and to convince him that he really had a voice (i.e., that his issues would be addressed). Case conferences were held with the school to better understand Ray's difficulties and to explore alternative programming. Communication and problem-solving skills were emphasized and considerable support was rallied at home and in school to help Ray learn and practice these skills.

The initial sessions focused on helping Ray to identify his own feelings about his parents and his school. Ray was asked to describe in detail incidents involving his father that upset him. As Ray spoke, the therapist reflected on Ray's feelings of anger and frustration. He focused on how Ray expressed these feelings and the reactions he received. Finally, Ray was asked to describe what he wanted and then he and the therapist explored ways to express his feelings that were morelikely to yield positive results. Ray and the therapist roleplayed these scenes and Ray was asked to play them out with his father and report back. Particular attention was given to helping Ray learn to empathize with others by examining the feelings that his behavior engenders in others.

Subsequent sessions were held with Ray and his parents to help them understand Ray's feelings and frustrations. These sessions focused on reinforcing their communications skills. The therapist acted as a referee, making sure that all communications were appropriately acknowledged by using traditional active listening skills (acknowledgment, paraphrasing, clarification, feedback). The family was instructed to emphasize these techniques at home during their everyday activities and conversations. These culminated in joint sessions that emphasized the constructive expression and acknowledgment of negative emotions.

Individual sessions with Ray's parents addressed their own issues, especially as they pertained to the children. Ray's parents were asked to give priority to the specific problem behaviors they would like to change. These sessions were followed by conjoint family problem-solving sessions during which they established guidelines and consequences for the behaviors they all agreed were most problematic. (Earlier sessions had been held with Robert to allow him to express his issues with the family and to feel an equal member in this process.)

During the course of treatment, Ray experienced a major setback. He became violent at home and some furniture was broken. Ray threatened his father and expressed suicidal wishes but did not act on this behavior. A psychiatric evaluation suggested Ray was depressed, and antidepressive medication was prescribed. The medication was very effective in altering Ray's behavior and allowed the family to carry on effectively with the therapeutic plan.

The family continued to make considerable progress. Both Ray and his parents reported improved relationships at home. During the problem-solving sessions, Ray and his father focused on their estranged relationship and decided to go skeet shooting together. This would allow Ray to use his gun with his father's approval and participation but did not include hunting, which was morally objectionable to his father. Case conferences continued with the school, resulting in the decision to transfer Ray to a program that was not as academically competitive. This led to Ray's becoming much more involved in school. Ray joined the football team the following fall.

Sessions were reduced to monthly contracts for support and successfully terminated after eight full months of treatment. The therapist agreed to call the family in six months to check on their progress. The police department would also notify the therapist if they had any contact. Treatment was very successful for this family. It needs to be emphasized that the case management performed by the therapist was an integral part of the treatment. Ongoing communication was maintained with the school, consulting psychiatrist, parents, and fire department. Regular phone contact was also maintained with the parents to provide support and guidance in implementing behavior management programs and mediating in family conflicts. At last report, Ray was doing well and there has been no additional fire use.

SUMMARY

Children's fire play and fire setting are much more prevalent than commonly thought. Over 50 percent of all children report having engaged in some form of fire play by the time they reach adolescence. Most often, fire play is the result of a mischievous curiosity, not an indication of serious psychopathology—a curiosity fueled by a false sense of security, easy access to ignition materials, exposure to or responsibility for activities involving fire, inadequate supervision and monitoring, and inconsistent punishment for detected fire play.

In a minority of cases, however, an involvement with fire is an attempt to draw attention to a more serious problem. A careful review of the incident, a thorough psychiatric evaluation of the child, and a careful assessment of the family will enable the clinician to distinguish between these two broad classifications.

Treatment always includes fire prevention education for both parents and children. If the fire setting is driven by something other than curiosity, treatment of the child is focused on identifying the antecedents of the fire setting, alternate ways to handle the frustration that might accompany these events, and communication and social skills training. Simultaneous parent counseling addresses contingency management, communication, and family problem solving.

REFERENCES

Achenbach, T. M., & Edelbrock, C. S. (1981). Behavioral problems and competencies reported by parents of normal and disturbed children aged four through sixteen. *Monographs of the Society for Research in Child Development*. Chicago: Society for Research in Child Development.

Bumpass, E. R., Fagelman, F. D., & Brix, R. J. (1983). Intervention with children who set fires. *American Journal of Psychotherapy, 37,* 328–345.

Carstens, C. (1982). Application of a work penalty threat in the treatment of a case of juvenile fire setting. *Journal of Behavior Therapy and Experimental Psychiatry, 13,* 159–161.

Cole, R. E., Grolnick, W. S., Laurenitis, L. R., McAndrews, M. M., Matkoski, K. M., & Schwartzman, P. I. (1986). *Children and fire: Rochester Fire-Related Youth Project progress report*. Rochester, NY.

Cole, R. E., Laurenitis, L. R., McAndrews, M. M. McKeever, J. M., & Schwartzman, P. (1983). *Juvenile firesetter intervention: Report of the Rochester Fire-Related Youth Program Project*. Rochester, NY.

Federal Emergency Management Agency. (1983). *Juvenile firesetters handbook: Dealing with children ages 7–14*. Washington, DC: U.S. Fire Administration.

Fine, S., & Louie, D. (1979). Juvenile firesetters: Do the agencies need help? *American Journal of Psychiatry, 136,* 433–435.

Fineman, K. R. (1980). Firesetting in childhood and adolescence. *Psychiatric Clinics of America, 3,* 483–500.

Geffen, M. (1991). *Juvenile firesetting*. Paper presented at Denver Children's Hospital, Denver.

Grolnick, W. S., Cole, R. E., Laurenitis, L., & Schwartzman, P. (1990). Playing with fire: A developmental assessment of children's fire understanding and experience. *Journal of Clinical Child Psychology, 19,* 128–135.

Gruber, A. R., Heck, E. T., & Mintzer, E. (1981). Children who set fires: Some background and behavioral characteristics. *American Journal of Orthopsychiatry, 51,* 484–488.

Hall, J. R. (1988). U.S. arson trends and patterns. *Fire Journal, 2,* 87–90.

Heath, G. A., Gayton, W. F., & Hardesty, V. A. (1976). Childhood firesetting. *Canadian Psychiatric Association Journal, 21,* 229–237.

Heath, G. A., Hardesty, V. A., Goldfine, P. E., & Walker, A. M. (1983). Childhood firesetting: Am empirical study. *Journal of the American Academy of Child Psychiatry, 22,* 370–374.

Holland, C. J. (1969). Elimination of firesetting behavior in a 7-year-old boy. *Behaviour Research and Therapy, 7,* 135–137.

Kafry, D. (1978). *Fire survival skills: Who plays with matches?* Technical Report for Pacific Southwest Fires and Range Service, Experimental Station, U.S. Department of Agriculture.

Kafry, D. (1980). Playing with matches: Children and fire. In D. Canter (Ed.), *Fires and human behavior* (pp. 47–61). Chichester, England: Wiley.

Kazdin, A. E. (1987). *Conduct disorders in childhood and adolescence*. Newbury Park, CA: Sage.

Kazdin, A. E., & Kolko, D. J. (1986). Parent psychopathology and family functioning among childhood firesetters. *Journal of Abnormal Child Psychology, 14,* 315–329.

Koles, M. R., & Jensen, W. R. (1985). Comprehensive treatment of chronic fire setting in a severely disturbed boy. *Journal of Behavior Therapy and Experimental Psychiatry, 16,* 81–85.

Kolko, D. J. (1983). Multicomponent parental treatment of firesetting in a six year old boy. *Journal of Behavior Therapy and Experimental Psychiatry, 14,* 349–353.

Kolko, D. J. (1985). Juvenile firesetting: A review and methodological critique. *Clinical Psychology Review, 5,* 345–376.

Kolko, D. J. (1990). Firesetting and pyromania. In C. G. Last and M. Hersen (Eds.), *Handbook of child psychiatric diagnosis*. New York: Wiley.

Kolko, D. J., & Ammerman, R. T. (1988). Firesetting. In M. Hersen & C. G. Last (Eds.), *Child therapy casebook*. New York: Plenum.

Kolko, D. J., Dorsett, P. G., & Milan, M. A. (1981). A total-assessment approach to the evaluation of social skills training: The effectiveness of an anger control program for adolescent psychiatric patients. *Behavioral Assessment, 3,* 383–402.

Kolko, D. J., & Kazdin, A. E. (1986). A conceptualization of firesetting in children and adolescents. *Journal of Abnormal Child Psychology, 4,* 49–61.

Kolko, D. J., Kazdin, A. E., & Meyer, E. C. (1985). Parent and reports. *Journal of Consulting and Clinical Psychology, 53,* 377–385.

Kuhnley, E. J., Hendren, R. L., & Quinlan, D. M. (1982). Firesetting by children. *Journal of the American Academy of Child Psychiatry, 21,* 560–563.

Macht, L. B., & Mack, J. E. (1968). The firesetter syndrome. *Psychiatry, 31,* 277–288.

Mash, E. J., & Dalby, J. T. (1979). Behavioral interventions for hyperactivity. In R. Trites (Ed.), *Hyperactivity in children: Etiology, measurement and treatment implications*. Baltimore: University Park Press.

McGrath, P., Marshal, P. T., & Prior, K. (1979). A comprehensive treatment program for a firesetting child. *Journal of Behavior Therapy and Experimental Psychiatry, 10,* 69–72.

Mieszala, P. (1981, August). Juvenile fire setters. *Rekindle,* pp. 11–13.

National Center of Health Statistics. (1984). Public Health Service, U.S. Department of Health and Human Services.

Ritchey, K., & Jankowski, J. (1989). Problems solving workshop for families. *Journal of Mental Health Counseling, 2,* 307–324.

Rutter, M., & Garmezy, N. (1983). Developmental psychopathology. In E. M. Hetherington (Ed.), *Carmichael's manual of child psychopathology (Vol. 4): Social and personality development*. New York: Wiley.

Sakheim, G. A., Vigdor, M. G., Gordon, M., & Helprin, L. M. (1985). A psychological profile of juvenile firesetters in residential treatment. *Child Welfare, 64,* 453–476.

Stawar, T. L. (1976). Fable mod: Operantly structured fantasies as an adjunct in the modification of firesetting behavior. *Journal of Behavior Therapy and Experimental Psychiatry, 7,* 258–287.

Stewart, M. A., & Culver, K. W. (1982). Children who set fires: The clinical picture and a follow-up. *British Journal of Psychiatry, 140,* 357–363.

Stewart, M. A., Meardon, J., & Cummings, C. (1980). Aggressive conduct disorder of children: The clinical picture. *Journal of Nervous and Mental Disease, 168,* 604–610.

Strachan, J. D. (1981). Conspicuous firesetting in children. *British Journal of Psychiatry, 138,* 26–29.

U.S. Department of Justice. (1989). A look at juvenile firesetter programs. *OJJDP Update on Research, Juvenile Justice Bulletin.*

U.S. Federal Bureau of Investigation. (1987). *Crime in the United States.* Washington, DC: U.S. Government Printing Office.

Vandersall, J. A., & Wiener, J. M. (1970). Children who set fires. *Archives of General Psychiatry, 22,* 63–71.

Welsh, R. S. (1971). The use of stimulus satiation in the elimination of juvenile firesetting behavior. In A. M. Graziano (Ed.), *Behavior therapy with children*. Chicago: Aldine.

West, D. J., & Farrington, D. P. (1973). *Who becomes delinquent?* London: Heinemann Educational.

Wolff, R. (1984). Satiation in the treatment of inappropriate firesetting. *Journal of Behavior Therapy and Experimental Psychiatry, 15,* 337–340.

Wooden, W. S., & Berkey, M. L. (1984). *Children and arson*. New York: Plenum.

Yarnell, H. (1940). Firesetting in children. *American Journal of Orthopsychiatry, 10,* 272–286.

CHAPTER 21

SEXUAL ABUSE

Judith A. Cohen   University of Pittsburgh
Anthony P. Mannarino   University of Pittsburgh

DESCRIPTION OF PROBLEM

Core Features

The core feature of child sexual abuse is the abusive act(s) perpetrated against the child. Unlike child psychiatric syndromes, sexual abuse is not a clinical disorder or diagnosis in itself. It is an event or, more accurately, it comprises a variety of events or experiences to which there may be a wide variety of behavioral and emotional responses. In this sense, sexual abuse is best conceptualized as a stressor, such as divorce or death of a family member, rather than a distinct clinical entity.

Sexual abuse has been defined in a number of different ways. Legally, the definition of sexual abuse varies somewhat from state to state. Surveys of mental health care providers have shown that there is little consensus regarding what acts constitute sexual abuse (Emery, 1989; O'Toole, Turbett, & Nalepka, 1983). Even among science researchers, there is no universally accepted definition of the term. For the purposes of this discussion, we will use one common operational definition: *Sexual abuse* is defined as sexual exploitation involving physical contact between a child and another person. Exploitation implies an inequality of power between the child and the abuser, on the basis of age, physical size, and/or the nature of the emotional relationship. Physical contact includes anal, genital, oral, or breast contact.

This definition obviously encompasses a number of different behaviors. It should be pointed out that this definition makes no mention of the number of times such behavior occurred, the presence or absence of physical force being used, or the identity of the perpetrator of the abuse. Thus, the term *child sexual abuse* can refer to a wide variety of experiences, and is far from being a unitary phenomenon.

Associated Features

Just as the event of child sexual abuse encompasses a wide variety of experiences, there is a great deal of variability in the behavioral, emotional, and social consequences of child sexual abuse. Empirical studies have consistently demonstrated that sexually abused children vary markedly in the behavioral and emotional symptoms they manifest. *As a group,* sexually abused girls have been found to manifest significantly more behavioral and emotional difficulties as rated by parents than do normal (nonabused) girls (Einbender & Friedrich, 1989; Friedrich, Beilke, & Urquiza, 1987; Mannarino, Cohen, & Gregor, 1989). It has also been demonstrated that these differences persist over time (Mannarino, Cohen, Smith, & Moore-Motily, 1990).

In the latter study, using the parent form of the Child Behavior Checklist, sexually abused girls differed from normal controls on the total behavior problems scale, internalizing scale, externalizing scale, and seven out of nine subscales at the initial evaluation and at 6- and 12-month followups. Despite these findings, however, there are still large numbers of sexually abused children who have *not* been found to display any significant psychological symptomatology by parent report. Gomes-Schwartz, Horowitz, and Sauzier (1985) found that nearly 60 percent of their sexual abuse sample did not exhibit significant behavioral or emotional problems on the Louisville Behavior Checklist parental rating form. Thus, according to parental reports, many sexually abused children have a wide range of significant psychological symptoms, but some sexually abused children are relatively free of observable symptomatology.

On self-report instruments, sexually abused children *as a group* have not typically demonstrated significantly more depressive symptoms or low self-esteem than nonabused normal controls (Einbender & Friedrich, 1989; Mannarino et al., 1989). One study found sexually abused girls to self-report significantly more state anxiety than either normal or psychiatric controls, but to not have increased levels of trait anxiety than the control groups (Mannarino et al., 1989). However, these researchers found that this elevated state anxiety did not persist at 6- and 12-month followup assessments (Mannarino et al., 1990). Thus, as a group, sexually abused children have not generally been found to endorse significant psychological symptoms on self-report instruments. (It should be emphasized that while these findings hold true for group comparisons, there were some sexually abused children who did endorse elevated levels of depression, anxiety, and/or poor self-esteem.)

What sexually abused children as a group do endorse are less global and less symptom-related problems, such as feeling different from their peers, having difficulty trusting others, feeling personally responsible for negative events, and feeling that other people do not believe them. Sexually abused children experience these problems significantly more than both nonabused normal and nonsexually abused psychiatric outpatient control groups (Cohen & Mannarino, 1990b). Thus, it appears that, in addition to a variety of nonspecific emotional and behavioral difficulties as reported by parents, there may be specific "abuse-related" issues such as those just mentioned, which characterize many child sexual abuse victims.

Special attention should be given to the issue of sexually inappropriate behavior. Most researchers who have examined this question have found that sexually abused children exhibit significantly higher rates of sexually inappropriate behavior than nonabused populations (Friedrich et al., 1987; Mannarino et al., 1989; White, Halpin, Strom, & Santilli, 1988). In fact, this is the one behavior that most consistently differentiates sexually abused children from psychiatric control groups. There are many theories as to why this behavior occurs in relation to sexual abuse, including learning of inappropriate behaviors through the abusive experience, the classical defense mechanisms of repetitive compulsion and identification with the aggressor, and that children with preexisting sexually inappropriate behavior are more likely to be targeted as victims of sexual abuse. Although the reasons for these behaviors are uncertain, it is clear that sexually inappropriate behavior is a frequently associated feature of child sexual abuse. (It should be noted that there may be other, nonabuse-related reasons for children to exhibit sexually inappropriate behaviors, and that these behaviors are not pathognomonic for sexual abuse.)

In summary, a wide variety of behavioral and emotional problems is associated with sexual abuse, but it should be clear from this discussion that there is no such entity as a "child sexual abuse syndrome." That is, there is no group of symptoms or a "characteristic" presentation that clinically distinguishes sexually abused children from nonsexually abused children.* Rather, sexual abuse may result in a variety of clinical presentations. Conversely, it should be clear that sexual abuse cannot be "diagnosed" by the clinical features present at evaluation. Such a determination depends on careful history taking and interviews with the child and significant others. (The one possible exception is in the case where a sexually transmitted disease is diagnosed in a child. Even in this situation, further information must be elicited to determine the identity of the perpetrator, etc.).

Epidemiology

Sexual abuse of children is a common occurrence in our society. Statistics suggest that approximately 25 percent of all girls and 10 percent of all boys in the United States are sexually abused by the age of 18 years (Finkelhor, 1979; Russell, 1983). Some researchers have suggested that these percentages are an underestimation of the frequency of sexual abuse, due to repression of traumatic memories and negative societal messages associated with disclosure of sexual abuse by male children in particular. One researcher has reported sexual asbuse rates as high as 30 percent for females and 18 percent for male children (Briere, 1990).

Although sexual abuse occurs across all religious, racial, and socioeconomic strats of society, there are several fctors that appear to put certain children at higher risk for sexual abuse. These have been identified by Finkelhor (1984). There is some controversy over the relationship between social class and child sexual abuse. Some researchers have found that reported cases of sexual abuse have come predominantly from families in the lower socioeconomic levels of society (Finkelhor, 1984; Strauss, Gelles, & Steinmetz,

1980). However, it appears that this may be due to a reporting phenomenon rather than a real socioeconomic status (SES) sexual abuse correlation (i.e., because lower SES families are more likely to be involved with social welfare agencies, public health care facilities, etc., identification and reporting of abuse in these families may be more likely). Indeed, other studies have found no relationship between sexual abuse and social class (Finkelhor & Barron, 1986; Russell, 1983).

Other risk factors for child sexual abuse that were identified by Finkelhor and Barron (1986) include a poor relationship between the child and parent; having a stepfather (which in itself appeared to more than double a girl's vulnerability to sexual abuse); having mothers who worked outside the home or were emotionally distant or often ill; and having a mother or father who did not live with the child for a period of time. As previously noted, gender is also a risk factor for child sexual abuse, with girls being at higher risk than boys.* Finkelhor also identified several factors that did *not* appear to be correlated with sexual abuse. Contrary to popular perception, physical abuse was not significantly associated with sexual abuse. Religion, ethnic background, family size, crowding, and alcohol abuse by either parent were also *not* found to be risk factors for sexual abuse in this study. It should be emphasized that despite the recognition of high-risk factors for child sexual abuse, this type of abuse is relatively common throughout U.S. society, and no subgroup of children can be considered immune.

DIAGNOSIS AND ASSESSMENT

Diagnostic Issues

Because child sexual abuse is an event (or events) rather than a clinical syndrome, and

---

*Some authors such as Green (1986) have proposed the existence of a "child sexual abuse syndrome," and have used this to differentiate true from false allegations of child sexual abuse. It should be emphasized that Green's hypothesized "syndrome" was not based on empirically sound research but only on clinical impressions.

*Because child sexual abuse victims are more often female, and to avoid cumbersome language, the female gender will be employed when refering to sexually abused children throughout this chapter. However, clinicians should be aware that substantial numbers of boys are also sexually abused.

psychological responses to this experience differ considerably, one would expect psychiatric diagnoses in sexually abused children to also vary considerably. This indeed has been the clinical experience. One study that examined this issue evaluated 207 consecutive cases seen in an outpatient clinic specifically treating sexually abused children (Sirles, Smith, & Kusama, 1989). The results indicated that the majority of victims did not have a DSM-III primary Axis I diagnosis of mental disorder. Most of these children (61.8 percent) were given V code diagnoses (indicating conditions not attributable to a mental disorder). Of those cases (38.2 percent) who did receive clinical diagnoses, by far the most common disorders diagnosed were Adjustment Disorders (22.7 percent of the total sample), indicating a variety of symptomatic reactions to the psychosocial stressor of the sexual abuse. More rarely seen were anxiety disorders (0.5 percent), psychiatric disorders with physical manifestations (3.4 percent), conduct disorder (5.3 percent), oppositional disorder (0.5 percent), attention deficit-hyperactivity disorder (2.9 percent), and mental retardation (2.9 percent). These findings indicate that there is not a particular psychiatric syndrome associated with sexual abuse in children. It also emphasizes the point that a considerable percentage of these children may not present with clinically significant emotional or behavioral symptoms.

Similar findings were demonstrated in 100 consecutive cases seen in another outpatient clinic for sexually abused children (Cohen & Mannarino, 1990a). All of these children had experienced or first disclosed sexual abuse within the six months prior to evaluation. In this group, the majority (61 percent) received a diagnosis of Adjustment Disorder; almost half of these (27 percent of the total sample) were diagnosed as having Adjustment Disorder with Anxious Mood. A Major Depressive Disorder was diagnosed in 12 percent, and Posttraumatic Stress Disorder was the diagnosis in 6 percent of these children. More chronic diagnoses such as Conduct Disorder (5 percent), Oppositional-defiant Disorder (6 percent), and Attention Deficit-Hyperactivity Disorder (5 percent) were also found in some proportion of this population. Unlike the Sirles and colleagues' (1989), virtually

all of these children presented with enough symptomatology to receive some DSM-III-R diagnosis. Part of this difference may be attributable to the fact that this population consisted entirely of cases with very recent abuse and/or disclosure, and all were involved in some sort of medical, legal, and/or child protective investigation. It is likely that this added to the level of psychosocial stress present for these children, resulting in more significant (if transient) symptomatology.

The process of determining accurate DSM-III-R psychiatric diagnoses in sexually abused children is similar to that used in nonabused populations. Diagnostic strategies for specific disorders have been addressed in earlier chapters of this book, and can be used with sexually abused children when appropriate. The issue of "diagnosing" whether or not a particular child has experienced sexual abuse is quite another topic. Making such a determination is a complex, medical, psychiatric, and legal process, which is beyond the scope of the present chapter. For detailed discussions of this issue, the reader may refer to Hindman (1987).

Assessment Strategies

The optimal assessment of sexually abused children involves more than a standard psychiatric evaluation and determination of diagnosis. Although these are necessary parts of the evaluation, there are several special areas of concern related to the sexual abuse experience that also must be addressed. These include possible legal involvement, child protective services interventions, medical issues related to the abuse, and other "abuse-related" issues of the child and family. These will be addressed separately in the following discussion.

Legal Involvement

Child sexual abuse is not only a psychosocial stressor but, in most cases, it is also a criminal act. For this reason, the legal system is frequently involved in investigation and prosecution of sexual abuse cases. Briefly, this includes the following activities: Typically a child is interviewed at least once by police detectives (hopefully specially trained in interviewing sexually abused children).

If a decision is made to prosecute the perpetrator, the child is interviewed at least once by a district attorney. If criminal charges are being pressed, the child is generally required to appear and testify at a preliminary hearing, where a decision is made either to dismiss the charge or hold a case over for trial. The subsequent trial may occur at any time up to several months after the charges are initially filed. If the perpetrator is a juvenile, a hearing before a juvenile court judge is held, with a possible adjudication of delinquency.

It is important for the assessing clinician to have an understanding of these complicated proceedings, and to be aware of what (if any) legal actions the child and family members are involved in. This often requires collaboration with the legal officers involved. One group of researchers (Runyan, Everson, Edelsohn, Hunter, & Coulter, 1988) have found that participation in these legal proceedings is in itself a significant stressor for sexually abused children, and that the waiting period between disclosure of abuse and going to trial is an especially difficult period. It is important for the clinician to assess the emotional reactions of the child and family members to ongoing legal activities and to try in therapy to minimize the traumatic nature of this involvement.

Child Protective Services Interventions

Because child sexual abuse is by definition a form of child abuse, child protective services (CPS) may be involved in investigating the case and possibly in custody and placement issues as well. Generally, this applies to cases where the perpetrator is a family member or where the caretaker adult failed to adequately protect the child from the sexual abuser. (CPS mandates vary somewhat from state to state.) A thorough evaluation must include information regarding the nature and extent of CPS involvement (whether a caseworker is involved; whether the report of abuse has been founded by CPS; what, if any, action regarding custody or placement is being pursued; etc.). Most likely this will require that the clinician discuss the case directly with the CPS worker involved.

Medical Issues Related to the Abuse

Many pediatric physicians specializing in the evaluation of sexually abused children maintain that *all* such children should receive a physical examination, even when the child's allegations do not involve the probability of sexually transmitted disease or physical trauma (e.g., digital fondling of the child's external genitalia). This is because physical examinastion in some of these cases reveals evidence of more extensive abuse than the child initially disclosed.* In general, clinics specializing in the treatment of sexually abused children routinely refer their clients for specialized medical evaluations. Medical evaluations are necessary to determine whether there is presence of a sexually transmitted disease, pregnancy, or physical trauma related to the sexual abuse; to gather medical-legal evidence; and to provide information and reassurances to the child and family regarding the child's physical health and "normality." The psychiatric evaluation should include these factors (by obtaining the medical information) and, more importantly, the child's and family's emotional reaction to the medical information.

"Abuse-Related" Issues of the Child and Family

In addition to assessing general emotional and behavioral symptoms, there are certain "abuse-related" issues that should be evaluated specifically during the assessment. This includes elucidating the nature and extent of the sexual abuse to some reasonable degree. (As will be discussed below, this is different from conducting a formal credibility evaluation for legal purposes.) The purpose for obtaining this information is to improve the clinician's insight into what clinical issues may

---

*Clinicians should be aware of the fact that in many cases of sexual abuse, including cases where the perpetrator has admitted to penile penetration of the vagina or anus, there is *no* physical evidence of such abuse (Muram, 1989).

be most salient to the child and family. Factors such as the type of sexual abuse experienced, how long it was going on, and the identity of the perpetrator may have direct effects on the child's and/or family's emotional reactions, attitudes, and concerns about the abuse. (For example, to some families it may be most traumatic that the abuse involved actual intercourse; whereas to other families this may be less relevant than the fact that the abuse was perpetrated by a trusted family member, etc.). This information in turn is essential to both define the family and child's current functioning and to prescribe appropriate therapeutic interventions.

Perhaps even more important than the *who, what,* and *where* details of the sexual abuse are the *hows* and *whys. How* the abuse occurred includes information as to whether the perpetrator used positive coercion such as promises or rewards, or negative coercion such as threats of harm or actual physical punishment or force. It also includes understanding whether the abuse consisted of a gradual process of breaking down the child's resistance (possibly fostering the illusion of the child "cooperating" with the abuse) or a sudden forceful violation of the child's bodily integrity. How the abuse occurred also entails insight into how the perpetrator gained access to the child: Was it through exploitation of a trusted position in the family (e.g., family member, babysitter, mother's paramour), through neglect of a caretaker (e.g., leaving the child with an obviously inappropriate sitter, intoxicated mother not cognizant of the perpetrator being in the child's bedroom, the caretaker ignoring or disbelieving the child's hints or disclosures regarding abuse), or during the child's normal activities of living (e.g., school bus driver abusing the child on the bus, child attacked while walking home from school, perpetrator breaking into the child's bedroom window while the child is sleeping, etc.)?

The child's and family's perceptions of *why* the sexual abuse occurred is also very relevant for assessment. Is it attributed to the perpetrator, the child, the parents, or some combination? Researchers have hypothesized that psychological symptom formation may be closely related to these attributions and to the child's and family's resultant responses to these attributions (National Children's Advocacy Center, 1987). For example, a child who attributes the abuse to something about herself rather than to perpetrator characteristics may be more likely to feel guilt and poor self-esteem; whereas a child who attributes the abuse to the violence and unpredictability of the perpetrator may have more difficulty with fear and anxiety symptoms. Similarly, parents who attribute the abuse in part to the child's behavior or appearance may be less likely to be supportive of the child, or even less likely to view the experience as abuse (as opposed to consensual sexual activity). These theories have yet to be examined empirically, but clinical experience suggests they have validity in many cases.

As noted earlier, issues such as feeling different from other children, having difficulty trusting others, feeling personally responsible for negative events, and feeling that others do not believe you have all been empirically identified as significant problems for many sexually abused children (Cohen & Mannarino, 1990b). Sgroi (1982) has described several other clinical issues that may be particularly relevant following sexual abuse. These include blurred role boundaries within the family, the "damaged goods" syndrome (feeling the abuse changed the child in some permanent and negative way), guilt about the abuse, fear regarding lack of safety and the possibility of future abuse, divided loyalties (i.e., ambivalent feelings toward the perpetrator), low self-esteem, and anger.

Many of these issues have been unified in the Traumagenic Dynamics Model as conceptualized by Finkelhor (1987) and Finkelhor and Browne (1985). This model suggests four basic dynamics or potential problematic issues that are relevant in many sexually abused children. These include experiences of traumatic sexualization, betrayal, stigmatization, and powerlessness. All of these issues and problems may arise either in direct response to experiencing sexual abuse, or secondarily in response to others' reactions to the disclosure of the abuse. The initial assessment should attempt to evaluate to what extent the child or family members are experiencing problems related to any of these clinical issues.

The Role of the Assessing Clinician

Because of the complex legal and child protective issues involved in cases of child sexual abuse, it is of paramount importance for the assessing clinician to clearly define his or her role in the case. It is assumed that most clinicians referring to this book are to be involved in the ongoing treatment of such children rather than being in a primarily investigative role. These roles are, and should be, separate and distinct as much as possible. Assessments for the purpose of treatment differ significantly from assessments for credibility or custody issues. As mentioned earlier, the latter types of evaluation are complex and beyond the scope of this chapter. However, it is generally considered a conflict of interest to evaluate a child for credibility of sexual abuse allegations, or to evaluate a child and parents for custody determination, and then to take that child and/or family as a treatment case. The objectivity of the treating clinician is typically considered to be compromised, due to the therapeutic relationship; whereas objectivity is a sine qua non in performing credibility and custody evaluations. The above discussion of assessment strategies applies to the clinical psychiatric evaluation of sexually abused children. *It does not describe an adequate credibility or custody evaluation.*

TREATMENT

Evidence for Prescriptive Treatments

Unfortunately, there have been virtually no adequately controlled empirical studies documenting the efficacy of any treatment modality for sexually abused children. This has resulted from many factors. Relatively few empirical researchers are involved in the field of child sexual abuse as opposed to other areas of child psychopathology such as depression, anxiety, and attention deficit-hyperactivity disorder. This is in part due to the complexities involved in working with the legal and child welfare systems.

Because child sexual abuse is not a clinical syndrome or diagnostic entity, it also does not lend itself to empirical study as easily as unitary disorders, which are clearly defined by specific behaviors, emotions, and/or symptoms. Standardized instruments have been developed to measure depression, anxiety, attentional problems, and so on in children, but there are to date no well-standardized instruments to adequately evaluate the very diverse symptomatology associated with sexual abuse. Finally, there has been a general lack of standardization in treatment protocols for this population. All of these factors have impeded the ability of researchers to conduct empirical treatment outcome studies with this population.

Despite these shortcomings, treatment of sexually abused children continues, with innovative therapeutic approaches being developed by many talented and experienced clinicians. Thus, although there is no empirical evidence for various prescriptive treatments, there is a great deal of clinical experience to suggest what types of interventions are most effective for different problems in this population. These will be discussed in the following sections.

Behavior Therapy

As discussed earlier, sexually abused children as as group have significantly more behavioral problems than normal children. The types of maladaptive behaviors vary. For example, some sexually abused children have difficulty with aggressive or sexually inappropriate behaviors, some have symptoms such as excessive clinginess and refusal to sleep alone, and others have problems with enuresis or similar age-inappropriate regressive behaviors.

Although some therapists believe that all of these behavioral problems are secondary to the sexual abuse and will spontaneously remit once the trauma of the abuse has been therapeutically resolved, many clinicians question such a conceptualization. First, a causative relationship between sexual abuse and behavioral problems has not been demonstrated. In addition, it is the experience of many therapists that behavioral symptoms respond to behavioral interventions regardless of the etiology of the symptoms. The argument is made, in effect, that even if a behavioral symptom is secondary to the abuse and even if therapy directed at the trauma of the abuse does eventually result in a remission of the behavioral symptom (both untested hypotheses), such therapy generally takes much longer than specific behavioral interventions and may prolong the behavioral symptom unnecessarily. It is further suggested that such behavioral problems over time may themselves result in poor self-esteem, feelings of powerlessness, and so on, which are already potential areas of vulnerability for these children, and therefore the intervention resulting in the most rapid behavioral improvement (i.e., behavioral therapy) is indicated.

Indeed, it has been the authors' experience that behavioral approaches have been clinically effective for symptoms such as enuresis, avoidant behaviors, sexually inappropriate behaviors, and oppositionalism in sexually abused children. Interventions such as systematic desensitization, progressive relaxation, and thought stopping have also been successful in treating symptoms such as anxiety, phobias, and intrusive thoughts (Berliner & Wheeler, 1988). Behavioral interventions such as contingency reinforcement programs, time-out procedures, and the like should be used *in conjunction* with treatment that focuses on the thoughts and feelings related to the sexual abuse, not as a replacement for the latter. Specific behavioral techniques should be determined by the presenting behavioral symptoms, and are discussed in earlier chapters of this book.*

A recent study has presented the first empirical evidence that cognitive-behavioral therapy is effective in treating certain sexually abused children (Deblinger, McLeer, & Henry, 1990). This study targeted various symptoms of Posttraumatic Stress Disorder, using modeling, skills training, gradual exposure to stressful stimuli, and education and prevention training interventions. The authors

reported significant symptom improvement as rated by parents and clinicians, as well as significant improvement of children's self-reported anxiety and depression. Although the study lacked an adequate control design, it is an important preliminary investigation of treatment outcome in this population.

In some cases, problematic behaviors may not respond readily to behavioral approaches in the context of outpatient treatment. If these behaviors are sufficiently severe or dangerous (such as sexually aggressive behavior toward other children), inpatient treatment may be necessary. Hospitalization in these cases serves the dual purposes of instituting more intensive behavioral (and other) therapy and protecting the child from endangering herself and other children.

Pharmacotherapy

Some percentage of sexually abused children also have disorders such as major depression or attention deficit-hyperactivity disorder, which are known to respond to phasrmacologic agents. As with behavioral symptoms, there are some therapists who view these syndromes in sexually abused children as resulting solely from the sexual abuse experience, and who therefore resist pharmacotherapy on the basis that these symptoms will remit once the core problem of the sexual abuse has been adequately addressed. Although sexual abuse as a stressor can certainly trigger the emergence of such symptoms, our current understanding of these disorders indicates that they are multifactorial in etiology and probably not caused solely by the abuse. Additionally, even if a biochemical imbalance had been triggered by stress alone, removal and resolution of the stressor would not necessarily guarantee reversal of the biochemical abnormality. For these reasons, it is believed that pharmacotherapy can be a useful adjunct to psychotherapy in cases where either very significant symptomatology exists or where such symptoms do not respond relatively quickly to therapeutic and psychosocial interventions.

It would be reasonable in most situations to begin appropriate nonpharmacologic interventions (such as removing the child from the perpetrator's access, correcting cognitive misconceptions, and

---

*One behavioral problem not specifically addressed elsewhere in this book is inappropriate sexual behavior. The reader is referred to MacFarlane and Cunningham (1988), who have designed a detailed cognitive-behavioral treatment program specifically for sexually abused children with sexually inappropriate behaviors.

enhancing familial support of the abused child) prior to considering a medication trial. In many instances, these interventions will result in significant remission of depressive and anxiety symptoms. In general, if these interventions fail to result in significant improvement of symptomatology, or these changes cannot be instituted and the symptoms persist, it would be reasonable to begin a trial of medication.

Medication is most commonly used in this population when a diagnosis of major depression or ADHD is present. In rare instances, anxiety disorders (particularly with phobic or panic symptoms) may require pharmacotherapy. However, since some degree of fear and anxiety are common symptoms following sexual abuse and are frequently short-term rather than ongoing symptoms for these children (Mannarino et al., 1990), adequate trials of behavioral and environmental interventions should be attempted prior to considering medication. Detailed discussions of pharmacotherapy for these disorders are provided in earlier chapters of this book and in general are equally applicable to sexually abused children.

Alternative Treatments

There are several treatment strategies that have been adapted specifically for use with sexually abused children. These include specialized forms of cognitive therapy, safety education and assertiveness training, group therapy, and family therapy. Each of these will be discussed briefly below.

Cognitive therapy. Frequently, sexual abuse victims have distorted cognitions asbout the abuse. Instruments such as the Burt Rape Myth Acceptance Scale (Burt, 1980) have been used in treating adult rape victims to identify specific cognitions that may distort the victims' understanding of what caused the rape to occur, who was responsible, and so on. Cognitive distortion and confusion is very common among child sexual abuse victims as well. This may be in part because many perpetrators present a distorted idea of the abuse to their victims (e.g., telling the child it's the child's fault, that tis is appropriate behavior, etc.); because of the child's cognitive developmental level; and/or because of children's lack of knowl-

edge and experience of adult sexuality. Cognitive therapy is aimed at identifying and correcting the particular cognitive distortions a child has related to the abuse. The process of identifying, challenging, and restructuring these distorted cognitions is similar to cognitive therapy in other settings and will not be described in detail here. Rather, the focus will be on specific distortions and appropriate responses.

Children have many misperceptions regarding different aspects of the sexual abuse. These commonly include ideas such as the following:

This was his way of loving me.
He did this because I was bad and I deserved it.
I must have done something to make him think I wanted him to abuse me.
He did it because he was drunk.
He did this with me because my mother wouldn't have sex with him.
If I had fought him, he wouldn't have done it.
If I tell about the abuse, he'll really do all the bad things he threatened to do.
Now that I've been sexually abused, I'll never really be a normal kid again.

Appropriate cognitive restructuring will educate the child about the self-centered behavior of the sexual offender (i.e., that the abuse was carried out for the perpetrator's gratification), that the adult's behavior was what was inappropriate in the abuse situation, and that the adult had more power in the situation than the child (and thus the abusing adult was the one responsible for the abuse). The child's cognitions should be restructured to recognize that hurting, frightening, and/or exploiting a child is not a loving act; that having sex with a child is not an appropriate punishment for *any* misbehavior, that in fct perpetrators pick their victims primarily on the basis of availability and their particular (aberrant) sexual arousal patterns rather than behaviors or feelings exhibited by the child herself; that being abused in a sexual way does not make a child into an adult, or have to permanently change anything about that child; that personal problems the perpetrator has such as alcoholism, loneliness, or difficulty with adult relationships are not appropriately dealt with by having sex with children; that children can rarely overpower or convince adults to change; and that no matter what the child did or said, responsibility for avoiding sexual contact still rests ultimately with the adult.

At the same time, actions of the child that may have perpetuated the abuse (such as the child repeatedly requesting the same babysitter who previously abused her, or actively seeking rewards in exchange for compliance with the abuse) need to be accurately identified and recognized by the child as factors that *were* within her control and that she can change in the future (Berliner & Wheeler, 1988; Janoff-Bulman, 1986). Realistic assessments of the perpetrator's present ability to hurt the child or family members should also be encouraged. Younger children such as preschoolers may not be able to understand these ideas, and sometimes must simply be reeducated regarding their cognitive misunderstandings (e.g., learning that private parts are private, that "it's not okay for anyone to touch you there," that they do not have to keep "bad secrets," etc.).

Cognitive therapy can occur in individual, group, and family therapy settings. The group may be particularly helpful when the child has distortions about herself in relation to peers. For example, many children believe they are different from other kids in some important way because of having been sexually abused. (Some children even believe that people can tell they were sexually abused just by looking at them.) In a group setting, children are confronted about these misperceptions by their peers, who are often more convincing than an adult therapist could be. The family setting may be the most appropriate in which to confront cognitive distortions when family members share or contribute to those distortions. For example, when a mother demands, "If the abuse really happened, why didn't you tell me sooner?", the entire family may need to be confronted regarding the degree of fear the sexually abused child may have been living with, and the frequency with which such children delay making the initial disclosure. Therapists frequently find that correcting cognitive distortions results in decreased guilt and improved self-esteem for sexually abused children, and that challenging these distortions in family members often leads to increased familial support of the abused child.

Safety education and assertiveness training. While correcting cognitive distortions in sexually abused children is designed to decrease the child's feeling of responsibility for the abuse, it may at the same time increase the child's sense of vulnerability to inappropriate adults. Every attempt should be made, using legal and CPS resources as indicated, to assure the abused child's actual safety (such as removing the perpetrator from the home, optimizing the quality of supervision, etc.). Learning general safety rules (such as not walking alone in deserted areas, avoiding strangers, etc.), recognizing sexually inappropriate behavior when it occurs, and knowing to report frightening or inappropriate situations to a trusted adult are important preventive lessons for all children to know. Learning and rehearsing assertive responses (saying "no," escaping, etc.) to inappropriate adult behavior are also valuable skills for any child. Many coloring books, board games, and similar aids have been devised to teach these lessons in enjoyable nonthreatening ways to children of all ages.

Sometimes adding concrete responses to a child's behavioral repertoire will succeed in decreasing her fear of reabuse and give her some sense of control over her fate. However, two caveats should be noted here. First, a child's sense of fear may have no relation to the degree of danger that actually exists in the situation. For some children whose fear seems out of proportion to the present circumstances, no amount of safety education or assertiveness training will be effective in alleviating the symptomatology. Other therapeutic approaches such as those described by Salter (1988, pp. 212–216) and Berliner and Wheeler (1988) may be more helpful in these situations. Second, the child, family, and therapist must all be realistic regarding the true degree of power and control a child can have in a threatening situation. Although many studies have examined how readily children learn preventive safety and assertiveness skills, ethical considerations prevent researchers from assessing how readily or effectively these skills would be used in an actual situation of threatened sexual abuse. Common sense, as well as experience, indicate that children can rarely physically resist or overcome adults intent on using physical force against them.

Similarly, it is unrealistic to think that a child's simply saying "no" will deter some adults from abusing the child. It is also unreasonable to expect most children to successfully escape or run away from a potential perpetrator, especially if the abuse is occurring in the child's own home. The therapist must be cautious not to create unrealistic expectations regarding the child's ability to protect herself; this may create more conflict and guilt if the child comes to believe she should have been able to prevent the original abuse, or if she later experiences reabuse.

Group therapy.   Various forms of group therapy have been devised for specific use with sexually abused children. Examples of these include brief time-limited psychotherapy groups (Friedrich, Berliner, Urquiza, & Beilke, 1988), groups for children with inappropriate sexual behavior (Johnson & Berry, 1989), and parallel parent and child groups for preschoolers (Damon & Waterman, 1986). An excellent general guide to running such groups has been written by Mandell and Damon (1989). Generally, these groups address similar issues to those discussed previously, which are believed to be particularly relevant to sexually abused children.

Usually in time-limited groups, a certain issue or therapeutic activity is focused on in each session. Open-ended groups may continue for several months and address issues as they are introduced by group members. One advantage of the group format over individual or family therapy is that children have the opportunity to meet and interact with peers who have experienced similar abuse. This allows them to establish positive images of other sexually abused children, which ultimately may improve their own self-perceptions. Children frequently accept challenges about their misperceptions more readily from peers than from adults; this is helpful in correcting cognitive distortions.

Groups also offer concrete support in terms of preparation for trial, visitations with the perpetrator, and so on, since members who have already gone through these events can share their experiences with other members of the group and offer advice. Often group members will even accompany each other to their trials, providing additional support at this stressful time. An additional advantage of group therapy is its time efficiency for the therapist or agency with limited resources. As with other types of groups, sexual abuse groups should be divided according to age (or developmental level) and gender, with group members being matched on these parameters.*

It is our clinical impression that most sexually abused children find the sexual abuse group therapy experience to be very positive and helpful; the optimal timing of when to begin this part of therapy may vary, however. Many children need some individual therapy prior to beginning group bedcause they are too uncomfortable or too acutely symptomatic to discuss their abuse and feelings with a group of unfamiliar peers. Some other children appear able to enter group therapy immediately. The decision of whether and when to start group treatment should be discussed with the child and parents; most children are eventually eager for the opportunity to meet other children who have been sexually abused. In general, a child who is able to verbalize feelings about the abuse to a reasonable degree, who does not have severe symptoms of withdrawal or panic or depression, and who is agreeable to trying group therapy is appropriate for referral to group. More refined decisions may need to be made on a case-by-case basis.

Family therapy.   In many cases of child sexual abuse, the parents and other family members appear to be more symptomatic than the victim herself. Feelings of responsibility and guilt related to not adequately protecting the child or not

---

*Although some therapists have run mixed gender groups, the sexual abuse experience tends to arouse gender-related ambivalence and conflict, which may create additional issues in groups. Whether this is beneficial or detrimental is debatable; nevertheless, most sexual abuse groups are single gender. For more details on specific group protocols, the reader is referred to the references cited above, as well as Sgroi (1982).

detecting the abuse earlier are common reactions of parents. Many parents also experience intense anger toward the perpetrator for the abuse. These feelings need to be explored, cognitive distortions should be challenged, and family members must be supported throughout the course of therapy.

Some family members may feel less than supportive of the sexually abused victim (Sgroi, 1982). Siblings may resent or blame the victim, especially if the perpetrator is a family member and disclosure of the abuse has resulted in a disruption of the family structure (by removal of the perpetrator from the home, placement of the children outside the parental home, marital separation of the parents, etc.). Some parents are also ambivalent toward the abused child, especially when there are divided loyalties between the victim and the perpetrator. In these situations, parents may minimize the extent of the abuse or even refuse to believe that it occurred. Familial coercion to recant the allegations of the abuse, not to press charges, or not to testify against the perpetrator may occur. Needless to say, such interactions may have very negative effects on the abused child and on overall family functioning, and require ongoing family interventions. Treatment of the intrafamilial perpetrator is an important topic, but beyond the scope of this discussion. (Salter [1988] provides an excellent review of this topic for the interested reader.)

Nonsupportive family members must be confronted regarding their reasons for disbelieving the abuse, their attributions regarding the abuse (i.e., who was responsible), their minimization of its negative impact on the victim, and their own roles in potentially revictimizing the abused child by their negative attitudes and behaviors. Groups for nonoffending spouses of perpetrators are available in many treatment centers and have been helpful in effectively confronting these issues in many cases. In extreme situations where, in spite of these types of interventions, the nonabusive parent is unable or unwilling to protect the child from further abuse, or where the negative familial attitudes are destructive to the victim's recovery, removal of the abused child from the home may be indicated. Unfortunately, this could be experienced as yet another negative event by the child, who

may feel that disclosing the abuse had worse results than the abuse itself. Such a child may truthfully say "I wish I had never told anyone" and, indeed, may be unlikely to report future abuse if it should occur. Fortunately, most families respond to some degree to family interventions, and the above scenario is not the typical outcome for most sexually abused children.

Selecting Optimal Treatment Strategies

Given the current lack of empirical support for any particular treatment modality for sexually abused children, most treatment decisions are based on presenting symptomatology and a clinical assessment of the most salient therapeutic issues in a given case. Many of the possible indicators for the various treatment strategies have been addressed in the previous sections. For example, children with significant behavioral problems should have some type of behavioral interventions as part of their treatment; children with cognitive distortions will probably benefit from cognitive therapy; children with nonsupportive or symptomatic family members will most likely need family interventions for optimal recovery; and so on.

Most sexually abused children will receive a combination of the various treatment strategies described. The exact sequence and timing of when to introduce which modality is at this time best determined by the problems that seem most significant at any given point, by relevant external considerations (such as an upcoming trial or custody battle), and ultimately by the therapist's clinical judgment and experience. Hopefully, empirical treatment outcome studies will better clarify optimal treatment strategies for individually sexually abused children in the near future.

Problems in Carrying Out Interventions

There are numerous potential problems in carrying out optimal treatment for sexually abused children; only a few can be discussed here. Briefly, three of the most daunting problems are the lack of familial cooperation with and support for therapy, the vagaries of the legal system, and the paucity of effective treatment facilities for the perpetrators of child sexual abuse. Some of the familial problems have been addressed in the section on family therapy. In addition to those issues, families can undermine treatment by missing appointments, giving the child subtle or overt negative messages about therapy ("it costs so much to see your therapist," "you don't need any more treatment," "that doctor wants to tear our family apart," etc.), or by simply withdrawing the child from treatment. At times the legal and CPS systems can provide leverage for keeping the child in treatment, but if the family remains opposed, it may be very difficult to effectively treat the child (who will often feel she is "betraying" her family by engaging in the therapeutic process).

The legal and CPS systems, although designed to protect the victimized child, also must protect the rights of the alleged perpetrator and family members. At times these interests collide, and the child is further traumatized (often referred to as *revictimization*), either by a destructive legal proceeding (such as a trial where the child is harassed, embarrassed, accused of lying, questioned about the irrelevant sexual activities, etc.) or by inappropriate placement (in a foster home where sexual abuse recurs, in a nonprotective home environment, or away from an appropriate home situation). Forming ongoing relationships with child protective service workers, district attorneys, and the specialized police units that investigate these cases can be helpful in minimizing these problems. However, even when these agencies work in total cooperation, detrimental outcomes do occur. Therapeutic interventions, no matter how effective, cannot be expected to fully counteract an ongoing destructive living situation.

Sexual abuse perpetrators most likely require a very specific, confrontive type of treatment to effectively change their behavior and to accept appropriate responsibility for the abuse (Pithers, Marques, Gibat, & Marlatt, 1983; Salter, 1988). Unfortunately, few communities have this type of treatment program readily available. Even where such programs exist, the vast majority of perpetrators are not compelled (either by court order or their own motivation) to enter and complete such treatment. Most perpetrators receive no treatment focused on their abusive behavior, do not accept responsibility for the abuse, and thus may prolong the child victim's struggle to accurately perceive the abuse. In situations where the perpetrator is not punished by the legal system and does not receive appropriate treatment, ongoing victim anxiety and confusion may be more difficult to change through therapy.

Most children who do not appear to respond positively to therapeutic interventions (admittedly this remains a subjective assessment at the present time) have had to cope with at least one of these problems. How to more effectively address these difficulties is an ongoing challenge for therapists who work with sexually abused children.

Relapse Prevention

Relapse prevention in this population refers to the prevention of future abuse. This would appear to be more dependent on perpetrator therapy and familial interventions regarding appropriate supervision than on any therapeutic interventions one could offer the child sexual abuse victim. However, there are some issues which, if effectively addressed with the victim, may decrease the likelihood of future sexual abuse.

First, although there are no empirical data to prove the following hypothesis, it would appear likely that children who exhibit sexually inappropriate behavior might be at higher risk for reabuse. Thus, effectively treating and eliminating such behaviors would seem to be one important aspect of relapse prevention. Second, although the limitations of safety education and assertiveness training have previously been addressed, these skills may have some significant impact at preventing future sexual abuse of the child, or at least in aiding in earlier disclosure if such reabuse should occur. Third, an accurate cognitive grasp of what constitutes inappropriate touching may prevent some children from experiencing another abusive episode. Finally, appropriate legal and CPS actions are essential in protecting sexually abused children from reabuse. More research is needed in all of these areas to determine the most effective treatment methods for optimal recovery from and prevention of future episodes of child sexual abuse.

CASE ILLUSTRATION

Case Description

Gabriella was a 10-year-old caucasian fifth-grade student who was referred for evaluation and treatment by her caseworker at Child Protective Services. Gabriella had recently disclosed to a friend that she was being sexually abused by her mother's boyfriend. This friend told his mother, who called the state child abuse reporting hot line. The case was then referred to the local CPS office.

At the time of evaluation, Gabriella was living with her 35-year-old mother, Carol, and her 14-year-old brother, Evan. Carol was employed full time as a nurse's aide. Gabriella's natural father had separated from Carol when Gabriella was an infant, and had had no contact with the family for several years. Carol's paramour, Thomas, had been living with the family for four years until his arrest two weeks prior to the evaluation. Thomas was currently in jail awaiting trial for the alleged sexual abuse.

Carol was interviewed individually to provide a developmental history as well as information regarding Gabriella's recent behavior. Carol reported that Gabriella's development was entirely normal, but that she had had problems such as lying, fighting with peers, stealing from mother, and being noncompliant with rules at home. Carol said that these problems had been going on for at least three years. Carol denied that Gabriella had ever experienced difficulty with sleep, appetite, energy level, sadness, paying attention in school, or self-destructive behaviors. She also denied that Gabriella was fearful, withdrawn, or avoidant of particular situations. Gabriella had always gotten along with her brother Evan, and had many friends at school and in the neighborhood. She was a B student and had no behavioral problems in school. Gabriella had never had any medical problems to Carol's knowledge.

Carol described Gabriella's natural father as violent; he had at times gotten into physical fights with Carol but had never been abusive to either of the children. He and Carol had been separated for 10 years and divorced for 8 years. Approximately 4 years prior to the evaluation, Carol met Thomas through mutual friends. They were romantically involved for two months prior to his moving in with the family. Carol reported that both children resented Thomas, and that they challenged his authority to tell them what to do. Carol said that she made it clear to the children that "Thomas could discipline them however he wanted to," and once he started to do so, their compliance improved. Carol was vague about whether Thomas ever used physical punishments with Gabriella. Thomas was often at home alone with Gabriella during the day, as Evan was involved in after-school activities and Carol was working full-time.

Carol reported that Gabriella and a girlfriend of hers had come to her the previous year, complaining that Thomas had "told them to pull down their pants." Carol confronted the girls with Thomas present; at that point, Gabriella's friend said she did not remember what had happened, but did not think Thomas had done anything wrong to the girls. Although Gabriella maintained her story, nothing more came of the incident at that time.

When asked whether she believed the present allegations of abuse, Carol said, "I don't know, I'm on the fence about that because Gabriella has lied about other things in the past." She was evasive when questioned about her present feelings toward Thomas, saying only, "He doesn't belong in jail."

Gabriella was also interviewed individually. She appeared very sad during the interview, with frequent tearfulness and downcast facial expressions. Gabriella admitted to occasionally taking money or clothes from her mother without asking, and was not sure whether this qualified as "stealing." Gabriella said she felt she was "ugly" and that other kids would not like her if they knew what Thomas had done to her. She said she felt "dirty" and "smelly" and that she frequently bathed to get rid of this feeling, but without success. Gabriella also described fearfulness at bedtime, with frequent difficulty falling asleep and frightening nightmares of Thomas chasing after her. She had not reported any of these symptoms to her mother. She denied suicidal thoughts or actions.

Gabriella described the first episode of sexual abuse as follows: One day when she was about 8 years old, she and Thomas were alone at home and Thomas told her to go into her mother's bedroom. He followed her into the room, locked the door, and then told her to take off her clothes. She said she was scared because Thomas had beaten her with belt and a whip in the past when she hadn't listened to him. She took off her clothes, and he put her on her mother's bed. He then inserted his middle finger into her vagina. Thomas told Gabriella not to tell, or he would punch her in the mouth.

Thomas did not approach Gabriella sexually for several months after that incident. When she was just past her ninth birthday, he again took her into mother's bedroom and told her to remove her clothes. This time he put his penis into her vagina and "jumped up and down on me and pulled it in and out of me." She saw liquid come out of his penis she described as being "white like snow." From that day on, Thomas did this to her almost every day her mother was at work. Thomas would frequently threaten to beat her up if she ever told anyone. Thomas also had anal intercourse with Gabriella on two occasions (both within the last four months).

The disclosure occurred when Gabriella told a male friend (aged 11 years) what Thomas had been doing to her. This friend told his mother, who reported the abuse to a hot line. CPS investigated and took Gabriella to the local University Children's Hospital the next day. Gabriella said that Thomas had had intercourse with her on the day of this examination. This was supported by the medical evidence from that examination, which found significant hymenal tearing and scars, as well as vaginal seminal fluid.

Gabriella stated that she was very mad at Thomas and that she wanted him to stay in jail. She wanted to testify against him at his trial and said she would "tell the cops" if anyone tried to stop her from doing this. She felt that the abuse

was Thomas's fault, but she wondered whether it happened partly because she was tall for her age and had experienced early menarche (at 9 years old). She thought that these things might have "made me look like I was sexy and like I wanted it." She said that Thomas often said these things while he was abusing her. Gabriella wanted to remain with her mother and wanted Thomas to stay in jail. Gabriella claimed that her mother did believe her with regard to the sexual abuse, but she became tearful when she said this and then admitted that she was not sure what Carol believed. Her one wish was "that Thomas would go away and never come back, and me and mom can stay together forever."

Differential Diagnosis and Assessment

The assessment included the above interviews, an interview with the CPS worker, and review of the medical records from Children's Hospital. In addition, Gabriella's teacher and Carol completed the teacher and parent forms, respectively, of the Child Behavior Checklist (CBCL) (Achenbach & Edelbrock, 1979). Gabriella also completed the Children's Depression Inventory (CDI) (Kovacs, 1983) because she had many symptoms suggestive of a major depressive episode.

There was a marked discrepancy between Carol's report of Gabriella's symptomatology and Gabriella's own reports. Carol's CBCL ratings showed elevation on the Externalizing, Delinquent, and Aggressive scales. Gabriella's teacher's CBCL ratings showed no elevations on these scales, but did demonstrate elevated scores on the Depression and Social Withdrawal subscales. Gabriella's score on the CDI was 22, indicative of clinically significant depression. The preponderance of evidence at the time of evaluation indicated that Gabriella had a diagnosis of Major Depressive Disorder (single episode). Although the teacher did not report conduct symptoms, Carol's information indicated that these were present. A rule-out diagnosis of conduct disorder, solitary aggressive type was made as well. DSM-III-R Axis III diagnosis was genital trauma secondary to sexual abuse (based on the medical report).

Assessment of the "abuse-related" issues indicated that Carol was neither fully believing nor supporting Gabriella with regard to her allegations. Carol seemed more focused on Gabriella's "always lying about things" than on Gabriella's obvious emotional distress or the medical evidence of sexual abuse. The evaluator's impression was that Carol at best was ambivalent in her loyalties, and at worst was actively undermining Gabriella's efforts to stop the abuse. It was also concluded that some of Gabriella's depressive symptoms could be in response to her perception that her mother did not really believe or fully support her. Gabriella's cognitions about the abuse experience were somewhat distorted in that she had accepted some of Thomas's inappropriate attributions for why it occurred. She also had negative self-perceptions and she was not accurately describing her mother's lack of support for her. Gabriella's immediate safety from ongoing sexual abuse by Thomas was not a concern, as he was being held in jail until the trial.

Treatment Selection

The most critical issues to address in this case appeared to be Gabriella's significant depressive symptoms and Carol's lack of support for Gabriella. It seemed that Gabriella's depression was in part due to her feeling different and isolated from her peers related to the abuse (feeling she would be socially ostracized if anyone found out), to her inaccurate attributions regarding the abuse, and to her apparent poor self-esteem (feeling "ugly," "dirty," and "smelly"). The decision was made to begin individual therapy with both Gabriella and her mother, and for Gabriella to begin group therapy as soon as a new group became available (in approximately one month). If she did not show symptomatic improvement within three to six weeks or if her depressive symptoms became worse, antidepressant medication would be started as well. The CPS worker was supportive of this plan, although she privately expressed to the evaluator great concern as to whether Carol could become adequately supportive of Gabriella.

Treatment Course and Problems in Carrying Out Interventions

Weekly individual therapy was begun for Gabriella and for Carol. In the first two weeks, Carol appeared somewhat open to the therapist's suggestions that Gabriella was telling the truth, and that Carol's difficulty in believing the abuse was related to her feelings toward Thomas. She agreed to stop interrogating Gabriella about "what *really* happened with Thomas," and she apparently did this for the first two weeks of treatment. Gabriella responded quickly to the therapist's support as well as to cognitive therapy directed at her partial self-blame for the abuse. She was able to openly express her confusion and pain that Carol "believes Thomas instead of me." During this time, Gabriella reported feeling less sad, sleeping better, and being more hopeful that things would be okay.

A crisis arose during the third week of treatment. Carol called the therapist and angrily stated, "Now I know that kid is lying." Carol had asked Gabriella to "go downtown" with her; she then took Gabriella to the county jail and insisted that Gabriella accompany her during her visit to Thomas (Carol had apparently been visiting him regularly in jail, although she had denied having any contact with him when asked about this during the first two therapy sessions). Carol then told Gabriella to "once and for all, tell Thomas to his face what you accused him of." Gabriella started to cry, and Carol took this to mean she had "made up the whole thing." Thomas said to Gabriella, "Wait 'til I get out of here," and Carol then took Gabriella home and sent her to her room. Carol was urged to come to see the therapist that same day, but she refused, saying she did not "need any more help with this."

The next day, Gabriella ran away to a friend's house. Carol called the therapist to report this, saying, "I don't care if she comes home or not; if she's going to be telling those lies, she can leave for all I care." The therapist called the CPS worker, who had Gabriella placed in an emergency shelter. When Gabriella was brought to see her therapist the following day, she was tearful during the whole session, saying, "Why does she love him more than me?" She wanted to return home to her mother, even though she recognized that Carol still did not believe the abuse occurred. She said, "I love my mother, even though she's mad at me new," and became very upset when it was suggested that returning home may not be the best decision. CPS determined that Gabriella should remain in shelter placement at this time.

Carol refused to return to therapy but told the CPS worker that Gabriella could come back home "whenever she's ready to tell the truth" (i.e., recant her allegations against Thomas). She also refused to let Gabriella have contact with her brother Evan. Gabriella continued to come to therapy weekly. Soon after she was placed in shelter, she began stealing from other children. The objects she stole were either of little material value (chewing gum or writing paper) or of no practical use to herself (another child's orthodontic retainer). When Gabriella was confronted by the shelter staff, she quickly confessed to stealing these objects. In therapy, Gabriella admitted that she had stolen with the hope that "they would kick me out and send me back home." It also appeared to serve an attention-getting purpose for Gabriella. She discussed alternative ways of getting attention from shelter staff, was rewarded by them for appropriate behaviors, and the stealing episodes soon stopped.

Gabriella's depressive symptoms also decreased somewhat following her placement in shelter. (Up to this point, antidepressant medication had been an active consideration. Had her symptoms not improved, this would probably have been started.) Although her sadness continued, her anxiety symptoms and sleeping improved markedly. In therapy she discussed her painful feelings about her mother not believing her, and focused on identifying positive qualities about herself, in an attempt to alter some of her negative distortions about herself. By this time, her attribution regarding the abuse had changed; she said that Thomas abused her "because he wanted to; he was old and ugly and mean, and I never did anything to 'ask for it' like he said."

The real turning point for Gabriella occurred once she began group therapy. She entered a time-limited (16 weeks) group with five other girls aged 10 to 12 years, all of whom had experienced sexual abuse. The protocol generally followed that described by Mandell and Damon (1989), with different sessions focusing on specific issues such as getting to know the other group members, identification and expression of feelings, telling the group members about the abuse, exploring cognitive distortions, dealing with familial issues, assertiveness and safety issues, appropriate and inappropriate types of intimacy, sexuality education, going to court, and closure issues.

Gabriella formed a strong attachment to two of the other girls in her group and responded very positively to their praise. (In one exercise, each group member was asked to write down words to describe another member; Gabriella was described as "pretty," "sweet," and "smart." In her next individual sessions, Gabriella said that for the first time she no longer felt ugly and dirty.) It was the group experience that helped her come to terms with her mother's behavior and to perceive her situation clearly.

During the sessions focusing on family reactions, Gabriella heard her friends describe supportive reactions by family members, and in the middle of one of these discussions, Gabriella started crying. The other group members initially did not understand her reaction (as Gabriella had been silent about her own mother's behavior), but they nonetheless gathered around her, asking what was wrong. Gabriella then described what her mother had done. The other girls reacted with shock and anger, calling Carol "evil" and "a witch." Gabriella initially came to her mother's defense, but the other group members challenged every excuse Gabriella came up with for Carol's actions. They continued to do this throughout the next few sessions as well, until Gabriella told the therapist in an individual session, "I still don't understand how my mother can do this to me, but she's wrong, not me. I know I'm telling the truth. . . . In fact, I tried to tell her the truth last year, and she wouldn't listen then either, so it's partly her fault I kept getting abused."

From this point on, Gabriella became less invested in reestablishing her relationship with Carol, and asked to be considered for a more permanent placement in a group home or foster home. This was done the following month. She continued to experience sadness at times in relation to her mother, and particularly with regard to Evan (who had believed her regarding the abuse but whom Carol prevented from having contact with Gabriella). Her other depressive symptoms did not recur, and she adjusted well to her foster home.

As part of the group process, a mock trial was performed by the group members. Gabriella played the role of the district attorney, and was very effective in assertively challenging the "perpetrator." By the time Thomas's trial occurred (seven months after beginning therapy), Gabriella was well integrated into her foster home, doing well in her new school, and was essentially symptom free. She continued to come to biweekly individual therapy after her group ended. Carol asked to have visits with Gabriella approximately two weeks prior to the scheduled trial. Gabriella agreed to this, and confided to her therapist that she still hoped that her mother "might change" and begin to support her. However, she was prepared for this to not be the case.

When Carol saw Gabriella (at insistence of the CPS worker, this visit occurred with her supervision), Carol brought her a new sweater as a gift and said how much she had missed Gabriella. Carol then asked if Gabriella wanted to come back and live "as a family," and Gabriella said, "Yes — with you and Evan." Carol then told Gabriella that if she did not testify against Thomas, Carol would make sure that Thomas would "leave you alone from now on." At that point, the CPS worker intervened, telling Carol not to discuss the trial if she could not be supportive of Gabriella. By the end of this meeting, Gabriella was tearful, telling Carol she loved her but she had to testify. Carol's last comment to Gabriella was, "It's not too late, you can change your mind any time."

For the next two weeks, Gabriella was very upset, alternating between wishing she had not visited with her mother and wishing she could return home. She did not waver about her decision to testify, however. At the trial, Carol insisted on sitting next to Gabriella, saying, "I'm her mother. My place is with her." Three of the girls from Gabriella's therapy group, as well as the

therapist and the CPS worker, were sitting on the other side of Gabriella. Several of them heard Carol whispering into Gabriella's ear, "Don't do it, baby, don't go through with it." Despite this, Gabriella gave testimony against Thomas, who was convicted of rape and involuntary deviate sexual intercourse and sentenced to several years in prison. After Gabriella's testimony, Carol refused to talk to her, but Gabriella received much support from her fellow group members. She was relieved to be finished with the trial and very glad that Thomas was sent to prison.

Outcome and Termination

Following the trial, Gabriella had five more individual sessions for posttrial evaluation and termination. Gabriella was resigned to her mother's "betrayal" of her (which was how she described Carol's behavior) and continued to do well in her foster home. When asked whether she had any regrets about disclosing the abuse or testifying against Thomas, she said, "I should have done it sooner." She was able to say that she was legitimately frightened by his threats and that it took a lot of courage on her own part to disclose at all. When asked whether being sexually abused had changed her, she said, "It made me stronger, even though it was bad." She still felt sadness related to her mother, but she also felt appropriate anger toward Carol, and believed that she was better off in her foster home than she had been with her own mother. Gabriella continued to be asymptomatic nine months after the initial evaluation, and termination occurred as agreed upon by her and the therapist.

Followup and Maintenance

Two years later, Gabriella continues to live in her original foster home. She is now 13 years old and doing well in all respects. She has had no further contact with her mother; she has requested visits with her brother (now 17 years old), which Carol has refused. Gabriella hopes that once Evan turns 18 years old, he will contact her and they can reestablish a relationship. She has had no depressive symptoms, although she feels passing sadness on holidays such as Mother's Day and her mother's birthday. Thomas remains in prison. Gabriella does not think about when he will be released but says, "He can't hurt me any more."

SUMMARY

Child sexual abuse encompasses a number of diverse experiences, and there is a great deal of variability in the behavioral, emotional, and social consequences of such experiences. A variety of psychological difficulties may be associated with sexual abuse, but there is no syndrome or group of symptoms that is "characteristic" of children who have been sexually abused. Sexually abused children may also have behavioral or emotional problems that preceded the abuse or are not directly related to the abuse experience. Clinicians working with sexually abused children must be aware of the multiple systems typically involved in such situations. These may include law enforcement agencies, child protective services, and medical care providers. Clinicians must also be sensitive to issues particularly relevant to the abusive experience such as feeling different from other children, loss of trust, inappropriate self-blame, and the impact of legal and child protective services actions on the child and her family.

To date there have been no adequately controlled empirical treatment outcome studies for sexually abused children, although a few such studies are currently under way. Behavior therapy, pharmacotherapy, cognitive therapy, safety education, assertiveness training, specialized group therapy, and family therapy are interventions that are frequently used in treating this population. Despite appropriate treatment, problems such as a lack of familial cooperation with treatment, unsatisfactory legal outcomes, or the lack of effective treatment available to sexual abuse perpetrators may undermine the effectiveness of therapy. It is important for clinicians working with sexually abused children to clearly define their role in these cases and to recognize the limitations of therapy in some situations. More research is needed to adequately demonstrate the efficacy of various intervention models in treating children who have experienced sexual abuse.

REFERENCES

Achenbach, T. M., & Edelbrock, C. S. (1979). The child behavior profile: II. Boys aged 12–16 and girls aged 6–11 and 12–16. *Journal of Consulting and Clinical Psychology, 47,* 223–233.

Berliner, L., & Wheeler, J. R. (1988). Treating the effects of sexual abuse on children. *Journal of Interpersonal Violence, 2*(4), 415–434.

Briere, J. (1990). *Research colloquium: Synopsis and bold debate.* Presented at the 1990 National Symposium on Child Victimization, Atlanta, GA.

Burt, M. R. (1980). Cultural myths and supports for rape. *Journal of Personality and Social Psychology, 38*(2), 217–230.

Cohen, J. A., & Mannarino, A. P. (1990a). *Psychiatric diagnoses in a child and adolescent sexual abuse clinic.* Unpublished manuscript, University of Pittsburgh, Pittsburgh, PA.

Cohen, J. A., & Mannarino, A. P. (1990b). *Measuring the unique problems manifested by sexually abused children: A new instrument.* Presented at the 1990 National Symposium on Child Victimization, Atlanta, GA.

Damon, L., & Waterman, J. (1986). Parallel group treatment of children and their mothers. In K. MacFarlane & J. Waterman (Eds.), *Sexual abuse of young children: Evaluation and treatment.* New York: Guilford.

Deblinger, E., McLeer, S. V., & Henry, D. (1990). Cognitive behavioral treatment for sexually abused children suffering post-traumatic stress: Preliminary findings. *Journal of the American Academy of Child and Adolescent Psychiatry, 29*(5), 747–752.

Einbender, A., & Friedrich, W. (1989). The psychological functioning and behavior of sexually abused girls. *Journal of Consulting and Clinical Psychology, 57,* 155–157.

Emery, R. E. (1989). Family violence. *American Psychologist, 44,* 321–328.

Finkelhor, D. (1979). *Sexually victimized children.* New York: Free Press.

Finkelhor, D. (1984). *Child sexual abuse: New theory and research* (pp. 24–32). New York: Free Press.

Finkelhor, D. (1987). The trauma of child sexual abuse: Two models. *Journal of Interpersonal Violence, 2*(4), 348–366.

Finkelhor, D., & Barron, L. (1986). Risk factors for

sexual abuse. *Journal of Interpersonal Violence, 1*(1), 43–71.

Finkelhor, D., & Browne, A. (1985). The traumatic impact of child sexual abuse: A conceptualization. *American Journal of Orthopsychiatry, 55*(4), 530–541.

Friedrich, W. N., Beilke, R. L., & Urquiza, A. J. (1987). Children from sexually abusive families: A behavioral comparison. *Journal of Interpersonal Violence, 2*(4), 391–402.

Friedrich, W. N., Berliner, L., Urquiza, A. J., & Beilke, R. L. (1988). Brief diagnostic group treatment of sexually abused boys. *Journal of Interpersonal Violence, 3*(3), 331–343.

Gomes-Schwartz, B., Horowitz, J. M., & Sauzier, M. (1985). Severity of emotional distress among sexually abused preschool, school-aged, and adolescent children. *Hospital and Community Psychiatry, 36,* 503–508.

Green, A. (1986). True and false allegations of sexual abuse in child custody disputes. *Journal of the American Academy of Child Psychiatry, 25*(4), 449–456.

Hindman, J. (1987). *Step by step: Sixteen steps toward legally sound sexual abuse investigations.* Ontario, OR: Alexandria Associates.

Janoff-Bulman, R. (1986). The aftermath of victimization: Rebuilding shattered assumptions. In C. Figley (Ed.), *Trauma and its wake: Study and treatment of post-traumatic stress disorder.* New York: Brunner-Mazel.

Johnson, T. C., & Berry, C. (1989). Children who molest: A treatment program. *Journal of Interpersonal Violence, 4*(2), 185–203.

Kovacs, M. (1983). *The Children's Depression Inventory: A self-rated depression scale for school-aged youngsters.* Unpublished manuscript, University of Pittsburgh, Pittsburgh, PA.

MacFarlane, K., & Cunningham, C. (1988). *Steps to healthy touching: A treatment workbook for kids 5–12 who have problems with sexually inappropriate behavior.* Mount Dora, FL: Kidsrights.

Mandel, J. G., & Damon, L. (1989). *Group treatment for sexually abused children.* New York: Guilford.

Mannarino, A. P., Cohen, J. A., & Gregor, M. (1989). Emotional and behavioral difficulties in sexually abused girls. *Journal of Interpersonal Violence, 4*(4), 437–451.

Mannarino, A. P., Cohen, J. A., Smith, J. A., &

Moore-Motily, S. (1990). *Six and twelve month follow-up of sexually abused girls.* Unpublished manuscript in submission, University of Pittsburgh, Pittsburgh, PA.

Muran, D. (1989). Child sexual abuse: Relationship between sexual acts and genital findings. *Child Abuse and Neglect, 13,* 211–216.

National Children's Advocacy Center. (1987). *Proceedings from the National Symposium on Assessing the Impact of Child Sexual Abuse: State of the art and future directions.* Huntsville, AL.

O'Toole, R., Turbett, P., & Nalepka, C. (1983). Theories, professional knowledge, and diagnosis of child abuse. In D. Finkelhor, R. J. Gelles, G. T. Hotaling, & M. A. Strauss (Eds.), *The dark side of families.* Beverly Hills: Sage.

Pithers, W. D., Marques, J. K., Gibat, C. C., & Marlatt, A. (1983). Relapse prevention with sexual aggressives. A self-control model of treatment and maintenance of change. In J. Greer & I. Stuart (Eds.), *The sexual aggressor: Current perspectives on treatment.* New York: Van Nostrand Reinhold.

Runyan, D. K., Everson, M. D., Edelsohn, G. A., Hunter, W. M., & Coulter, M. L. (1988). Impact of legal intervention on sexually abused children. *The Journal of Pediatrics, 113*(4), 647–653.

Russell, D. (1983). *Intrafamilial child sexual abuse: A San Francisco survey.* Final report to the National Center on Child Abuse and Neglect.

Russell, D. E. H. (1983). The incidence and prevalence of intrafamilial and extrafamilial sexual abuse of female children. *Child Abuse and Neglect, 7,* 133–146.

Salter, A. C. (1988). *Treating child sex offenders and victims: A practical guide.* Newbury Park, CA: Sage.

Sgroi, S. (1982). *Handbook of clinical interventions in child sexual abuse.* Lexington, MA: Lexington Books.

Sirles, E. A., Smith, J. A., & Kusama, H. (1989). Psychiatric status of intrafamilial child sexual abuse victims. *Journal of Child and Adolescent Psychiatry, 28*(2), 225–229.

Strauss, M. A., Gelles, R., & Steinmetz, S. (1980). *Behind closed doors: Violence in the American family.* New York: Doubleday.

White, S., Halpin, B. M., Strom, G. A., & Santilli, G. (1988). Behavioral comparisons of young sexually abused, neglected, and nonreferred children. *Journal of Clinical Child Psychology, 17,* 53–61.

CHAPTER 22

PHYSICAL ABUSE AND NEGLECT

Sandra T. Azar   Clark University

Renée Pearlmutter   Clark University

DESCRIPTION OF PROBLEM

Core Features

Consensus regarding the behaviors that constitute child abuse and neglect does not exist. Until recently, attempts at definition were guided by a goal of case identification and prosecution, not treatment planning. Consequently, *physical abuse* has sometimes been described in terms of the *intent* of the parent (e.g., intentional use of force aimed at injuring or destroying a child) and at other times in terms of the *effect* a parental action has on the child (e.g., bruises that last more than 48 hours).* Similarly, *neglect* has been defined in terms of the *omission* of actions that lead to harm or endangerment of children's health or well-being. While such concrete definitions have utility in systems where black and white delineations are required for action (e.g., courts), children sustaining a bruise or not being adequately fed may result from a variety of causal factors and lead to multiple psychological outcomes. Such definitions, therefore, do not provide a useful framework for treatment planning.

Recently, a new view has emerged that places such parental responses at one end of a continuum of other parenting behaviors that result in poor child outcome (Azar, 1986; Azar & Wolfe, 1989; Cicchetti & Rizley, 1981). At the other end are modes of responding that promote children's development and welfare. Such a framework leads more directly to treatment choices. For example, Wolfe (1987) defined *abuse* and *neglect* as the degree to which a parent uses aversive or inappropriate control strategies with his or her child (e.g., beatings, consistent use of coercive responses) or fails to provide minimal standards of care giving and nurturing in the areas of

---

*Other dimensions are also present, including definitions that differ along a narrow to broad continuum (e.g., "demonstrable harm" versus "endangerment") and a continuum of actions (e.g., "threw something" to "used a gun or knife"; Straus & Gelles, 1986). It also has been noted that what we consider abusive is "socially mediated," (i.e., dependent on what a given community or society determines is unacceptable behavior toward a child).

medical care, education, nutrition, supervision, emotional contact, and safety, as well as providing little in the way of environmental stimulation and structure.

Azar (1986; 1989) further emphasized the lack of positive care-giving responses in such families as crucial in defining the disorder (e.g., lack of developmentally sensitive care giving, positive affect) and cognitive disturbances that may underlie both types of responses (e.g., disturbed information processing) Maladaptive parenting, of which abuse and neglect are exemplars, therefore occurs when parents cease to function as facilitators of children's physical, social, and cognitive development (i.e., fail as socialization agents).* This view argues for a developmental focus in defining core treatment targets (Azar & Siegel, 1990). Some of these targets will be period specific (e.g., inability to deal with crying infants) and others may apply across different developmental periods (e.g., inaccurate identification of children's capabilities.

Associated Features

No one set of factors distinguish maltreating parents (Wolfe, 1987). A number of cognitive and behavioral characteristics, however, are worthy of consideration. Family interaction patterns for both types of maltreatment appear to be marked by low levels of parent-initiated stimulation, with neglectful parents providing the lowest rates (Bousha & Twentyman, 1984). Positive interaction rates also appear to be depressed, and negative transactions occur at high levels. While the former may be distinctive, the latter apparently does not distinguish maltreaters from their nonabusive spouses nor parents drawn from child clinics (Loeber, Felton, & Reid, 1984; Reid, 1985). Empirically based typologies of interaction patterns are beginning to appear that ultimately may define

groups with different treatment needs and trajectories (Oldershaw, Walters, & Hall, 1989)

Parental skill deficits have also been implicated, including poor parenting skills (e.g., a narrow and negative repertoire of solutions to child-rearing problems); poor impulse control; lack of social skills; stress management problems; and cognitive disturbances that lead to faulty information processing in parenting situations (Azar & Twentyman, 1986). The last of these may underlie the other four. Maltreating parents appear to have unrealistic expectations about what is appropriate to expect from children. When the child consistently violates these standards, a negative attributional bias toward him or her may evolve (e.g., blaming the child for what may be developmentally appropriate behavior). Ultimately, this sequence of events may lead to lowered parental self-efficacy and inappropriate parenting responses (e.g., avoidance of child needs; aversive reactions).

Other psychological problems may be present, including substance abuse, psychoses, personality disorders, and mental retardation. The last may be most common among neglectful parents. These problems, however, do not account for large numbers of maltreaters.

Data regarding abused and neglected children are limited (Ammerman, Cassisi, Hersen, & VanHasselt, 1986; Azar, Barnes, & Twentyman, 1988; Conaway & Hansen, 1989), especially on the consequences of maltreatment during specific developmental eras (e.g., adolescence; Azar & Siegel, 1990). The paucity of data on neglect is particularly noteworthy, given it effects more children. Children raised in neglectful environments may in some ways be exposed to greater risk than those experiencing abuse alone. Lack of supervision, for example, endangers them by exposure to fires, falls, poisons, and unsuitable peers, as well as a whole host of health and educational problems (Cantwell, 1980).

As with their parents, abused and neglected children do not exhibit a single distinct clinical picture. Four major areas should concern the clinician. First, physicl problems have been noted. These children appear to suffer disproportionately from central nervous system damage — showing

---

*Although this view has utility, it should be noted that some theorists continue to view both abuse and neglect as distinct entities and not on a continuum with normal parenting, and they might argue for different treatment considerations.

everything from verbal deficits to mental retardation. Second, cognitive delays and deficits appear to be common, as do language and academic problems. And last, externalized and internalized behavioral symptoms also appear to be common, including heightened aggressive behavior, impulsivity, conduct problems, including heightened aggressive behavior, impulsivity, conduct problems, and noncompliance, as well as depression, low self-esteem, and self-destructive behavior. Interpersonal skill deficits are also beginning to be documented (e.g., deficits in affective recognition skills). Finally, these children are overrepresented in handicapped, special education, and institutionalized samples.

It is unclear whether these symptoms predate maltretment or are a consequence of it. Given that similar problems have been found in the siblings of abused children (Salzinger, Kaplan, Pelcovitz, Samit, & Krieger, 1984), they may be more indicative of the generally poor socialization environment in such families (Azar et al., 1988). Attempts to protect children may also account for symptoms found (e.g., the impact of foster care placements).

Epidemiology

Child maltreatment is a private event and as such it presents problems in discussing prevalence and incidence. Consequently, figures vary depending on definitions chosen and who is making the judgment. Physical abuse figures vary from 4.9 to 19.0 per 1,000 children, depending on whether reports are by professionals (Burgdorf, 1988) or represent results from surveys of the general population (Straus & Gelles, 1986). For neglect, population survey data are not available, but professional reports indicate that 7.9 per 1,000 children are affected.

Both forms of maltreatment vary with family size and income levels, but not by race and ethnicity. Children in families with incomes under $15,000 experience more abuse and neglect than those in homes with incomes over this figure (54.0 versus 7.9 per 1,000; Burgforf, 1988). Families with over four children appear to exhibit more maltreatment than do smaller ones. Rates also appear to increase with age, with some studies showing peaks during specific periods (e.g., age 4 and in adolescence; Wauchope & Straus [1987]). Overall, gender does not appear to be a factor, but boys tend to be victims more frequently during younger years and girls in older ages.

Once maltreatment is identified, recidivism appears to be high (e.g., between 20 and 70 percent; Williams, 1983). Since estimates are based on samples receiving some form of treatment, actual rates may be much higher. Even if abuse does not recur, excessive punishment and emotional abuse may continue. Neglectful behavior may also persist, except in cases where specific stressors or episodic drug abuse are precipitants.

Reported case figures indicate increases in abuse and neglect over the last decade, whereas a population survey reports a decline. The former may represent an increase in reporting due to mandatory reporting laws, whereas the latter may be due to greater public awareness.

DIAGNOSIS AND ASSESSMENT

Diagnostic Issues

As noted earlier, abusive and neglectful parents have not been shown to come from any one diagnostic group. When they do receive a diagnosis, a number of DSM-III-R categories may be applied. By most estimates, only a small percentage (5 to 10 percent) warrants a diagnosis involving psychotic symptoms or severe pathology. More often, those who do receive diagnoses are personality disordered or developmentally disabled. The latter may be more common in neglectful parents. Another problems that has received attention recently is substance abuse. Only small percentages of incidents of maltreatment, however, have been associated with alcohol use. Less information is available on drug use (e.g., cocaine and its derivatives). While psychiatric diagnoses may account for only a small minority of maltreaters, careful screening should still be carved out to identify those who require treatment for such disturbances.

As with adults, no consistent diagnostic picture

characterizes maltreated children. The clearest evidence for diagnostic categorization comes from work with adolescents, but this work must be viewed with caution in that most of the samples studied are drawn from troubled youth (e.g., delinquents). Higher levels of antisocial behavior appear within maltreated samples, and violent delinquents are distinguished from nonviolent ones based on their experience of physical abuse (Deykin, Alpert, & McNamarra, 1985; Livingston, 1987). Depression also may be found (Kazdin, Moser, Colbus, & Bell, 1985).

Assessment Strategies

Because of the heterogeneity of these cases, a broad spectrum assessment process will be outlined, with attention to those issues unique to these populations. First and foremost, a determination of immediate risk to the child is required. It may be so great that removal of the child must occur before treatment can proceed safely. Given recidivism rates, risk assessment should be ongoing. Models of risk assessment have been developed for evaluating reports to social agencies, but assessing risk in the therapeutic context has not received much attention.

Ideally, the assessment model chosen should combine family system elements with cognitive behavioral ones. That is, the clinician should assess both the family as a system embedded in a larger community context (e.g., availability of social supports) and the individual skills of its members. The McMaster model of family functioning is a useful framework for structuring the systems assessment (Epstein, Bishop, & Baldwin, 1982). In this model, the family's ability to accomplish three important tasks must be examined: the capacity to provide for the basic needs of its members (e.g., food, housing, etc.); the capacity to adjust to the changing developmental needs of children; and the capacity to handle emergency situations. System-based mechanisms in six areas are required to accomplish these tasks: problem solving, behavioral control, affective responsiveness, affective involvement, communication, and adequate distribution of family roles. Evi-

dence should be present that the system has such mechanisms and that they operate effectively both within the family (e.g., marital relationship) and within larger social systems (e.g., work).

As a starting point for individual assessment, traditional cognitive, academic, and personality evaluations of both the parent and children are useful to rule out psychiatric disturbance requiring simultaneous intervention and to identify obstacles to treatment (e.g., intellectual limitations, learning disabilities). For example, an intellectually low-functioning client treated by one of the authors was seen as noncompliant by previous treatment providers because she missed appointments. In a carefully done assessment, however, it was found she could not tell time.

Physical and neurological examinations might also be useful. Children who are malnourished may suffer from apathy in a classroom setting, lowering their performance. Head injuries and neurological disturbances have also been linked with aggressive behavior and are worth investigating. With children, assessment for sexual abuse might also be done, in that there is often overlap between types of maltreatment.

Background history can also aid treatment. Parents' own care-taking history may provide clues regarding learned child-rearing strategies and may uncover the origins of distorted beliefs regarding children. Past events can also act as obstacles to parents' attempts at new strategies. For example, one parent linked the use of time out to her own parent locking her in closets as a child, and she therefore resisted efforts to utilize it. Understanding this allowed the therapist an opportunity to highlight distinctions and institute more "acceptable" approaches. Similarly, a developmental history done on the children will not only uncover problems but also allow exploration of events surrounding pregnancies and children's births, providing insights into the parent-child relationship.

Contact with significant others may provide additional useful information. Teachers may provide independent data about child behavior problems and also help to uncover patterns of maltreatment. Prolonged absences, for example, may indicate periods when the child was recovering from injuries. Caseworkers may also provide data regarding chronicity and previous interventions that failed.

A cognitive and behavioral skills assessment should also be undertaken with both parent and child. For the parent, the skill areas outlined earlier might serve as a framework (i.e., parenting, cognitive disturbances, impulse control, social skills, and stress management) and may be examined using structured interviews or instruments with family members and significant others, behavioral observation, and reviewing of record data. Paper-and-pencil measures may include stressful event questionnaires, social contact instruments, anger inventories, marital assessment scales, and instruments assessing knowledge regarding children, parental belief systems, attributional style toward children, and problem-solving skills (e.g., see Azar & Twentyman, 1986; Wolfe, 1987). Observations of family interactions are crucial. Structured activities in the home may provide the best picture of skill deficits (e.g., command situations like picking up toys).

Similarly, a skills-based assessment of the child might be undertaken, starting with his or her interactions with the parent, as well as other adults (e.g., nonmaltreating parent, teachers) and peers. Behavior problem checklists might also be completed. Given that the parent may have distorted views of the child, more than one source should be utilized. Instruments assessing social cognitive skills (empathy), depression, anxiety and fear symptoms, and anger might also be utilized with older children. An evaluation of the child's social resources might also be undertaken (e.g., relatives who play a compensatory role in the child's life).

TREATMENT

Evidence for Prescriptive Treatments

Evidence supporting the efficacy of treatments for maltreating parents has been growing over the last decade, but information is still limited and suffers from many methodological problems (Azar, 1988). The best evidence at this point comes from the application of behavioral interventions. The need for adjunct services has also been emphasized and the evidence for these will be outlined. In contrast, there is almost no literature addressing treatment efficacy for abused and neglected children (Ammerman, 1989; Azar & Wolfe, 1989). Strategies that might be considered, however, can be outlined based on typical presenting problems.

Behavior Therapy

Behavioral and cognitive behavioral strategies have shown positive effects with maltreating parents (for detailed reviews, see Azar, 1989, or Isaacs, 1982). The most work has been done with families with preschool or school-aged children, with more recent attempts being aimed at families of infants and adolescents. A developmental framework has been advocated (i.e., treatments tailored to the developlmental requirements of the different phases of parenting (Azar & Siegel, 1990).

In treating parents, the major modes of presentation have been therapist modeling, coaching, behavioral rehearsal, and feedback. Technology has also been employed (e.g., one-way mirrors and bug-in-the-ear transmitters). Group work can be very helpful, in that it informally works on breaking up parents' social isolation, allows for a wider range of problems for discussion, and provides multiple sources of modeling.

For parents of nursery and elementary school-aged children, child management training has been commonly employed, including training in positive reinforcement and appropriate punishment techniques (e.g., time out, response costs, etc.), use of clear commands, charts, and behavioral contracts. Films and various parenting texts (e.g., Becker's [1971] *Parent's Are Teachers*) have also been used.

Work with parents of infants and toddlers might most fruitfully be directed at common triggers for abuse within this age group (e.g., infant crying) and on developmental stimulation. Studies have successfully used desensitization techniques to increase parental tolerance for crying and to increase physical contact (Gilbert, 1976; Sanders, 1978; Sanford & TGustin, 1974). Training has also been carried out with at-risk parents using modeling, visual and verbal prompts, and rehearsal to promote positive and responsive parent-infant interactions (Wolfe, Edwards, Manion, & Koverola, 1988).

Abused and neglected adolescents are the least likely age group to be reported to authorities and often are identified because of their *response* to maltreatment (e.g., truancy, runaway behavior). This may explain the lack of attention to their treatment needs. Societal reaction is typically punishment (i.e., they are labeled "persons in need of supervision" or status offenders and placed in foster care).

Adolescence is marked by a number of major developmental tasks, including separation from family, shifting allegiance to peers, and adjusting to emerging sexuality. These tasks may be particularly difficult for abusive parents. For example, given their social isolation, such parents may want teenagers to stay at home and not go out with friends or perceive their desire to be with friends as a direct attack on them. By adolescence, the child may have also adopted some of the parent's interpersonal biases (e.g., negative attributional style) and begun to model similar skill deficits (e.g., poor problem solving and impulsive behavior), further increasing potential for conflict. Schellenbach and Guerney (1987) suggested a multicomponent intervention for families with this age child that includes developmental education and training in empathic listening, goal setting, problem solving, negotiation skills, and use of reinforcement and alternative discipline techniques. Data for the efficacy of this approach, however, are needed.

The most recent strategies applied to maltreatment have been cognitive ones. These approaches target parental disturbed schema regarding children, negative attributional biases in assigning causality to child behavior, poor problem-solving skills, and a lowered sense of parenting self-efficacy (Azar, 1989). Imagery techniques and films of aversive parent-child interactions are helpful to facilitate parents to generate their own personalized dysfunctional thoughts. Therapist modeling is also helpful in increasing parents comfort level with sharing thoughts. Then, cognitive restructuring and training in problem-solving skills may be focused on those cognitions that act to trigger abuse (e.g., unrealistic expectations, misattributions).

A myriad of other care-taking behaviors labeled as neglected can be targeted in behavioral interventions, including failing to provide enough nutrients to children, failure to supervise young children by leaving them unattended in an apartment or by allowing them to roam the streets past a reasonable hour, and inappropriate responses to child medical needs. Operant approaches have been used to train meal planning and budgeting to improve child nutrition (Sarber, Halasz, Messmer, Bickett, & Lutzker, 1983), to teach parents to identify and respond appropriately to medical illnesses (Delgado & Lutzker, 1985), and to train home safety skills (Tertinger, Green, & Lutzker, 1984).

Along with parenting skills, parental impulsive behavior has also been a target. Anger-control strategies developed by Novaco (1975) have been applied to help parents handle their affective responses to aversive child behavior and other sources of stress. These strategies are designed to help parents identify the sources and cues for their anger (situational, physiological, and cognitive) and decrease their affective responses (e.g., training in relaxation techniques and cognitive strategies such as problem solving and use of calming self-statements). Self-control and stress management training have also been undertaken. Here, the targets are a broad range of affective and behavioral responses that are maladaptive for the parents' sense of well-being and that interfere with appropriate interpersonal and parenting responses. Examples of treatments aimed at nonparenting targets that are sources of stress have included work on migraine headaches, marital discord, and lack of leisure skills.

Efforts to improve parents' social skills might also be undertaken. There is considerable literature in training adults in social skills, indicating the efficacy of modeling, rehearsal, and feedback, in conjunction with self-monitoring and self-reinforcement. Low-functioning neglectful parents in particular may require training in such skills. A board game that requires parents to provide social responses which the therapist can then reinforce has been successfully employed with such parents (Fantuzzo, Wray, Hall, Goins, & Azar, 1986).

Behavioral treatment outcome work has primarily involved single case design studies or small samples and has not employed control groups or comparative treatments, making it difficult to speak definitively about differential treatment efficacy. In addition, most studies have not assessed recidivism; instead, they focus on the impact on intermediate outcome variables believed to mediate abuse and neglect (e.g., positive parenting strategies). Some exceptions exist. Wolfe, Sandler, and Kaufman (1981) and Azar and Twentyman (1984) both found no recidivism at one-year followup with group treatments employing short-term package approaches (e.g., child management training, cognitive strategies, etc.) and adjunct home training. Some evidence for differential treatment effects between behavioral strategies and between behavioral and nonbehavioral approaches have also been found on intermediate variables (Egan, 1983; Brunk, Henggeler, & Whelan, 1987). At this point, behavioral approaches to treating the parents who abuse and neglect their children appear promising. Some evidence exists, however, that such approaches may work with less severe cases, but not the more chronic ones who are dysfunctional across a range of responses (Szykulas & Fleischman, 1985). Clearly, more research is needed.

As noted earlier, our knowledge base regarding interventions with maltreated children is poor. This may be due to a greater emphasis by clinicians on safety issues than on long-term social and emotional consequences. Indeed, findings from one study indicate that sexually abused children are more likely to be referred to services than other types of maltreatment (Vitulano, Lewis, Doran, Nordhaus, & Adnopoz, 1986). Clinicians should be alert to this bias.

Based on what is known about symptoms in such populations, a number of intervention suggestions are possible (Ammerman, 1989; Azar & Twentyman, 1986). Given that these children have undergone trauma and lived in chaotic, understimulating and punitive home environments, certain common elements of intervention should be employed no matter what other dispositional choices are made. These include attention to nutritional and health issues, developmental stimula-

tion, opportunities for socializing with peers and positive adult figures, and safeness (e.g., a warm, nurturing environment, low punitiveness; Martin, 1976).

Specific target behaviors might include developmental and cognitive delays (especially in language and speech), motor delays, lack of appropriate utilization of social cues (e.g., perspective taking, emotional cue identification, interpersonal problem solving, etc.), and behavioral deviations in peer/adult relations, including affective withdrawal and aggression. Behavioral interventions with children and adolescents in each of these areas has shown some success. For example, operant techniques have been used to work with severe speech deficits (Rigley & Wolfe, 1967; Steven-Long, Schwarz, & Bliss, 1976) and presumably would be helpful with the less severe deficits found in abused children. Behavioral approaches have also been utilized to increase social skills in both young children and adolescents. For instance, peer prompting has been used successfully with maltreated children to work on social withdrawal (Fantuzzo et al., 1990). Impulsive and aggressive behavior have also been dealt with successfully using cognitive behavioral strategies and operant approaches (Kendall & Braswell, 1985).

Pharmacotherapy

Almost no attention has been given to pharmacotherapy with abusive and neglectful parents or their children. Some features associated with these problems may respond to such therapy (e.g., depressive symptoms). Only one study could be located that utilized drug therapy (Sanders, 1978), but unfortunately it included other treatment strategies, precluding a determination of its impact alone. For the small percentages of parents who suffer from psychotic behavior, drug therapy's impact on parenting is yet to be determined. In practice, such parents may lose custody of their children by virtue of their disorder, and thus, no data have been collected.

Alternative Treatments

Psychodynamic approaches to treating child abuse and neglect were the first to appear in the literature, and while efficacy was claimed, little data supporting their use have been collected (Parke & Collmer, 1975). A recent comparative outcome study included a short-term insight-oriented group treatment condition that had some positive impact on intermediate variables for this approach, but did not show decreases in abuse and neglect itself. Therefore, the efficacy of such approaches still remains in question. "Systemic" approaches have also been advocated, and in one study, such an intervention was shown to decrease parental social problems. Impact on parenting, however, was not demonstrated, suggesting that this approach alone is insufficient to produce the kind of broad spectrum changes required for such families.

Lay therapists and family support volunteers have also been used. In probably the best demonstration of a preventive intervention, Olds (1986) successfully used nurses as home visitors over a one- or two-year period to provide developmental education, family support, health advice, and care and other support services to at-risk young mothers. More typically, adjunct workers have been used to assist parents in day-to-day crises while the family is working on more long-term issues in treatment. Home visitors provide a social network from which a parent may gain strength to make changes and can provide opportunities for modeling of new behaviors. Indeed, the findings in one study indicated that adjunct home-based training may be crucial to success to behaviorally based office work (Azar & Twentyman, 1984).

Other efforts targeted at breaking up the social isolation of parents and providing new sources of parenting knowledge include use of self-help groups, like Parents Anonymous. It has been the authors' experience that group work without outside professional input or monitoring may not be useful, as parents may share inappropriate parenting techniques. For example, one abusive parent in a parent training program was overheard telling another one how she tied her son to the toilet when he failed to be toilet trained quickly!

Other kinds of support services have been provided to parents alone or while they were involved in treatment, such as homemakers, daycare, respite care, and hot lines. The goal of such ser-vides is typically to reduce parental stress. The interactive effects of such services with treatments, however, is not known. For example provision of such services may adversely affect a parent's attributions for treatment gains. Daycare may also have some unanticipated negative side effects. Observations within caycare settings indicate that such children are difficult to handle, and this may result in their further rejection by adult staff and peers. Also, placing a child who has lived within a very rigid and perhaps restrictive environment into one that is responsive and sensitive may produce behaviors at home that are not tolerated (e.g., the child may make new demands on the parent). Further research is needed to evaluate the impact of such services.

Selecting Optimal Treatments

Given the paucity of outcome data, decision rules about selecting optimal treatments are difficult to present. Clearly, in training parenting skills, there should be attentiveness to potential for increasing child risk when selecting order of presentation. For example, teaching extinction techniques (e.g., ignoring tantrums) may result in what have been called *extinction bursts* (i.e., an increase in the level of the tantrum before a decrease is seen). Failure to provide a priori stress management strategies for dealing with such aversive behavior may increase risk of abuse. Similarly as just noted, providing the child with an alternative context that is positive and has different "rules" than his or her home environment may result in behaviors that may be perceived as provocative. Finally, problems in substance abuse and other psychiatric problems may require attention before parenting can be addressed.

Problems with Carrying Out Assessments and Interventions

Work with maltreating families presents unique difficulties. The first of these involves the clinician's own values and feelings regarding parents who have maltreated children. Two opposite responses can act as obstacles to treatment—

clinicians may either deny that the maltreatment occurred or may find it difficult to identify a parent who would engage in such behavior. The first stance increases the risk that signs of reabuse or reneglect will be ignored; and the latter may preclude making a therapeutic alliance with the parent, reducing the potential for positive changes in the child's life. This stance may also make any future therapist's work that much harder. A middle ground must be achieved of being vigilant about child risk and developing an alliance with the parent. No clinician can do this in all cases; generous use of consultation with colleagues or a treatment team approach in such cases is suggested.

It should be noted that there may be some parents who ultimately will be deemed "untreatable." Such cases have only recently received discussion and may bring the clinician in contact with the legal system (i.e., termination of parental rights proceedings), which present a new set of difficult issues that are beyond the scope of this chapter (see Azar [1992] for such a discussion).

The legal mandate to report maltreatment also presents difficulties. Given the recidivism rates cited earlier, such a need is likely to arise. Reporting biases have been well documented (e.g., decreased reporting of middle-class parents) and care must be taken to consider them in one's own decision making. The possibility of reporting should be raised early in therapy and plans for how it might be handled should be devised in conjunction with the client. Contracting may also be used to solicit a promise from a client not to engage in physical means of discipline while in a treatment program. Discussing this issue models open communication and planning, both of which are difficult for such families. If the need should arise to report, the client might be given the opportunity to make the report himself or herself with the therapist's assistance. This may act to reduce the view that the therapist is "punishing" and may help to preserve the relationship.

The characteristics of abusing families make assessment and treatment more difficult. First, parents are often poorly educated. Thus, paper-and-pencil instruments must be administered with care. The authors typically read all items to clients,

clearly adding considerable time to the assessment. In addition, lack of norms for disadvantaged and minority groups warrant caution in interpreting findings.

Caution must also be exhibited in the use of behavioral strategies with clients who may not have well-developed interpersonal skills. For example, they may require therapists' modeling or film presentations initially to make them comfortable in attempting to engage in roleplays. Use of predetermined scripts have also been utilized (Barth, Blythe, Schinke, Stevens, & Schilling, 1983). Again, caution must be exhibited, as these clients may have difficulty reading, and asking them to read aloud may induce resistance.

In conducting child management training, particular caution must be exhibited that the parents are not misapplying techniques. Careful roleplaying of time-out procedures and detailed discussion regarding its use are necessary. This strategy may be overused by the parent, thus decreasing its efficacy. In addition, because they may exhibit poor judgment and/or have a punitive style, parents may lock children in closets or other inappropriate or unsafe areas (e.g., a bathroom where dangerous medicines are kept).

Maltreating families typically enter treatment involuntarily, thus introducing the potential for motivational problems. High attrition rates have been found. Suggestions regarding incentives have been made, including provision of babysitting, contracting, movie tickets, and so on. Empirical data regarding their efficacy are still lacking.

Another problem area has to do with the chaotic lifestyle of such families. Many competing stressors occur that disrupt the treatment process. The clinician can get caught up with these stressors and not consistently follow-through on treatment goals. If target skills are kept in mind, even crises present places for skill building.

Maltreated children also present unique problems that may interfere with the collecting of accurate information and the development of a therapeutic relationship (Martin, 1976). Given their history with punitive adults, these children may approach testing with fear and anxiety and may be uncomfortable being alone in a therapy room. For example, in one of the author's cases, a child periodically opened the door in the midst of a session to "feed" an imaginary dog. Abused children also have been observed to be hyper-vigilant in contact with adults and to seek approval, which may distract from completing assessments. Indeed, one study suggests that use of peers as "therapeutic agents" under some circumstances may be a better choice than adults (Fantuzzo et al., 1990). Children may also have difficulty attending to instructions, be verbally inhibited, and resistant. Modifications in treatment structure and testing presentation may be needed to increase effectiveness.

Relapse Prevention

As noted earlier, high rates of relapse have been found. Relapse prevention work, however, has been quite limited in the literature. Stokes and Baer (1977) have outlined a number of strategies for improving maintenance in behavioral and cognitive behavioral training that might be applied to interventions with abusive and neglectful parents, including fading of sessions, self-control training, booster sessions, and training in multiple exemplars. It is noteworthy that the two studies that found reduced recidivism both employed some form of self-control training and home trainers who adapted parenting strategies to naturally occurring examples in the home setting. More systematic examinations of relapse prevention efforts need to occur.

CASE ILLUSTRATION

This case provides an opportunity to illustrate the many treatment issues encountered in abusive and neglectful families.*

Case Description

Louise was a 23-year-old single welfare mother who had two sons, aged 3 and 5. The family had multiple reports of physical abuse and neglect,

_____
*This case is a hypothetical one, combining elements from a number of families seen by the authors.

including Louise's failure to adequately care for her younger son's diaper rash, the children being found wandering the streets unattended late at night, and Louise's beating her elder child with a belt, leaving bruises.

Louise had her first child as a teenager and lived with her mother during his early years. She had no further contact with the baby's father. She describes her mother during this time as continually finding fault with her parenting. Shortly after meeting her younger son's father, she moved in with him. At the time she was seen, however, she was no longer living with him, but he would visit fairly regulary.

Differential Diagnosis and Assessment

Assessment was conducted in two home visits for observations and two angency visits for more formal evaluations. A system's-based evaluation indicated that, for the most part, Louise was able to provide housing, cloth her children, and provide them with adequate food, occasionally drawing on the younger son's father for financial help.

The family evidenced many problems with developmental tasks. Louise failed to meet the children's needs for age-appropriate guidance and supervision. For example, she had no standard bedtime for the children and would allow them to stay up all night watching television. She also did not provide supervision of their outdoor play activities. On one early home visit, the 5-year-old was found on the roof of the house. These situations were indicative of difficulties in problem solving (failure in the identification stage) and inadequate mechanisms for behavioral control in the family system.

On the other hand, there was some evidence of affective responsiveness and involvement between the mother and children (e.g., Louise was affectionate with the children and would hang pictures they drew on the wall). Her communication with the children was quite direct, but often consisted of yelling, which suggested some difficulties here as well.

Louise's relationship with the outside world was marked by problems. She appeared to have a conflictual relationship with her family of origin and almost no social relationships aside from occasional contacts with her younger child's father and other men she met. These relationships were also conflict riddenand often involved her being verbally abused. She also experienced difficulties with her caseworker and missed scheduled appointments, which led to a threatened loss of custody.

Traditional assessment of Louise indicated some strengths and a number of skill deficiencies. Her intellectual ability placed her in the average range and no major personality difficulties were noted in her MMPI profile, although some indications of depressive symptoms and potential substance abuse were present. Although alcohol abuse was denied, over the course of treatment it unfolded that Louise would drink small amounts of beer to "make" herself "feel better."

Cognitive assessment of the children indicated low average abilities. Developmental assessment of the 3-year-old showed severe delays in language and fine motor skills. The older boy was highly distractible during testing and had trouble attending to tasks. A potential diagnosis of attention deficit-hyperactivity disorder was considered. Problems in preacademic skills were also noted (e.g., knowledge of colors).

The cognitive/behavioral assessment performed with Louise showed problems in each of the five areas described earlier. An assessment of her expectations regarding children using the Parent Opinion Questionnaire (Azar, Robinson, Hekimian, & Twentyman, 1984) indicated many unrealistic beliefs. She responded with agreement to statements such as: "Parents can expect even a child as young as 2 and 1/2 to be able to comfort them when they are sad and crying"; "A 3-year-old child usually knows when his mom or dad is upset and that he should stay out of the way at those times"; and "It's OK to leave a 3-year-old who is soundly sleeping in a bed, alone in the house or apartment while the parent walks a friend to the corner bus stop."

Her solutions to a set of hypothetical parenting problems indicated a narrow repertoire of child-rearing strategies that were often not age appropriate (e.g., talking to a 2-year-old to get him to stop hitting his infant brother instead of removing the 2-year-old from within range of the baby). Louise's parenting was further assessed by using a structured diary that asked her to record discipline incidents and her cognitive and behavioral responses. Her entries indicated a high rate of coercive responses and a negative attributional bias toward her elder son. For example, she described one incident where he spilled milk. When asked why the incident occurred, she wrote: "He's a brat. He never listens and likes to make work for me." Her response to this incident was "screamed at him and told him how stupid he was."

Observations of the parent-child interactions further indicated that Louise had a poor ability to give clear commands and utilized a high frequency of coercive responses (e.g., threats, yelling, criticism). Similarly, the children also responded with high rates of noncompliance and negative behavior. For example, a task of getting the children to pick up toys was assigned. The older son noncomplied in a "clowning" manner and elicited Louise's laughter in the midst of her attempts to get him to comply. Given Louise's negative bias toward him, her positive response was a very powerful reinforcer and, of course, increased the noncompliance. At a certain point, however, without warning, Louise attempted to "get serious" and became angry. The boy tried harder to elicit his mother's laughter, which infuriated her and led her to threaten him with a physical response. On other occasions, Louise ignored the boys' misbehavior. Since it was often designed to elicit attention, the behavior would escalate until she responded, typically in an extreme, negative way.

Maternal anger control was poor, and Louise described herself as "having a short fuse," with no specific triggers to her anger, saying, "I just lose it." However, questioning revealed that incidents typically occurred in the context of other life stressors (e.g., after a negative transaction with her boyfriend). When a life event scale was administered, maternal life stress was found to be significant. Many of the events, however, were controllable (e.g., arguments with family members). Thus, Louise's interpersonal skills seemed to play a role. She reported few social contacts on a social network instrument and indicated dissatisfaction with the ones she did have.

Although Louise's alcohol use was a concern, it was felt that it was secondary to depressive symptoms. Her depression appeared to have a cognitive base (i.e., it was marked by negative and self-deprecatory statements) and centered around her worth as a parent and social isolation; therefore, it might lessen if these other issues were addressed.

Treatment Selection

A multimodal treatment was planned. Since the agency in which Louise was seen had a number of modalities available, over the course of the nine months of treatment she received multiple forms. First, the children were placed in the agency daycare program to reduce Louise's child-rearing stress and to work on their cognitive and academic delays (e.g., speech therapy for the youngest). Given the children's ages, it was felt that therapy would most fruitfully be directed at Louise, although, as will be discussed later, some behavioral work was done with the children's teacher with respect to management problems.

Louise was provided with both individual home-based treatment and short-term parenting group work. Treatment was administered in the form of a 10-week group cognitive behavioral package that included standard child management training (e.g., use of positive reinforcement, time-out procedures), cognitive work (e.g., cognitive restructuring), anger control, and stress masnagement training and communication training (e.g., teaching perspective taking and listening skills.)

Individual home visits were also carried out to help apply newly acquired parenting skills and to make modifications where needed. This home-based treatment later took a broader focus (with fading of sessions in the last two months), working on other intrapersonal (depression) and interpersonal (social) problems, as well as continuing to fine-tune parenting responses. Goals included decreasing her cognitive disturbances, increasing her parenting skills, improving her supervision of the children's activities, increasing her

ability to modulate anger, and expanding her social network.

Treatment Course and Problems in Carrying Out Interventions

In cognitive parent training, any child problem elicited should be explored for its interpretive meaning. Even commonly cited difficulties may be associated with misattributions that must be changed before the parent will be willing to utilize new strategies. For example, as is typical of the age, Louise's 3-year-old would occasionally refuse to do something requested. Cognitive techniques were utilized to elicit Louise's attributions for the behavior. She initially said she felt he was "trying to get to me", to "tell me he's the boss." When this was questioned further, she responded with a self-deprecatory response (e.g., "He thinks I'm stupid"). When asked if there were others in her life who felt this way, she responded by listing her mother or the boy's father. She elaborated on the latter: "He's just like his dad, always trying to push me. . . . He thinks I'm dumb and laughs at me."

This internal dialogue indicated some discrimintion training was needed before training in parenting strategies could be undertaken. that is, before Louise could choose an appropriate socialization response, she had to see her child as in need of "education" — not as malevolent in intent and not the same as the other adults in her life.

This negative attributional style may be limited to parents' children, but in this case seemed more generalized. For example, vocational training was set as a goal for the mother as an alternative source of self-efficacy (to decrease depressive symptoms). The first step in achieving this goal was enrollment in a GED program. Unfortunately, Louise wanted to quit the program after only a week despite an initial positive response. The teacher had used a mistake she had made on a quiz for illustrative purposes in class and Louise felt she was being "made fun of" and ridiculed.

As cognitive responses were challenged, new strategies for child management were instituted. For example, Louise was provided with alternatives to physical punishment (e.g., time out, response cost) as well as positive strategies. Video feedback and roleplays were used to help to formulate clearer commands and avoid the delivering of "mixed" messages (e.g., laughing when trying to solicit compliance).

Her lack of supervision was the most difficult to treat. Such situations required anticipatory skills that seemed lacking in this client's repertoire. The first element in such skills is a recognition of children's limited capacity to anticipate risks. Louise clearly believed that the children "knew" what they were doing and "could take care of themselves" and only got into difficulties because they were "being stupid" or "trying to get her in trouble." Cognitive challenging was undertaken. This was done in a number of ways. First, the mother was encouraged to think about what her ideas were like at her children's age, with examples that would illustrate children's limited thinking capacity. For example, children's different conception of time was illustrated by asking her to reflect on how long Christmas seemed in coming when she was little and how it seems to come so quickly for her as an adult, or how far away her school seemed to her as a child and how in reality it was quite close.

Experiments were also undertaken. Piagetian conservation tasks were done with the boys to illustrate the fact that children look at the world differently and make mistakes because of this. Louise's own needs for safety and security were discussed. Once elicited, these feelings were linked to her children's needs. Examples from her own childhood of being left alone for days or being in situations where she did not feel safe were accessed to bring this point home.

Louise's "short fuse" was also targeted. She was provided with strategies for dealing with anger. As in other areas, cognitive factors that might "fan the fire of anger" were elicited first. As noted earlier, Louise denied signs that she was about to "lose it," saying that "it just happens." Imagery techniques and roleplays were useful. Using examples she provided, cognitive, physiological, and situation cues were identified. These factors were labeled as cues to engage in strategies to "dampen the response," including calming self-statements and preventive relaxation responses before high-

risk situations. When these failed, avoidant responses (e.g., counting to 10, leaving the scene) were suggested as alternatives.

Louise indicated a desire (although ambivalent—"friends hurt you") to increase her social network. Each day as she waited with her children for the daycare bus, Louise saw another mother whom she indicated a desire to meet. The therapist engaged her in problem solving as to how she might approach beginning an acquaintance with this women. The therapeutic relationship was itself used as a model of the difficulties in the initial phases of meeting someone (e.g., "It was tough at first for us to talk" and "What did I do that made it easier for you to talk to me?"). The therapist also modeled cognitive strategies to decrease obstacles to forming a new relationship (e.g., dealing with fears that the other person will not talk). Initial contact was roleplayed and the possible alternative ways the transaction might go were considered. Louise made an attempt to make contact and invited this person for coffee one morning. This contact was utilized as an example, and the therapist went over the parts that went well with the client and problems solved the parts that had felt awkward. A similar strategy was utilized for transactions with the GED teacher and the men in her life.

Many difficulties arose during the course of treatment. These situations, while interfering with treatment gains, presented opportunities for further skill building. At one point, Louise was evicted from her apartment, and gains made in the use of parenting strategies disappeared as she dealt with this crisis. The episode was used in treatment as an example of how stress interfered with Louise's parenting skills and how she might cope better. There appeared some capriciousness on the landlord's part, therefore problem solving was used to generate potential ways to change his decision. The therapist happened to be present during one of the landlord's visits and was able to monitor this transaction to fine-tune Louise's skills. For example, Louise immediately became passive when the landlord made an unreasonable demand as to when she should leave. Work on assertive responses were undertaken. In addition, this episode appeared to act as an antecedent to irritable and coercive responses toward the children, and the therapist pointed out the spillover.

Outcome and Termination

Over the nine months of treatment, Louise made steady improvements in her transactions with the boys. Her involvement with child protective services was terminated by the end of treatment. She increased her social network slightly and completed the GED program. Alcohol use appeared to decrease, as did her depressive symptoms. Her relationship with her son's father continued to be marked by conflict, but he refused to participate in sessions. Ultimately, Louise became involved with another man. This relationship, while far from ideal, was an improvement over her previous ones. The younger son's speech problems improved significantly, and both boys' preacademic skills showed marked gains. Unfortunately, the 5-year old's behavior problems continued. When he entered kindergarten, behavioral work in the classroom was instituted with his teacher's help with some limited success.

Followup and Maintenance

At one-year followup, Louise had still not become reinvolved with child protective services. She had terminated the relationship with the man she was seeing during treatment and had formed another relationship, which appeared to be headed toward marriage. The 5-year old's behavior problems had worsened, however, and in first grade he was placed in a special classroom. Medication was used to control his attentional problems, and Louise was receiving further professional help with parenting around his behavior.

SUMMARY

Despite their heterogeneity, abusive and neglectful families present many common features that are amenable to intervention. The numerous stresses experienced by these families and the clinician's response to the chaotic and sometimes violent nature of such cases can act as major obstacles to treatment success. Careful assessment is required to identify all problems within the family, and a consistent goal-directed approach is needed.

REFERENCES

Ammerman, R. T. (1989). Child abuse and neglect. In M. Hersen (Ed.), *Innovations in child behavior therapy* (pp. 353–394). New York: Springer.

Ammerman, R. T., Cassisi, J. E., Hersen, M., & VanHasselt, V. B. (1986). Consequences of physical abuse and neglect in children. *Clinical Psychology Review, 6,* 291–310.

Azar, S. T. (1986). A framework for understanding child maltreatment: An integration of cognitive behavioral and developmental perspectives. *Canadian Journal of Behavioral Science, 18,* 340–355.

Azar, S. T. (1988). Methodological considerations in treatment outcome research in child maltreatment. In J. T. Hotaling, D. Finkelhor, J. T. Kirkpatrick, & M. Straus (Eds.), *Coping with family violence. Research and policy perspectives* (pp. 288–298). Beverly Hills, CA: Sage.

Azar, S. T. (1989). Training parents of abused children. In C. E. Shaefer & J. M. Briesmeister (Eds.), *Handbook of parent training: Parents as cotherapists for children's behavior problems* (pp. 414–441). New York: Wiley and Sons.

Azar, S. T. (1992). Legal issues in child abuse. In R. Ammerman & M. Hersen (Eds.), *Assessment of family violence. A clinical and legal handbook* (pp. 47–70). New York: Wiley and Sons.

Azar, S. T., Barnes, K. T., & Twentyman, C. T. (1988). Developmental outcomes in abused children: Consequences of parental abuse or a more general breakdown in caregiver behavior? *The Behavior Therapist, 11,* 27–32.

Azar, S. T., Robinson, D. R., Hekimian, E., & Twentyman, C. T. (1984). Unrealistic expectations and problems solving ability in maltreating and comparison mothers. *Journal of Consulting and Clinical Psychology, 52,* 687–691.

Azar, S. T., & Siegel, B. R. (1990). Behavioral treatment of child abuse: A developmental perspective. *Behavior Modification, 14,* 279–300.

Azar, S. T., & Twentyman, C. T. (1984, November). *An evaluation of the effectiveness of behaviorally versus insight oriented group treatments with maltreating mothers.* Paper presented at the annual meeting of the Association for the Advancement of Behavior Therapy, Philadelphia.

Azar, S. T., & Twentyman, C. T. (1986). Cognitive-behavioral perspectives on the assessment and treatment of child abuse. *Advances in cognitive-behavioral research* (Vol. 5, pp. 237–267). New York: Academic Press.

Azar, S. T., & Wolfe, D. A. (1989). Child abuse and neglect. In E. J. Mash & R. A. Barkley (Eds.), *Treatment of childhood disorders* (pp. 451–489). New YOrk: Guilford Press.

Barth, R. P., Blythe, B. J., Schinke, S. P., Stevens, P., & Schilling, R. F. (1983). Self control training with maltreating parents. *Child Welfare, 62,* 313–323.

Becker, W. C. (1971). *Parents are teachers.* Champaign, IL: Research Press.

Bousha, D., & Twentyman, C. T. (1984). Abusing, neglectful, and comparison mother-child interactional style: Naturalistic observations in the home setting. *Journal of Abnormal Psychology, 93,* 106–114.

Brunk, M., Henggeler, S. W., & Whelan, J. P. (1987). Comparison of multisystemic therapy and parent training in the brief treatment of child abuse and neglect. *Journal of Consulting and Clinical Psychology, 55,* 171–178.

Burgdorf, K. (1988). *Study of national incidence and prevalence of child abuse and neglect: 1988.* Washington, DC: NCCAN.

Cantwell, H. B. (1980). Child neglect. In C. H. Kempe & R. E. Helfer (Eds.), *The battered child* (pp. 183–197). Chicago: University of Chicago Press.

Cicchetti, D., & Rizley, R. (1981). Developmental perspectives on the etiology, intergenerational transmission, and sequelae of child maltreatment. *New Directions for Child Development, 11,* 31–56.

Conaway, L. P., & Hansen, D. J. (1989). Social behavior of physically abused and neglected children: A critical review. *Clinical Psychology Review, 9,* 627–652.

Delgado, A. E., & Lutzker, J. R. (1985, November). *Training parents to identify and report their children's illness.* Paper presented at the annual convention of the Association for Advancement of Behavior Therapy, Houston.

Deykin, E. Y., Alpert, J. J., & McNamarra, J. J. (1985). A pilot study of the effect of exposure to child abuse or neglect on adolescent suicidal behavior. *American Journal of Psychiatry, 142,* 1299–1303.

Egan, K. (1983). Stress management and child management with abusive parents. *Journal of Clinical Child Psychology, 12,* 292–299.

Epstein, N. B., Bishop, D. S., & Baldwin, L. M. (1982). McMaster model of family functioning. In F. Walsh (Ed.), *Normal family processes* (pp. 115–141). New York: Guildord.

Fantuzzo, J. W., Jurecic, L., Stovall, A., Hightower, A. D., Goins, C., & Schachtel, D. (1990). Effects of adult and peer social initiations on the social behavior of withdrawn, maltreated preschool children. *Journal of Consulting and Clinical Psychology, 56,* 34–39.

Fantuzzo, J. W., Wray, L., Hall, R., Goins, C., & Azar, S. T. (1986). Parent and social skills training for mentally retarded parents identified as child maltreaters. *American Journal of Mental Deficiency, 91,* 135–140.

Gilbert, M. T. (1976). Behavioral approach to the treatment of child abuse. *Nursing Times, 72,* 140–143.

Isaacs, C. D. (1982). Treatment of child abuse: A review of the behavioral interventions. *Journal of Applied Behavioral Analysis, 15,* 273–294.

Kazdin, A. E., Moser, J., Colbus, D., & Bell, R. (1985). Depressive symptoms among physically abused and psychiatrically disturbed children. *Journal of Abnormal Psychology, 94,* 298–307.

Kendal, P. C., & Braswell, L. (1985). *Cognitive behavioral therapy for impulsive children.* New York: Guilford.

Loeber, R., Felton, D. K., & Reid, J. B. (1984). A social learning approach to the reduction of coercive processes in child abusive families. A molecular analysis. *Advances in Behaviour Research and Therapy, 6,* 29–45.

Livingston, R. (1987). Sexually and physically abused children. *Journal of American Academy of Child Psychiatry, 26,* 413–415.

Martin, H. P. (1976). *The abused child.* Cambridge, MA: Ballinger.

Novaco, R. W. (1975). *Anger control: The development and evaluation of an experimental treatment.* Lexington, MA: Lexington Books.

Oldershaw, L., Walters, G. C., & Hall, D. K. (1989). A behavioral approach to the classification of different types of abusive mothers. *Merrill-Palmer Quarterly, 35,* 255–279.

Olds, D. L. (1986). Preventing child abuse and neglect: A randomized trial of nurse home visitation. *Pediatrics, 78,* 65–78.

Parke, R. D., & Collmer, C. W. (1975). Child abuse: An interdisciplinary analysis. In E. M. Hetherington (Ed.), *Review of child development research* (Vol. 5, pp. 509–590). Chicago: University of Chicago Press.

Reid, J. B. (1985). Behavioral approaches to intervention and assessment of child abusive families. In P.

H. Bornstein & A. E. Kazdin (Eds.), *Handbook of clinical behavior therapy with children* (pp. 772–802). Homewood, IL: Dorsey.

Risley, T., & Wolfe, M. (1967). Establishing functional speech in echolalic children. *Behaviour Research and Therapy, 5,* 73–88.

Salzinger, S., Kaplan, S., Pelcovitz, D., Samit, C., & Krieger, R. (1984). Parent and teacher assessment of children's behavior in child maltreating families. *Journal of the American Academy of Child Psychiatry, 23,* 458–464.

Sanders, R. W. (1978). Systematic desensitization in the treatment of child abuse. *American Journal of Psychiatry, 135,* 483–484.

Sandford, D. A., & Tustin, R. D. (1974). Behavioral treatment of parental assault on a child. *New Zealand Psychologist, 2,* 76–82.

Sarber, R. E., Halasz, M. M., Messmer, M. C., Bickett, A. D., & Lutzker, J. R. (1983). Teaching menu planning and grocery shopping skills to a mentally retarded mother. *Mental Retardation, 21,* 101–106.

Schellenbach, C. J., & Guerney, L. F. (1987). Identification of adolescent abuse and future intervention. *Journal of Adolescence, 10,* 1–12.

Steven-Long, J., Schwarz, J. L., & Bliss, D. (1976). The acquisition and generalization of compound sentence structure in an autistic child. *Behavior Therpy, 7,* 397–404.

Stokes, T. F., & Baer, D. M. (1977). An implicit technology of generalization. *Journal of Applied Behavioral Analysis, 16,* 349–367.

Straus, M. A., & Gelles, R. J. (1986). Societal change in family violence from 1976 to 1985 as revealed by two national survey. *Journal of Marriage and the Family, 48,* 465–479.

Szykulas, S. A., & Fleischman, M. J. (1985). Reducing out-of-home placement of abused children: Two controlled studies. *Child Abuse and Neglect, 9,* 277–284.

Tertinger, D. A., Greene, b. F., & Lutzker, J. R. (1984). Home safety: Development and validation of one component of an ecobehavioral treatment program for abused and neglected children. *Journal of Applied Behavior Analysis, 17,* 150–174.

Vitulano, L. A., Lewis, M., Doran, L. D., Nordhaus, B., & Adnopoz, J. (1986). Treatment recommendations, implementation, and follow-up in child abuse. *American Journal of Orthopsychiatry, 56,* 478–480.

Wauchope, B. A., & Straus, M. A. (1987, July). *Age, class, and gender differences in physical punishment and physical abuse of American children.* Paper presented at the National Conference of Family Violence Research, Durham, NH.

Williams, G. (1983). Child abuse reconsidered: The urgent need for authentic prevention. *Journal of Clinical Child Psychology, 12,* 312–319.

Wolfe, D. A. (1987). *Child abuse: Implications for child development and psychopathology.* Newbury Park, CA: Sage.

Wolfe, D. A., Edwards, B., Manion, I., & Koverola, C. (1988). Early intervention for parents at risk of child abuse and neglect: A preliminary investigation. *Journal of Consulting and Clinical Psychology, 56,* 40–47.

Wolfe, D. A., Sandler, J., & Kaufman, K. (1981). A competency based parent training program for abusive parents. *Journal of Consulting and Clinical Psychology, 49,* 633–640.

CHAPTER 23

CHILDREN OF DIVORCE

Daniel S. Shaw   University of Pittsburgh
Katherine Dowdell Hommerding   University of Pittsburgh

DESCRIPTION OF PROBLEM

Divorce is one of the most common environmental stressors experienced by children. As more has been learned about children's adjustment to divorce and response to treatment, researchers have come to view it as a complex series of transitions and adaptations, rather than a simplistic, unitary event. Within this process framework, a greater appreciation for the differential effects of divorce and application of treatment has been achieved. This chapter will review present conceptualizations of the impact of divorce on children's adjustment, literature pertinent to treatment outcome, and suggestions to optimize intervention. At the conclusion of the chapter, a case illustration is provided to demonstrate the multifaceted issues involved in clinical work with this population of children.

Core Features and Epidemiology

Within the last two decades, the divorce rate in the United States has increased substantially. Since 1958, when there were 2.1 divorces per 1,000 population, a gradual increase in the number of divorces has occurred, reaching 2.5 per 1,000 in-

dividuals in 1965 and peaking at 5.3 per 1,000 population in 1979 and 1981 (Glick & Lin, 1986). According to projections based on 1983 census data, 40 percent of all children can expect to spend "some meaningful length of time" in a single-parent household because of divorce (Norton, 1983). Although a gradual decline in the divorce rate took place in the 1980s, a combination of counterbalancing forces makes the probability of dramatic changes in the divorce rate unlikely.

Population growth, increases in the employment and status of women, and a high rate of cohabitation outside of marriage are all factors related to higher divorce rates. However, the rising age at which people marry, the scarcity of eligible women (due to the lower birth rate after the Baby Boom), and fears about the effects of divorce on children may mitigate any major rise in divorce (Glick, 1989). Based on the dramatic increase of divorces over the last two decades and the prospect that a similarly high number of families will continue to be affected by divorce in the future, it remains imperative to understand the effects of parental separation on children's adjustment.

At a basic level, it can be stated with assurance that all divorces involve change for children. Some of these changes might occur prior to the parental separation. Similarly, some might produce improved rather than worsened conditions. Whatever the outcomes, these changes require that children adapt to new environmental conditions. Despite the growing commonality of divorce in the United States, the transitions that are typically involved in the family adaptation to divorce should not be minimized. Divorce involves significant changes in daily living for parents *and* children. On the other hand, to assert that these changes will necessarily result in a pathological outcome for children would also be an inaccurate representation of our current knowledge base.

In this section, important issues related to children's adjustment to divorce will be examined. This will include a review of family process factors that have been found to increase or decrease children's vulnerability to the effects of marital dissolution and a review of children's outcome to divorce in specific domains.

Types of Problems Experienced by Divorced Children

Though many children from divorced families will never show signs of severe psychopathology, a substantive body of research indicates that divorce does place children at an increased risk for three different types of adjustment difficulties (Atkeson, Forehand, & Rickard, 1982; Emery, 1988; Long & Forehand, 1987): (1) externalizing problems, (2) internalizing problems, and (3) cognitive deficits.

Externalizing Problems

Perhaps the most robust and consistent finding in the divorce literature relates to the association between divorce and children's externalizing problems. These include such behaviors as delinquency, aggression, and disobedience. Although early research on this relationship did not attempt to control for such variables as the reason for the parental separation and socioeconomic status (SES) (Glueck & Glueck, 1950; Nye, 1957), later more sophisticated research designs have repeatedly replicated this result (Hetherington, Cox, & Cox, 1978; Shaw & Emery, 1987).

Using data from the National Survey of Children (NSC), a nationally representative sample of 1,423 7- to 11-year-olds, children's adjustment was evaluated in 1976 and 1981 (Furstenberg & Allison, 1989). The majority of families remained married during this five-year duration. However, a large minority experienced a parental separation before or during the course of the study, permitting investigators to examine the effects of age and divorce on children's short- and long-term functioning at home and school. Children of divorced parents were reported to be more aggressive than children from two-parent families according to mothers, teachers, and their own self-report, at both initial and five-year followup assessments (Zill, 1978).

Hetherington and associates (1978), in their comparison of children from divorced and married families, also found children from divorced families to demonstrate more disobedient and aggressive behavior than peers from two-parent families. In addition, children from divorced families have been overpresented among delinquents according to the self-reports of boys (Goldstein, 1984) and girls (Kalter, Riemer, Brickman, & Chen, 1985), and official delinquency statistics (Wadsworth, 1979). Recent reviews of this association all concur that divorced children are more likely to show externalizing behaviors, particularly boys (Emery, 1982, 1988; Felner, Farber, & Primavera, 1980; Lamb, 1977).

Internalizing Problems

The relation between divorce and internalizing problems has been less compelling than for externalizing problems. Scattered evidence suggests that there might be such a relation (Peterson & Zill, 1986), particularly for girls (Furstenberg & Allison, 1989). However, despite the voluminous theoretical literature relating the experience of parental loss through divorce or death to children's susceptibility to internalizing problems, relatively few investigators have found such a relation to exist. This lack of association can be partly attributed to difficulties in operationalizing the precise meaning of internalizing disorders in childhood (e.g., depression) and to the lack of observability of internalizing when compared with externalizing behaviors. Still, the evidence remains equivocal.

In two studies of samples of 200 children, consisting of middle school and high school students, respectively (Raschke & Raschke, 1979; Slater & Haber, 1984), no differences were found in the reported self-concepts of children from divorced and two-parent families. Berg and Kelly (1979) also found no differences between the same two groups in a sample of boys ranging from grammar to high school age. However, in a study of *recently* divorced families of 11- to 13-year-old children, significant differences were found between divorced and married families (Forehand, McCombs, Long, Brody, & Fauber, 1988). Two other studies also found differences between groups on the dimension of self-concept as long as the divorced mothers had yet to remarry (Parrish & Taylor, 1979; Young & Parish, 1977). Finally, results from the NSC database indicated an increase in self-reported distress among girls from disrupted marriages (Furstenberg & Allison, 1989). And at five-year followup, more depressed/withdrawn behavior was found among girls and boys from divorced families (Peterson & Zill, 1986). This increase in internalizing symptomatology was also more pronounced among high-conflict, married families.

Cognitive Deficits

Like much of the research on divorce and children's adjustment in general, the majority of investigations in this area have not partitioned out the effects of "third variables" in explaining children's functioning. Single-parent status and lowered family income—two common consequences of divorce—are two factors that need to be ruled out before attributing changes in child functioning exclusively to the parental separation. For example, there is agreement that children raised in *single*-parent families perform more poorly than children from two-parent families in a number of academic areas, though the magnitude of these differences tends to be small. In reviews by Hetherington, Camera, and Featherman (1981) and Shinn (1978), children from single-parent families show deficits in (1) IQ scores, ranging between 1 and 7 points; (2) lower school achievement scores averaging less than one year in school; and (3) lower grade attainment of three-quarters of a year. However, not all of these families attained single-parent status via divorce.

Socioeconomic status (SES) also has been related to poor achievement and correlated with single-parent status. However, when the effects of social class are taken into account, though academic differences are less, children from single-parent families still show significantly poorer academic functioning than children from two-parent families (Featherman & Hauser, 1978; Ferri, 1976; Guidubaldi, Perry, & Cleminshaw, 1984; Lambert & Hart, 1976; Zill, 1978). Moreover, when both the effects of SES and the reason for single-parent status are accounted for, investigators have generally found that children from divorced families to *more* poorly on academic tasks than children from other types of single-parent families (Ferri, 1976; Gregory, 1965; Santrock, 1972; Zill, 1978). Children from non-divorced, single-parent families, in turn, appear to experience more academic difficulties than children from two-parent families.

Guidubaldi and colleagues' (1984) study of 699 children from 38 states provided some insight as to how children from divorced families might differ from children from other types of single-parent and two-parent families. Again, we know from other research that children from single-parent families show small, but significant differences on measures of intellectual capacity and school achievement compared with two-parent families. However, these differences are much larger, according to the Guidubaldi and colleagues' data, if measured by teacher behavior ratings, grade point averages, school attendance, and number of years in school. Divorced children in particular were found to be significantly more dependent, noncompliant, and unpopular with peers according to teacher reports. They also had a history of lower grades in history and math, and were more likely to have repeated a grade.

If children are having problems with adjusting to the transition of divorce, particularly in the first two years following the separation, it is probable that their poorer school performance could be mediated by their behavior problems at school.

The disequilibrium at home may make school a low priority, especially given the inconsistent parenting practices known to follow divorce. Data from teachers' reports of child behavior and lowered child attendance support this interpretation of why children from divorced families would perform more inadequately than children from other types of single-parent families.

ASSESSMENT

Although children from divorced families show a wide array of behavioral difficulties at home and in school, the criteria used for diagnosis of these problems do not differ considerably from children of two-parent families. What does differ for children from divorced families are the issues that may precipitate problems. This section will review factors that have been related to poorer outcomes for divorced children.

As previously stated, divorce in and of itself is not a reliable indicator of child psychopathology. As research on divorce and children's adaptation has accumulated, there has been a gradual shift in emphasis from family structure to family process (Emery, 1988; Emery, Hetherington, & DiLalla, 1984). That is, events that accompany marital dissolution, rather than the event of divorce per se, have been identified as potentially more salient correlates of children's adjustment (Berg & Kelly, 1979; Emery, 1982, 1988; Shaw & Emery, 1987, 1988; Shaw, 1989). Longitudinal investigations of divorced families (Hetherington, Cox, & Cox, 1978, 1981; Wallerstein & Kelly, 1980, 1983) have provided particularly strong support for this focus on family process. Rather than discuss how "the" divorced child will adapt to divorce, investigators have redirected their attention to mediating factors that might account for the heterogeneity of child outcomes to divorce.

Within this family process perspective, Emery (1988) and Hetherington (1979) have suggested that the psychological impact of divorce on children needs to be divided into at least two levels. The first level relates to the short-term effects of the parental separation on the children's adjustment—a process that all children must undergo. Hetherington (1981) has conceptualized this initial transition in terms of a crisis model. From this perspective, children and adults must adapt to stresses associated with parental separation, including marital conflict, loss, and uncertainty.

The second level is related to the long-term psychological impact of divorce on children's adjustment. In the long-term, children's functioning reflects the family's adaptation to the changes necessitated by the divorce. As we shall see, children's long-term adjustment to divorce may be better, worse, or merely different than their predivorce adjustment, but appears to be mediated by several interrelated family process variables. These process variables include changes and adaptations in the following areas: (1) interparental conflict; (2) separation from an attachment figure; (3) temporal influences, including the passage of time and the child's age at the time of divorce; (4) parenting practices and nature of the relationship between the residential parent and children; (5) the relationship between children and their non-residential parents; (6) remarriage; and (7) family economics.

Interparental Conflict

Although clinicians have postulated an association between parental conflict and maladjustment in children for many years (Baruch & Wilcox, 1944; Minuchin. 1974), empirical attention to the effects of parental discord on children has increased only in the last decade. From these recent controlled studies and from earlier reports of so-called broken families, interparental conflict has been consistently identified as a major source of behavior problems in children across a wide array of family structures and settings (Christoupolus et al., 1987; Emery & O'Leary, 1982; Hetherington, Cox, & Cox, 1985; Porter & O'Leary, 1980; Shaw, 1989; Wolfe, Jaffe, Zak, & Wilson, 1986), including divorced and separated families (Hetherington, 1979; Kurdek, 1981; Shaw & Emery, 1987; Wallerstein & Kelly, 1983).

In fact, results from two types of between-family comparisons suggest that separation is not necessarily as important to children's later development as the quality of the parents' relationship with one another (Hetherington, Cox, & Cox,

1979; Jacobson, 1978; Lowenstein & Koopman, 1978; Rosen, 1979). First, research efforts that have compared maritally intact, conflictual homes with conflict-free, single-parent families consistently have reported that children in the latter group have fewer emotional difficulties (Gibson, 1969; Hetherington et al., 1979; McCord, McCord, & Thurber, 1962; Nye, 1957; Power, Ash, Schoenberg, & Sorey, 1974; Rutter, 1979).

The second type of between-family comparison has been conducted with different types of single-parent families. Although research on attachment has found evidence that separation from a parent in and of itself may be a salient factor in children's later adjustment (Bendiksen & Fulton, 1975; Bowlby, 1963, 1980; Rutter, 1966), several investigators have reported children from divorced families to experience more behavioral problems than children from families where a father has died (Douglas, Ross, Hammond, & Mulligan, 1966; Glueck & Glueck, 1950; Gibson, 1969; Gregory, 1965; Rutter et al., 1975a, 1975b).

Separation from an Attachment Figure

Despite the evidence implicating the greater importance of interparental conflict than separation from an attachment figure in mediating children's adjustment to divorce, literature from other areas of child development suggests that children's separation from, and loss of, attachment figures relates to difficulties in interpersonal relationships (Ainsworth, 1979; Bowlby, 1951). Unfortunately, there is a dearth of research that examines how divorce per se affects children's attachment to their parents and their other interpersonal relationships. Clinical experience and research from other contexts (i.e., children's reactions to parental death, separation due to military service) indicate that the short-term consequences of separation from an attachment figure follow a three-stage "acute distress syndrome" of upset/protest, followed by apathy/despair, and subsequent loss of interest/detachment (Bowlby, 1980; Rutter, 1981). Less is known about the long-term adjustment of children who experience such a loss, particularly in the context

of divorce, where visitation schedules and custody arrangements are subject to change.

Thus, it is difficult to ascertain if problems are directly related to the separation, to other family process variables, or to a combination of factors. It appears likely that the latter case would be the norm, with the loss of the attachment figure being more of a cause for concern to the child when the divorce has taken place recently. Other family process variables may also exacerbate the child's sense of loss and provide him or her with little sense of security to function in the postdivorce environment.

Temporal Influences

One temporal influence is the passage of time since the parental separation. There is an adage, "Time heals all wounds." In understanding children's adjustment to divorce, the maxim has proven to be quite accurate. From a theoretical perspective, the healing properties of time have been conceptualized within Hetherington's (1981) crisis model of the short-term adaptation to divorce. As time passes, many of the stressors associated with divorce are lessened in intensity as adults and children adapt to new living situations. Thus, an 8-year-old child whose parents were divorced six years ago will most likely appear different from a child of the same age whose parents separated last year.

Unfortunately, from an empirical perspective, many investigators have failed to consider how long it has been since the parental separation took place when presenting their findings. Yet Kurdek (1981), Hetherington (1981), and Wallerstein and Kelly (1983) have all found that children's adjustment improves with time, as family members learn to cope with new living arrangements. Though this evidence is not conclusive, we do know that more children experience greater adjustment difficulties in responding to divorce in the short run rather than the long run. In the more methodologically rigorous of the three studies cited above, Hetherington (1979) found that most children were showing improved functioning after two years following the parental separation, provided that other family process variables were not interfering with the adaptation process (e.g., continued conflict between parents).

Another temporal issue of considerable practical significance is the child's age at the time of the divorce. Parents often wonder whether they should stay together "for the sake of the child" until a certain age. There are several theoretical viewpoints on this topic that suggest children will differentially interpret the parental separation according to their stage of cognitive and emotional development (Ainsworth, 1979; Bowlby, 1980; Goldstein, Freud, & Solnit, 1973; Meissner, 1978). However, relatively little empirical data have been gathered to answer this question, particularly studies that control for *both* the children's age at the time of divorce and the length of time since the parental separation occurred. Moreover, the research that has been carried out in this area has typically compared children who were younger than 5 or 6 years old when their parents separated with children whose parents separated after that age, making the task of drawing inferences between school-age and adolescent children difficult. In general, there are reasons to believe that many age groups might be more vulnerable to the effects of divorce.

Some investigators have hypothesized that preschoolers may be the most vulnerable group in dealing with a divorce because of their limited cognitive capacity (Hetherington, 1979; Kurdek, 1981; McDermott, 1968; Wallerstein & Kelly, 1980). Preschool-aged children often report feeling they are to blame for their parents' troubles due to an inability to fully appreciate the complexity of their parents' feelings and behavior (Hetherington, 1979).

Although school-aged children have been found to be more aware of the reasons and rationales for their parents' emotional difficulties, some of these children have exhibited marked signs of distress and depression (Hetherington, 1981). Wallerstein and Kelly (1980) found children in the 5- to 8-year range overcome by pervasive sadness and a yearning for their parents' reconciliation. Children ages 9 and 10, while sharing some of the same feelings of sadness, displayed a greater capacity for worry and genuine empathy for their parents (Wallerstein & Kelly, 1974).

Some investigators have argued that adolescents should have fewer emotional problems in coping with divorce because of their advanced cognitive maturity and their increased likelihood for having social support outside of the nuclear family (Hetherington, 1981). However, others have hypothesized that these children should be the most affected due to their longer exposure to the conflict (Sorosky, 1977; Wallerstein & Kelly, 1974, 1980) and their more pronounced feelings of responsibility for their parents' separation.

Kurdek, Blisk, and Siesky (1981) have completed a longitudinal study of upper middle-class adolescents whose parents had separated within the last one to seven years, and found children's levels of interpersonal reasoning and locus of control to be important mediating variables in predicting their adjustment later in time. Other researchers have found similar components important in mediating adolescents' divorce experience, including the development of heterosexual relations, self-identity, and independence (Hetherington, 1972; Sorosky, 1977; Wallerstein & Kelly, 1980).

The Relationship Between the Residential Parent and the Child

The term *change* was used to describe children's adaptation to divorce at the beginning of this chapter. Nowhere are these changes more apparent than in the relationships children have with their parents following the marital dissolution. Although this is true for both nonresidential and residential parents, disruptions in the latter's child-rearing activities are so frequent and dramatic in the first few years following divorce that Wallerstein and Kelly (1980) have termed it a time of "diminished parenting." Since mothers continue to dominate as primary residential parents (i.e., the rate of father-custody families continues to be about 10 percent), even in families that share legal custody, the discussion that follows will pertain to issues faced in mother-headed divorced families. For the residential parent, many of these changes reflect the challenges of single-parent family status. As homeostatic balances in the family are disrupted, new equilibriums must be achieved in at least three substantive areas: (1) affectional relationships, (2) family authority structure, and (3) household task completion (Emery, 1988).

First, affectional relationships may be drawn closer or more distant due to the parent's own emotional needs, the parent's perception of the child's needs, or loyalty dilemmas in the parent-child-parent triad. Since Hetherington's (1986; Hetherington, Cox, & Cox, 1985) longitudinal study of mother-custody families is the most detailed empirical investigation of parenting practices in divorcing families, these findings will be the primary source of reference in this area. In the first year following divorce, compared with always-married women, Hetherington found divorced mothers to be less affectionate with their children, particularly boys. However, by two years following the divorce, there was an increase in maternal nurturant behavior towards children.

Hetherington also found the same disorganization-reorganization pattern of events in the domains of family structure and household task completion. Both processes appear to undergo dramatic change in the first year following divorce as children assume a greater amount of independence and number of responsibilities. This transformation, however, is not particularly smooth in the first year. Hetherington and others (Burgess, 1978; Colletta, 1979) report that custodial mothers make fewer maturity demands, communicate less well, and generally show more negative and inconsistent parenting practices than do married mothers. At the two-year followup, Hetherington's mothers had become more consistent and better able to control their children, though overall, children divorced families remained less compliant than children from two-parent families. Finally, at the six-year followup, divorced mothers were just as nurturant as nondivorced mothers, but continued to be more negative and less competent in disciplining their sons.

Though there is little empirical evidence to document other dysfunctional patterns of parent-child relationships following divorce, clinical experience suggests that problems at the opposite extremes also occur. For example, some mothers might become overly permissive, rigid, or emotionally dependent on their children. When parents lack a supportive other, discipline policies might be compromised because of the increased emotional dependence on the child, changing the nature of the hierarchical parent-child relationship to one where parent and child are confidantes. Unfortunately, parents who share this type of relationship with their children are more likely to use permissive parenting strategies for fear of loss of the child's willingness to play the role of friend. Similarly, it is likely that some parents react to adverse changes in emotional and financial resources associated with the divorce with a more rigid type of parenting style.

In sum, long-term disturbances in parenting are probably mediated by a number of factors, including the mother's emotional well-being, the social and economic support available to her, and the number, ages, and sex of the children (Emery, 1988). This has been demonstrated empirically, as mothers who are depressed, who are cut off from family and friendship support networks, who have more severe economic difficulties, or who have a number of young children are more likely to have parenting difficulties with their children (Emery et al., 1984).

The Relationship Between the Nonresidential Parent and the Child

The relationship between children and their nonresidential parents also must undergo a great transformation following divorce. The frequency of contact obviously changes as nonresidential parents, typically fathers, establish a new homeostatic balance with their children. However, before we review how this variable might affect children's adjustment, it is important to understand how frequent such visitations are on the average.

Using the NSC data based on a nationally representative sample (Furstenberg, Peterson, Nord, & Zill, 1983), it is illuminating to note that 50 percent of children did not see their fathers in the past year, and only 16.4 percent saw them as frequently as once a week or more. Contact with nonresidential mothers is substantially higher, with only 13 percent of children not seeing their non-residential mothers in the past year and 31 percent seeing their mothers on at least a weekly basis. Several factors are related to frequency of visitation for fathers. They include (1) time: as it passes, contact decreases; (2) education: more highly educated fathers spend significantly more time with their children; (3) race: black fathers spend significantly less time with their children than do whites or other minorities; and (4) distance to the residential parent's house: the closer the distance, the greater the amount of visitation.

Perhaps even more surprising than the lack of time nonresidential parents spend with their children is the lack of consensus regarding how frequency of contact with the nonresidential parent affects child adjustment. Hetherington and colleagues (1978) and Wallerstein and Kelly (1980) found that frequency of visitation was positively related to child adjustment except when the father was emotionally disturbed or interparental conflict was high. Similarly, Hess and Camera (1979) reported visitation duration, but not frequency, to be related to improved child adjustment.

However, several studies have failed to establish this link. In fact, using the NSC data, Furstenberg, Morgan, and Allison (987) found few significant relations between frequency of contact and child adjustment covering a wide variety of domains. Other researchers have also failed to replicate Hetherington's and Wallerstein and Kelly's results (Kurdek et al., 1981; Luepnitz, 1982). In fact, Hodges, Wechsler, and Ballantine (1979) found that greater contact was associated with increased aggression according to mother's and teacher's reports. Again, frequency of contact and child adjustment is probably mediated by other factors, including the quality of both the father-child and father-mother interaction. Indeed, there is some research to suggest that having a good relationship with one parent can buffer the adverse effects of divorce (Hetherington et al., 1979; Peterson & Zill, 1986; Rutter, 1971). However, given the influence and interaction of other family process variables, such as interparental conflict, it remains unclear whether the frequency of contact by the nonresidential parent is related to long-term child adjustment to divorce.

Remarriage

Remarriage is another environmental stressor many children from divorced families must face. The nationally representative NSC data indicate that within five years of a marital disruption, four of seven white children and one of eight black children will enter stepfamilies (Furstenberg et al., 1983). Thus, for at least the majority of children from white families, living in a single-parent family will not be a long-term circumstance. For children from black families, single-parent status is likely to be more of an enduring condition. Though space does not permit a thorough investigation of how this transition affects children's functioning, a few pertinent findings will be discussed.

First, though this area of literature is fraught with even more methodological problems than research on children's adjustment to divorce, there is some preliminary evidence to suggest that boys from divorced families experience benefits from remarriage (Chapman, 1977; Oshman & Manosevitz, 1976), whereas girls respond unfavorably (Clingempeel, Brand, & Ievoli, 1984; Santrock, Warshak, Lindbergh, & Meadows, 1982). The sex difference is believed to be a function of children's relationships with the custodial parent. Since most children reside with their mothers following divorce, this transition typically involves the addition of a stepfather. For boys, the addition of a same-sex parent may serve to buffer the strained mother-son relationship that typically follows divorce (Hetherington, 1986). But for girls, who tend to draw closer to mothers following divorce, the stepfather may be viewed as an intruder (Peterson & Zill, 1986).

Remarriage may also produce other changes for children, including a decrease of visitation with the nonresidential parent (Furstenberg et al., 1983), increased parental conflict between the children's biological parents (Wallerstein & Kelly, 1980), and an additional parental divorce (Furstenberg & Spanier, 1984). With regard to this latter finding, the presence of children from a previous marriage is associated with an increased risk of divorce (Emery, 1988). In the NSC study, 37 percent of children who entered a stepfamily later experienced an additional parental divorce, with 10 percent experiencing three or more marital changes.

Family Economics

Loss of family income is a reality of divorce, particularly for mothers. Since mothers are generally the primary custodians of children following divorce, most children experience a lowered standard of living. In analyzing the effects of loss of income on children's adjustment to divorce, it has been a difficult task to partition out the effects of low-income and single-parent status (which occurs for a number of reasons other than divorce) from divorce in particular (Emery, 1988). However, using data from the Michigan Panel Study of Income Dynamics (MPSID) based on the changing incomes of 2,400 women, Hoffman (1977) found that the real income of couples who divorced decreased 19.2 percent for men and 29.3 percent for women between 1968 and 1974. The fact that women were more likely to be responsible for the primary care of children was the single factor most responsible for the difference. Although many fathers are required to pay child support as a part of the divorce settlement, compliance with support orders is the exception, not the rule (Emery, 1988). In 1981, only 47 percent of mothers who were ordered to receive child support received the full amount; 28 percent received no payment at all (National Institute for Child Support Enforcement, 1986).

What does a loss of income mean to a child from a divorcing family? The impact is likely to include several changes that cumulatively appear to have the effect of debilitating children's coping resources. Some of the consequences include moving the family home, changing schools, losing contact with friends, spending more time in daycare settings while mother is working, and dealing with the parent's concerns over financial pressures (Emery, 1988). These factors might, in turn, affect the quality and quantity of interactions children have with their residential parent. Though very few investigators have attempted to identify how economic factors might be related to increased psychological impairment, divorced working mothers do provide less cognitive and social stimulation to their children than both married nonworking and married working mothers (MacKinnon, Brody, & Stoneman, 1982). Thus, children might be affected psychologically by the loss of income at two levels: (1) indirectly through poorer parenting, as residential parents have less time and energy to give to their children because of the increased demands necessitated by the loss of income; and (2) directly through the changes in environmental circumstances such as lower-quality schools and neighborhoods, and the loss of friends.

TREATMENT

Evidence for Prescriptive Treatments

Despite the multitude of modalities and techniques, there is a paucity of empirical evidence for prescriptive treatments with children of divorce. To date, there have been *no* systematic investigations of the efficacy of individual or family interventions designed specifically for divorced families. The majority of well-controlled treatment outcome research has been conducted with school-based, group interventions. These findings are limited because the children were not identified as *clinically* disturbed. Nevertheless, many of the studies demonstrated statistically significant positive results on pre- and posttreatment measures of adjustment.

Stolberg and colleagues (Stolberg, Cullen, & Garrison, 1982; Stolberg & Garrison, 1985) developed a preventive program, the Divorce Adjustment Project (DAP), intended for psychologically *healthy* children facing divorce. The DAP consisted of school-based, children's support groups (CSG) and community-based single-parent's support groups (SPSG). The children's support group treatment consisted of 12 sessions. The first part of each 60-minute session was devoted to discussion of divorce-related topics; the second part focused on teaching problem-solving, anger control, communication, and relaxation skills. The parent's group—a 12-week support and skills-building program for divorced, custodial mothers—was expected to indirectly influence children's adjustment by enhancing parenting skills and the postdivorce adjustment of their parents.

Some 82 children (aged 7 to 13 years) and their mothers participated in one of four treatment groups: child intervention alone, parent intervention alone, concurrent child and parent intervention, and no intervention. At posttreatment and five-month followup, subjects in the children's support group reported statistically significant improvements in self-concept and adaptive social skills. When parents participated in the support group, treatment prevented the deterioration in parent adjustment found in the other groups at posttesting, but had no demonstrable effect on children's adjustment. The concurrent child and parent intervention yielded no significant improvements for either children or parents. The authors suggest that this lack of effect may be related to the nonrandom group assignment, which resulted in significant between-groups differences. Mothers in the concurrent parent-child treatment groups had been separated longer, had lower employment status, and reported less time spent by noncustodial fathers with their children.

As an outgrowth of the DAP, Pedro-Carroll and Cowen (1985) created the Children of Divorce Intervention Project (CODIP), a group program consisting of 10 sessions, with a focus on mutual support and cognitive-behavioral skills. Additionally, the program included an affective component and involved activities designed to enhance child self-esteem. In two investigations of the efficacy of CODIP with fourth- to sixth-grade suburban school children (Pedro-Carroll & Cowen, 1985; Pedro-Carroll, Cowen, Hightower, & Guare, 1986), the experimental groups demonstrated greater improvement on child, parent, and teacher ratings of adjustment relative to comparison and control groups. Similar positive effects were reported with younger, urban school children, using an age-appropriate version of the program (Alpert-Gillis, Pedro-Carroll, & Cowen, 1989).

A few caveats concerning the Pedro-Carroll and colleagues' studies are worthy of mention. First, the level of child disturbance was limited to subjects who were not currently in therapy or receiving mental health services. Although the children of divorce showed more problems than the intact comparison group on many measures (Alpert-Gillis et al., 1989; Pedro-Carroll et al., 1986), it is not clear that these differences were clinically significant. Second, parents and teachers were aware of the children's group status, which indicates a potential for bias and a need for caution in interpreting results.

Although parental conflict has been identified as an important influence on children's adjustment (Emery, 1982, 1988), only one intervention study has considered this component directly as it affects child outcome. Bornstein, Bornstein, and Walters (1985) developed and investigated a six-session, group treatment program focusing on identification of feelings, communication skills, and anger control skills. The first five sessions involved only the children (aged 7 to 14 years). The sixth session also included their recently separated or divorced parents. Subjects were assigned to one of two experimental groups or a delayed treatment control group, matched for age, sex, and parent ratings of parent-parent conflict.

The results of the investigation were ambiguous. Parents in the experimental condition indicated substantially improved relationships with their ex-spouses. Whether this change was a function of time, treatment effect, or the knowledge that their child had participated in a divorce adjustment program was unclear. Although teachers reported a decrease in child problem behavior in the experimental group, overall child adjustment was judged unchanged by both parent and child reports. Despite the apparent lack of improvement, both child and adult consumer satisfaction questionnaires revealed high levels of satisfaction with the treatment program.

These data suggest that affective sharing in a supportive group environment, as well as instruction in interpersonal skills, problem solving, and anger management, are effective in improving the adjustment of *non*disturbed children. Whether such programs are beneficial to children presenting with clinically significant levels of pathology is unknown. The only two studies of the efficacy of such treatments on levels of depression in children did not make criterion-based diagnoses, and report conflicting results (see Crosbie-Burnett & Newcomer, 1990; Roseby & Deutsch, 1985).

One additional area of intervention deserves mention because of its *potential* for improving the adjustment of children from divorced families — divorce mediation. Given the established relation between postdivorce parental acrimony and child behavior problems, divorce mediation represents an indirect means of providing assistance to children caught in the middle of their separated parents' conflict. To date, it appears to be the only type of divorce therapy that has received "considerable" empirical attention (Gurman, Kniskern, & Pinsoff, 1986; Sprenkle & Storm, 1983). Though the most obvious goal of divorce mediation is to negotiate a mutually acceptable divorce settlement, it provides a chance for couples to address areas of disagreement and possibly decrease the amount of acrimony for future relations (Emery & Shaw, 1989; Emery, Shaw, & Jackson, 1987).

Thus far, research on divorce mediation has demonstrated that it represents a viable alternative to the antagonistic climate of traditional divorce court proceedings, and an especially more appealing alternative for fathers who often feel dissatisfied with adversarial procedures (Emery & Wyer, 1987). However, no data are yet available to assess whether mediation's hypothesized potential for decreasing parental conflict also may have long-term benefits for children's psychological well-being.

CASE ILLUSTRATION

Case Description

This case study represents a compilation of several real cases seen by the coauthors. Its intent is to illustrate the challenges associated with treating children from divorced families.

Initially, Mrs. Joanne Pilbus, age 32, contacted the Psychology Department Clinic because of the problematic behavior of her 11-year-old son, Reggie. At the time of the phone intake, Mrs. Pilbus mentioned that she had separated from her husband, Jim Pilbus, age 35, nine months ago. Reggie's behavior had begun deteriorating a few months prior to the separation. Mrs. Pilbus noted that her other child, Alicia, age 8, had shown few behavior problems since the separation, though Alicia did speak of missing her father about once every two weeks.

According to Mrs. Pilbus, Reggie was currently demonstrating externalizing behavior problems at home and at school. At home, Reggie had developed a pattern of noncompliance and defiance toward his mother, including refusing to complete daily chores and consistently challenging Mrs. Pilbus's authority to make family decisions. Reggie had also developed an "attitude" toward Alicia, regularly starting fights and acting aggressively toward her. At school, Reggie's grades had fallen from A's and B's to C's and D's in the past six months, and he had been suspended from school twice during the same period of time for fighting with peers during recess. According to Mrs. Pilbus, Reggie had only begun having behavior problems at home and school shortly prior to the parental separation. Previously, though he showed an occasional temper tantrum at home, he completed chores regularly, questioned Mrs. Pilbus's authority only once every month or two, and had never engaged in fighting at school.

During the phone intake, Mrs. Pilbus described her relationship with Mr. Pilbus as "horrible," commenting that the divorce had become "messier and messier" during the past year. According to Mrs. Pilbus, the marriage had dissolved because Mr. Pilbus had engaged in several extramarital affairs. Mr. Pilbus was now living with Ms. Sylvia Duncan, age 24, whom he had begun seeing prior to the Pilbus's separation. Mrs. Pilbus stated that she was still extremely angry at Mr. Pilbus concerning the affairs and the dissolution of the marriage. She noted that she only talks to Mr. Pilbus when "it is absolutely necessary." When asked if

Mrs. Pilbus thought Mr. Pilbus would be interested in helping with Reggie's problems, Mrs. Pilbus responded, "Probably not," and that she would prefer as little contact as possible with Mr. Pilbus.

When asked if and how often the two children were seeing their father, she commented that Mr. Pilbus's visitation was "irregular at best." During the first few months after the initial separation, he had seen the children at least once every two weeks, but during the past four to five months, his contact had become sporadic. In the past two months, he had seen Reggie and Alicia only once. Mr. Pilbus had also been negligent in making child support payments, following the same pattern as visitation, wavering from an initially consistent record.

The initial intake session included Mrs. Pilbus and the two children. Based on Mrs. Pilbus's information about Mr. Pilbus's behavior and the couple's willingness to work together, he was not included in the initial intake. During the intake, Mrs. Pilbus was very adamant about both Reggie's and Mr. Pilbus's misbehavior. Though Alicia spoke only when spoken to, Reggie articulately defended his own *and* his father's behavior, challenging Mrs. Pilbus's competency to make decisions for the family, especially his own behavior. He suggested that Mrs. Pilbus had become extremely inconsistent in establishing and enforcing rules in the past year. When Reggie was asked about his behavior at school, he was less forthcoming, stating only that he would be "okay if people just left him alone." When asked to describe the quality of his relationship with his father, Reggie said it was "good," and that he would very much like to see his father more often than he had recently.

Differential Diagnosis

The Pilbus family was dealing with several of the most problematic issues facing recently separated families. These include highly acrimonious relations between the separating parents, disturbed relations between the residential parent and her son (including problems in parenting), and problematic relations between the nonresidential parent and the two children. It was also clear that both children missed seeing their father on a regular basis, especially Reggie. Finally, though Mr. Pilbus had not yet remarried, he was now living with another woman. The children had only met Ms. Duncan twice and were not forthcoming with positive or negative opinions about her.

Though Mr. and Mrs. Pilbus had been separated for nine months, the family still appeared to be in the midst of Hetherington's (1981) crisis phase in adapting to the separation. For the family to make the successful adjustment, several unresolved issues would need to be addressed. Based on the cross-sectional and longitudinal research conducted in the area along with the limited number of intervention studies, the following goals were suggested for effective intervention: (1) decreasing the amount of parental acrimony between Mr. and Mrs. Pilbus; (2) improving the relationship between Mrs. Pilbus and her children, particularly Reggie; (3) working with Mrs. Pilbus to empower her parenting and establish a more consistent, authoritative style; (4) exploring ways to improve the children's contacts with Mr. Pilbus, especially working to enhance the frequency and consistency of visitation; and (5) finding an outlet for the children, particularly Reggie, to vent some of their hurt and frustration in dealing with the loss of their parents' marriage and daily contact with their father.

Treatment Selection

Treatment was planned to address as many of the aforementioned issues as possible. First, to improve the parenting of Mrs. Pilbus and relations between her and Reggie, family sessions were held. Second, an attempt was made to contact Mr. Pilbus, despite Mrs. Pilbus's objections, to explore ways of improving the couple's relationship as well as Mr. Pilbus's relationship with his children. Finally, an attempt was made to find a group for children from divorced families, for both Reggie and Alicia, to help cope with the complex transitions of the divorce process.

Treatment Course and Problems in Carrying Out Interventions

A multifaceted treatment package was designed and implemented based on the goals detailed above. In the first few months, treatment was marked by variability in Reggie's behavior and by problems in implementing specific components of intervention. Family meetings with Mrs. Pilbus and the two children were initiated immediately following the first intake session. Family work was aimed at improving the quality of communication between the children and Mrs. Pilbus, particularly Reggie and his mother. The therapist also worked to improve the consistency of Mrs. Pilbus's parenting, encouraging her to provide and uphold a firm set of rules for the children.

Both Reggie and Alicia were encouraged to help Mrs. Pilbus design family regulations. However, Mrs. Pilbus was treated as the higher voice of authority in resolving disputes. Though Reggie's behavior showed dramatic improvement during the first few weeks of therapy, there were two weeks in the second and third months of treatment in which he showed signs of regression. On one occasion, Reggie was involved in a fight at school, while on another occasion he refused to complete chores at home for a full week. Overall, Mrs. Pilbus was showing greater consistency in setting and enforcing rules, while Reggie's behavior was marked by inconsistency.

While "family" treatment was initiated without delay, involving Mr. Pilbus in therapy was a more difficult task. Although Mr. Pilbus sounded eager to be more involved with his children and resolve disputes with Mrs. Pilbus during the initial phone contact, he was less cooperative in his attendance at sessions. An initial session with Mr. Pilbus alone was scheduled to discuss his past experiences and present goals for improving family relations. After two cancellations, Mr. Pilbus met with the therapist. At this session, Mr. Pilbus agreed with many of the goals expressed by Mrs. Pilbus and the children. He concurred with the children's wishes to spend more time together and not let the quality of his relationship with Mrs. Pilbus get in the way of his relationship with Reggie and Alicia.

He added to these goals a desire for the children to get to know Ms. Duncan. Conjoint sessions were planned with the children and with Mrs. Pilbus separately.

After the children had reestablished contact with Mr. Pilbus, plans were made to include Ms. Duncan in family meetings with the children. Mr. Pilbus repeatedly needed to cancel family sessions during the first month of work. However, during the second and third month of treatment, sessions were held three out of every four weeks. Sessions focused on reestablishing positive relations between Mr. Pilbus and the children. Mr. Pilbus was able to explain his frustration in having enough time for Reggie and Alicia, while at the same time maintaining his relationship with Ms. Duncan. The children, especially Reggie, were permitted to vent their anger and hurt concerning their parents' divorce and their father's perceived abandonment of them since the separation.

At the end of three months of treatment, although some goals of therapy were beginning to become actualized (e.g., improved parenting of the residential parent, reestablishment of relations between the children and nonresidential parent), several issues remained unresolved. First, no children's divorce group was located for Reggie or Alicia. Despite efforts to find such a treatment modality throughout the course of treatment, these were unsuccessful. Second and most notably, the parents' level of conflict continued to be elevated. To treat this latter issue, the next phase of intervention involved conjoint sessions with Mr. and Mrs. Pilbus *without* the children. Though these sessions were not intended as mediation, many of the goals of mediation were achieved.

Mrs. Pilbus was reluctant to attend sessions with Mr. Pilbus, but the therapist was able to convince her of the importance of the sessions for the children's well-being, if not for herself. Although the first two of these sessions were marked by hostile comments from Mrs. Pilbus and bitter counterattacks by Mr. Pilbus, both sessions were productive in establishing a structured medium for the parents to discuss time-sharing issues. The therapist played an active role to minimize open conflict by structuring most of the sessions closely (see Emery, Shaw, & Jackson, 1987). Both Mr. and Mrs. Pilbus were permitted to vent their anger, but only in a controlled manner (e.g., when tempers flared, the therapist intervened to literally stop the interaction). Discussions were focused on plans for changing the present circumstances concerning visitation and support. Mr. Pilbus was encouraged to visit more frequently, but at times all parties found acceptable. Mr. Pilbus also was encouraged to provide consistent child support payments.

By the end of the second session, both Mr. and Mrs. Pilbus had agreed in principle to these proposed changes. The parents were encouraged to think of visitation plans that would be mutually acceptable during the week. In the meantime, a visit with the children was arranged for Mr. Pilbus. After four more sessions, firm plans were laid for visitation and support. Though Mr. and Mrs. Pilbus were not particularly friendly to one another during most of the meetings, they "agreed to disagree" and work out their disagreements over time sharing for the children's welfare.

While the work with Mr. and Mrs. Pilbus was taking place in months 4 to 6 of therapy, Reggie and Alicia also were meeting with the therapist each week. Some of these sessions were held with Mrs. Pilbus in order to continue working on parenting and mother-child relationship issues. Other sessions involved Mr. Pilbus and sometimes Ms. Duncan in order to discuss parent-child issues and relations with Ms. Duncan, respectively. Though the children initially were not pleased with the introduction of Ms. Duncan into sessions, once rapport with their father had been improved, her presence was tolerated and even appreciated at times (e.g., when she stood up for the children's point of view in discussing rules at Mr. Pilbus's residence). Finally, once a month the children met with the therapist alone to discuss intrapersonal issues surrounding the divorce process. Though these sessions were not viewed as a replacement for the children's group, they did allow both Reggie and Alicia to explore and vent feelings relating to the divorce process.

Outcome and Termination

All phases of therapy were terminated seven months after the initial intake. Many of the in-

itial goals of therapy were attained. At termination, relations between Mr. and Mrs. Pilbus, as well as relations between the children and their parents, had showed great improvement. Reggie's behavior at home and school had returned to levels approaching his status prior to the parental separation. Fighting with peers at school and at home with Alicia had diminished dramatically. Reggie's school work had also improved, though he did receive two C's on his report card prior to termination.

Mr. and Mrs. Pilbus continued to minimize contact with one another but were successful in establishing a consistent visitation schedule for their children. Mr. Pilbus also was more consistent with support payments. He was two weeks late on one payment during the course of therapy, but this issue was raised and discussed without altercation in therapy. Though Mrs. Pilbus was not pleased with the incident, she tolerated the delay without retribution toward Mr. Pilbus (e.g., withholding visitation privileges).

Followup and Maintenance

At termination, all parties were informed that the therapist would be available for further consultation should the need arise. A "check-up" session was scheduled with Mr. and Mrs. Pilbus and the children four months following termination to ensure that gains achieved in therapy were maintained. One month prior to the scheduled session, Mrs. Pilbus called the therapist to request a session alone with the therapist concerning Mr. Pilbus's behavior. After reviewing the impetus for the call, it was suggested that Mr. Pilbus also attend this meeting. According to Mrs. Pilbus, though relations with the children and Mr. Pilbus were generally going well, Mr. Pilbus had become more lax in picking up and returning the children at scheduled times. Mr. Pilbus agreed to attend the meeting.

At the session, the therapist began by complimenting the parents on their success during the last few months, but quickly moved to discuss the current reason for meeting. Mr. Pilbus admitted he had become less conscientious in the past few months, but did not appreciate the extent to which this had bothered Mrs. Pilbus. She was given time to explain to Mr. Pilbus how the change in scheduling affected her routine. Plans were made for altering times to make it easier for Mr. Pilbus to return the children on time. All parties agreed to cancel the session scheduled one month from now. One year following the initial termination, no more sessions were required. Mrs. Pilbus made one additional call to the therapist nine months after termination, but was able to resolve the issue concerning Reggie's behavior without additional assistance.

SUMMARY

This chapter has outlined the complex issues involved in treating children from divorced families. Several core diagnostic issues were described that are often related to child behavior problems in divorced families. These include interparental conflict, parenting practices and nature of the relationship between the residential parent and children, loss of contact and relationship with the children's nonresidential parent, remarriage, and loss of family income. Though few empirical investigations have provided data that relate improvement in these factors to clinically significant gains in child behavior, it is suggested that clinicians pay close attention to these variables when intervening with troubled children from divorced families. A case example illustrated how successful intervention might be implemented. It is recommended that a multifaceted treatment package be used to deal with the complex issues facing families adapting to changes necessitated by divorce.

REFERENCES

Ainsworth, M. D. S. (1979). Infant-mother attachment. *American Psychologist, 34,* 932–937.

Alpert-Gillis ,L., Pedro-Carroll, J., & Cowen, E. (1989). The children of divorce intervention program: Development, implementation, and evaluation of a program for young urban children. *Journal of Consulting and Clinical Psychology, 57,* 583–589.

Atkeson, B. M., Forehand, R., & Rickard, K. M. (1982). The effects of divorce on children. In B. B. Lahey & A. E. Kazdin (Eds.). *Advances in clinical child psychology* (Vol. 4, pp. 255–281). New York: Plenum.

Baruch, D. W., & Wilcox, J. A. (1944). A study of sex differences in preschool children's coexistent with interpersonal tensions. *Journal of Genetic Psychology, 64,* 281–303.

Bendiksen, R., & Fulton, R. (1975). Death and the child: An anterospective test of the childhood bereavement and later behaviour disorder hypothesis. *Omega, 6,* 45–59.

Berg, B., & Kelly, R. (1979). The measured self-esteem of children from broken, rejected, and accepted families. *Journal of Divorce, 2,* 363–369.

Bornstein, M., Bornstein, P., & Walters, H. (1985). Children of divorce: A group-treatment manual for research and application. *Journal of Child and Adolescent Psychotherapy, 2,* 267–273.

Bornstein, M., Bornstein, P., & Walters, H. (1988). Children of divorce: Empirical evaluation of a group-treatment program. *Journal of Clinical Child Psychology, 17,* 248–254.

Bowlby, J. (1951). *Maternal care and child health.* Geneva: World Health Organization.

Bowlby, J. (1963). Pathological mourning and childhood mourning. *Journal of the American Psychoanalytic Association, 11,* 500–541.

Bowlby, J. (1980). *Loss: Sadness and depression.* New York: Basic Books.

Burgess, R. L. (1978). *Project interact: A study of patterns of interaction in abusive, neglectful, and control families* (Final Report). Washington, DC: National Center on Child Abuse and Neglect.

Chapman, M. (1977). Father absence, stepfathers, and the cognitive performance of college students. *Child Development, 48,* 1155–1158.

Christoupolus, C., COhen, D. N., Shaw, D. S., Joyce, S., Sullivan-Hanson, J., Kraft, S. P., & Emery, R. E. (1987). Children of abused women I: Adjustment at time of shelter residence. *Journal of Marriage and the Family, 49,* 611–619.

Clingempeel, W. G., Brand, E., & Ievoli, R. (1984). Stepparent-stepchild relationships in stepmother and stepfather families: A multimethod study. *Family Relations, 33,* 465–473.

Colletta, N. D. (1979). The impact of divorce: Father absence or poverty? *Journal of Divorce, 3,* 27–35.

Crosbie-Burnett, M., & Newcomer, L. (1990). Group counseling children of divorce: The effects of a multimodal intervention. *Journal of Divorce, 13,* 69–78.

Douglas, J. W. B., Ross, T. M., Hammond, W. A., & Mulligan, D. G. (1966). Delinquency and social class. *British Journal of Criminology, 6,* 294–302.

Emery, R. E. (1982). Interparental conflict and the children of discord and divorce. *Psychological*

Bulletin, 92, 310–330.

Emery, R. E. (988). *Marriage, divorce, and children's adjustment.* Beverly Hills: Sage.

Emery, R. E., Hetherington, E. M., & DiLalla, L. F. (1984). Divorce, children, and social policy. In H. W. Stevenson & A. E. Siegel (Eds.), *Child development research and social policy.* Chicago: University of Chicago Press.

Emery, R. E., & O'Leary, K. D. (1982). Children's perceptions of marital discord and behavior problems of boys and girls. *Journal of Abnormal Child Psychology, 10,* 11–24.

Emery, R. E., & Shaw, D. S. (1989). Child custody mediation. *The Behavior Therapist, 12,* 81–84.

Emery, R. E., Shaw, D. S., & Jackson, J. A. (1987). A clinical description of a model of child custody mediation. In J. P. Vincent (Ed.), *Advances in family intervention, assessment, and theory* (Vol. 4, pp. 309–337). New York: Sage.

Emery, R. E., & Wyer, M. M. (1987). Child-custody mediation and litigation: An experimental evaluation of the experience of parents. *Journal of Consulting and Clinical Psychology, 55,* 179–186.

Featherman, D. L., & Hauser, R. M. (1978). *Opportunity and change.* New York: Academic.

Felner, R. D., Farber, S. S., & Primavera, J. (1980). Children of divorce, stressful life events and transitions: A framework for preventive efforts. In R. H. Price, R. F. Ketterer, B. C. Bader, & J. Monohan (Eds.), *Prevention in mental health: Research, policy, and practice* (Vol. 1, pp. 81–108). Beverly Hills: Sage.

Ferri, E. (1976). *Growing up in a one-parent family: A long-term study of child development.* London: National Foundation for Educational Research.

Forehand, R., McCombs, A., Long, N., Brody, G., & Fauber, R. (1988). Early adolescent adjustment to recent parental divorce: The role of interparental conflict and adolescent sex as mediating variables. *Journal of Consulting and Clinical Psychology, 56,* 624–627.

Furstenberg, F. F., & Allison, P. D. (1989). How marital dissolution affects children: Variations by age and sex. *Developmental Psychology, 25,* 540–549.

Furstenberg, F. F., Morgan, S. P., & Allison, P. D. (1987, April). *Paternal participation and children's well-being after marital disruption.* Paper presented at the annual meeting of the Population Association of America, Chicago.

Furstenberg, F. F., Peterson, J. L., Nord, C. W., & Zill, N. (1983). The life course of children of divorce: Marital disruption and parental contact. *American Sociological Review, 48,* 656–668.

Furstenberg, F. F., & Spanier, G. B. (1984). *Recycling the family: Remarriage after divorce.* Beverly Hills, Sage.

Gibson, H. B. (1969). Early delinquency in relation to broken homes. *Journal of Child Psychology and Psychiatry, 10,* 195–204.

Glick, P. C. (1989). The role of divorce in the changing family structure. In S. A. Wolchik & P. Karoly (Eds.), *Children of divorce: Empirical perspectives on adjustment.* New York: Gardner.

Glick, P. C., & Lin, S. (1986). Recent changes in divorce and remarriage. *Journal of Marriage and the Family, 48,* 737–747.

Glueck, S., & Glueck, E. T. (1950). *Unraveling juvenile delinquency.* New York: Commonwealth Fund.

Goldstein, H. S. (1984). Parental composition, supervision, and conduct problems in youths 12 to 17 years old. *Journal of the American Academy of Child Psychiatry, 23,* 679–684.

Goldstein, J., Freud, A., & Solnit, A. J. (1973). *Beyond the best interests of the child.* New York: Free Press.

Gregory, I. (1965). Anterospective data following childhood loss of a parent. *Archives of General Psychiatry, 13,* 110–120.

Guidubaldi, J., Perry, J. D., & Cleminshaw, H. K. (1984). The legacy of parental divorce: A nationwide study of family status and selected mediating variables on children's academic and social competencies. In B. B. Lahey & A. E. Kazdin (Eds.), *Advances in child clinical psychology* (Vol. 7, pp. 109–155). New York: Plenum.

Gurman, A. S., Kniskern, D. P., & Pinsoff, W. M. (1986). Research on marital and family therapies. In S. L. Garfield & A. E. Bergin (Eds.), *Handbook of psychotherapy and behavior change* (pp. 565–626). New York: Wiley.

Heffs, R. D., & Camera, K. A. (1979). Post-divorce family relationships as mediating factors in the consequences of divorce for children. *Journal of Social Issues, 35,* 79–96.

Hetherington, E. M. (1972). Effects of father absence on personality development in adolescent daughters. *Developmental Psychology, 7,* 313–326.

Hetherington, E. M. (1979). Divorce: A child's perspective. *American Psychologist, 34,* 851–858.

Hetherington, E. M. (1981). Children and divorce. In R. Henderson (Ed.), *Parent-child interaction: Theory, research, and prospect* (pp. 35–58). New York: Academic Press.

Hetherington, E. M. (1986). Family relations six years after divorce. In K. Palsey & M. Ihinger-Tallman

(Eds.), *Remarriage and stepparenting today: Research and theory* (pp. 185–205). New York: Guilford.

Hetherington, E. M., Camera, K. A., & Featherman, D. L. (1981). Achievement and intellectual functioning of children in one-parent households. In J. Spence (Ed.), *Assessing achievement*. New York: Freeman.

Hetherington, E. M., Cox, M., & Cox, R. (1978). The aftermath of divorce. In J. H. Stevens, Jr., & M. Mathews (Eds.), *Mother-child, father-child relations*. Washington DC: National Association for the Education of Young Children.

Hetherington, E. M., Cox, M., & Cox, R. (1979). Family interaction and the social, emotional, and cognitive development of children following divorce. In V. Vaughn & T. Brazelton (Eds.), *The family: Setting priorities* (pp. 89–128). New York: Science and Medicine.

Hetherington, E. M., Cox, M., & Cox, R. (1981). Effects of divorce on parents and children. In M. E. Lamb (Ed.), *Nontraditional families*. Hillsdale, NJ: Erlbaum.

Hetherington, E. M., Cox, M., & Cox, R. (1985). Long-term effects of divorce and remarriage on the adjustment of children. *Journal of the American Academy of Child Psychiatry, 24,* 518–530.

Hodges, W. F., Wechsler, R. C., & Ballantine, C. (1979). Divorce and the preschool child: Cumulative stress. *Journal of Divorce, 3,* 55–68.

Hoffman, L. (1977). Marital instability and the economic status of women. *Demography, 14,* 67–76.

Jacobson, D. S. (1978). The impact of marital separation/divorce on children. II: Interparental hostility and child adjustment. *Journal of Divorce, 2,* 3–19.

Kalter, N., Riemer, B., Brickman, A., & Chen, J. W. (1985). Implications of parental divorce for female development. *Journal of the American Academy of Child Psychiatry, 24,* 538–544.

Kurdek, L. (1981). An integrative perspective of children's divorce adjustment. *American Psychologist, 36,* 856–866.

Kurdek, L., Blisk, D., & Siesky, A. E. (1981). Correlates of children's long-term adjustment to their parents' divorce. *Developmental Psychology, 17,* 565–579.

Lamb, M. E. (1977). The effects of divorce on children's personality development. *Journal of Divorce, 1,* 163–174.

Lambert, L., & Hart, S. (1976). Who needs a father? *New Society, 37,* 80.

Long, N., & Forehand, R. (1987). The effects of parental divorce and parental conflict on children: An overview. *Journal of Developmental and Behavioral Pediatrics, 8,* 292–296.

Lowenstein, J. S., & Koopman, E. J. (1978). A comparison of the self-esteem between boys living with single-parent mothers and single-parent fathers. *Journal of Divorce, 2,* 195–208.

Luepnitz, D. A. (1982). *Child custody: A study of families after divorce*. Lexington, MA: Lexington Books.

MacKinnon, C. E., Brody, G. H., & Stoneman, Z. (1982). The effects of divorce and maternal employment on the home environments of preschool children. *Child Development, 53,* 1392–1399.

McCord, J., McCord, W., & Thurber, E. (1962). Some effects of paternal absence on male children. *Journal of Abnormal and Social Psychology, 64,* 361–369.

McDermott, J. (1968). Parental divorce in early childhood. *American Journal of Psychiatry, 10,* 1424–1432.

Meissner, W. W. (1978). Conceptualization of marriage and family dynamics from a psychoanalytic perspective. In T. J. Paolino & B. S. McCrady (Eds.), *Marriage and marital therapy* (pp. 25–88). New York: Brunner/Mazel.

Minuchin, S. (1974). *Families and family therapy*. Cambridge, MA; Harvard University Press.

National Institute for Child Support Enforcement (NICSE). (1986). *History and fundamentals of child-support enforcement* (2nd ed.). Washington, DC: U.S. Government Printing Office.

Norton (1983). Recent statistics on divorce and remarriage. Unpublished raw data.

Nye, F. I. (1957). Child adjustment in broken and unhappy homes. *Marriage and Family Living, 19,* 356–361.

Oshman, H. P., & Manosevitz, M. (1976). Father absence: Effects of stepfathers upon psychosocial development in males. *Developmental Psychology, 12,* 479–480.

Parrish, T. S., & Taylor, J. (1979). The impact of divorce and subsequent father absence on children's and adolescent's self-concepts. *Journal of Youth and Adolescence, 8,* 427–432.

Pedro-Carroll, J. L., & Cowen, E. L. (1985). The Children of Divorce Intervention Program: An investigation of the efficacy of a school-based prevention program. *Journal of Consulting and Clinical Psychology, 53,* 60.

Pedro-Carroll, J. L., & Cowen, E. L. (1987). The Children of Divorce Intervention Program: Implementation and evaluation of a time-limited group approach. In J. P. Vincent (Ed.), *Advances in family intervention, assessment and theory* (Vol. 4, pp. 281–308). Greenwich, CT: JAI.

Pedro-Carroll, J., Cowen, E., Hightower, A., & Guare, J. (1986). Preventive intervention with latency-aged children of divorce: A replication study. *American Journal of Community Psych., 14,* 277–290.

Peterson, J. L., & Zill, N. (1986). Marital disruption, parent-child relationships, and behavior problems in children. *Journal of Marriage and the Family, 48,* 295–307.

Porter, B., & O'Leary, K. D. (1980). Marital discord and childhood behavior problems. *Journal of Abnormal Child Psychology, 80,* 287–295.

Power, M. J., Ash, P. M., Schoenberg, E., & Sorey, E. C. (1974). Delinquency and the family. *British Journal of Social Work, 4,* 17–38.

Raschke, H. J., & Raschke, V. J. (1979). Family conflict and children's self-concepts: A comparison of intact and single-parent families. *Journal of Marriage and the Family, 4,* 367–374.

Roseby, V., & Deutsch, R. (1985). Children of separation and divorce: Effects of a social role-taking group intervention on fourth and fifth graders. *Journal of Clinical Child Psychology, 14,* 55–60.

Rosen, R. (1979). Some crucial issues concerning children of divorce. *Journal of Divorce, 3,* 19–26.

Rutter, M. (1966). *Children of sick parents.* London: Oxford University Press.

Rutter, M. (1971). Parent-child separation: Psychological effects on the children. *Journal of Child Psychology and Allied Disciplines, 12,* 233–260.

Rutter, M. (1979). Maternal deprivation 1972–1978: New findings, new concepts, new approaches. *Child Development, 50,* 283–305.

Rutter, M. (1981). *Maternal deprivation reassessed* (2nd ed.). Harmondsworth: Penguin Press.

Rutter, M., Cox, A., Tupling, C., Berger, M., & Yule, W. (1975a). Attainment and adjustment in two geographical areas: 1. The prevalence of psychiatric disorder. *British Journal of Psychiatry, 126,* 493–509.

Rutter, M., Yule, B., Quinton, D., Rowlands, O., Yule, W., & Berger, M. (1975b). Attainment and adjustment in two geographical areas: 3. Some factors accounting for area differences. *British Journal of Psychiatry, 126,* 520–533.

Santrock, J. W. (1972). Relation of type and onset of father absence to cognitive development. *Child Development, 43,* 455–469.

Santrock, J. W., Warshak, R. A., Lindbergh, C., &

Meadows, L. (1982). Children's and parents' observed social behavior in stepfather families. *Child Development, 53,* 472–480.

Shaw, D. S. (1989, April). *The effects of divorce and parental conflict on children's adjustment: A prospective study.* Paper presented at the biennial meeting of the Society for Research in Child Development, Kansas City, MO.

Shaw, D. S., & Emery, R. E. (1987). Parental conflict and other correlates of the adjustment of school-age children whose parents have separated. *Journal of Abnormal Child Psychology, 15,* 269–281.

Shaw, D. S., & Emery, R. E. (1988). Multiple family adversity and school-age children's adjustment. *Journal of the American Academy of Child Psychiatry and Adolescence, 27,* 200–206.

Shinn, M. (1978). Father absence and children's cognitive development. *Psychological Bulletin, 85,* 295–324.

Slater, E. J., & Haber, J. D. (1984). Adolescent adjustment following divorce as a function of family conflict. *Journal of Consulting and Clinical Psychology, 52,* 920–921.

Sorosky, A. D. (1977). The psychological effects of divorce on adolescents. *Adolescence, 12,* 123–136.

Sprenkle, D. H., & Storm, C. L. (1983). Divorce-therapy outcome research: A substantive and methodological review. *Journal of Marital and Family Therapy, 10,* 239–258.

Stolberg, A., Cullen, P., & Garrison, K. (1982). The Divorce Adjustment Project: Preventive programming for children of divorce. *Journal of Preventive Psychiatry, 1,* 365–368.

Stolberg, A. L., & Garrison, K. M. (1985). Evaluation a primary prevention program for children of divorce: The Divorce Adjustment Project. *American Journal of Community Psychology, 13,* 111–124.

Wadsworth, J. (1979). *Roots of delinquency.* New York: Barnes and Noble/Harper and Row.

Wallerstein, J. S., & Kelly, J. B. (1974). The effects of parental divorce: The adolescent experience. In E. J. Anthony & C. Koupernik (Eds.). *The child and his family: Children at psychiatric risk.* New York: Wiley.

Wallerstein, J. S., & Kelly, J. B. (1980). *Surviving the breakup.* New York: Basic Books.

Wallerstein, J. S., & Kelly, J. B. (1983). Children of divorce: Stress and developmental tasks. In N. Garmezy & M. Rutter (Eds.), *Stress, coping, and development in children* (pp. 265–302). New York: McGraw-Hill.

Wolfe, D. A., Jaffe, P. J., Zak, L., & Wilson, S. (1986).

Child witnesses to violence between parents: Critical issues in behavioral and social adjustment. *Journal of Abnormal Child Psychology, 14,* 95–104.

Young, E. R., & Parrish, T. S. (1977). Impact of father absence during childhood on the psychological adjustment of college females. *Sex Roles, 3,* 217–227.

Zill, N. (1978, February). *Divorce, marital happiness, and the mental health of children: Findings from the FCD national survey of children.* Paper presented at the NIMH Workshop on Divorce and Children, Bethesda, MD.

CHAPTER 24

CHRONIC MEDICAL ILLNESS

Jan L. Wallander   University of Alabama at Birmingham
Daniel S. Marullo   University of Alabama at Birmingham

DESCRIPTION OF PROBLEM

Core Features

For centuries, infectious diseases were the primary threat to children's health, but with these now being more successfully controlled, chronic medical diseases have become of greater concern. Improvements in the management of chronic conditions have further prolonged life. For example following the discovery of insulin in 1922, children with insulin-dependent diabetes now have more reasonable life expectancies, approximating 75 percent of normal (Craig, 1981). Whereas the median survival in children with acute lymphoblastic leukemia was less than two years in 1967, some 60 percent of children diagnosed in 1983 will survive five years or longer (Miller & Miller, 1984).

There is a large variety of chronic medical illness affecting children, of which asthma, diabetes mellitus, seizure disorder, congenital heart disease, and arthritis are the most common. As a group, they differ from acute physical conditions in several important respects (Johnson, 1988). First, although a chronic illness is usually treatable, it is not curable, and thus it must be "managed" in some way for long periods of time. Second, because of this ongoing need to manage the disease, medical responsibility is transferred from the physician to the patient, and, in the case of children, the child's family. For most, this means a lifelong commitment often to complex and sometimes painful procedures for managing their disease. Third, the family almost always becomes involved, especially when a child has a chronic illness. Because the child-patient may be too young to be responsible for his or her medical management, parents must assume this responsibility.

For these and other reasons, there has long been a concern about how a chronic medical illness affects a child's psychosocial development and adjustment. This chapter will primarily deal with assessment and treatment of *general psychosocial adjustment problems in children with a chronic medical illness. Psychosocial adjustment* is defined herein as the behavioral, emotional, and social well-being of the child and is indexed typically by

Preparation of this chapter was supported in part by NIH-NICHD grants K04 HD00867, R01 HD25310, and R01 HD24322.

a consideration of the child's behavior. Indications of psychosocial maladjustment includes anxiety, depression, aggressiveness, acting out, social withdrawal, or peer difficulties.

Views on the psychosocial development of children with chronic medical illness have changed over time (Drotar, 1981; Johnson, 1980). However, most recent epidemiological surveys have shown that there is considerable variation in psychosocial adjustment within the chronic illness child population. At the same time, these surveys report a frequency of adjustment problems in children with chronic physical diseases of nearly double the rate observed in the general population (cf. Haggerty, 1986). This has led to the position that children with a chronic medical illness represent a population at risk for psychosocial adjustment problems. On average, they may display more psychosocial problems than expected in healthy peers, although few evidence clinically significant problems or psychopathology.

We have proposed a conceptual model that partially explains the observed variation in the adjustment of children with chronic medical illness (Wallander, Varni, Babani, Banis, & Wilcox, 1989). The various factors hypothesized to play a role in adjustment of children with chronic medical illness are organized into a risk-and-resistance framework (see Figure 24–1). Disease/disability parameters, functional independence, and psychosocial stress are considered factors primarily responsible for causing adjustment problems in children with chronic medical illness. However, since children with similar risk factors display differences in adjustment, resistance factors are thought to influence the risk-adjustment relationship, both through a moderation process and direct influences on adjustment (see Figure 24–1). The model distinguishes between intrapersonal factors, social ecology factors, and stress processing as resistance factors. We will rely on this model in discussing assessment and treatment of psychosocial adjustment problems in children with chronic medical illness.

Associated Features

Although we will not deal directly with these, there are several associated features common to childhood chronic medical illnesses that must be noted. Some specific disorders cause physical pain as a primary symptom (e.g., arthritis, hemophilla), whereas for others, there are painful medical procedures that must be administered with some frequency (e.g., lumbar puncture and bone marrow aspirations associated with acute lymphocytic leukemia, chest physiotherapy for cystic fibrosis) (Varni, 1983). Frequent hospitalizations and surgery are needed by some children with chronic medical illness (Jay, 1988).

Furthermore, a chronic medical illness often carries with it the burden of managing a complex treatment regimen. This is illustrated by the daily requirements for managing insulin-dependent diabetes mellitus (e.g., blood glucose testing, insulin injections, maintaining a restrictive diet and a constant level of physical activity, and engaging in various health and safety behaviors). Consequently, adherence to treatment recommendations becomes a salient issue in chronic medical illness (e.g., La Greca, 1988).

Given that children with chronic medical illness most often live in a family, family issues become germane. The family has to be involved in the management of the child's illness, including learning about the illness, communicating with the child's physician, and managing the treatment regimen. The family is also involved in helping the chronically ill child cope with the direct and indirect effects of the illness. At the same time, the youngster's illness likely will have an impact on the family. Interactions within the family, the relationships of family members to individuals outside the family, and the well-being of family members are affected by the child's medical illness and the demands associated with managing it (e.g., Johnson, 1985).

Epidemiology

Any specific chronic illness is relatively rare, but the overall rate of children with any chronic condition is estimated at 10 to 20 percent (Gortmaker & Sappenfield, 1984). Most chronic conditions are physiologically relatively benign. However, 10 percent of children with chronic illnesses, or over 1,000,000 of the total childhood

Figure 24–1. Conceptual model for research on children with handicaps or chronic medical illnesses.

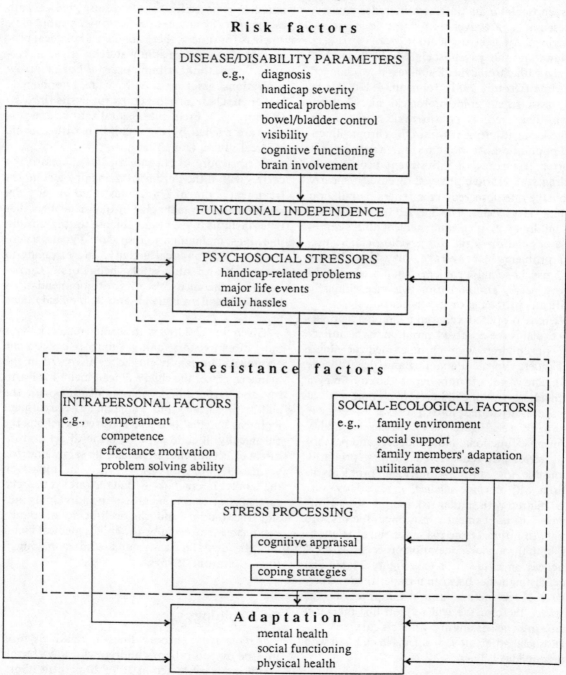

Source: Wallander, J. L., et al., (1989). Family resources as resistance factors for psychological maladjustment in chronically ill and handicapped children. *Journal of Pediatric Psychology, 14.* Reprinted by permission of Plenum.

population, have physiologically severe conditions (Gortmaker & Sappenfield, 1984). These conditions interfere on a regular or daily basis with their ability to go to school, play with other children, perform household chores, or do other things that children their age are expected to do. Cystic fibrosis, juvenile onset diabetes, certain congenital heart diseases, sickle-cell anemia, juvenile arthritis, and leukemia are examples of more severe conditions.

It is difficult to estimate the number of children with chronic medical illness who have psychosocial adjustment problems. However, when information from the same informant is compared (e.g., all teachers or all parents), children with chronic physical diseases are typically found to have nearly double the rate observed in the general population of children (Haggerty, 1986). Whereas epidemiological surveys from several sites show that 5 to 15 percent of all children are reported by parents to display behavior problems, the rate for children with severe chronic conditions (e.g., cystic fibrosis, spina bilfida) ranges between 20 and 37 percent (Haggerty, 1986). In our own research on volunteer samples of children with different chronic conditions, between 9 and 12 percent of children were reported by their parents as maladjusted on the Child Behavior Checklist (i.e., they obtained a total score > 2 SD above norm sample M), compared with an expected rate in the population of 2 percent (Wallander, Varni, Babani, Banis, & Wilcox, 1988).

DIAGNOSIS AND ASSESSMENT

Diagnostic Issues

It is important to determine what causes psychosocial adjustment problems. One concern must be whether psychosocial problems are a direct effect of the medical illness. Some physiological processes are known to link physical disease and psychological well-being. For example, the relationship between brain damage and behavior problems is well established (Rutter, 1977). Consequently, disorders such as seizure disorder or cerebral palsy, where a dysfunctional brain is a central feature, may produce behavioral difficulties in children. A neuroendocrine process is exemplified in the case of insulin-dependent diabetes, in which transient behavioral irritability may be observed during periods of hypoglycemia (Ryan, Vega, & Drash, 1985). Knowledge about the physiological processes involved will facilitate a determination of the role of the medical illness in the psychosocial status of the child. Identification of such relationships may make it feasible to improve psychosocial status through medical interventions (e.g., change in seizure medication, adjustment of insulin dosage).

Furthermore, some medical treatments are known to cause negative behavioral reactions. First, the medical intervention may directly affect brain functioning, which may in turn cause behavioral changes and psychosocial adjustment problems. For example, radiation and chemotherapy for various cancers have been known to change neuropsychological functioning and behavior in some children. Furthermore, many medical treatments are acutely stressful or put a chronic level of low or moderate stress on a child. Examples of the former are the lumbar puncture and bone marrow aspirations common in the treatment of leukemia, which can cause significant behavioral reactions, such as anxiety, depression, and acting out (Jay, 1988). Other treatments have an effect over the long run because of their insistent demands for a lifestyle that may be incompatible with normal child behavior. The treatment of insulin-dependent diabetes is a prime example of this.

Another diagnostic issue is the sometime temporary nature of psychosocial adjustment problems in chronically ill children. For example, in childhood cancer, to the extent that the child is cognitively developed enough to understand the ramifications of being diagnosed with a cancer, it is likely that negative adjustment reactions may occur to this serious revelation. This may be further exacerbated by the initiation of intensive treatment of the cancer, involving traumatic and painful medical procedures, which may have major side effects, such as nausea, hair loss, and general malaise. Because these treatments and their effects may be time limited, psychosocial adjustment may improve once the child is removed from these significant invasions in his or her life. This does not imply, however, that intervention should not be attempted to help a child in this highly stressful phase. Knowledge that the phase is likely to be temporary may indicate the use of certain interventions over others. Moreover, a positive expectation may be communicated to the child and his or her family for psychosocial improvement in relatively short order.

Assessment Strategies

Psychological assessment of chronic medical illness will rely to a great extent on procedures developed for children in general. To this generally available body of assessment procedures must be added procedures specific to the task. (Discussion of both general and specific assessment procedures for children with chronic medical illness can be found in Johnson [1988] and Karoly [1988]). Assessment of psychosocial adjustment in children with chronic medical illness must progress from a conceptual basis that may guide the psychologist as to what constructs to assess and how to relate the various pieces of obtained information. Unfortunately, there has not been much conceptual model development in this field. However, Johnson (1988) and Wallander and Varni (see Figure 24–1; Wallander et al., 1989; Wallander & Varni, in press) are examples of models that may facilitate the assessment process. Using Wallander and Varni's model, we highlight some assessment strategies herein.

Disease/disability parameters are specific to each illness in question. The medical diagnosis of the child is, of course, paramount because each diagnosis has very unique implications. The severity of the condition is typically indexed through some medical test. For example, metabolic functioning of insulin-dependent diabetes is measured by a chemical assay that provides an average glycosylated hemoglobin level for the past two months for the child. The severity of hemophilia is indexed by percent of clotting factor remaining in the blood and the individual's ability to contribute to the clotting of the blood and inhibition of a bleed.

The notion that more visible conditions puts more stress on the child is common, but it is not uniformly supported (Wallander et al., 1988). However, it may be an important consideration in the assessment of a given child. The extent of brain involvement may have to be determined, as much to learn about its possible role in the child's psychosocial adjustment as implications for cognitive and behavioral functioning generally. When brain involvement is suspected, it is advisable to administer an intelligence test suitable for the child's age and developmental level. Further comprehensive neuropsychological assessment may also be indicated.

A second risk factor closely related to disease/disability parameters is the functional independence displayed by the child in relation to age expectations. A chronic medical illness may, to varying degrees, impair the child's ability to function independently in an age-appropriate fashion. A well-developed set of instruments for assessing this with excellent norms and psychometric properties is the Vineland Adaptive Behavior Scales (Sparrow, Balla, & Cicchetti, 1984). This instrument will help identify strengths and weaknesses in the child's functional ability in such areas as everyday responsibilities, communication, social behavior, community functioning, and, for younger children, motor skills.

The third risk factor identified in our conceptual model is psychosocial stressors. Generally construed major and minor life events may be assessed using the Life-Events Checklist (Johnson & McCutcheon, 1980) or the Adolescent Perceived Events Scale (Compas, Davis, & Forsythe, 1985). However, all existing life-events measures were developed to address stress experienced by middle-class children and adolescents (Johnson & Bradlyn, 1988). Events more commonly experienced by youth residing in the inner city and of lower SES are typically absent (e.g., witnessing violence, being offered illicit drugs). To improve on this, we have developed the Adolescent Life Events Survey, which attempts to be more sensitive to the experience of disadvantaged youth (Hale, Cole, & Wallander, 1991). Stressful events experienced by the family may be assessed with the Family Inventory of Life Events (McCubbin,

Patterson, & Wilson, 1981). In addition to general life events, it may be helpful to assess medically related events in more detail, but there are few instruments established for this purpose. We are aware of the Diabetes Hassles Scale (Kanner & Jacobson, 1984), and we are currently developing an inventory of stressful events related to having a physical disability (Wallander & Hardy, 1991).

Our conceptual model also identifies three clusters of resistance factors. The impact of the noted risk factors on adjustment should be influenced by personal characteristics of the child or intrapersonal style. Based on research on adjustment in children in general, it is beneficial to assess temperament, effectance motivation, and social problem-solving ability (Wallander & Varni, in press). The Dimensions of Temperament Survey (Lerner, Palermo, Spiro, & Nesselroade, 1982) is useful for assessing temperament because of its empirical foundation and comparable scales for different ages, including adults. Effectance motivation subsumes several more specific dimensions, including perceived competence, self-efficacy, and locus of control. Given the concern about self-esteem of children with a chronic medical illness, the Self-Perception Profile (Harter, 1987) provides information about perceived competence across several important domains (e.g., cognitive, social, physical). A pictorial version has also been developed for use with preschoolers (Harter & Pike, 1984). Finally, social problem-solving ability can be assessed in a variety of ways following Spivak and Shure's (1974) development of this construct.

The social ecology represents another cluster of resistance factors generally recognized as important for adjustment of children with chronic medical illness. Among these, we have emphasized the psychosocial relationships within the family, adjustment of other family members, practical resources available to the family, and social support as being especially important for the child's adjustment. Much information is now available on the assessment of the family (e.g., Grotevant & Carlson, 1989). For practical reasons, one is often restricted to administering simple instruments to family members to obtain any information about family variables. Common choices to assess general psychosocial relationships within the family are the Family Environmental Scale (Moos & Moos, 1981) and the Family Adaptability and Cohesion Evaluation Scale (Olson, Portner, & Bell, 1978).

There are also a few available measures to assess illness impact on the family, such as the Impact-on-Family Scale (Stein & Riessman, 1980). This latter instrument provides information on financial burden, family/social impact, personal strain, and mastery from the perspective of a parent informant. The adjustment of family members, in particular parents, is well known to be associated with child adjustment (cf. Heatherington & Martin, 1986). Parents of children with chronic medical illness are better viewed as members of the general population rather than a pathological group. Thus, instruments appropriate for population assessment and that can discriminate the relatively minor variation to be expected in this group should be used. Examples are the Mental Health Inventory (Veit & Ware, 1983) and the Symptom Checklist-90-R (Derogatis, 1983), which provide a broad survey of individual adjustment.

Practical resources available to the family may make it easier for it to care for the special needs of a child with a chronic medical illness. A related construct is the financial burden experienced by the family members. The Family Inventory of Resources for Management (McCubbin, Comeau, & Harkins, 1981) can be used to assess such aspects. Finally, the child's perceived social support may be assessed with the Social Support Scale for Children (Harter, 1985).

Stress processing represents the third resistance factor in our model. This includes the distinct yet related constructs of cognitive appraisal and coping strategies that have been identified by Lazarus and Folkman (1984) as quite dependent on one another and paramount to an understanding the stress-adjustment relationship. However, assessment of children's appraisals has not advanced sufficiently, and the literature is only slightly further along regarding the assessment of coping strategies.

The assessment procedures currently available are best characterized as research tools. Compas,

Malcarne, and Fondocaro (1988) developed a procedure where children are interviewed about their use of different coping strategies in relation to specific and idiosyncratic stressful events. Spirito, Stark, and Williams (1988) developed a brief paper-and-pencil instrument for use in assessing which of 10 coping strategies a child has used to manage a particular stressful event. Our own efforts exemplify yet another approach, as we have attempted to develop a behavioral test to elicit samples of how adolescents cope with, in this case, disability-related stressors (Wallander & Hardy, 1991). Focusing on children with a gross motor physical disability, we present them with 25 concrete vignettes describing a particularly stressful problem related to their disability. They are then asked to describe how they would deal with this particular problem. Their responses are coded into different coping strategies (e.g., direct problem solving, avoidance, support seeking).

The assessment of adjustment in these children should be done with instruments that cover a broad range of problem behaviors, that are suitable for a broad range of ages to facilitate followup, and that have well-developed norms for how children in general score. In our own research and clinical work, we have primarily used the different forms of the Child Behavior Checklist (Achenbach & Edelbrock, 1983). With its hierarchical structure, it provides information at the most general level about overall behavior problems, as well as at a more specific level internalizing and externalizing behavioral problems, and at its most specific level finer domains of problem behaviors (e.g., depression, withdrawal, aggressive, delinquent). It also provides information about the social competence of the child in such areas as activities, peer functioning, and school performance. It has norms on 1,300 children from randomly selected homes fairly representative of the population in terms of race and socioeconomic status. In addition, information is available on 2,300 clinic-referred children from various public and private mental health centers. It has excellent psychometric properties and a voluminous research literature available now on many different types of children, including children with chronic medical illness.

TREATMENT

Evidence for Prescriptive Treatment

Pediatric psychology has not been blessed with many comparative treatment outcome studies. A few specific areas, such as preparation for medical procedures and hospitalization (see reviews by Jay, 1988; Peterson & Mori, 1988), have advanced to the point where some preliminary prescriptive statements can be made about interventions that are expected to work better than others. However, this is not the case with intervention for psychosocial maladjustment in children with chronic medical illness. There are several reasons for this underdeveloped state. As noted earlier, specific chronic medical illnesses are not very common, making it difficult to conduct studies while controlling for type of illness. The idea of combining children with different medical illnesses when studying interventions for psychosocial maladjustment has not been carried out (Pless & Perrin, 1985). Second, traditional pediatric medicine has not placed sufficient priority on helping children who evidence psychosocial maladjustment. It is still relatively rare that pediatric psychologists or other professionals interested more broadly in children's development are integral members of the treatment team.

Third, there continues to be a controversy present even within the pediatric psychology field whether psychosocial adjustment in children with chronic medical illness is a significant issue. A number of studies were published in the late 1970s and early1980s suggesting tht children with chronic medical illness were indistinguishable from healthy peers in their adjustment (e.g., Drotar et al., 1981; Gayton, Friedman, Tavormina, & Tucker, 1977). We have pointed out some possible explanations for the discrepancy between these studies and the epidemiological surveys (Wallander et al., 1988). These include (1) difficulties in determining adjustment in children, (2) the use of different sources for measurement of adjustment, (3) the use of much smaller samples in those studies reporting no differences, and (4) investigation of children with different chronic physical disorders in different studies making comparisons difficult.

We think that the large-scale population surveys are sounder and better represent the current state of affairs. With this in mind, there is a significant need for comparative treatment outcome studies that can lead to prescriptive statements regarding the relative efficacy of different types of interventions.

It should also be noted that clinical efforts at improving psychosocial adjustment in children with chronic medical illness tend not to be compartmentalized into those involving behavior therapy versus pharmacotherapy. First, psychosocial maladjustment in children with chronic medical illness is rarely treated with pharmacotherapy. Aside from the potential complications inherent in relying on pharmacological agents for improving psychosocial adjustment in children who may already be receiving multiple drugs to manage their medical illness, psychosocial maladjustment is typically not manifested in severe enough degrees to consider pharmacotherapy. More common are broadly construed adjustment reactions, low-grade depression and anxiety, and social withdrawal. One may also see more externalizing problems, such as conduct disorder and aggressive behavior, as reactions to living with a chronic medical illness and its demands.

This is not to say that a child or adolescent with a chronic medical illness may not benefit from pharmacotherapy. There may certainly be significant depression or anxiety disorders, for example, that can benefit from drug therapy. In those cases, pharmacological intervention for psychosocial problems must be coordinated carefully with the medical regimen already in place.

Selecting Optimal Treatment Strategies

Given the absence of evidence for prescriptive treatments for psychosocial maladjustment in children with chronic medical illness, the selection of an optimal treatment strategy for a given child is best accomplished from a conceptual basis and a careful individual assessment of the child in question. We have proposed such a conceptual model (see Figure 24–1) that may aid in this process. At this point, there are no clear indications of how to intervene with identified targets in children who have a chronic medical disorder and experience psychosocial maladjustment. Rather, one's general clinical knowledge and borrowing from the general literature on intervention with child problems have to guide this endeavor.

A variety of treatment strategies may be employed as thought to be suitable for the particular child and his or her circumstances. However, given that a child is the identified "problem," intervention will typically involve the family. This may take the form of educating parents as to the disease itself as well as its effects on normal development, and working with parents to provide the child with a less stressful situation and more support within the family. Consultation with the child's school may also be indicated. This may take the form of educating the teacher and classmates about the child's condition (Katz & Varni, 1988). Educating members of the health team about the psychosocial aspects of the chronic illness may also be required (Johnson, 1988).

An overriding concern in selecting optimal treatment strategies must be the child's developmental level. This is not unique to the consideration of the child with chronic medical illness, but influences all child treatment. Although much of the clinical work is similar in its specific techniques to that dealing with traditional mental disorders, the core features of a chronic medical illness discussed earlier must be considered throughout. In addition, the various associated features also discussed earlier need to be considered in planning and implementing treatment. It is these core and associated features that make working with a child with a chronic medical illness unique.

Problems in Carrying Out Interventions

There are several problems in carrying out interventions with children with chronic medical illness that are relatively specific to this population. It may be more common in this population that the therapist will experience resistance from the family in agreeing to be seen by a mental health professional as well as following through on treatment recommendations. The family may be more adamant than families in general that they are a "normal" family, not needing mental health intervention — their perspective may be that they have a child with a *medical* illness. Furthermore, less enlightened colleagues in the medical professions may be less than supportive of the family and the child being seen by a mental health professional. Both the family and other members of the treatment team may see any psychosocial problems as simply "natural consequences" of being diagnosed with or living with a chronic medical disease. This less than enthusiastic welcoming of the mental health professional may be exacerbated by the very real and significant stress experienced by the family with a child with a chronic medical illness.

On top of attempting to deal with the often devastating fact that one's child has a chronic, possibly life-threatening, illness, the family has to deal with its usual demands, such as work, home, and care of other children. There simply may not be much energy left to mobilize for working with a mental health professional. A key in overcoming this common problem is to gain the support of the entire treatment team for the role of the mental health professional. This may be provided up front, but if not, a significant effort often has to be expanded over a period of time to overcome this negative perspective. A few "successes" in improving the situation of some children can go a long way. If the family senses that the medical personnel (who probably have a higher perceived value) encourage and support treatment of the *whole* child, they are more likely to follow up on any recomendation to work with the mental health professional. Otherwise, overcoming resistance from a family may require initial focus on helping to improve some very practical problems in the life of the family and the care of the child with the chronic medical illness. Providing education may also be helpful before moving on to more intensive work.

Another problem unique to working with children with chronic medical illness is the environment in which this work often needs to be carried out. The child is seen in the medical clinic with its own physical and functional structure, which typically requires the mental health professional to integrate his or her efforts in this structure. For example, rather than being able to consult with the family in the comfort of his or her office suitably equipped with couches, tables, and the like, the consultation often has to take place in a physical exam room, hallway, or the waiting room. Furthermore, the consultation often has to be done on a catch-as-catch-can basis rather than on a schedule. Stealing 10 or 15 minutes prior to or following a medical procedure may be a common mode of operating. Thus, traditional methods often have to be considerably altered or abbreviated. Working effectively under these conditions becomes a special challenge for the pediatric mental health professional.

Relapse Prevention

Preventing a relapse of problems may be the significant challenge in traditional mental health work. In working with children with chronic medical illness, however, this problem may be less significant for several reasons. First a child with a chronic medical illness is typically part of a care system. A chronic medical illness requires repeated contact with a medical professional or a treatment team. This can provide the mental health professional with opportunities for reinforcing improvements already achieved and identifying adjustment problems before they become significant. Second, the mental health professional can sensitize both the family and medical professionals to high-risk periods for psychosocial adjustment problems. These high-risk periods may be related to the course of the illness or its treatment or be more generally developmental in nature. Children with chronic medical illness may experience problems especially at significant changes in their development, such as the beginning of regular schooling, transfer to junior high school, or initiation of puberty. Concerned individuals can then be alerted both to prevent negative experiences during these high-risk periods and observe for development of adjustment problems.

CASE ILLUSTRATION

Case Description

The following is a hypothetical account of the Samuals family based on a composite of several families seen in a children's hospital outpatient endocrinology clinic. Ben is a 10-year-old boy with insulin dependent diabetes mellitus (IDDM) of two years' duration. Since diagnosis, he has experienced a number of medical complications due to his inability to maintain appropriate metabolic control of his diabetes. He also appears to experience psychosocial difficulties, as does his family.

Ben often experiences nausea and bouts of vomiting. He becomes quite irritable at times and has difficulty concentrating on tasks. Ben's poor metabolic control has resulted in frequent diabetic ketoacidosis (DKA), a condition in which the body breaks down body fats into fatty acids. Consequently, he has had frequent emergency room visits and has required four hospitalizations in a recent one-month period. Thus, Ben is at greater risk for long-term complications of IDDM (e.g., myocardial infarction, gangrene in the extremities, renal failure, blindness). The short-term consequences of his poor control are that he spends an inordinate amount of time at home or in the hospital. He has missed a significant amount of school and has showed a decrease in school performance since his diagnosis. Ben has now also become socially isolated from peers. Possibly as a result of decreased contact with peers and exposure to potentially positive experiences, Ben appears to feel distressed and has low self-esteem.

Ben's uncontrolled diabetes also has had implications for the family, which consists of Ben's mother, Ellen, father, Gene, and 6-year-old brother, Todd. Gene, who works the night shift in the city garage, often experiences interrupted sleep during the day by calls from the school because Ben is ill. He must then pick Ben up from school and care for him during the day. Eileen is often required to leave work early or miss work in order to share the care of Ben. Gene and Eileen have been married for 11 years. They have experienced marital discord and have engaged in extremely vocal arguments in the past. They currently do not spend much time together due to their work schedules, the demands of caring for their children, and especially Ben's illness. When asked, both parents report that their main concern is Ben's welfare and their own needs must come second. While it initially appears that each parent is vigilant and active in Ben's treatment, the fact remains that Ben's medical condition is deteriorating. Compounding the situation is Ben's problematic psychosocial adjustment, as well as the stress experienced by the family as a whole. For these reasons, the Samuals were referred by the Diabetologist to the Pediatric Psychologist.

Differential Diagnosis and Assessment

The suspected difficulties implied by the history may include more disease-specific factors, such as nonadherence to the medical regimen. However, other problems may be present, which are of concern in their own right and also could adversely affect the disease course. Consequently, the following DSM-III-R diagnoses were initially considered: noncompliance with medical treatment; adjustment disorder with mixed emotional features; marital problem (parents); and parent-child problem. The following assessment was initiated to rule out these diagnoses.

An evaluation of the parents' and Ben's knowledge of diabetes and its treatment was undertaken to rule out noncompliance with medical treatment. This was accomplished using the Test of Diabetes Knowledge (Johnson et al., 1982) and a 24-hour recall of IDDM treatment (Johnson, Silverstein, Rosenbloom, Carter, & Cunningham, 1986) administered to Ben and each of his parents. Actual skill levels for preparation of insulin and injections were also assessed using a behavioral observation task, the Skills Test of Insulin Injection (Johnson, 1985). The parents' behaviors relevant to various areas of diabetes treatment and psychosocial adaptation to IDDM that may affect adherence was assessed with the Parent Diabetes Behavior Test (Marullo & Wallander, 1991). Although primarily a research instrument, this structured interview utilizes vignettes of situations judged to be relevant to parents to determine trends in their behavior in diabetes specific situations.

Results of this assessment suggested that Ben and his parents had poor knowledge about IDDM, which likely hampers their efforts to manage it effectively. Daily adherence behaviors by the family were also found to be inadequate. Diet was a particular problem; specifically, Ben and his parents frequently made inappropriate food choices, resulting in Ben consuming inadequate calories. This was complicated by Ben missing scheduled morning and afternoon snacks, as well as his inconsistent timing of insulin injections and meals, resulting in peak blood insulin levels not corresponding to peak blood sugar levels.

Ben also skipped some insulin injections. Both he and his parents were observed to prepare injections and mix the insulin incorrectly. This would have a tremendous impact on the efficacy of the insulin injections that were administered. The parenting style of Eileen and Gene in diabetes-specific situations was determined to be inconsistent and rather noninvolved. The majority of the responsibility for Ben's management of IDDM was left to 10-year-old Ben himself. The information obtained from this evaluation suggested that the diagnosis of noncompliance with medical treatment was appropriate.

An assessment of general family environment and parental marital status was undertaken to rule out marital problems and parent-child problems. The Family Environment Scale (FES; Moos & Moos, 1981) was used to determine general interactions among family members (including family cohesion, expressiveness, and conflict) and the Dyadic Adjustment Scale (DAS; Spanier, 1976) was used to assess the Samuals's marital satisfaction. In conjunction with information obtained from interviews, findings suggested that the family experienced conflict and poor cohesion. Gene and Eileen each indicated that they were not satisfied with their marriage. Conflict between them, however, was often suppressed.

Assessment to rule out adjustment disorder with mixed emotional feature was initiated by obtaining a behavioral profile, based on parent and teacher reports using the Child Behavior Checklist

(CBCL; Achenbach & Edelbrock, 1983). Also, depression, anxiety, and self-esteem were each assessed more specifically using the Children's Depression Inventory (CDI; Kovacs, 1981), State-Trait Anxiety Inventory for Children (STAIC; Spielberger, 1973), and Self-Perception Profile (Harter, 1985). Results indicated that Ben experienced adjustment problems. Both teacher and parent reports on the CBCL suggested that he displayed more internalizing behavior problems, such as anxiety, depression, somatic complaints, and social withdrawal, than externalizing problem behaviors. Depressed and anxious affect and negative self-perception in most domains were also reported on the CDI, STAIC, and SPP. By both parent and teacher report, he also had difficulties with peers. Thus, a diagnosis of adjustment disorder with mixed emotional features was determined to be appropriate.

Treatment Selection

To adress noncompliance with medical treatment, Ben and his parents were referred to the diabetes nurse educator for further education about diabetes and its treatment skills (e.g., proper procedure for insulin injections, timing of meals and snacks with insulin injection). The family was also referred to the clinical dietician for counseling regarding appropriate food types, calorie intake, and meal planning. The parent-child problem and marital problem were addressed by giving Eileen and Gene feedback about the role of the family in maintaining metabolic control in children with IDDM. They were also referred for marital therapy. Ben's adjustment disorder was addressed by recommending individual therapy for Ben. A support group for children with IDDM was also recommended to enhance his own self-perception by interacting with others with similar difficulties.

Treatment Course and Problems in Carrying Out Interventions

Ben and his parents received counseling from the diabetes nurse educator and clinical dietician initially for just a couple of sessions. Reassessment of their general level of knowledge concerning diabetes and problem-solving skills one week after completing these sessions determined their skills to be adequate. The family was then given spot checks on specific skills on their return appointments every two to three months. Use of 24-hour recall and diet diaries suggested that Ben and his parents, although improved, continued to have difficulty choosing appropriate types of food. Ben also continued to skip snacks, although meal times became more consistent. The family was constantly reinforced by the clinic staff for their efforts and improvement. Ben's school was also contacted, with permission of Ben and his parents, to establish some mechanism to ensure snacks during the day. Education about IDDM was also provided to Ben's teachers and school staff.

Gene and Eileen chose not to follow through with marital therapy because they maintained that their difficulties were mainly a consequence of Ben's IDDM. However, in response to counseling by the staff, they began assuming more control of Ben's daily treatment management, as evidenced by sporadic 24-hour recall interviews. Ben still maintained a large amount of control of his treatment behavior, particular in regard to his choice of foods and snacks and injecting himself with insulin. The staff continued to struggle with helping the family establish more appropriate roles for the parents and Ben in the treatment for IDDM.

The parents did follow through on the recommendations for individual therapy for Ben and for enrolling him in the support group for children with IDDM, as this met their perception that Ben was "the one with a problem." However, consistent with the difficulties they had in adhering to the medical recommendations, Ben attended therapy sessions and support meetings irregularly. The clinic staff, who enjoyed a good working relationship with the Samuals, were able to encourage the family to take advantage of the therapy offered. Individual therapy focuses on helping Ben identify his feelings about having diabetes and correcting misperceptions about the disease. It also involved helping Ben get into age-appropriate activities he would find reinforcing, such as soccer

and scouting. The overriding theme of this intervention was to normalize Ben's life and development such that the diabetes became a relatively less important and routine aspect of his everyday life.

Outcome and Termination

While Ben and his family still struggled with adhering to the diabetes treatment protocol, and he continued to experience blood glucose levels significantly outside the normal range, the number of hospitalizations for DKA declined from an average of one per month to two admissions during the last year. Ben did not miss school or leave school early as often as before, although his absences were still high when compared with classmates. The results of his remaining in school longer was improvement in grades and peer interactions. Ben also showed general improvement in his adjustment to IDDM. This was evidenced by his becoming more socially active, expressive, and projecting a more positive self-image. With time, he also displayed less depressed and anxious affect. When focused individual therapy was terminated about eight months later, parents' and teacher's reports on the CBCL were within normal limits. Ben reported less distress and better self-perception on the CDI, STAIC, and SPP as well.

Followup and Maintenance

Of course, Ben continues to be followed by the diabetes clinic staff due to the chronic nature of IDDM. He has a regular appointment every two months. Ben and his parents continue to receive spot checks on the medical management of IDDM. The clinic staff reinforces the Samuals's and correct any problems. They also generally check informally on Ben's psychosocial status and lets the psychologist know of any concerns. In this manner, the treatment team has been able to anticipate potential problems. For example, when Ben began puberty a couple of years after the initial treatment phase described above, the psychologist and diabetologist were able to prepare Ben and his family, psychologically as well as medically, for the disruptive effects of increased hormonal activity on Ben's metabolic control. Treatment outcome and maintenance are thus facilitated in the clinic by frequent contacts and establishment of long-term relationships between the staff and the family. Efforts are continuously made to bolster this family's ability to manage IDDM.

SUMMARY

There are concerns about the effects of chronic illness on the child's psychosocial development and adjustment. Children with chronic medical illness are considered to be at greater risk for adjustment problems than healthy peers, although few actually evidence clinically significant levels of psychopathology. Variations in the adjustment of children with chronic medical illness may be explained by the proposed conceptual presented in Figure 24–1. Assessment strategies to determine psychosocial adjustment in children with a chronic medical illness are relatively underdeveloped at this time. Therefore, reliance must be placed on more general or traditional tools of child assessment. Assessment utilizing the proposed conceptual model should emphasize disease/disability parameters, functional independence of the child, psychosocial stressors, and resistance factors in the areas of personal characteristics, social ecology, and stress-processing capabilities of the child.

Similarly, even though optimal treatment strategies for psychosocial maladjustment related to specific chronic medical conditions are in the nascent stage, general treatment strategies may be employed and chosen based on assessment using this conceptual model, with the goal of normalizing the child's experience and development. To this end, strategies such as support groups, enhancing competencies, and exposing the child to normal developmental experiences may be used. In addition, education of the family about the disease and its effect on development and adjustment is necessary, as is similar communication with schools. However, the medical setting in which chronically ill children are most typically seen often presents special challenges for implementing psychosocial interventions. These include resistance on the part of both the parents and the medical staff, as well as the heavy emotional and practical burden experienced by the family resulting from the child's chronic illness. On the brighter side, relapse prevention may be facilitated by the child's and family's regular contact with the clinic. Thus, progress may be monitored, support given, and rapport maintained over a long period of time.

REFERENCES

Achenbach, T. M., & Edelbrock, C. S. (1983). *Manual for the Child Behavior Checklist and Revised Child Behavior Profile.* Burlington: University of Vermont, Department of Psychiatry.

Compas, B. E., Davis, G. E., & Forsythe, C. J. (1985). *Assessment of major and daily life events during adolescence: The Adolescent Perceived Events Scale.* Unpublished manuscript, University of Vermont.

Compas, B. E., Malcarne, V. L., & Fondocaro, K. M. (1988). Coping with stressful events in older children and young adolescents. *Journal of Consulting and Clinical Psychology, 56,* 405–411.

Craig, O. (1981). *Childhood diabetes and its management* (2nd ed.). Boston: Butterworths.

Derogatis, L. R. (1983). *SCL-90-R administration, scoring & procedures manual—II for the Revised version* (2nd ed.). Townson, MD: Clinical Psychometric Research.

Drotar, D. (1981). Psychological perspectives of chronic childhood illness. *Journal of Pediatric Psychology, 6,* 211–228.

Drotar, D., Doershuk, C. F., Stern, R. C., Boat, C. F., Boyer, W., & Matthes, L. (1981). Psychosocial functioning of children with cystic fibrosis. *Pediatrics, 67,* 338–343.

Gayton, W. F., Friedman, S. B., Tavormina, J. F., & Tucker, F. (1977). Children with cystic fibrosis: I. Psychological test findings of patients, siblings, and parents. *Pediatrics, 59,* 888–894.

Gortmaker, S. L., & Sappenfield, W. (1984). Chronic childhood disorders: Prevalence and impact. *Pediatric Clinics of North America, 31,* 3–18.

Grotevant, H. D., & Carlson, C. I. (1989). *Family assessment: A guide to methods and measures.* New York: Guilford.

Haggerty, R. J. (1986). The changing nature of pediatrics. In N. A. Krasnegor, J. D. Arasteh, & M. F. Cataldo (Eds.), *Child health behavior: A behavioral pediatrics perspective* (pp. 9–16). New York: Wiley.

Hale, C., Cole, J., & Wallander, J. L. (1991).

Measurement of life events stress in adolescents with special sensitivity to those from low SES, inner-city families. Research in progress. University of Alabama at Birmingham.

Harter, S. (1985). *Manual for the Self-Perception Profile for Children.* University of Denver.

Harter, S. (1987). The determinants and mediational role of global self-worth in children. In N. Eisenberg (Ed.), *Contemporary topics in developmental psychology* (pp. 219–242). New York: Wiley.

Harter, S., & Pike, R. (1984). The Pictorial Scale of Perceived Competence and Social Acceptance for Young Children. *Child Development, 55,* 1969–1982.

Heatherington, E. M., & Martin, B. (1986). Family factors and psychopathology inchildren. In H. C. Quay & J. S. Werry (Eds.), *Psychopathological disorders of childhood* (3rd ed., pp. 332–390). New York: Wiley.

Jay, S. M. (1988). Invasive medical procedures: Psychological intervention and assessment. In D. K. Routh (Ed.), *Handbook of pediatric psychology* (pp. 401–425). New York: Guilford.

Johnson, J. H., & Bradlyn, A. S. (1988). Assessing stressful life events in childhood and adolescence. In P. Karoly (Ed.), *Handbook of child health assessment: Biopsychosocial perspectives* (pp. 303–331). New York: Wiley Interscience.

Johnson, J. H., & McCutcheon, S. M. (1980). Assessing life stres in older children and adolescents: Preliminary findings with the Life Events Checklist. In I. G. Sarason & C. D. Spielberger (Eds.), *Stress and anxiety* (Vol. 7, pp. 111–124). Washington, DC: Hemisphere.

Johnson, S. B. (1980). Psychosocial factors in juvenile diabetes: A review. *Journal of Behavioral Medicine, 3,* 95–116.

Johnson, S. B. (1985). The family and the child with chronic illness. In D. Turk & R. Kerns (Eds.), *Health, illness and families: A life span perspective* (pp. 220–254). New York: Wiley.

Johnson, S. B. (1988). Chronic illness and pain. In E. J. Mash & L. G. Terdal (Eds.), *Behavioral assessment of childhood disorders* (2nd ed., pp. 491–527). New York: Guilford.

Johnson, S. B., Silverstein, J. H., Rosenbloom, A. L., Carter, R., & Cunningham, W. (1986). Assessing daily management in childhood diabetes. *Health Psychology, 5,* 545–564.

Kanner, A. D., & Jacobson, A. (1984). *Diabetes Hassles Scale.* Palo Alto, CA: Stanford University, Department of Psychiatry.

Karoly, P. (Ed.). (1988). *Handbook of child health assessment: Biopsychosocial perspectives.* New York: Wiley.

Katz, E. R., & Varni, J. W. (1988). *The impact of social skills training on coping and adjustment in newly diagnosed children with cancer.* American Cancer Society, Grant No. PBR-31.

Kovacs, M. (1981). Rating scales to assess depression in school-aged children. *Acta Paedospychiatrica, 46,* 305–315.

La Greca, A. M. (1988). Adherence to prescribed medical regimens. In D. K. Routh (Ed.), *Handbook of pediatric psychology* (pp. 299–320). New York: Guilford.

Lazarus, R. S., & Folkman, S. (1984). *Stress, appraisal, and coping.* New York: Springer.

Lerner, R. M., Palermo, M., Spiro, A., & Nesselroade, J. R. (1982). Assessing the dimensions of temperamental individuality across the life span: The Dimensions of Temperament Survey (DOTS). *Child Development, 53,* 149–159.

McCubbin, H. I., Comeau, J., & Harkins, J. (1981). Family Inventory of Resources for Management (FIRM). In H. McCubbin & A. Thompson (Eds.), *Family assessment inventories for research and practice* (pp. 59–75). Madison: University of Wisconsin, Madison.

McCubbin, H. I., Patterson, J. M., & Wilson, L. R. (1981). Family inventory of life events and changes. In D. Olson, H. I. McCubbin, H. Barnes, & A. Larsen (Eds.), *Families Inventories* (pp. 59–75). St. Paul, MN: Author.

Miller, L. P., & Miller, D. R. (1984). The pediatrician's role in caring for the child with cancer. *Pediatric Clinics of North America, 31,* 119–131.

Moos, R., & Moos, B. (1981). *Family Environment Scale manual.* Palo Alto, CA: Consulting Psychological Press.

Olson, D. H., Portner, J., & Bell, R. Q. (1978). *Family Adaptability and Cohesion Evaluation Scales.* St. Paul, MN: Family Social Science, University of Minnesota, St. Paul.

Peterson, L. J., & Mori, L. (1988). Preparation for hospitalization. In D. K. Routh (Ed.), *Handbook of pediatric psychology* (pp. 460–491). New York: Guilford.

Pless, I. B., & Perrin, J. M. (1985). Issues common to a variety of illness. In H. Hobbs & J. M. Perrin (Eds.), *Issues in the care of children with chronic illness: A sourcebook on problems, services, and policies* (pp. 41–60). San Francisco: Jossey-Bass.

Rutter, M. (1977). Brain damage syndromes in childhood: Concepts and findings. *Journal of*

Clinical Child Psychology and Psychiatry, 18, 1–21.

Ryan, C., Vega, A., & Drash, A. (1985). Cognitive deficits in adolescents who developed diabetes early in life. *Pediatrics, 75,* 921–927.

Sparrow, S. S., Balla, D. A., & Cicchetti, D. V. (1984). *Vineland Adaptive Behavior Scales.* Circle Pines, MN: American Guidance Service.

Spielberger, C. D. (1973). *State-Trait Anxiety Inventory for Children.* Palo Alto, CA: Consulting Psychological Press.

Spirito, A., Stark, L. J., & Williams, C. (1988). Development of a brief coping checklist for use with pediatric populations. *Journal of Pediatric Psychology, 13,* 555–574.

Spivack, G., & Shure, M. B. (1974). *Social adjustment of young children.* San Francisco: Josey-Bass.

Stein, R. E., & Reissman, C. K. (1980). The development of an impact-on-family scale: Preliminary findings. *Medical Care, 18,* 465–472.

Varni, J. W. (1983). *Clinical behavioral pediatrics: An interdisciplinary biobehavioral approach.* New York: Pergamon.

Veit, J. E., & Ware, C. T. (1983). The structure of psychological distress and well-being in general populations. *Journal of Consulting and Clinical Psychology, 51,* 730–742.

Wallander, J. L., & Hardy, D. (1991). *Adolescents coping with stress related to physical disability.* Research in progress. University of Alabama at Birmingham.

Wallander, J. L., & Varni, J. W. (in press). Adjustment in children with chronic physical disorders: Programmatic research on a disability-stress-coping model. In A. M. La Greca, L. Siegel, J. L. Wallander, & E. C. Walker (Eds.), *Advances in pediatric psychology: 1. Stress and coping with pediatric conditions.* New York: Guilford.

Wallander, J. L., Varni, J. W., Babani, L., Banis, H. T., & Wilcox, K. T. (1988). Children with chronic physical disorders: Maternal reports of their psychological adjustment. *Journal of Pediatric Psychology, 13,* 197–212.

Wallander, J. L., Varni, J. W., Babani, L., Banis, H. T., & Wilcox, K. T. (1989). Family resources as resistance factors for psychological maladjustment in chronically il and handicapped children. *Journal of Pediatric Psychology, 14,* 157–173.

AUTHOR INDEX

SUBJECT INDEX